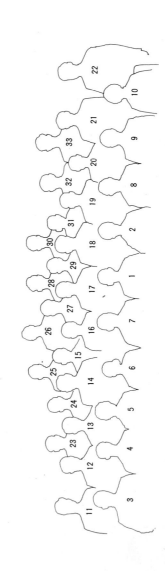

PARTICIPANTS

1.	H.I.H. Prince Takamatsu	2.	H.I.H. Princess Takamatsu	3.	Dr. Bock	4. Dr. Dawe
5.	Mrs. Dawe	6.	Mrs. Bock	7.	Dr. Druckrey	8. Dr. Magee	9. Dr. Sanders
10.	Mrs. Heidelberger	11.	Dr. Narisawa	12.	Dr. Odashima	13. Dr. Takayama	14. Dr. Lawley
15.	Dr. Nishizuka	16.	Dr. Tomatis	17.	Dr. Krüger	18. Dr. Ivankovic	19. Dr. Preussmann
20.	Dr. Weisburger	21.	Dr. Mirvish	22.	Dr. Sander	23. Dr. Nagata	24. Dr. Hirono
25.	Dr. Sugimura	26.	Dr. Higginson	27.	Dr. Ito	28. Dr. Hashimoto	29. Dr. Hayashi
30.	Dr. Nagasaki	31.	Dr. Nakahara	32.	Dr. Ishidate	33. Dr. Kawazoe	

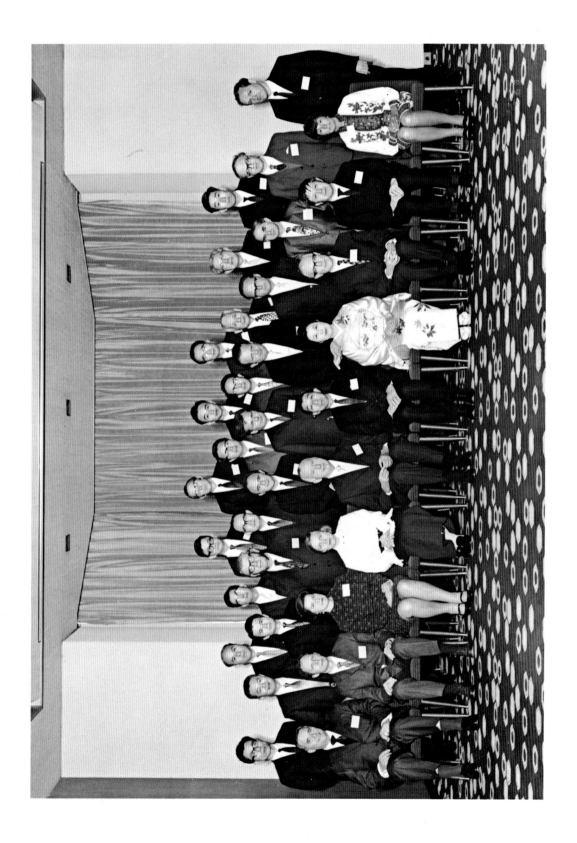

TOPICS IN
CHEMICAL CARCINOGENESIS

Proceedings of the 2nd International Symposium of
The Princess Takamatsu Cancer Research Fund

TOPICS IN CHEMICAL CARCINOGENESIS

Edited by

**WARO NAKAHARA, SHOZO TAKAYAMA,
TAKASHI SUGIMURA,** and
SHIGEYOSHI ODASHIMA

UNIVERSITY PARK PRESS

UNIVERSITY PARK PRESS
Baltimore · London · Tokyo

Library of Congress Cataloging in Publication Data
Main entry under title:

Topics in chemical carcinogenesis.

1. Carcinogenesis—Congresses.   I. Nakahara,
Warō, 1894–   ed.   II. Takamatsu no Miya Hi Gan
Kenkyū Kikin. [DNLM: 1. Carcinogens—Congresses.
2. Neoplasms, Experimental—Congresses. QZ 202
T674 1972]
RC268.6.T66   616.9'94'071   72-11781
ISBN 0-8391-0748-X

© UNIVERSITY OF TOKYO PRESS, 1972
UTP No. 3047-67771-5149
Printed in Japan.

Originally published by
UNIVERSITY OF TOKYO PRESS

Princess Takamatsu Cancer Research Fund

Organizing Committee of the 2nd International Symposium

Waro NAKAHARA
    National Cancer Center Research Institute, Tsukiji, Tokyo, Japan
Takashi SUGIMURA
    National Cancer Center Research Institute, Tsukiji, Tokyo, Japan
Shigeyoshi ODASHIMA
    National Institute of Hygienic Sciences, Setagaya-ku, Tokyo, Japan
Shozo TAKAYAMA
    Cancer Institute, Japanese Foundation for Cancer Research, Toshima-ku,
    Tokyo, Japan

Participants

Bock, Fred G.
Orchard Park Laboratories, Roswell Park Memorial Institute, Orchard Park, New York 14127, U.S.A.

Dawe, Clyde J.
Comparative Oncology Section, National Cancer Institute, National Institutes of Health, Bethesda, Maryland 20014, U.S.A.

Druckrey, H.
Forschergruppe Praeventivmedizin, am Max-Planck-Institut für Immunbiologie, 78 Freiburg, Stefan-Meier-Str. 8, Germany

Hashimoto, Yoshiyuki
Tokyo Biochemical Research Institute, Takada 3–41–8, Toshima-ku, Tokyo, Japan

Hayashi, Yuzo
Shionogi Research Laboratory, Shionogi and Co., Ltd., Fukushima-ku, Osaka, Japan

Heidelberger, Charles
McArdle Laboratory for Cancer Research, University of Wisconsin, Madison, Wisconsin 53706, U.S.A.

Higginson, John
International Agency for Research on Cancer, 16, Avenue Maréchal Foch, 69, Lyon (6 ème), France

Hirono, Iwao
Department of Pathology, Gifu University School of Medicine, Tsukasa, Gifu, Japan

Ishidate, Morizo
Tokyo Biochemical Research Institute, Takada 3–41–8, Toshima-ku, Tokyo, Japan

ITO, NOBUYUKI
Cancer Center, Nara Medical University, Shijo 840, Kashihara, Nara, Japan

IVANKOVIC, S.
Institute of Experimental Toxicology and Chemotherapy, 69 Heidelberg, Berliner Str. 27, Germany

KATSUTA, HAJIM
Department of Cancer Cell Research, Institute of Medical Science, University of Tokyo, Shirokanedai, Minato-ku, Tokyo, Japan

KAWAZOE, YUTAKA
Chemotherapy Division, National Cancer Center Research Institute, Tsukiji 5–1–1, Chuo-ku, Tokyo, Japan

KRÜGER, F. W.
Institute of Experimental Toxicology and Chemotherapy, 69 Heidelberg, Berliner Str. 27, Germany

LAWLEY, P. D.
Chester Beatty Research Institute, Pollards Wood Research Station, Nightingales Lane, Chalfont St. Giles, Buckinghamshire, England

MAGEE, P. N.
Courtauld Institute of Biochemistry, Middlesex Hospital Medical School, London, W. 1, England

MIRVISH, SIDNEY
The Eppley Institute for Research in Cancer, University of Nebraska Medical Center, 42nd and Dewey Avenue, Omaha, Nebraska 68105, U.S.A.

NAGASAKI, HIROSHI
Department of Hygiene, Nara Medical University, Shijo 840, Kashihara, Nara, Japan

NAGATA, CHIKAYOSHI
Biophysics Division, National Cancer Center Research Institute, Tsukiji 5–1–1, Chuo-ku, Tokyo, Japan

NAKAHARA, WARO
National Cancer Center Research Institute, Tsukiji 5–1–1, Chuo-ku, Tokyo, Japan

NARISAWA, TOMIO
Department of Surgery, Akita University School of Medicine, Senshukubota 6–10, Akita, Japan

NISHIZUKA, YASUAKI
Laboratory of Experimental Pathology, Aichi Cancer Center Research Institute, Tashiro, Chigusa-ku, Nagoya, Japan

ODASHIMA, SHIGEYOSHI
Department of Chemical Pathology, National Institute of Hygienic Sciences, Kamiyoga, Setagaya-ku, Tokyo, Japan

PREUSSMANN, R.
Institute of Experimental Toxicology and Chemotherapy, 69 Heidelberg, Berliner Str. 27, Germany

SANDER, J.
Institute of Hygiene, University of Tübingen, 74 Tübingen, Germany

SANDERS, F. K.
Division of Cell Biology, Sloan-Kettering Institute for Cancer Research, 410 East 68 Street, New York, N.Y. 10021, U.S.A.

SCHMÄHL, D.
Institute of Experimental Toxicology and Chemotherapy, 69 Heidelberg, Berliner Str. 27, Germany

STICH, H. F.
The University of British Columbia, Cancer Research Center, Vancouver 8, Canada

SUGIMURA, TAKASHI
Biochemistry Division, National Cancer Center Research Institute, Tsukiji 5-1-1, Chuo-ku, Tokyo, Japan

TAKAYAMA, SHOZO
Department of Experimental Pathology, Cancer Institute, Kami-Ikebukuro 1-37-1, Toshima-ku, Tokyo, Japan

TOMATIS, L.
International Agency for Research on Cancer, Lyon, France

WEISBURGER, JOHN H.
American Health Foundation, 2 East End Ave., New York, N.Y. 10021, U.S.A.

Observers

H. I. H. Prince Masahito Hitachi, Cancer Institute

Go Akagi, Tokushima University School of Medicine

Kaneyoshi Akazaki, Aichi Cancer Center Research Institute

Toshio Andoh, Institute of Medical Science, University of Tokyo

Tsuneo Baba, Kyushu University Cancer Research Institute

Hideya Endo, Kyushu University Cancer Research Institute

Makoto Enomoto, Institute of Medical Science, University of Tokyo

Ryo Fukunishi, Kagoshima University School of Medicine

Fumiko Fukuoka, National Cancer Center Research Institute

Masaru Hayakawa, Tohoku University School of Medicine

Hidematsu Hirai, Hokkaido University School of Medicine

Takeshi Hirayama, National Cancer Center Research Institute

Hiroshi Hoshino, National Cancer Center Research Institute

Hidehiko Isaka, Sasaki Institute

Toshisada Ishido, National Cancer Center Administration Department

Takeo Kakunaga, Institute of Microbial Diseases, Osaka University

Shozo Kamiya, National Institute of Hygienic Sciences

Masayoshi Kanisawa, Institute of Food Microbiology, Chiba University

Hiroshi Kurata, National Institute of Hygenic Sciences

Masanori Kuratsune, Kyushu University School of Medicine

Toshio Kurokawa, Cancer Institute Hospital

Toshio Kuroki, Institute of Medical Science, University of Tokyo

Masao Marugami, Nara Medical University Cancer Center

Mutsushi Matsuyama, Aichi Cancer Center Research Institute

Toru Miyaji, Osaka University School of Medicine

Norikazu Morita, Kagoshima University Faculty of Medicine

Takeo Nagayo, Aichi Cancer Center Research Institute

Shinsaku Natori, National Institute of Hygienic Sciences

Kusuya Nishioka, National Cancer Center

Research Institute

MASASHI OKADA, Tokyo Biochemical Research Institute

EIGORO OKAJIMA, Nara Medical University

TEISUKE OKANO, Tohoku University School of Medicine

YOSHIHITO OMORI, National Institute of Hygienic Sciences

TETSUO ONO, Cancer Institute

MAMORU SAITO, Institute of Medical Science, University of Tokyo

TAKAO SAITO, Kyushu University School of Medicine

YOSHIO SAKURAI, Cancer Institute

HARUO SATO, Research Institute for Tuberculosis, Leprosy and Cancer, Tohoku University

SHIGEAKI SATO, Institute of Medical Science, University of Tokyo

CHIKEN SHIBUYA, Gifu University School of Medicine

HAYASE SHISA, Aichi Cancer Center Research Institute

HARUO SUGANO, Cancer Institute

KEIZO TADA, Kyoritsu Pharmaceutical College

MITSUHIKO TADA, Aichi Cancer Center Research Institute

MICHIHITO TAKAHASHI, Nagoya City University Medical School

TOSHIKO TAKAOKA, Institute of Medical Sciece, University of Tokyo

NOZOMI TAKEMURA, Jikei University School of Medicine

SHOICHI TAKIZAWA, Research Institute for Nuclear Medicine and Biology, Hiroshima University

AKIRA TANAKA, National Institute of Hygienic Sciences

TATSUYA TANAKA, Aichi Cancer Center Research Institute

KIYOSHI TERAO, Chiba University School of Medicine

HIROSHI TERAYAMA, Faculty of Science, University of Tokyo

REIKO TOKUZEN, National Cancer Center Research Institute

YOSHIHIKO TSUBURA, Nara Medical University

KEMPO TSUKAMOTO, National Cancer Center

MAKOTO UMEDA, Yokohama City University School of Medicine

TADASHI UTAKOJI, Cancer Institute

MITSUO WATANABE, National Institute of Hygienic Sciences

SUSUMU WATANABE, National Cancer Center Research Institute

TADASHI YAMAMOTO, Institute of Medical Science, University of Tokyo

YUICHI YAMAMURA, Osaka University School of Medicine

KENJIRO YOKORO, Research Institute for Nuclear Medicine and Biology, Hiroshima University

TOMIZO YOSHIDA, Cancer Institute

Opening Address

H.I.H. Princess KIKUKO TAKAMATSU

I am very pleased that this opening meeting has afforded me the opportunity of personally greeting all the scientists gathered together here to participate in the symposium on " Topics in Chemical Carcinogenesis."

This is the second of a series of international symposia to be held as a part of the projects of the Cancer Research Fund which bears my name. The first symposium took place last year on virology and immunology of human tumors, in which Burkitt's lymphoma, nasopharyngeal carcinoma, and the specific virus associated with them formed the central theme. It was such a success that we have been encouraged to hope that a second symposium of similar scale on another aspect of cancer research may be worthwhile.

As the subject for this second symposium, my scientific advisers suggested that experimental cancer production by chemical agents, especially nitro and nitroso compounds, might be highly desirable. They pointed out to me that a considerable amount of knowledge has been accumulated on the chemistry and cancer producing activity of nitroquinolines and other carcinogens, such as nitrosoguanidines and nitrosamines, and the studies carried out in different laboratories are converging upon the fundamental point that these various carcinogens may function through metabolic intermediates common to them all. They also referred to the possibility of the production of carcinogenic nitrosamine in the animal body and also to the possible existence of nitrosamines in natural products. These recent developments in the field of experimental cancer research, I am informed, are giving some grounds for suspecting that nitroso compounds may actually play a causative role in human cancer.

The purpose of this symposium is, then, to bring together those scientists who are actively working on various aspects of this important problem, that each may learn from the others, first-hand, what has been accomplished so far, in order that suggestions may develop as to what should be investigated in the future.

The Organizing Committee of the present symposium spent a great deal of time and energy on the work of arranging the program, for which my appreciation is due. I think they are to be congratulated on getting so many distinguished participants from abroad.

I wish to express to you my sincere hope that your discussions here, which are so important scientifically, will be very successful and to bid you all a very warm welcome.

Prof. HERMAN DRUCKREY

Your Imperial Highness, it is for me an honored as well as welcome duty to express grateful thanks for the generous invitation of your Imperial Highness. The same appreciation is due to our Japanese colleagues, who, under your patronage, prepared so wonderfully this second Symposium of the Princess Takamatsu Cancer Research Fund.

The whole world is watching with high respect the endeavors of your Imperial Highness in the fight against cancer. Here we face something that is more than research on some scientific problems. Each year some 3 million people die of this dread disease; almost no family being spared. Our sympathy for the people suffering from the disease in general and from personal loss of a beloved individual is a decisive reason for us to dedicate our modest power to this task. The solution of the problems demands the close cooperation of all mankind.

Epideminological research in recent years has clearly shown that cancer has its cause in the human environment and that chemical carcinogens in our environment have the greatest practical significance. At the same time, experimental research discovered many carcinogenic substances, with which almost every kind of cancer can be produced in experimental animals in a specific manner. In this way reliable models for studies in all areas have become available. Of special significance is the knowledge that such substances exist in our environment or can generate in the human body, as in the case of some nitro and N-nitroso compounds, to which the present symposium is devoted.

In all these fields Japanese researchers have played decisive pioneering roles: Tomizo Yoshida, Waro Nakahara, Takashi Sugimura, and many others are among the foremost. Their names enjoy the highest scientific regards throughout the world. It is an honor for me that have had friendly connections with them for many years.

The process of research is, however, not possible without unselfish encouragement by influential personalities. In this sense I wish your Imperial Highness the best success for the blessed work of the Princess Takamatsu Cancer Research Fund. May this Second International Symposium become a milestone toward the great objective of the conquest of cancer, for which we are all united.

Prof. P. N. Magee

Your Imperial Highness, it is a very great privilege and honor for me to reply to your gracious opening address on behalf of all the participants in the Symposium on " Topics in Chemical Carcinogenesis " which your Fund for Cancer Research has so generously sponsored.

It is, of course, highly appropriate that a symposium on chemical carcinogenesis should be held in your country because, as every student in the world knows, the experimental study of this subject was initiated by the two great Japanese scientists Yamagiwa and Ichikawa, and workers in Japan have remained in the forefront of research in this field until the present day. An outstanding recent advance has been the discovery of the carcinogenic action of 4-nitroquinoline N-oxide by Dr. Nakahara, as mentioned by your Highness, and there have been rapid advances in knowledge of the properties of this group of carcinogenic compounds to which so may Japanese colleagues have contributed—including, of course, Dr. Sugimura.

As is well known, all branches of science vary greatly in their speed of advance, and it is perhaps true to say that, at the present moment, viral and immunological aspects of carcinogenesis are receiving greater public interest than chemical carcinogenesis. This shift of emphasis is, of course, closely related to the outstanding recent advances in the molecular biology of viruses and in knowledge of the immunology of tissue and organ transplantation. It is, nevertheless, sometimes overlooked that there is indisputable evidence that some human cancers can be and have been caused by chemicals in our environment, and many informed workers believe that the greater number of human cancers are so caused. As far as I am aware, there is no such convincing evidence for a viral causation of human cancer, and even if such evidence is forthcoming there will still remain the question of how the chemical agents act to induce cancer and whether, as is strongly suggested by some scientists, they do really act by activation of latent cancer viruses in more than a minority of cases. It is therefore most admirable that you, your Highness, and your scientific advisers have chosen chemical carcinogenesis as the subject of this symposium.

I have so far spoken mainly of research efforts aimed at the elucidation of the mechanisms of tumor induction, and these will always provide a fascinating intellectual challenge. It must be admitted, however, that the problems involved are truly formidable and that progress is slow. The same can be said of research on the treatment of cancer, including cancer chemotherapy, although there have been remarkable successes, notably with chorioncarcinoma and Burkitt's lymphoma. It may therefore be, for the time being at any rate, that the greatest promise of cancer control may lie in its prevention, by the elimination—as far as is possible—of potential carcinogens from the human environment. Your Highness has mentioned the possibility of the production of carcinogenic nitrosamines in the animal body and of their existence in natural products, and there may well be other chemicals with similar carcinogenic properties which remain to be discovered.

On behalf of all my fellow participants I would like to express the hope that the formal presentations and informal discussions at this symposium will lead to better understanding of the problems of chemical carcinogenesis and to the formulation of new approaches to their solution.   We also hope very much indeed that the second Princess Takamatsu Cancer Symposium will be as successful as the first.

Finally, I would like to express the great appreciation of all of us from foreign countries for the opportunity to visit, or revisit, Japan and to meet old and new friends.   For all these things, your Highness, we are truly grateful.

Dr. Waro Nakahara

On behalf of the entire audience I have the honor of gratefully acknowledging the gracious words of Your Highness.   Your Highness felicitated the Organizing Committee for obtaining the attendance of so many distinguished participants from abroad.   I wish to say that we have Dr. Heidelberger, representing that powerful McArdle group from the United States, Dr. Higginson of the International Agency for Cancer Research, Lyon, France, and many other well-known experts in the study of carcinogenesis.   We are especially fortunate in having with us the strong German group, headed by Professor Druckrey, who has done an enormous amount of work on nitrosamine carcinogenesis, and Dr. Magee from England, who was the first to discover the carcinogenicity of a nitroso compound.   With the cooperation of these able participants, I feel quite sure that this second symposium will be a great success.

We may now consider the Second International Symposium of the Princess Takamatsu Cancer Research Fund open, and proceed to the scientific sessions.

Contents

Chemical Aspects of Carcinogenesis by 4-Nitroquinoline 1-Oxide

Yutaka KAWAZOE, Misako ARAKI, and Guang-Fu HUANG

Chemotherapy Division, National Cancer Center Research Institute, Tokyo, Japan

The first part of this paper is on the relationship between the carcinogenicities and chemical structures of 4-nitroquinoline 1-oxide (4NQO) and related compounds, and the second part is on the chemical profiles of the proximate carcinogens thought to be related to this type of carcinogenesis.

Relationship between Carcinogenicity and Chemical Structure

We synthesized more than one hundred compounds thought to be related to 4NQO carcinogenesis and tested their carcinogenicities by subcutaneous injection into mice (*3, 13, 15, 19*). Histologically, the tumors induced at the site of injection were diagnosed as mainly fibrosarcomas and squamous-cell carcinomas. These compounds were classified into three groups on the basis of their carcinogenicities: potent carcinogens, weak carcinogens, and noncarcinogens, as shown in Fig. 1. The noncarcinogenic compounds may include derivatives which were too weakly carcinogenic to induce tumors under our experimental conditions.

The results are summarized as follows.

1) The only compounds found to be carcinogenic were 4-nitro and 4-hydroxy-amino derivatives. The position-isomers of 4NQO, *i.e.*, 3-, 5-, 6-, 7-, and 8-nitroquinoline 1-oxides, were all noncarcinogenic, and none of the derivatives with groups other than nitro and hydroxyamino groups at the 4-position were carcinogenic.

2) Most 4NQO derivatives with substituted alkyl and halogeno groups in various positions of the 4NQO molecule were potent carcinogens. In addition, the hydroxyamino derivatives of the carcinogenic 4NQO derivatives were also potent carcinogens.

3) 6-Carboxy-4NQO, the most hydrophilic derivative, was weakly carcinogenic, and 6-*n*-hexyl and 6-cyclohexyl-4NQO, the most lipophilic derivatives, were not carcinogenic when injected at the standard dose.

1

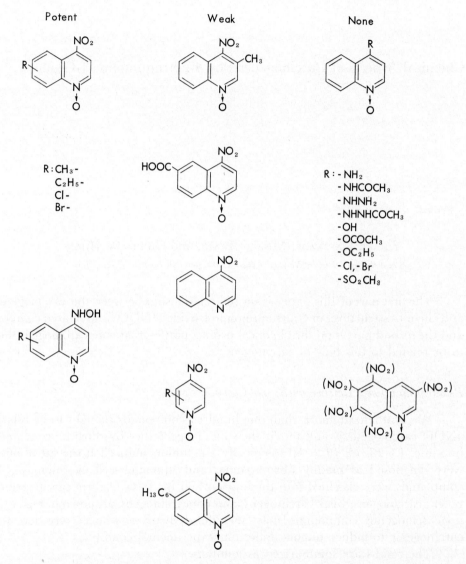

Fig. 1. Carcinogenicity.

4) None of the 4-nitropyridine derivatives tested were potent carcinogens.

5) 4-Nitroquinoline, a deoxygenated derivative of 4NQO, was weakly carcinogenic.

6) 3-Methyl-4NQO, in which the nitro group is twisted out of the plane of the aromatic ring, was weakly carcinogenic, and 3,5-dimethyl-4-nitropyridine 1-oxide, which has a similar steric structure to 3-methyl-4NQO, was noncarcinogenic.

These results lead us to tentative conclusions on the structural requirement for the carcinogenicity of this group of nitro compounds, as follows (Fig. 2).

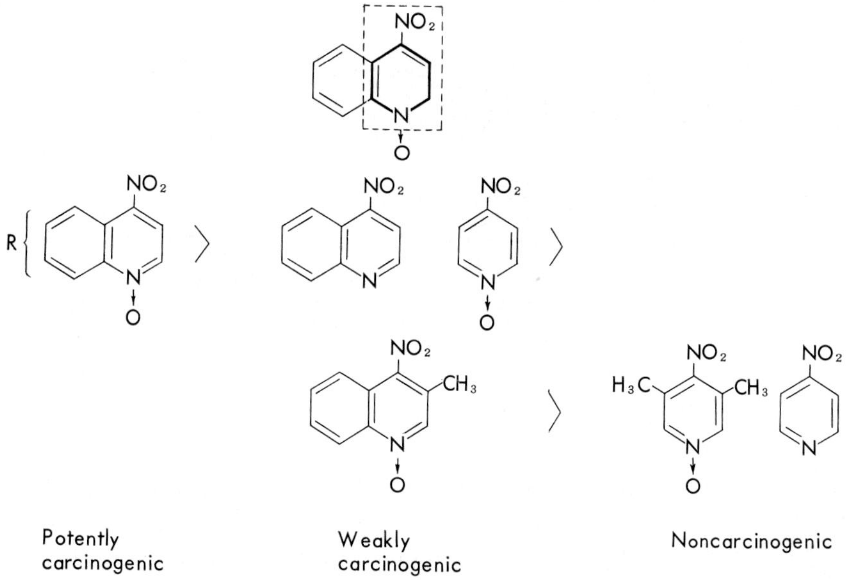

FIG. 2.   Structure-carcinogenicity relationship.

Structural Requirement for 4NQO Carcinogenesis

Fundamental Skeleton must be
  4-nitropyridine (an electron-deficient nitro compound).
Carcinogenicity is enhanced by the presence of
  1)   a fused benzene moiety (such as 4NQO).
  2)   an N-oxide group.
Carcinogenicity is reduced by the presence of substituents
  1)   making the derivative too hydrophilic or too lipophilic for carcinogenesis.
  2)   twisting the nitro group out of the plane of the aromatic ring.

  Now, let us consider how one can characterize 4-nitropyridine, which is supposed to have the fundamental structure of this class of carcinogens.   The nitro group in this compound is more electron-deficient than other types of nitro groups, such as those in nitro-benzenes and -naphthalenes, due to the strong electron-withdrawing effect of the pyridine ring nitrogen.   In other words, this nitro group is distinguished in terms of higher susceptibilities to attack by nucleophiles, leading to nucleophilic replacement, and to attack by an electron, leading to reduction of the nitro group.

  Attention should be given to the fact that among these derivatives these reactivities are enhanced by introduction of a fused benzene moiety into the molecule and also by N-oxygenation of the ring nitrogen.   In addition, these reactivities are reduced by twisting the nitro group out of the plane of the aromatic pyridine ring. These facts are evidenced by many chemical data (*26*).   We wish to emphasize that these chemical features fit the order of carcinogenicity of this group of carcinogens. Therefore, we tentatively conclude that 4NQO carcinogenesis is attributable to the reactivity of the electron-deficient nitro group.   This leads us to expect that the

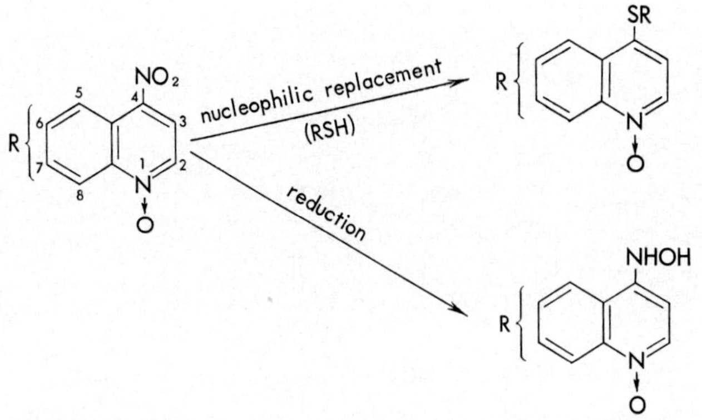

Fig. 3.   Reactivity of 4NQO.

mechanism of carcinogenesis of the 2-nitro derivative of quinolines, in which the 2-nitro group is as electron-deficient as the 4-nitro one, is the same as that involved in 4NQO carcinogenesis.   2-Nitroquinoline 1-oxide has not yet been synthesized, but Mori *et al.* (*24*), found that 2-nitroquinoline was weakly carcinogenic.   This gives additional support to the above tentative conclusion.

The next question to be considered is which reaction is actually involved in 4NQO carcinogenesis, nucleophilic replacement or reduction to the hydroxyamino derivative (Fig. 3).

We have almost conclusive evidence for the latter, *i.e.*, that the 4-hydroxyamino structure is the proximate form in 4NQO carcinogenesis.   This evidence is as follows:

1)   All the 4-hydroxyaminoquinoline 1-oxides which can be derived chemically from the carcinogenic 4NQO derivatives are also potently carcinogenic (*19*).

2)   4-Hydroxyaminoquinoline 1-oxide (4HAQO) is one of the main stable metabolites in mice (*20*) and rats (*6, 22, 32*) and also in cultured cells (*1*).

3)   When 4NQO is injected subcutaneously into mice, the resulting concentration of 4HAQO is much higher in the lungs, which are more susceptible to 4NQO carcinogenesis than other organs, whereas the concentration of 4HAQO is negligible in the liver, which is very resistant to malignant transformation by 4NQO treatment (*20*).

4)   Data on the polarographic reduction of 4NQO derivatives indicate that all the carcinogenic derivatives are stabilized at the reduction stage of the 4HAQO structure in the reduction media (*19, 33*).   That is, the carcinogenic derivatives readily undergo reduction to hydroxyamino derivatives and, at the same time, resist further reductions to amino and deoxygenated products.

5)   Both 4NQO and 4HAQO show similar behavior in interacting with DNA in cells.   Evidence was obtained that they induce the unscheduled DNA repair synthesis in synchronously cultured Syrian hamster cells.   In the case in which a nitro derivative has a capacity for induction of the repair synthesis, the corresponding 4-hydroxyamino derivative also has this capacity to a similar extent (*30*).

6)   More evidence was obtained from a study of the chemical binding of 4NQO

and 4HAQO with DNA in AH-130 and Ehrlich carcinoma cells.   After treatment of the cells with ^{3}H-labeled 4NQO or 4HAQO, the DNA was isolated.   Then the nucleic acid bases bound with the labeled chemicals were analyzed by paper and thin-layer chromatographies, and two or more of the same kinds of quinoline-bound nucleic acid bases were isolated from either 4NQO or 4HAQO treatment (*35*).

Those results show that 4NQO and 4HAQO may induce tumors through the same mechanism.   In other words, 4HAQO is the proximate carcinogen in 4NQO carcinogenesis.   Therefore, this carcinogenesis is related to those of aromatic amines, and all these carcinogenesis constitute so called *arylhydroxylamine carcinogenesis* (Fig. 4).

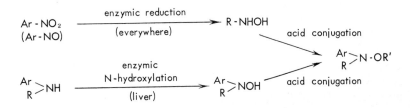

Ar , aryl; R , alkyl, acyl, or H; R' , acid residue

FIG. 4.   Enzymic activation of the precursers in carcinogenesis by arylhydroxylamines.

On the basis of this conclusion, the structural requirement for 4NQO carcinogenesis may be written in a general form as being *"An electron-deficient (i.e., readily reducible) nitro or nitroso group which is present in the molecule and its reduced from with a hydroxyamino structure which is stabilized in reduction media."*   The capacities of the derivatives for carcinogenesis may, therefore, be governed by the following capacities: 1) to be incorporated in cell nuclei (an appropriate hydrophilic-lipophilic character), 2) to be metabolized to the hydroxyamino derivatives, 3) to resist further reductive metabolism, and probably, 4) to induce a certain DNA lesion through the hydroxyamino form itself or its acidconjugate form.   All the chemical and biological profiles so far observed in this carcinogenesis are satisfactorily explained on the basis of this conclusion.

Chemical Profiles of Proximate Carcinogens Thought to Be Related to 4NQO Carcinogenesis

Next we would like to examine what chemical behaviors of 4NQO and its metabolites may constitute major or minor factors in the mechanism of 4NQO carcinogenesis.   These chemical considerations and speculations should be of help in understanding the chemical basis not only of 4NQO carcinogenesis, but also of chemical carcinogenesis in general.

4NQO itself is a very reactive compound undergoing nucleophilic reactions with biological materials under physiological conditions.   The active metabolite, 4HAQO, is also a very labile compound undergoing free radical reactions through an

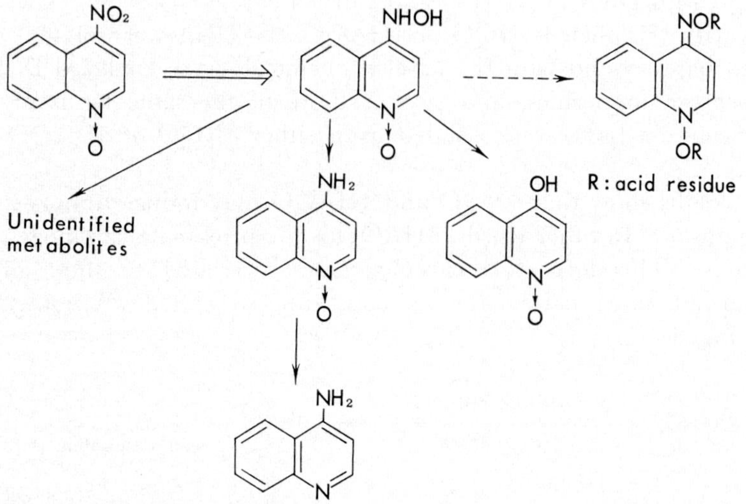

Fig. 5.   Metabolism of 4NQO in mice and rats.

oxidative process.   4HAQO should also undergo a further metabolic change to an acid-conjugate such as the acetate, phosphate, or sulfate.   The reason why such a conjugate is considered is that both the heterolytic and homolytic reactivities of the hydroxyamino group should be greatly increased by conjugation with an electron-withdrawing acid residue.   Other metabolites which have been examined experimentally are all noncarcinogenic, so it seems unnecessary to consider them.   We would, therefore, like to present the chemical profiles of these three types of presumed carcinogens (Fig. 5).

Reactivity of 4-Nitroquinoline 1-Oxide (4NQO) (13)

   4NQO may undergo replacement reactions with nucleophiles, such as the SH-groups of proteins, leading to binding with protein, as illustrated in Fig. 6.   Endo

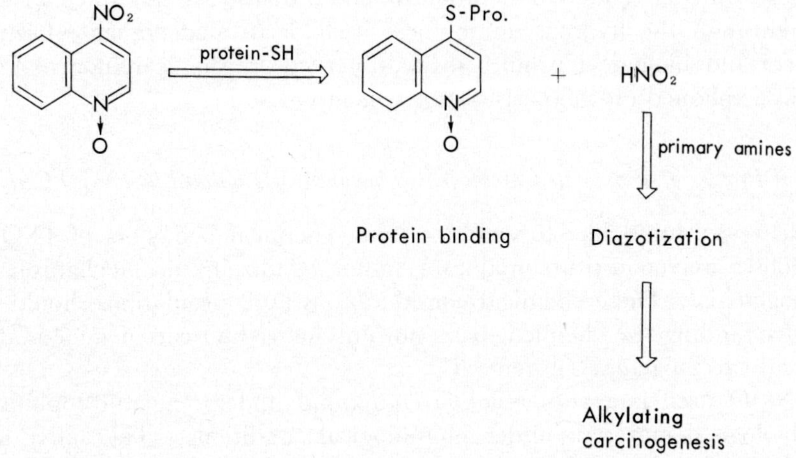

Fig. 6.   Nucleophilic replacement of NO₂ group.

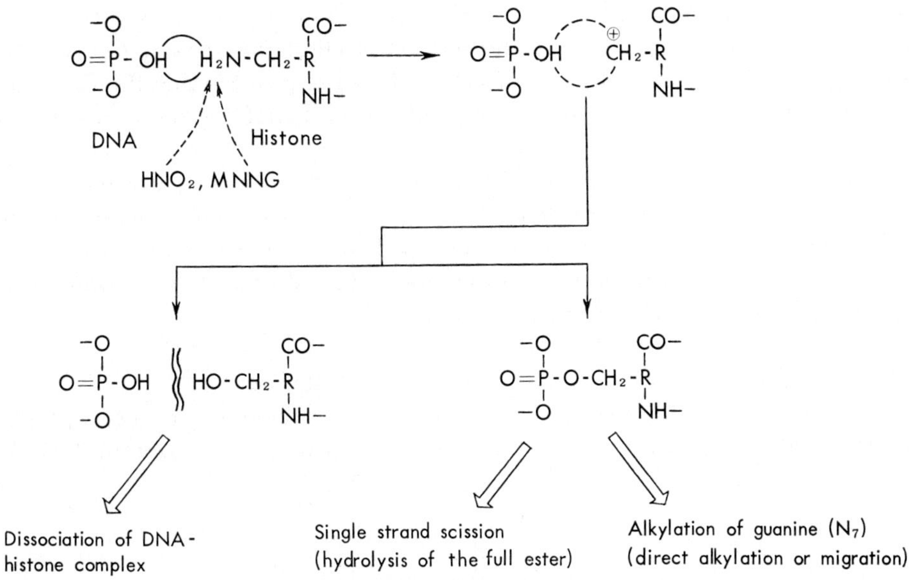

FIG. 7. An imaginary reaction scheme for DNA damage induced by nitroso compounds.

et al. (*4*) and Okamoto *et al.* (*27, 28*) found a good parallelism between the carcino-genicities and reactivities toward nucleophiles of this group of nitro derivatives. It is possible, although unlikely, that this protein-binding may be important in carcinogenesis.

In this replacement reaction of 4NQO, nitrous acid is always liberated, as shown in Fig. 6.   Nitrous acid can react with primary amines of biological materials in the cell to produce diazonium ions, leading to decomposition to carbonium ions which are thought to be the active intermediate in alkylating carcinogenesis.   How-ever, this is not likely to be the carcinogenic process, because nitrous acid requires acidic conditions for diazotization of primary amines.   However, a more likely mechanism of carcinogenesis may be deduced from this kind of mechanism.   That is intermolecular migration of a nitroso group from a certain nitroso compound to the primary amino group of biological materials such as histones in the cell nucleus. Figure 7 shows an example of a possible reaction pathway of N-methyl-N'-nitro-N-nitrosoguanidine (MNNG).   It may transfer its nitroso group to an amino group, in a kind of ammonolysis, to produce the diazonium ion.   The diazonium ion thus produced is readily decomposed to the carbonium ion shown in Fig. 7.   Recently, Sugimura *et al.* (*31*) studied the enzymic hydrolysis of MNNG.   The reaction mechanism may be as follows.   The nitroso group is transferred to some group of protein, probably an amino group of the enzyme protein with evolution of nitrogen gas.   After administering MNNG, Sugimura *et al.* (*31*) found that the only metab-olite in the urine was denitrosated methylnitroguanidine.   These results are strong indications that the type of nitroso migration suggested here may occur in the cell.

If the carbonium ion thus produced reacts with a hydroxide ion, dissociation of the DNA-histone complex may result through interruption of an electrostatic interaction between DNA and histone. If the carbonium ion reacts with a phosphate moiety in its vicinity, a single strand scission of DNA may result, due to the ready hydrolysis of full ester of phosphoric acid. It is also possible that the full ester or the carbonium ion itself reacts with the basic nitrogen of guanine to produce an alkylated product of DNA.

If this is so, as one part of the nitroso carcinogenesis, one group of chemical carcinogens may be incorporated into the cell and then transfer its nitroso group to other molecules, such as the amino group of histones. For instance, alkylnitrites may be involved in this category of compounds. We are now examining the carcinogenicity of this type of nitroso compound.

Reactivity of 4-Hydroxyaminoquinoline 1-Oxide (4HAQO) (13)

4HAQO is readily oxidized to produce a free radical, the structure of which was determined by electron spin resonance spectroscopy, as shown in Fig. 8. This

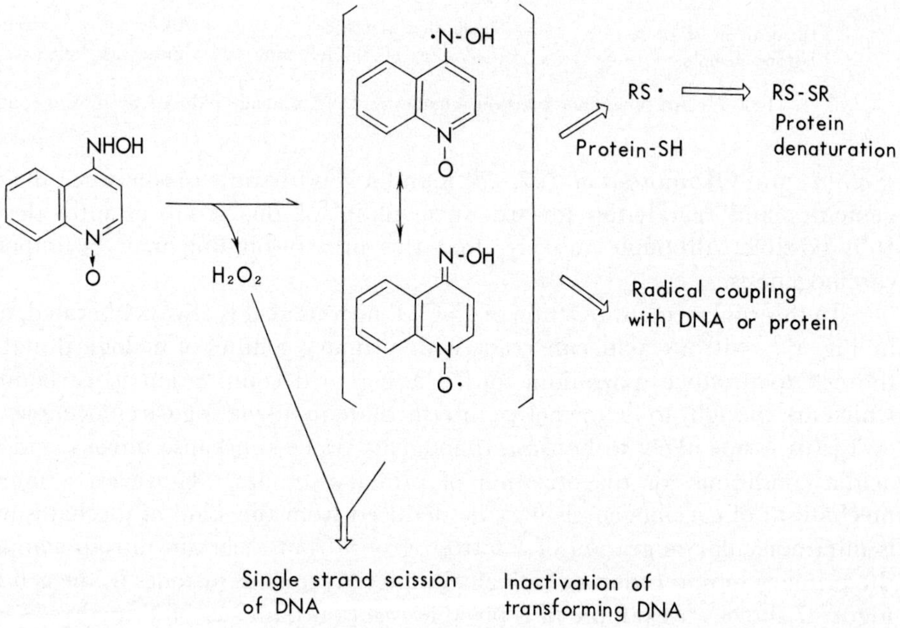

FIG. 8. Free radical reaction of 4HAQO. Similar to mutagenesis by H_2O_2, NH_2OH or NH_2NH_2.

process is accompanied by production of hydrogen peroxide, as shown by Hozumi (*8*). The free radical produced readily removes hydrogen from SH, for example, through a homolytic reaction process, to produce the free radical RS·, and this forms the dimer R-S-S-R *in vitro* (*7, 9*). 4HAQO induces single strand scission of DNA *in vitro* through a similar process involving a free radical (*16*). This reaction mechanism seems to operate in inactivation of transforming DNA of *B. subtilis* (*29, 36*).

If the reactivity of this free radical is involved in this type of carcinogenesis, then the mechanism is similar to that in the mutagenesis caused by hydrogen peroxide, hydroxylamines, or hydrazine, because the chemical reactivity of 4HAQO with DNA described above is involved in the reactions of these types of mutagens.

It seems unlikely, however, that a single strand scission actually occurs *in vivo* through this type of free radical process, because a single strand scission *in vitro* is completely prevented by the presence of radical scavengers, such as organic molecules and bromide ions (*16, 36*).   DNA is completely surrounded by protein molecules in the cell.

Ionic Reactivity of the Acid-conjugate of 4HAQO

4HAQO also undergoes another reaction, namely, heterolytic cleavage of the N-O bond.   This type of ionic reaction of hydroxyamino derivatives in general must be greatly enhanced by conjugation with an electron-withdrawing acid residue. Assuming that 4HAQO conjugated in this way is the proximate carcinogen, we prepared the diacetyl derivative of 4HAQO as a model compound.   This compound is potently carcinogenic (*15*), and its structure was determined as O,O'-diacetyl 4HAQO by infrared spectroscopy, as shown in Fig. 9 (*12*).   This acyl derivative should react in electrophilic reactions through a mechanism similar to that of N-acetoxyacetylaminofluorene (AcO-AAF) studied by Miller *et al.* (*21, 23*).   If so, three types of intermediates may be expected, as shown in Fig. 9 (I, II, and III). These may react with electron-rich carbons of the aromatic compounds, such as position-8 of guanine, as demonstrated experimentally with AcO-AAF by Miller *et al.* (*21, 23*).   On the basis of AcO-AAF carcinogenesis, products I', II', and III' should be produced from the intermediates I, II, and III, respectively.

Tada *et al.* (*34*) demonstrated that 4-aminoquinoline 1-oxide is liberated by treatment of the bound DNA with alkali.   This is strong evidence of the presence of I' in the bound DNA *in vivo*.

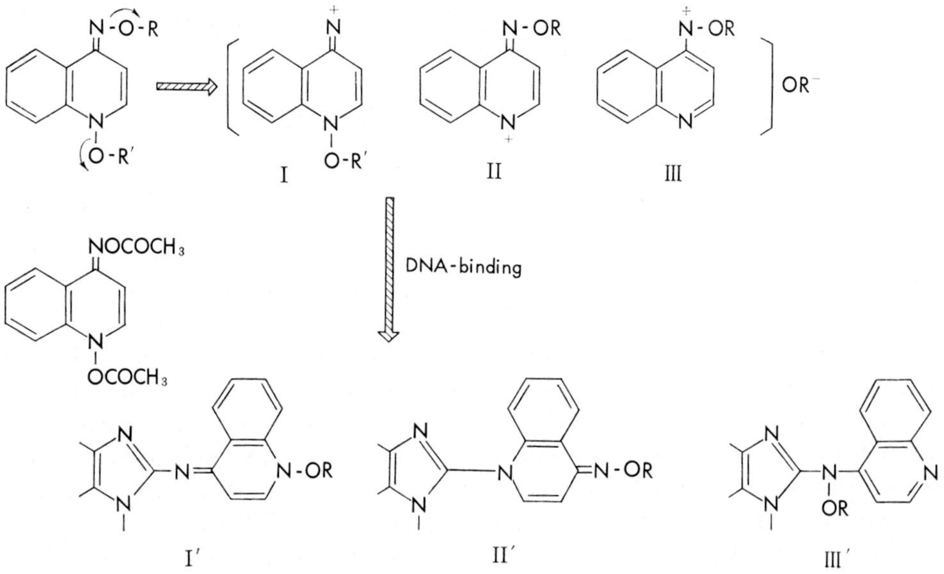

FIG. 9.   Ionic reaction of acid-conjugated 4HAQO.

In chemical binding with DNA *in vivo*, the ultimate reactant in 4NQO carcinogenesis must be this type of cationic nitrogen intermediate (*34, 35*).

Free Radical Reactivity of the Acid-conjugate of 4HAQO (13)

Another reaction of the acid-conjugate of 4HAQO is N-O bond homolytic fission. This produces a free radical and the RO· radical, as shown in Fig. 10.

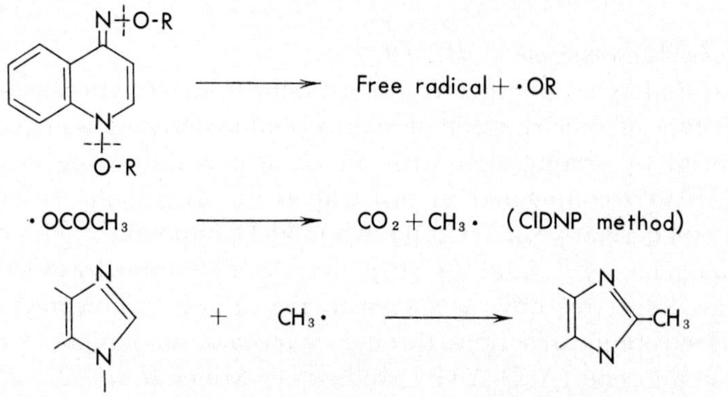

FIG. 10. Free radical reaction of acid-conjugated 4HAQO.

We will only mention the role of the RO· radical. When the acetyl derivative is used, the acetoxy radical is produced, which immediately decomposes to the methyl radical and carbon dioxide. This process has been fully studied by the chemically induced dynamic nuclear polarization method using nuclear magnetic resonance spectroscopy (*3, 14*). We found that the methyl radical reacts with purine bases, such as guanine, to give 8-methylguanine at room temperature (*17*). The methyl radical also reacts with pyrimidine bases of DNA to give addition products and methylated pyrimidine bases, probably through a free radical process (*1*). Details of the mechanism are now under investigation.

Reactivity of Alkyl-free Radical Produced from Alkylhydroperoxides

The alkyl-free radical is generally produced from organic peroxides as well as from diacetyl 4HAQO, so we will mention briefly the possible mechanism of carcinogenesis by peroxides.

One of the simplest organic peroxides is *t*-butylhydroperoxide, which is weakly carcinogenic (*5*). This is decomposed to the butoxy radical and the OH· radical in the presence of a metal catalyst. The butoxy radical is immediately transformed to the methyl radical. It is, therefore, possible that carcinogenesis by organic peroxides may involve a new type of alkylation of the carbon atom, although the possibility that the OH· radical is essential has not been eliminated. On this assumption, it is speculated that purine bases in DNA might be modified at position-8 by C-alkylation with alkyl-free radical intermediates in organic peroxide carcinogenesis, whereas they may be modified by amination with cationic nitrogen intermediates in AcO-AAF carcinogenesis, and probably also 4NQO carcinogenesis. C-alkylation may be distinguished from N-alkylation induced by so-called alkylating

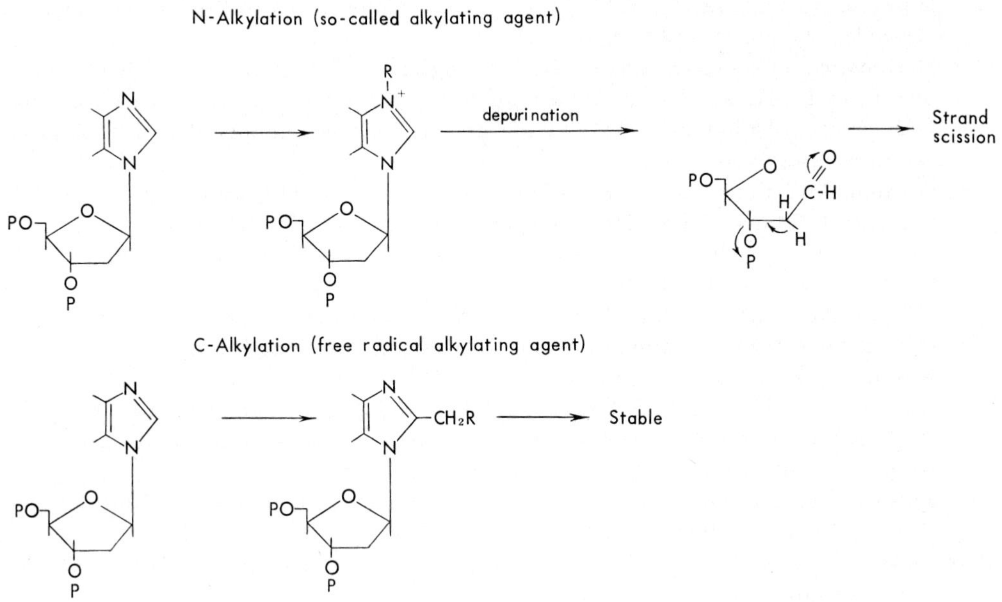

N-Alkylation (so-called alkylating agent)

C-Alkylation (free radical alkylating agent)

FIG. 11.   Difference between N-alkylation and C-alkylation of purine bases.

agents by the fact that N-alkylation produces a quaternary salt of a purine base which may undergo depurination reaction, followed by single strand scission of DNA through a β-elimination mechanism, whereas C-alkylation at position-8 of the base may produce a stable product in DNA, like the amination product formed on treatment with AcO-AAF (Fig. 11).

In the latter part of this paper we have discussed from consideration of the chemical reactivity of the carcinogen possible mechanisms of carcinogenesis which only seem to be related to 4NQO carcinogenesis.   I hope that these chemical considerations and speculations may be of some help in producing a working hypothesis for studies on chemical carcinogenesis.

We are greatly indebted to Dr. Waro Nakahara, Director of National Cancer Center Research Institute (Tokyo), for his great cooperation and valuable discussion throughout this work.

REFERENCES

1. Araki, M., and Kawazoe, Y.   To be published.
2. Araki, M., Kawazoe, Y., and Nagata, C.   Homolytic Degradation of O, O'-Diacetyl-4-hydroxyaminoquinoline 1-Oxide.   Chem. Pharm. Bull., Tokyo, *17*: 1344, 1969.
3. Araki, M., Koga, C., and Kawazoe, Y.   Carcinogenicity of 4-Nitroquinoline 1-Oxide Analogs.   Pyridine Series. Gann, *62*: 325, 1971.
4. Endo, H.   On the Relation between Carcinogenic Potency of 4-Nitroquinoline 1-Oxides and the Reactivity of Their Nitro Group with SH-Compounds.   Gann, *49*: 151, 1958.

5. Hoshino, H., Chihara, G., and Fukuoka, F.   Carcinogenicity of Tertiary Butylhydro-peroxide.   Gann, *61*: 121, 1970.

6. Hoshino, H., Fukuoka, F., Okabe, K., and Sugimura, T. Metabolism of 4-Nitroquino-line 1-Oxide. II. *In vivo* Conversion of Subcutaneously Injected 4-Nitroquinoline 1-Oxide to 4-Aminoquinoline 1-Oxide and 4-Hydroxyquinoline 1-Oxide in Rats. Gann, *57*: 71, 1966.

7. Hozumi, M.   Reaction of the Carcinogen 4-Hydroxyaminoquinoline 1-Oxide with Sulfhydryl Groups of Proteins.   Biochem. Pharmacol., *17*: 769, 1968.

8. Hozumi, M.   Production of Hydrogen Peroxide by 4-Hydroxyaminoquinoline 1-Oxide.   Gann, *60*: 83, 1969.

9. Hozumi, M., Inuzuka, S., and Sugimura, T.   Oxidation of Sulfhydryl Compounds *in vitro* by 4-Hydroxyaminoquinoline 1-Oxide, a Carcinogenic Metabolite of 4-Nitroquinoline 1-Oxide.   Cancer Res., *27*: 1378, 1967.

10. Kataoka, N., Imamura, A., Kawazoe, Y., Chihara, G., and Nagata, C.   The Structure of the Free Radical Produced from Carcinogenic 4-Hydroxyaminoquinoline 1-Oxide.   Bull. Chem. Soc. Japan, *40*: 62, 1967.

11. Kawachi, T., Hirata, Y., and Sugimura, T.   Carcinogenic Activity of 6-Carboxy-4-nitroquinoline 1-Oxide.   Gann, *56*: 415, 1965.

12. Kawazoe, Y., and Araki, M.   O,O'-Diacetyl-4-hydroxyaminoquinoline 1-Oxide. Gann, *58*: 485, 1967.

13. Kawazoe, Y., and Araki, M.   Chemical Problems in 4NQO Carcinogenesis. *In*; Nakahara, W. (ed.), Chemical Tumor Problems, pp. 45–104, Japanese Society for the Promotion of Science, Tokyo, 1970.

14. Kawazoe, Y., and Araki, M.   Chemically Induced Dynamic Nuclear Polarization during Pyrolysis of O,O'-Diacetyl-4-hydroxyaminoquinoline 1-Oxide.   Chem. Pharm. Bull., Tokyo, *19*: 1278, 1971.

15. Kawazoe, Y., Araki, M., and Nakahara, W.   The Structure-Carcinogenicity Relationship among Derivatives of 4-Nitro- and 4-Hydroxyamino-quinoline 1-Oxides (Supplement).   Chem. Pharm. Bull., Tokyo, *17*: 544, 1969.

16. Kawazoe, Y., Huang, G.-F., Araki, M., and Mita, T.   To be published.

17. Kawazoe, Y., Maeda, M., and Nushi, K.   Homolytic C-Methylation of Guanine, Guanosine, and Guanylic Acid.   Chem. Pharm. Bull., Tokyo, *20*: 1341, 1972.

18. Kawazoe, Y., and Tachibana, M.   Synthesis of Some Derivatives of 4-Nitro- and 4-Hydroxyamino-quinoline 1-Oxides.   Chem. Pharm. Bull., Tokyo, *15*: 1, 1967.

19. Kawazoe, Y., Tachibana, M., Aoki, K., and Nakahara, W.   The Structure-Carcinogenicity Relationship among Derivatives of 4-Nitro and 4-Hydroxyamino-quinoline 1-Oxides.   Biochem. Pharmacol., *16*: 631, 1967.

20. Kawazoe, Y., Uehara, N., Araki, M., and Tamura, M.   Metabolism of Tritiated Carcinogenic 4-Nitroquinoline 1-Oxide and Distribution of Its Metabolites in Mouse. Gann, *60*: 617, 1969.

21. Kriek, E., Miller, A. J., Juhl, U., and Miller, E. C.   8-(N-2-Fluorenylacetamido) guanosine, an Arylamidation Reaction Product of Guanosine and the Carcinogenic N-Acetoxy-N-2-fluorenylacetamide in Neutral Solution.   Biochemistry, *6*: 177, 1967.

22. Matsushima, T., Kobuna, I., Fukuoka, F., and Sugimura, T.   The Quantitative Determination of *in vivo* Conversion of 4-Nitroquinoline 1-Oxide at Subcutaneous Tissue of Rat.   Gann, *59*: 247, 1968.

23. Miller, E. C., Juhl, U. and Miller, A. J.   Nucleic Acid Guanine: Reaction with the Carcinogen N-Acetoxy-2-acetylaminofluorene.   Science, *153*: 1125, 1966.

24. Mori, K., Kondo, M., Tamura, M., Ichimura, H., and Ohta, A. A New Carcinogen, 2-Nitroquinoline. Induction of Lung Cancer in Mice. Gann, *60*: 609, 1969.

25. Mori, K., Kondo, M., Tamura, M., Ichimura, H., and Ohta, A. Induction of Sarcoma in Mice by a New Carcinogen, 4-Nitroquinoline. Gann, *60*: 663, 1969.

26. Ochiai, E. "Aromatic Amine Oxides," Elsevier, Amsterdam, 1967.

27. Okamoto, T., and Itoh, M. Reaction Mechanism in Aromatic Heterocyclic Compounds. V. Kinetics of the Reaction of 4-Nitroquinoline 1-Oxide and Related Compounds with Thioglycolic Acid. Chem. Pharm. Bull., Tokyo, *11*: 785, 1963.

28. Okamoto, T., and Mochizuki, M. Kinetics of the Reaction of Carcinogenic 4-Nitroquinoline 1-Oxide and Its Derivatives with Sodium Ethoxide. Chem. Pharm. Bull., Tokyo, *17*: 987, 1969.

29. Ono, T. The Effect of Carcinogens on the Biological Activity of Nucleic Acids (in Japanese). Tanpakushitsu Kakusan Koso, *9*: 1122, 1964 (Chem. Abstr., *64*: 2323, 1966).

30. Stich, H. F., San, R. H. C., and Kawazoe, Y. DNA Repair Synthesis in Mammalian Cells Exposed to a Series of Oncogenic and Non-oncogenic Derivatives of 4-Nitroquinoline 1-Oxide. Nature, *229*: 416, 1971.

31. Sugimura, T. Kawachi, T., Kogure, K., Nagao, M., Tanaka, N., Fujimura, S., Takayama, S., Shimosato, Y., Noguchi, M., Kuwabara, N., and Yamada, T. Induction of Stomach Cancer by N-Methyl-N'-nitro-N-nitrosoguanidine: Experiments on Dogs as Clinical Models and the Metabolism of this Carcinogen. *In*; Nakahara, W. (ed.), Topics in Chemical Carcinogenesis, pp. 105–120, Univ. of Tokyo press, Tokyo, 1972.

32. Sugimura, T., Okabe, K., and Nagao, M. An Enzyme Catalyzing the Conversion of 4-Nitroquinoline 1-Oxide to 4-Hydroxyaminoquinoline 1-Oxide in Rat Liver and Hepatomas. Cancer Res., *26*: 1717, 1966.

33. Tachibana, M., Sawaki, S., and Kawazoe, Y. Polarographic Reduction Potentials of Nitroquinoline Derivatives. Chem. Pharm. Bull., Tokyo, *15*: 1112, 1967.

34. Tada, M., and Tada, M. Interaction of a Carcinogen, 4-Nitroquinoline 1-Oxide, with Nucleic Acids: Chemical Degradation of the Adducts. Chem.-Biol. Interactions, *3*: 225, 1971.

35. Tada, M., Tada, M., Huang, G.-F., Araki, M., and Kawazoe, Y. To be published.

36. Tanooka, H., Kawazoe, Y., and Araki, M. Reaction Mechanism of 4-Hydroxyaminoquinoline 1-Oxide and Related Compounds in Inactivation of the Transforming Activity of Deoxyribonucleic Acid. Gann, *60*: 537, 1969.

Discussion of Paper by Drs. Kawazoe et al.

Dr. NAKAHARA: I did not hear the first part of your presentation.   Some years ago when I first started working on 4NQO, I did test the effect of 4NPO and obtained negative results.   By increasing doses and prolonging the observation period Kawazoe and his collaborators found several pyridine derivatives to be carcinogenic.   I am very glad of this discovery, since it seems to me to open up the possibility of comparing the structure-activity relationship between the two closely allied quinoline and pyridine series.   This may help toward the eventual elucidation of the carcinogenic mechanism on the basis of what I call " chemical reaction " biology.

Dr. HEIDELBERGER: I think we must keep an open mind about the reactivity of carcinogens with proteins as important in the mechanism of carcinogenesis.   I am sure that Dr. Kawazoe will agree that all the reactive intermediates, both ionic and free radical, could react with proteins, as easily as with the purines that he showed on his slides.   Also I cannot agree that the fact that fluorodinitrobenzene is not carcinogenic is relevant to the protein-binding of 4NQO, because structure-activity specificity is always encountered.

Dr. MIRVISH: Is the compound with those rings (*i.e.*, with two benzene rings, one on either side of the nitroquinoline oxide ring) carcinogenic?

Dr. KAWAZOE: 9-Nitroacridine N-oxide was not carcinogenic.

Dr. HEIDELBERGER: We must not oversimplify structure-activity relationships to interaction with intracellular targets, because these will also affect the metabolism, the distribution in the body, the permeability at the cell surface—as well as the intracellular target.

Dr. KAWAZOE: I know that.   Metabolism is another important factor for carcinogenicity.   What I have told you is just an apparent relationship between carcinogenicity and chemical structure but not reactivity.

Dr. MAGEE: How were these compounds tested for carcinogenicity?

DR. KAWAZOE: Carcinogenicity was tested by subcutaneous injection in mice.

DR. DRUCKREY: Dr. Kawazoe, Did you test the 5- or 8-hydroxy derivative of 4-nitroquinoline-N-oxide?

DR. KAWAZOE: No, we did not.

The Link between Oncogenicity of 4NQO and 4NPO Derivatives, Induction of DNA Lesions and Enhancement of Viral Transformation

H. F. Stich

Cancer Research Centre, University of British Columbia, Vancouver, British Columbia, Canada

It has become fashionable to view all biological phenomena through the eyes of biochemists. I would like to apologize for departing from this tendency and for supporting a genetic approach to carcinogenesis. I would also like to deviate from the well-established custom of reviewing the literature by citing only a few old, mostly German papers from the last century and restricting all other quotations to articles published in U.S. journals. Since virtually all contributions in the exciting field of nitroquinoline and pyridine 1-oxide carcinogenesis were done by our Japanese colleagues, and since I do not like to be accused of carrying coal to Newcastle, it may suffice to mention the comprehensive monograph on 4NQO and its derivatives (*13*), the recent review (*22, 23*), the journal Gann, which abounds with papers covering a multitude of studies with 4-nitroquinoline 1-oxide, and last but not least Drs. Nakahara and Fukuoka, who introduced 4NQO to the scientific community (*29, 30*).

DNA Repair Synthesis and the Oncogenicity of N-Oxide Compounds

Recent studies on various bacteria revealed an efficient mechanism for correcting DNA alterations induced by physical and chemical mutagens (*4, 17, 19, 41, 46, 49*). A similar, if not identical, repair system seems to operate in mammalian cells irradiated with UV (*7, 33, 36, 37*) or exposed to various chemicals (*9, 38, 44*) including nitroquinoline 1-oxides (*43, 45*). Since the correction of DNA lesions involves the synthesis of short DNA pieces which can occur at any stage of the mitotic cycle, the terms " DNA repair synthesis " and " unscheduled DNA synthesis " were introduced (*33, 36*). The repair synthesis which follows single-strand breaks and excision of short nucleotide chains can be measured by estimating the incorporation of radioactive precursors into the two DNA strands separated by equilibrium centrifugation (*6, 8, 33*), by enumerating the incorporation of ^{3}H-TdR with auto-

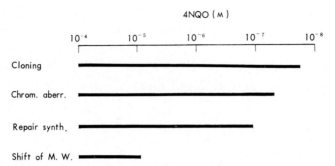

FIG. 1.   Relative sensitivity of various techniques for estimating damage to the genome of mammalian cells.   The black lines indicate the concentrations of 4NQO which produced a damage detectable by measuring the cloning efficiency, counting chromatid breaks or exchanges, estimating DNA repair synthesis and applying centrifugation in alkaline sucrose gradients.

radiographic techniques (*6, 36, 43*), by using alkaline sucrose gradients to study the shifts in molecular weights of DNA (*18, 38, 47*) or by sensitizing the repairing DNA strands with 5-bromodeoxyuridine to a subsequent exposure to light (*37*).

The DNA repair synthesis can be used as a relatively simple tool to measure the extent of DNA lesions.   Particularly the autoradiographic detection of ^{3}H-TdR incorporated into DNA during repair synthesis proved a highly sensitive technique as compared to various centrifugation procedures (Fig. 1).   Although it is somewhat cumbersome and tedious, the technique provides data on individual nuclei and reveals the variations in DNA repair efficiency in a cell population.

The experimental design was based on a simple idea.   If mutations are involved in the transformation of normal cells into neoplastic ones, then carcinogens

TABLE 1.   DNA Repair Synthesis in Syrian Hamster Cells Exposed to High, Weak and Non Oncogenic 4NQO Derivatives and Related Compounds

Compounds	Oncogenicity[a]	Grains per nucleus at concentrations (M)[b]				
		6×10^{-5}	8×10^{-6}	4×10^{-6}	2×10^{-6}	1×10^{-6}
4NQO	++	11	62	50	31	18
4HAQO	++	57	43	13	6	0
Di-Ac-HAQO[c]	++	8	2	0	0	0
6-Methyl-4NQO	++	9	55	27	16	9
3-Methyl-4NQO	+	8	4	1	0	0
6-Carboxy-4NQO	+	12	5	1	0	0
6NQO	−	0	0	0	0	0
4HAQ	−	0	0	0	0	0
QO	−	0	0	0	0	0

[a]   Relative oncogenicity was determined by *in vivo* studies.

[b]   Prior to the onset of experiments secondary cultures of embryonal Syrian hamster cells were kept for two to three days in arginine-deficient culture medium (ADM) to arrest cell division and entry into S-phase. Therafter they were treated for 90 min with the various compounds and then exposed for further 90 min to ^{3}H-TdR (10 μCi/ml).   Autoradiographs were prepared in the usual way.

[c]   A significantly elevated unscheduled ^{3}H-TdR incorporation occurs at higher concentrations, *e. g.*, 48 grains/nucleus at 5×10^{-4}M.

should interfere directly or indirectly with the genome of cells.   Assuming that this is accomplished by altering DNA molecules, the treated cells should respond with a DNA repair synthesis.   The level of the latter which can be accurately measured should reflect the oncogenic potentiality of a compound.

In cooperation with Dr. Kawazoe (National Cancer Center Research Institute, Tokyo) 30 isomeric 4-nitroquinoline 1-oxides, substituted 4NQO derivatives and related compounds were examined for their capacity to elicit DNA repair synthesis in secondary cultures of embryonal Syrian hamster cells, BHK-21 cells and human fibroblasts.   Four compounds were discarded because of their low solubility in water. The results based on the examination of 26 compounds indicate a strict association between oncogenicity of a nitroquinoline 1-oxide and its capacity to produce a type of DNA alteration which leads to an extensive DNA repair synthesis.   The few examples given in Table 1 show that aliquot concentrations of strong, weak and nononcogenic 4NQO derivatives elicit intensive, moderate or no DNA repair synthesis. The weakly carcinogenic ones must be applied at concentrations up to 200 times that of the strongly oncogenic 4NQO derivatives in order to achieve a comparable level of repair synthesis.   The results are strongly influenced by toxicity, solubility and stability of the compound.   High concentrations of the oncogenic 4NQO derivatives " poison " cells, thus leading to a reduced repair synthesis.   Compounds which are only slightly soluble in the tissue culture medium can give negative results in spite of their oncogenic capacity.   Unstable derivatives such as di-Ac-HAQO

TABLE 2. Frequency of Chromatid Breaks and Exchanges in Cultured Syrian Hamster Cells (BHK-21) Exposed to 4NQO and Related Compounds

Compounds	Onco-genicity	Frequency of metaphase plates with chromosome aberrations at concentrations[a]									
		1×10^{-4}	5×10^{-5}	2.5×10^{-5}	1×10^{-5}	5×10^{-6}	2.5×10^{-6}	1×10^{-6}	5×10^{-7}	2.5×10^{-7}	1×10^{-7}
4NQO	++	×[b]	×	×	×	×	×	91.7	63.1	25.8	11.1
4HAQO	++	×	×	×	×	84.0	19.6	5.8	4.7	3.8	2.4
Di-Ac-HAQO	++	39.5	29.5	10.0	3.1	0.0	0.4	0.1	0.4	0.4	0.3
6-Methyl-4NQO	++	×	×	×	×	×	83.3	34.8	11.6	1.3	1.5
3-Methyl-4NQO	+	83.9	52.6	12.0	1.6	0.5	0.0	0.3	0.4	—	—
6-Nitro-4NQO	+	18.8	4.7	3.8	2.1	1.9	1.9	0.4	0.3	—	—
6-Carboxy-4NQO	+	29.6	1.2	0.2	0.7	0.0	0.4	0.4	0.0	—	—
6NQO	—	0.2	0.0	0.7	0.9	0.1	—	—	—	—	—
4HAQ	—	0.9	0.7	0.2	0.3	0.0	—	—	—	—	—
QO	—	1.1	0.5	0.1	0.4	0.5	—	—	—	—	—

[a]   The proliferation of BHK-21 cells was arrested by placing them in ADM for two days prior to the onset of the experiment.   The arrested cells were exposed for 90 min to the various chemical compounds and were transferred thereafter into MEM to stimulate their entry into a mitotic cycle.   The metaphase plates were accumulated by colchicine which was applied 18 to 22 hr post treatment.   Definite chromosome breaks (as charaterized by dislocated distal fragments) and chromatid exchanges were counted to establish the frequency of chromosome aberrations.   Under the experimental conditions used, up to 92% of all chromosome aberrations are represented by single or multiple chromatid exchanges.

[b]   The symbol × indicates a lethal effect of a compound.   The symbol — is used to show that the concentration has not been used.

must be applied at relatively high concentrations to elicit DNA repair synthesis. These factors must be considered when interpreting DNA repair synthesis.

The induction of DNA lesions, mistakes at DNA repair synthesis, a reduced repair capacity, and the entry of unrepaired DNA molecules into replication increase considerably the mutation rates in bacteria (49). If this pattern also applies to mammalian cells, then the DNA alterations and the DNA repair synthesis induced by the oncogenic 4NQO derivatives reflect their mutagenic capacity. More direct evidence was obtained by exposing cultures of hamster cells to nitroquinoline 1-oxides and estimating the increased frequency of mutants to 8-azaguanine according to Chu's method (5). A strict correlation between oncogenicity of a compound and its capacity to induce mutations at the chromosome level was observed (Table 2). Thus the oncogenic 4NQO derivatives are not only mutagenic for bacteria (31) and yeast (14, 15) but also for mammalian cell cultures, in which they cause neoplastic transformation.

DNA Repair Synthesis as a Monitoring System

Bioassays for carcinogens which use mice are costly, need large holding facilities and last for one or two years. Their relevance is questionable because the concentrations and amounts of chemicals administered greatly exceed those found in nature. The examination of lower, more realistic levels of a compound is virtually impossible because it would require a prohibitively large number of animals. Thus the search for sensitive and relevant assays is an urgent matter actively pursued in many laboratories. The use of microbiological systems has been repeatedly suggested. Large numbers of bacteria, yeast and fungi can be kept in a small area; they can be exposed to minute quantities of chemicals and analyzed within a very short time span. Undoubtedly a vast amount of interesting data can be readily obtained. Whether the results can be transferred to mammalian systems remains, however, in doubt.

Considering the link, just described, between oncogenicity of a nitroquinoline 1-oxide and its capacity to elicit DNA lesions, the question was raised whether DNA repair synthesis would lend itself as a fast, economic and reliable monitoring system. The idea appeared an attractive one because cells of patients with various congenital anomalies, of tumor-prone families and of persons with a high risk for leukemia could be readily employed and their response to carcinogens compared. Probably the greatest advantage of measuring DNA repair synthesis must be sought in the small number of cells required. Between 100 and 200 diploid cells suffice to give a fairly accurate value of unscheduled DNA synthesis when analyzed by the autoradiographic technique. The few cells emigrating from skin biopsies can be used within a couple of days after having been placed into tissue cultures. This number of cells compares very favorably with the 100,000 to 500,000 cells required for estimating single-strand breaks by centrifugation in an alkaline sucrose gradient or for counting the frequency of chromosome aberrations. Furthermore DNA repair synthesis can be measured in nondividing cells, whereas the other procedures depend on a rapidly proliferating cell population.

The time required to complete and analyze DNA repair synthesis by the auto-radiographic procedure is comparable to that of the two other techniques. The application of mutagens or carcinogens followed by the addition of ³H-TdR, fixation of cells and coating with the emulsion can be easily accomplished in one day. The exposure time of the standard autoradiographic emulsions varies between 14 to 21 days but can be reduced to a few hours by applying a newly developed procedure (48). The enumeration of grains is the most time-consuming part but can be readily semimechanized. Thus the autoradiographic procedure could be applied in a large-scale screening program.

The sensitivity of DNA repair synthesis was compared with that of a few other well-established methods: the counting of chromosome aberrations, the estimation of cells entering into DNA replication at S-phase, the evaluation of clone-forming capacity and the determination of shifts in molecular weights. The results are shown schematically in Fig. 1. Although the sensitivity does not surpass most of the other procedures, it would appear acceptable for a bioassay. A restriction of the DNA repair synthesis as a screening procedure for all types of mutagens lies in its specificity. Only DNA alterations which initiate DNA repair synthesis can be detected by the above-mentioned techniques.

DNA Repair Synthesis and Susceptibility

Numerous genetic and nongenetic factors influence the susceptibility of cells, tissues and animals to carcinogenic agents. For example, point mutations are responsible for the strain differences among mice. The age dependent frequency of several virus-induced tumors appears due to the developing immunological competence after birth of the host. In cultured tissues the transformation frequency is greatly affected by the degree of cell division. The organ-specific responses for carcinogens may be influenced by their distribution within the body and the activation or inactivation of potential carcinogens in particular tissues. In spite of these numerous biological observations, the basic cellular mechanism controlling the level of susceptibility is only poorly understood.

Insight into this problem may be gained by applying the results obtained on microbiological systems to cells of higher organisms. Several different mutants of *Escherichia coli* with a greatly increased sensitivity to UV irradiation were shown to be deficient in correcting DNA lesions (19, 41, 49). These mutants either lack a normal endonuclease activity, have a reduced polymerase function or possess a faulty recombination mechanism. Some of the UV-sensitive mutant strains are also deficient in the repair of DNA lesions induced by chemical mutagens including N-methyl-N'-nitro-N-nitrosoguanidine (MNNG), methylmethanesulfonate (MMS) or nitrogen mustard. These observations indicate a strict association between deficient repair capacity and increased lethality and mutability (41, 49).

Cleaver was the first to demonstrate repair-deficient mutants in man (6–9). An extension of the original observations revealed various levels of repair deficiencies among patients afflicted with *Xeroderma pigmentosum* (XP) (2, 24). Mild, moderately severe and extremely severe forms of *Xeroderma pigmentosum* seem to be

TABLE 3. DNA Repair Synthesis in Fibroblasts of a *Xeroderma pigmentosum* Patient (XP_H) and an Unafflicted Person (An) Exposed to UV, N-Oxides or MNNG

		Grains per nucleus[a]				
	UV	4NQO 1×10^{-5}M	4HAQO 5×10^{-5}M	2-M-4NQO 1×10^{-5}M	3-M-4HAPO 1×10^{-5}M	MNNG
XP_H	16.8	15.4	12.2	13.9	9.1	58.6
An	98.3	108.2	99.7	114.8	43.9	54.6

[a] All the chemical compounds were applied for 90 min, followed by 90 min of ^{3}H-TdR (10 μCi/ml). For technique see footnote in Table 1.

correlated with a minor, mediocre and large defect in DNA repair capacity following UV irradiation.

The question of the specificity of this lesion in XP patients must be raised. The response of *Xeroderma pigmentosum* cells exposed to various chemical mutagens should provide an answer to this problem. Cultured XP cell strains (XP_H, XP_K and XP_V) which originated from three patients were chosen. Their unscheduled DNA synthesis following a single UV dose was about 15%, 32% and 55% of that seen in 8 different fibroblast cultures obtained from unafflicted persons unrelated to the XP patients. They also show a reduced DNA repair synthesis when challenged with the oncogenic 4NQO, 4HAQO, 2-methyl-4NQO or 3-methyl-4HAPO. An example is given in Table 3. The level of DNA repair synthesis in the 4NQO-treated XP_H, XP_K and XP_V cells corresponds to that found following UV irradiation. The extent of DNA repair synthesis in the XP fibroblasts does not differ from that in normal cells when exposed to MNNG or MMS.

The simplest interpretation of these results is to assume that 4NQO does not induce by itself scissions in DNA strands in spite of its complex formation with DNA (*21, 32, 34, 35*) and a possible charge transfer with deoxyguanosine and adenine. The actual initiation of repair processes in normal quinoline N-oxide-treated cells is probably due to enzymatically induced strand breaks. Since the activity or level of scission-producing enzymes is reduced in XP cells, the DNA repair synthesis following 4NQO application starts at a subnormal level. On the other hand, MNNG and MMS seem to lead to strand breakage without involvement of an endonuclease. This may explain the absence of a difference in repair synthesis between XP cells and normal ones when treated with MNNG or MMS.

DNA Repair Synthesis and Viral-induced Transformation

The genetic concept of carcinogenesis and the viral theory of oncogenesis were considered to be mutually exclusive ideas. The various arguments usually led to a dilemma, because neither can one easily disprove a claim of " hidden " or " latent " viruses nor can one refute the presence of mutations in neoplastic cells. This old controversy was renewed by the recent observation indicating a synergistic effect between chemical carcinogens and oncogenic viruses (*10, 16, 42*).

In cooperation with Dr. B. Casto we initiated a series of experiments to reveal an effect of 4NQO on neoplastic transformation induced by the Simian adenovirus

SA7. The method of estimating the frequency of SA7-transformed cells has been previously described in great detail (3). Primary cultures of embryonal Syrian hamster cells were exposed for 90 min to nitroquinoline 1-oxides, thereafter repeatedly washed, inoculated with 2×10^6 PFU of SA7 (3-hr absorption) and then subcultured. Foci of densely packed, piled up cells were counted about 4 weeks after virus inoculation. The cells of these colonies contain viral neoantigen and produce tumors when inoculated into Syrian hamsters (3). They are considered to be SA7-transformed neoplastic cells. The loss of cells due to a lethal effect of the chemical carcinogens was estimated by measuring the colony-forming capacity of the treated cells. The data obtained were used for adjusting the transformation frequency.

The three experiments which bear on our topic are summarized.

1)   Primary cultures of Syrian hamster cells were treated with the highly oncogenic 4NQO, the weakly oncogenic 3-methyl-4NQO and the non-oncogenic 6NQO prior to the addition of SA7. These compounds induce high, weak and no detectable DNA repair synthesis, respectively (45). A pretreatment of cells with 4NQO and 3-methyl-4NQO significantly increases the frequency of SA7-induced transformation, whereas 6NQO has no stimulating or retarding effects. The levels of enhancement evoked by 4NQO and 3-methyl-4NQO also differ. The weakly oncogenic derivative must be applied at considerably higher concentration than 4NQO to increase the transformation frequency.

2)   If DNA scissions, single-strand breaks and/or synthesis of single-strand segments are involved in viral-induced cell transformation then the time period between 4NQO treatment and SA7 inoculation should be of utmost importance. Information on this problem was obtained by exposing primary cultures of Syrian hamster cells to 4NQO for 90 min and adding the virus preparations at different intervals thereafter. As previously shown the DNA repair synthesis following a single 4NQO application is mainly completed by 8- to 10-hr post treatment (43). To see the effect of an ongoing and completed repair synthesis, SA7 was added immediately after 4NQO treatment, or 12 to 24 hr later. The results shown in Table 4 clearly demonstrate that a significantly increased transformation frequency occurs only when the virus was added immediately after the 90 min-long 4NQO application.

TABLE 4.   Frequency of Transformed Syrian Hamster Cells Exposed to Simian Adenovirus SA7 at Different Intervals Following 4NQO Treatment

Time between 4NQO application and SA7	Transformation frequency[a]	
	SA7[b] only	4NQO $(2 \times 10^{-6}$M$)$ +SA7
0 hr	17	435
12	17	26
24	17	12
48	17	7

[a]   Transformation frequency is expressed as number of colonies per 2×10^6 inoculated cells.

[b]   To facilitate a comparison the frequency of transformed clones was adjusted to the average figure of 17.

3)   The observations described above lead to the question whether a 4NQO pretreatment of cells would also render them more susceptible to chromosome aberrations elicited by adenoviruses.   Secondary subcultures of embryonal hamster cells were placed in ADM for 3 days, exposed for 90 min to various concentrations of 4NQO, inoculated thereafter with various cases of human adenovirus type 12 (AD12), changed into MEM to stimulate cell division, sampled 18 to 27 hr later, and analyzed for chromatid breaks and exchanges.   The extent of chromosome damage produced by these two agents is strictly additive.

COMMENTS AND OUTLOOK

Many forms of congenital anomalies have a genetic basis involving changes at the chromosomal or subchromosomal level.   The correlation between particular biochemical, morphological or behavioral defects and particular karyotypic aberrations is of considerable value to the clinician and is of great help in family counselling. Compared to these gratifying successes the genetic approach to the cancer problem is quite disappointing (1).   More than half a decade has passed since the genetic concept of neoplasia was proposed, and we are still unprepared to accept or discard this idea.

The same dilemma is met when an interpretation of 4NQO carcinogenesis is attempted.   The close link between degree of oncogenicity of nitroquinoline 1-oxide compounds and degree of mutagenicity for lower organisms and mammalian cells cannot be completely ignored.   A similar relationship has been previously reported for a series of high, weak and nononcogenic derivatives of butter yellow (27) and acetylaminofluorenes (25, 26).   With the increasing understanding of the intracellular activation or inactivation of carcinogens the restriction of many widely used bioassays for mutagenicity have become only too obvious (28).   Negative results obtained on one particular test system cannot, therefore, be taken too seriously. To my knowledge there is no evidence of a single properly examined chemical carcinogen which has not also a mutagenic property in one or another of the bioassays.

The absence of a consistent genetic change in neoplastic cells is a source of considerable controversy.   Retinoblastomas, neurofibromas and other relatively rare tumors (1) are transmitted according to the Mendelian laws and exemplify the involvement of recessive or dominant mutations in neoplastic transformations. Abnormal chromosome complements are a feature common to primary sarcomas and carcinomas of man and appear to be the rule in chemically induced solid tumors of rodents.   The transcription of the viral genome or part of it seems mandatory for at least an early stage in neoplastic transformation if not for the maintenance of a neoplastic state induced by DNA-containing viruses.   Do we actually deal with three unrelated ways leading to neoplastic transformation, or do we glimpse only various aspects of one phenomenon?

To decide which one of the above-mentioned phenomena plays the crucial part in 4NQO-induced carcinogenesis is a herculean task.   The breaks of single DNA strands, followed by repair synthesis and a premature entry of unrepaired DNA molecules into replication, should greatly increase the frequency of altered

DNA molecules, thus giving rise to mutations and a genetically heterogeneous cell population. The latter may comprise the source from which a transformed cell arises. Similarly one could argue that the various nonlethal chromosome aberrations following 4NQO application contribute to the pool of genetically abnormal cells. A sufficiently large number of mutated cells will then include one with neoplastic properties. If the mutagenic effect of 4NQO follows a random pattern then one can hardly expect each neoplastic cell to be endowed with the same genetic anomaly.

The interpretation given above can be seriously challenged by pointing to the increased transformation frequency in cell populations exposed to the oncogenic nitroquinoline N-oxides and thereafter inoculated with SA7. The main contribution of the carcinogen could be sought in the production of single-strand breaks which may facilitate the incorporation of viral DNA. If this interpretation is the correct one, then the main if not the only role of chemical carcinogens must be sought in their effect on cell DNA. Mutations resulting from the action of carcinogens would not be actually involved in neoplastic transformation, although they must necessarily appear when 4NQO and DNA interact. These contradictory opinions could be easily resolved if the apparent difference between DNA molecules act as genes and DNA molecules that function as viruses should disappear. The oncogene concept may hopefully provide such an unifying basis (20).

These speculations and interpretations of the molecular and cellular events should not detract from some of the more practical implications of our results. The increasing intentional and unintentional introduction of chemicals with potential mutagenic and carcinogenic properties into our environment makes the search for sensitive and relevant assays an urgent matter. DNA repair synthesis as a screening procedure for detecting all types of mutagens or carcinogens appears to be of limited value because only agents which cause DNA breaks in resting cells can be detected. However, this method may prove to be extremely useful in the identification of persons deficient in the DNA repair process and thus more susceptible to the detrimental action of DNA damaging agents. Patients variably deficient in the correction of UV-induced DNA changes can be readily recognized. The degree of repair deficiency and the risk of developing skin tumors in areas exposed to sun seem to be linked (8). Since cells of these persons do not respond with a normal DNA repair synthesis to the challenge of several N-oxides, they could also be prone to neoplastic transformation by these oncogens.

The question must be raised whether a " tolerable " or " safe " dose of a mutagen or carcinogen can ever be proposed. If this is at all possible then it can surely only apply to " normal " persons with an " efficient " DNA repair synthesis. The " tolerable " and " permissible " dose must be lowered for all those persons with reduced levels of DNA repair synthesis. Unfortunately nobody is at present in a position to even guess the proportion of persons with deficient repair in the population. They may be unable to correct one or more different types of DNA alterations. The idea cannot be completely discarded that patients with various levels of repair deficiencies to various obnoxious agents may represent a susceptible group in which most neoplasms may be concentrated.

This investigation was supported by grants from the National Cancer Institute of Canada and the National Research Council of Canada.

REFERENCES

1. Anderson, D. E.   *In*; " Genetic Concepts and Neoplasia," 23rd Ann. Symp. on Fundamental Cancer Research.   The Williams and Wilkins Company, 1969.
2. Bootsma, D., Mulder, M. P., Pot, F., and Cohen, J. A.   Different Inherited Levels of DNA Repair Replication in Xeroderma Pigmentosum Cell Strains after Exposure to Ultraviolet Light.   Mutation Res., *9*: 507–516, 1970.
3. Casto, B. C.   Adenovirus Transformation of Hamster Embryo Cells.   J. Virol., *2*: 376–383, 1968.
4. Cerda-Olmedo, E., and Hanawalt, P. C.   Repair of DNA Damaged by N-Methyl-N′-nitro-N-nitrosoguanidine in *Escherichia coli*.   Mutation Res., *4*: 369–371, 1967.
5. Chu, E. H. Y., and Malling, H. V.   Mammalian Cell Genetics.   2.   Chemical Induction of Specific Locus Mutations in Chinese Hamster Cells *in vitro*.   Proc. Natl. Acad. Sci., *61*: 1306–1312, 1968.
6. Cleaver, J. E.   Defective Repair Replication of DNA in Xeroderma Pigmentosum.   Nature, *218*: 652–656, 1968.
7. Cleaver, J. E.   DNA Repair and Radiation Sensitivity in Human (Xeroderma Pigmentosum) Cells.   Int. J. Radiation Biol., *18*: 557–565, 1970.
8. Cleaver, J. E.   DNA Damage and Repair in Light-sensitive Human Skin Disease.   J. Invest. Derm., *54*: 181–195, 1970.
9. Cleaver, J. E.   Repair of Alkylation Damage in Ultraviolet-sensitive (Xeroderma Pigmentosum) Human Cells.   Mutation Res., *12*: 453–462, 1971.
10. Coggin, J. H.   Enhanced Virus Transformation of Hamster Embryo Cells *in vitro*.   J. Virol., *3*: 458–462, 1969.
11. De Lucia, P., and Cairns, J.   Isolation of an *E. coli* Strain with a Mutation Affecting DNA Polymerase.   Nature, *224*: 1164–1166, 1969.
12. Endo, H., and Kume, F.   Comparative Studies on the Biological Actions of 4-Nitroquinoline 1-Oxide and Its Related Compound, 4-Hydroxyaminoquinoline 1-Oxide.   Gann, *54*: 443–453, 1963.
13. Endo, H., Ono, T., and Sugimura, T., editors.   Chemistry and Biological Actions of 4-Nitroquinoline 1-Oxide.   Springer-Verlag, Berlin, 1971.
14. Epstein, S. S., and St. Pierre, J. A.   Mutagenicity in Yeast of Nitroquinolines and Related Compounds.   Toxicol. Appl. Pharmacol., *15*: 451–460, 1969.
15. Epstein, S. S., and Saporoschetz, I. B.   On Association between Lysogeny and Carcinogenicity in Nitroquinolines and Related Compounds.   Experientia, *24*: 1245–1248, 1968.
16. Freeman, A. E., Price, P. J., Igel, H. J., Young, J. C., Maryak, J. M., and Huebner, R. J.   Morphological Transformation of Rat Embryo Cells Induced by Diethylnitrosamine and Murine Leukemia Virus.   J. Natl. Cancer Inst., *44*: 65–77, 1970.
17. Hanawalt, P. C., and Haynes, R. H.   Repair Replication of DNA in Bacteria: Irrelevance of Chemical Nature of Base Defect.   Biochem. Biophys. Res. Commun., *19*: 462–467, 1965.
18. Horikawa, M., Nikaido, O., Tanaka, T., Nagata, H., and Sugahara, T.   Comparative Studies on Rejoining of DNA-Strand Breaks Induced by X-Irradiation in Mammalian Cell Lines *in vitro*.   Expl. Cell Res., *63*: 325–332, 1970.

19. Howard-Flanders, P., and Boyce, R. P. DNA Repair and Genetic Recombination: Studies of Mutants of *Escherichia coli* Defective in These Processes. Radiation Res., Suppl., *6*: 156–184, 1966.

20. Huebner, R. J., and Todaro, G. J. Oncogenes of RNA Tumor Viruses as Determinants of Cancer. Proc. Natl. Acad. Sci., *64*: 1087–1094, 1969.

21. Karreman, G. Electronic Aspects of Quantum Biology. Ann. N.Y. Acad. Sci., *96*: 1029–1051, 1962.

22. Kawazoe, Y., and Araki, M. Chemical Problems in 4NQO Carcinogenesis. *In*; Nakahara, W. (ed.), Chemical Tumor Problems, pp. 45–104, Japanese Society for the Promotion of Science, Tokyo, 1970.

23. Kawazoe, Y., Araki, M., Aoki, K., and Nakahara, W. Structure-carcinogenicity Relationship among Derivatives of 4-Nitro and 4-Hydroxyaminoquinoline 1-Oxides. Biochem. Pharmacol., *16*: 631–636, 1969.

24. Kleijer, W. J., Lohman, P. H. M., Mulder, M. P., and Bootsma, D. Repair of X-Ray Damage in DNA of Cultivated Cells from Patients Having Xeroderma Pigmentosum. Mutation Res., *9*: 517–523, 1970.

25. Maher, V. M., Miller, E. C., Miller, J. A., and Szybalski, W. Mutations and Decreases in Density of Transforming DNA Produced by Derivatives of Carcinogens 2-Acetylaminofluorene and N-Methyl-4-aminoazobenzene. Mol. Pharmacol., *4*: 411–426, 1968.

26. Maher, V. M., Miller, J. A., Miller, E. C., and Summers, W. C. Mutations and Loss of Transforming Activity of *Bacillus subtilis* after Reaction with Esters of Carcinogenic N-Hydroxy Aromatic Amides. Cancer Res., *30*: 1473–1480, 1970.

27. Maini, M., and Stich, H. F. Chromosomes of Tumor Cells. II. Effect of Various Liver Carcinogens on Mitosis of Hepatic Cells. J. Natl. Cancer Inst., *26*: 1413–1427, 1961.

28. Miller, E. C., and Miller, J. A. *In*; Hollaender, A. (ed.), Chemical Mutagens, Vol. 1, pp. 83–119, Plenum Press, New York, 1971.

29. Nakahara, W., Fukuoka, F., and Sakai, S. The Relation between Carcinogenicity and Chemical Structure of Certain Quinoline Derivatives. Gann, *49*: 33–41, 1958.

30. Nakahara, W., Fukuoka, F., and Sugimura, T. Carcinogenic Action of 4-Nitroquinoline 1-Oxide. Gann, *48*: 129–137, 1957.

31. Okabayashi, T., Ide, T., Yoshimoto, A., and Otsubo, M. Mutagenic Activity of 4-Nitroquinoline 1-Oxide and 4-Hydroxyaminoquinoline 1-Oxide on Bacteria. Chem. Pharm. Bull., Tokyo, *13*: 610–611, 1965.

32. Okano, T., Niitsuma, A., Takadate, A., and Uekama, K. Charge Transfer in Molecular Interaction of 4-Nitroquinoline 1-Oxide and Related Carcinogens with DNA and Deoxyribonucleosides. Gann, *60*: 97–106, 1969.

33. Painter, R. B., and Cleaver, J. E. Repair Replication Unscheduled DNA Synthesis and Repair of Mammalian DNA. Radiation Res., *37*: 451–466, 1969.

34. Paul, J. S., Montgomery, P. O. B., Jr., and Louis, J. B. A Proposed Model of the Interaction of 4-Nitroquinoline 1-Oxide with DNA. Cancer Res., *31*: 413–419, 1971.

35. Pullman, B., and Pullman, A. "Quantum Biochemistry," Interscience, New York, 1963.

36. Rasmussen, R. E., and Painter, R. B. Radiation-stimulated DNA Synthesis in Cultured Mammalian Cells. J. Cell Biol., *29*: 11–19, 1966.

37. Regan, J. D., Setlow, R. B., and Ley, R. D. Normal and Defective Repair of

Damaged DNA in Human Cells-Sensitive Assay Utilizing Photolysis of Bromode-oxyuridine.   Proc. Natl. Acad. Sci., *68*: 708–712, 1971.

38.   Roberts, J. J., Crathorn, A. R., and Brent, T. P.   Repair of Alkylated DNA in Mammalian Cells.   Nature, *218*: 970–972, 1968.

39.   Setlow, R. B., Regan, J. D., German, J., and Carriers, W. L.   Evidence that Xero-derma Pigmentosum Cells Do Not Perform the First Step in the Repair of Ultraviolet Damage to Their DNA.   Proc. Natl. Acad. Sci., *64*: 1035–1041, 1969.

40.   Shirasu, U.   Further Studies on Carcinogenic Action of 4-Hydroxyaminoquinoline 1-Oxide.   Gann, *54*: 487–495, 1963.

41.   Smith, K. C., and Hanawalt, P. C.   " Molecular Photobiology, Inactivation and Recovery," Academic Press, New York, 1969.

42.   Stich, H. F., and Laishes, B. A.   DNA Repair and Chemical Carcinogens. Patho-biology Annual, In press.

43.   Stich, H. F., and San, R. H. C.   DNA Repair and Chromatid Anomalies in Mam-malian Cells Exposed to 4-Nitroquinoline 1-Oxide.   Mutation Res., *10*: 389–404, 1970.

44.   Stich, H. F., and San, R. H. C.   Reduced DNA Repair Synthesis in Xeroderma Pigmentosum Cells Exposed to the Oncogenic 4-Nitroquinoline 1-Oxide and 4-Hydroxyaminoquinoline 1-Oxide.   Mutation Res., *13*: 279–282, 1971.

45.   Stich, H. F., San, R. H. C., and Kawazoe, Y.   DNA Repair Synthesis in Mammalian Cells Exposed to a Series of Oncogenic and Non-oncogenic Derivatives of 4-Nitro-quinoline 1-Oxide.   Nature, *229*: 416–419, 1971.

46.   Strauss, B., and Robbins, M.   DNA Methylated *in vitro* by a Monofunctional Alkylating Agent as a Substrate for a Specific Nuclease from Micrococcus Lysodeik-ticus.   Biochim. Biophys. Acta, *161*: 68–75, 1968.

47.   Sugimura, T., Otake, H., and Matsushima, T.   Single Strand Scissions of DNA Caused by a Carcinogen, 4-Hydroxylaminoquinoline 1-Oxide.   Nature, *218*: 392, 1968.

48.   Weingrad, D., Folkman, J., and Sade, R. M.   A Method for Rapid Autoradio-graphy.   Expl. Cell. Res., In press.

49.   Witkin, E. M.   Ultraviolet-Induced Mutations and DNA-repair.   Ann. Rev. Genetics, *3*: 525–552, 1969.

Discussion of Paper by Dr. Stich

DR. SANDERS: What is your criterion of viral transformation? Is stimulation by 4NQO a real enhancement of viral transformation or hyperconversion as described by Sanders and Burford (1968)? If this is a true enhancement of viral transformation does it necessarily take place at the DNA level? What is the DNA repair capacity of Xeroderma pigmentosum heterozygotes?

DR. STICH: Fibroblasts obtained from skin biopsies of 6 persons heterozygous for Xeroderma pigmentosum (parents of 3 unrelated XP patients) were examined. The cultured cells were exposed for 90 min to various concentrations of 4NQO or 4HAQO and for a further 90 min to ^{3}H-TdR (10 μCi/ml). The unscheduled incorporation of ^{3}H-TdR was measured by the autoradiographic procedure. The DNA repair synthesis in the heterozygous cells did not differ significantly from that observed in fibroblasts of 16 unafflicted persons. It is possible that an excessive stress on the repair system by a prolonged application of oncogenic N-oxides may reveal a difference between normal cells and XP-heterozygous ones.

There are many different ways to explain the stimulating effect of 4NQO on the viral-induced transformation. The involvement of DNA changes and repair is suggested by the observation that an enhancement is obtained only when SA7 is added to the cells within the period of DNA repair synthesis following a single 90-min application of 4NQO.

DR. HIGGINSON: In *Xeroderma pigmentosum*, presumably the defect involves DNA in all organs especially as the tumors in this condition are epithelial skin tumors. Is there evidence for a diffuse increase in tumors in other organs in this condition?

In the general population with a relatively few minor exceptions, there is little evidence of a group of individuals with markedly increased susceptibility at several organ sites.

DR. STICH: I am not aware of a reliable study on the frequency of carcinomas or sarcomas in various tissues of persons homozygous or heterozygous for *Xeroderma pigmentosum*. A reduced DNA repair synthesis has been revealed only in fibroblasts, epithelial cells of the skin, lymphocytes and monocytes exposed to UV, 4NQO or 4HAQO. However, it is very likely that cells of all tissues show a repair deficiency. If we assume a higher susceptibility of repair deficient cells to N-oxides,

N-acetoxy-AAF or N-hydroxy-AAF, then XP patients should show an elevated frequency of neoplasms when exposed to these types of oncogenic agents.

Groups consisting of persons who are heterozygous for a "tumor-prone" gene may easily escape detection. This is particularly the case when the heterozygous carrier cannot be identified. The recent study by Swift on the frequency of neoplasms among relatives of patients afflicted with Fanconi's anaemia may exemplify this pattern. The heterozygous persons show about a five-fold increase of tumors at various sites as compared to the average frequency in the U.S. population. This field will rapidly advance when tests for the recognition of the heterozygous carriers are introduced.

DR. HEIDELBERGER: I suggest that your correlation with extent of repair and carcinogenesis may in fact represent toxicity, not carcinogenicity. In order to establish such a relationship it would be necessary to present data on toxicity, neoplastic transformation and DNA repair in the same experiments. We now have such studies under way.

DR. STICH: There is a link between the oncogenic property of an N-oxide compound and its capacity to "kill" cells or prevent their proliferation. This relationship is not unexpected, because the highly or weakly oncogenic compounds induce severe or moderate damage to the chromosomes and DNA as measured by DNA repair synthesis. The various levels of injuries to the genome are then reflected in various degrees of cell survival. The nononcogenic 4NQO derivatives, which do not reduce the cloning efficiency, have neither a detectable effect on the DNA nor chromosome complement. I believe that all potent chemical or physical carcinogens will also be potent cytotoxic agents.

In this connection it is of interest to note that DNA repair synthesis can be detected in virtually all cells (primary cultures of Syrian hamster cells or human cells) when exposed to nonlethal concentrations of 4NQO, 4HAQO or 2-methyl-4NQO.

DR. NAKAHARA: In connection with the question raised by Dr. Heidelberger I wish to call attention to the fact that 4-nitroquinoline N-oxide is a powerful cytotoxic agent. The compound is so fixed in our mind as a powerful carcinogen, but we should not lose sight of the toxicity. I am glad that Dr. Stich brought up the question of injury to DNA.

DR. KATSUTA: I would like to emphasize from the side of cell biologists that the term "transformation" should be critically used, e.g., malignant transformation, morphological transformation, or others. They have been too often confused.

DR. STICH: In my presentation and paper the term "transformation" means neoplastic transformation.

Dr. Kakunaga: Pretreatment of 3T3 cells with 4NQO for 30 min immediately before viral infection enhanced the morphological cell transformation by SV40. Enhancement was also observed when 4NQO was added one day before or immediately after the viral infection.   The treatment with 4NQO alone induced no transformation.

A subclone which I selected from A-31 cells was transformed quantitatively by chemical carcinogens.   From the results with experiments which were carried out by using these cells, it was indicated that one cycle of cell division was required for the fixation of cell transformation by chemical carcinogens.   DNA lesions and their repair mechanisms may be involved in the phenomena described above.

Dr. Sugimura: I would like to inform you that we have a mutant of yeast which is more sensitive to UV and also more sensitive to 4NQO.   But as Dr. Stich indicated in the case of *Xeroderma pigmentosum*, this mutant yeast has just the same sensitivity to MNNG.   Possibly the lesion in the DNA repairing system in *Xeroderma pig-*

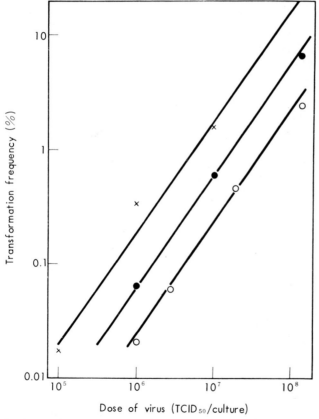

Fig. I.   Enhancement of SV40 transformation by 4NQO.   Twenty-four hours after plating the cultures were treated with 4NQO for 30 min.   The cells were infected immediately after the treatment with 4NQO.   Number of surviving colonies was determined on the 7th day after the treatment, and number of transformed colonies on the 14th day.   Transformation frequency was estimated on the basis of surviving colonies.

mentosum and in our mutant yeast might be the same.   This enzymatic lesion is now being studied.

DR. KAKUNAGA: I would like to show you four slides.

The first slide indicates the enhancing effect of 4NQO on cell transformation by simian virus 40 (SV40), and the other three indicate the requirement of DNA synthesis for fixation of transformation by chemical carcinogens.

A mouse embryonic cell line, 3T3 cells, can be transformed quantitatively by SV40.   These cells were treated with 4NQO for 30 min before or after the infection of SV40.   Pretreatment with 4NQO at the final concentration of 1 or 3×10^{-6} M immediately before the viral infection increased the efficiency of transformation by SV40 (Fig. I).   Enhancement was also induced by the treatment with 4NQO either one day before or immediately after the virus infection.   Treatment with 4NQO alone induced no transformation in these cells.   There was no difference in the sensitivity to the cytotoxic effects of 4NQO between untransformed and transformed cells.   By examination with fluorescent antibody against SV40 T antigen, all the transformed cells proved to contain SV40 T antigen in their nuclei.   These results indicate that the treatment with 4NQO enhances the transformation by SV40.

On the other hand, I have found that a subclone which I selected from A31 cells, originate from BALB/c mouse embryonic cells, are transformed quantitatively by chemical carcinogens.   Figure II shows the dose-response curves of induction of transformation and of reduction of plating efficiency by 4NQO.   4NQO was added to the culture medium for 30 min.   Number of foci per plate increased as 4NQO concentration was increased, although capacity of cells to form colony decreased.

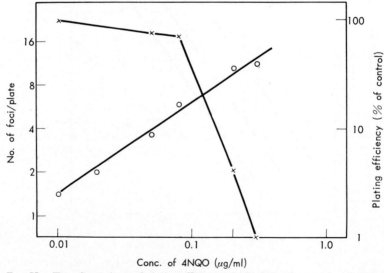

FIG. II.   Transformation and plating efficiency of A31-714 cells treated with 4NQO.   Twenty-four hr after plating the cultures were treated with 4NQO for 30 min.   Plating efficiency ($\times$———$\times$) was determined on the 7th day after the treatment, and number of transformed foci per plate (O———O) on the 28th day.

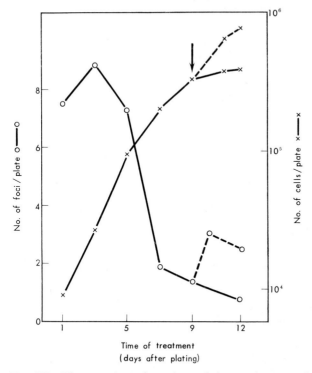

FIG. III. The rate of transformation and the growing state of cells after the treatment with 3-methylcholanthrene. The cultures were treated with 3-MC for 24 hr at daily intervals. Number of transformed foci was determined on the 27th day after the treatment. Broken lines show the values of which concentration of serum was increased to 30% on the day after plating.

Figure III shows the growth curve of cells and number of transformed foci induced by 3-methylcholanthrene (3MC). These cells were well contact-inhibited, and therefore ceased to synthesize DNA when they reached the saturation density. Treatment of the growing cells with 4 μg/mg of 3MC for 24 hr resulted in the formation of about 8 foci per plate. But when the carcinogen was added to the cells in the nongrowing state, the transformation frequency was markedly low. At the time indicated by the arrow, serum concentration was increased to 30% and about one cell division was induced. Serum addition did not enhance markedly the transformation rate.

The cultures treated with carcinogen at nongrowing state were transferred to new dishes at four-fold dilution at daily intervals, and the transformation assayed. As shown in Fig. IV, by transferring the culture within one day after the carcinogen treatment, the frequency of transformation increased to the level of that in growing cultures. But the frequency of transformation was not elevated when the cultures were transferred after the inoculation for four days under the nongrowing state. On the other hand, nongrowing cultures kept the capacity to induce transformed foci if the cells were forced to divide once immediately after the carcinogen treatment by addition of serum.

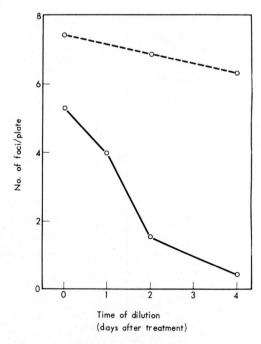

Time of dilution
(days after treatment)

Fɪɢ. IV.   The time of transfer of nongrowing cultures treated with 3-methylcholanthrene and the rate of transformation.

O————O, Twelve days after seeding 10^4 cells per plate were treated with 3MC (1 μg/ml) for 24 hr and transferred at daily intervals at a ratio of 1 : 4 of the original cell content.   Transformed foci were counted after further incubation of 28 or 29 days.   O·······O, As described above, except that serum concentration in culture medium was increased to 30% at 9 days after seeding and reversed to 10% at the end of the 3MC-treatment.

    Theses results seem to suggest the requirement of DNA synthesis for the fixation of transformation by chemical carcinogens.

    DNA lesions and their repair mechanisms may be involved in the phenomena described above.

Detection of the Unstable Intermediate, 4-Nitrosoquinoline 1-Oxide

Akio MATSUYAMA and Chikayoshi NAGATA

Biophysics Division, National Cancer Center Research Institute, Tokyo, Japan

It is now generally accepted that many chemical carcinogens are converted metabolically to active intermediates *in vivo*. These active intermediates are often called proximate carcinogens, and their attack on target molecules is, in the true sense, responsible for production of tumors. It is therefore very important for understanding of the mechanism of carcinogenesis to clarify the chemical properties and biological actions of the active intermediates.

A potent carcinogen, 4-nitroquinoline 1-oxide (4NQO), is reduced to 4-hydroxyaminoquinoline 1-oxide (4HAQO) and further to 4-aminoquinoline 1-oxide (4AQO) both *in vivo* and *in vitro* (20, 22). The formation of an intermediate, 4-nitrosoquinoline 1-oxide, during reduction from 4NQO to 4HAQO has been inferred by analogy with the reductive reactions of 4-nitropyridine 1-oxide and other nitro compounds. Kosuge *et al.* (*11, 13*) deduced that the nitroso compound was formed from the fact that a characteristic diazonium compound was produced on addition of aniline or hydroxylamine to the reaction mixture during oxidation of 4HAQO. 4-Nitrosoquinoline 1-oxide, however, has never been detected directly or isolated during either the reduction or oxidation of 4NQO and 4HAQO, probably because it has a short life and is extremely reactive.

Nitroso compounds are, in general, known to be very reactive both biologically and chemically. For example, 2-nitrosofluorene, dialkylnitrosamine, N-methyl-N′-nitro-N-nitrosoguanidine and nitrosobutylurea are carcinogenic, and the nitroso group is thought to be essential for their carcinogenicity. Ishizawa and Endo (*6*) found that the T4 phage-inactivating capacity of 4HAQO was much greater under aerobic conditions than under nonaerobic conditions, and from this they concluded that 4HAQO itself is not directly responsible for the inactivation of the phage but that an oxidative product, such as a nitroso intermediate or free radical, is responsible for this. These facts indicate that the nitroso compound may be closely related to the carcinogenic processes and other biological actions of 4NQO and

4HAQO.   Thus it is desirable to prove that the nitroso compound is formed in the metabolic pathway of 4NQO or 4HAQO and to examine its reactions with various biological substances.

The present report is chiefly on the direct detection of the nitroso compound produced during nonenzymatic and enzymatic oxidation of 4HAQO.   As stated above, 4-nitrosoquinoline 1-oxide is very unstable, so it was difficult to find a method for its detection.   In this work we tried to follow the reactions spectroscopically using a rapid scan spectrophotometer.

In addition to the nitroso intermediate, a free radical was found to be produced during alkaline oxidation of 4HAQO (*8, 18*).   The present paper also describes the formation of another type of free radical produced during enzymatic oxidation of 4HAQO.   Formation of free radicals from other carcinogenic compounds has been described by one of the present authors and co-workers (*17, 19*), and it has been suggested that they may be important in chemical carcinogenesis.   The enzymatic production of the free radical is of special interest from this point of view, as mentioned briefly in this paper.

MATERIALS AND METHODS

Chemicals

4HAQO hydrochloride, kindly given by Dr. Y. Kawazoe of the Chemotherapy Division of our institute, was used throughout the present experiments. H_2O_2 and ascorbic acid of guaranteed reagent grade were purchased from Mitsubishi Edogawa Chemicals Co., Tokyo, and Daiichi Pure Chemicals Co., Tokyo, respectively.   Horseradish peroxidase (EC I.II.1.7.), purity grade II, was obtained from Boehringer, Mannheim, Germany.

Spectroscopic Measurements

Absorption spectra of stable molecules were recorded with a JASCO model ORD/UV-5 spectrophotometer.   Spectral changes in the course of the oxidative reactions of 4HAQO were followed by a stopped-flow method with a Hitachi Rapid Scan spectrophotometer, model RSP-2, equipped with a mixing cell, flow generator and mixing controller.   This spectrophotometer is a double-beam instrument, and can record an absorption spectrum from 220 mμ to 700 mμ within about 150 msec and also follow the time course of the change in absorption at a selected wavelength.   The mixing cell of this apparatus is a four-jet type with a light path of 10 mm.   The structure of the cell and the method of mixing compounds are shown schematically in Fig. 1.   For examination of alkaline oxidation an aqueous solution of 4HAQO was placed in syringe 1 and an alkaline solution (NaOH) or a suitable buffer solution in syringe 2.   For examination of enzymatic oxidation syringe 1 contained an aqueous solution of 4HAQO and peroxidase, and syringe 2 contained H_2O_2 dissolved in a suitable buffer solution.   In the both cases, when a highly con-

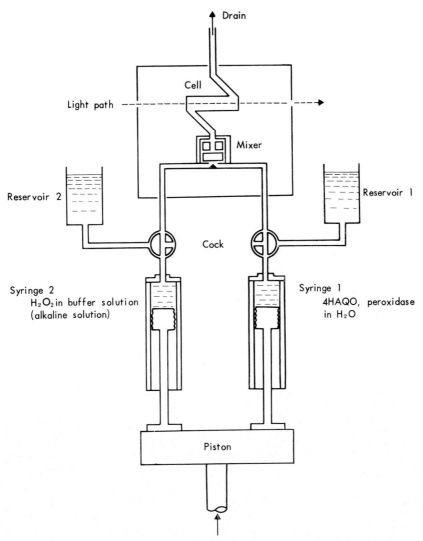

FIG. 1.   Mixing apparatus and method.   Solutions were prepared and placed in the reservoirs immediately before measurements.

centrated solution of 4HAQO was needed, a very small amount of ethyl alcohol (less than 2%) was added to increase the solubility of 4HAQO.   Absorption spectra at the selected times after mixing the two solutions from the syringes were stored in a memoriscope, Hitachi, model V-108, and then photographed with a Polaroid land camera, model 180.   The mixing speed of the solutions was usually adjusted to about 30 msec/mm.

ESR Measurements

ESR spectra were obtained with a Japan Electron Optics Laboratory spectro-meter, model JES-3BX with a 100 kc/s field modulation.   For ESR measurements the reaction was started in a test tube, and the reaction mixture was then rapidly transferred to an ESR tube with an inside diameter of 1 mm, and ESR spectra were recorded as quickly as possible.   In this way it was possible to follow the time course of an ESR signal in the order of 1 min.

RESULTS

Alkaline Oxidation of 4HAQO

In our previous paper (*18*) it was shown that 4HAQO is readily oxidized by oxygen in an alkaline medium to produce a relatively stable free radical.   Kosuge and Yokota (*11*) suggested that an unstable intermediate may be produced during the reaction, although the product could not be detected and isolated because of its lability and short life.   To obtain definite and direct information on the transient intermediates, we first examined the spectral changes in the early stage of the oxidative reaction in an alkaline medium using the rapid scan spectrophotometer.   Figure 2 shows the changes in absorption spectra of 4HAQO in the ultraviolet and visible regions.   In reaction mixture at pH 12.5 the rate of the oxidative reaction was very fast.   The figure shows that within about 30 msec* after mixing the absorption maximum of 4HAQO (355 mμ) disappeared completely and a new absorption maximum appeared at around 420 mμ.   This is probably that of an anion of 4HAQO by

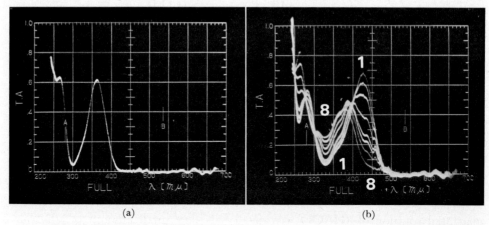

(a)   (b)

Fig. 2.   Changes in absorption spectra of 4HAQO in the ultraviolet and visible regions (200–700 mμ) caused by alkaline oxidation.   Light source, xenon lamp.   Jagged lines seen from 450 to 700 mμ in both photographs indicate noise originating from the light source and other parts of the instrument.   One division of the ordinate scale represents 0.2 absorbance.   a) Absorption spectrum of 4HAQO in distilled water.   b) Spectral changes of 4HAQO after mixing with sodium hydroxide solution.   Concentration of 4HAQO, 13 μg/ml; pH of the reaction mixture, 12.5.   The numbers on the absorption spectra indicate that the spectra were taken at the following times: 1) <1/3 sec, 2) 3 sec, 3) 6 sec, 4) 12 sec, 5) 20 sec, 6) 30 sec, 7) 60 sec, 8) 120 sec.

---

* This time was estimated from another experiment on the time course of the absorption change at a selected wavelength.

analogy with the spectral changes during reactions of other aromatic molecules with a hydroxyl group.   These results indicate that almost all the 4HAQO molecules were first converted to anions at an early stage of the reaction.   Then the new band gradually decreased in intensity and shifted to a shorter wavelength.   During the change, a transient absorption band with a vibrational structure at 435 and 456 mμ appeared about 10 sec after mixing, reached its maximum intensity after 15 sec and disappeared after 2 min.   This absorption band corresponds exactly to the free radical described previously (8).   The present experiment clearly indicates that the radical is produced *via* the anion of 4HAQO.   The subsequent changes in the spectra are due to formation of various reaction products, that is, azo compounds, 4NQO and other compounds (see other compounds below).

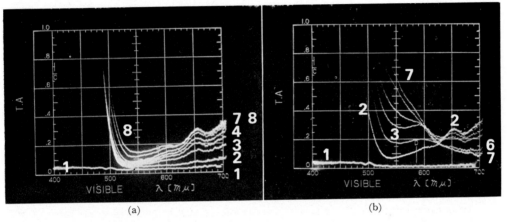

Fig. 3.   Changes in absorption spectra of 4HAQO in the visible region caused by alkaline oxidation; (a) within 15 sec, (b) from 10 sec to 300 sec.   Light source, tungsten lamp.   Concentration of 4HAQO, 400 μg/ml; pH of the reaction mixture, 12.5.   (a) 1) base line, 2) <1/3 sec, 3) 1 sec, 4) 2 sec, 5) 3 sec, 6) 5 sec, 7) 10 sec, 8) 15 sec.   (b) 1) base line, 2) 10 sec, 3) 30 sec, 4) 60 sec, 5) 90 sec, 6) 180 sec, 7) 300 sec.

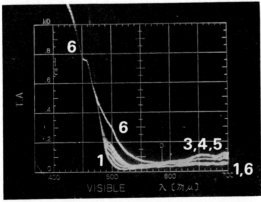

Fig. 4.   Changes in absorption spectra of 4HAQO in the visible region caused by alkaline oxidation.   Concentration of 4HAQO, 120 μg/ml; pH of the reaction mixture, 11.0.   1) 1 sec, 2) 5 sec, 3) 10 sec, 4) 15 sec, 5) 20 sec, 6) 180 sec.

Next, the spectral changes in a concentrated solution of 4HAQO were measured in the visible region from 400 to 700 mμ*, since the unstable intermediate, nitroso compound, is known to have a characteristic absorption band in the near infrared region (*10*).   As shown in Fig. 3, a new absorption band with a maximum at about 650 mμ appeared within 1 sec after mixing, increased and reached maximum intensity after 10 sec.   Then the band gradually decreased in intensity and disappeared completely within 1–2 min.   Many nitroso compounds exhibit a weak absorption in this region, so the transient absorption band observed at 650 mμ is probably that of 4-nitrosoquinoline 1-oxide.   The short lifetime of the compound is also consistent with the lability of the nitroso intermediate during the reduction of 4NQO.

Figure 4 shows the spectral changes observed at a concentration of 4HAQO intermediate between those used in the above two experiments (Figs. 2 and 3).   These results show that the new band at the longer wavelength (650 mμ) disappeared more rapidly than the transient band at the shorter wavelength (456 mμ), clearly indicating that the former does not correspond to the free radical.

When a high concentration of 4HAQO was used (Fig. 3), the reaction mixture became turbid within 1 to 2 min after the start of the reaction, and then a reddish precipitate formed.   The absorption spectra of the precipitate dissolved in chloroform agreed with those of 4,4′-azodiquinoline 1,1′-dioxide and other azo compounds (*11, 12*).

Enzymatic Oxidation of 4HAQO

In connection with the *in vivo* reactivity of 4HAQO, it was of great interest and importance to see whether the reaction described above could be achieved enzymatically.   Accordingly, we examined the oxidation of 4HAQO with horseradish peroxidase and H_2O_2 and observed the formation of 4-nitrosoquinoline 1-oxide as a transient intermediate.

Figure 5 shows the spectral changes of 4HAQO at longer wavelengths during enzymatic reactions at various pH values.   Solutions of 4HAQO in buffers at these pH values were stable, and no spontaneous oxidative reaction occurred.   Furthermore, when the enzyme or H_2O_2 was omitted from the reaction mixture, no spectral changes were observed.   These facts show that the observed spectral changes were definitely due to enzymatic oxidation of 4HAQO.   The reaction mixture became turbid during the enzymatic reactions, and the base lines of the spectra increased considerably during the reactions.   Therefore, the spectra were probably less reliable than those recorded during the alkaline oxidation.   Nevertheless, a transient absorption band was observed in the vicinity of 675 mμ.   It was located at a slightly longer wavelength than that in the alkaline oxidation, but was definitely due to the nitroso intermediate.   Thus the nitroso compound can be produced enzymatically under physiological conditions.   The intensity of the new band

---

* The absorption band of the nitroso compound in this region was expected to be very weak, so a concentrated solution was used for its detection.

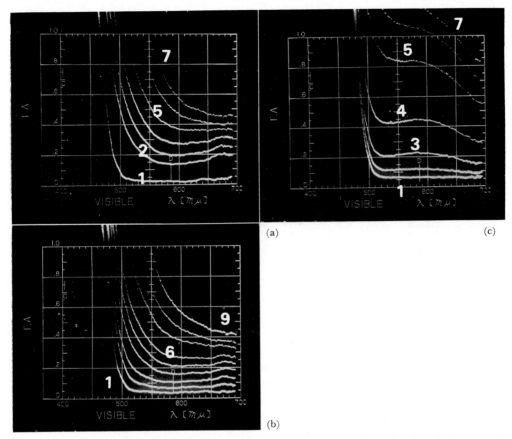

FIG. 5.   Changes in absorption spectra of 4HAQO in the visible region caused by enzymatic oxidation.   (a) pH 7.3 (0.025 M phosphate buffer).   Concentration of 4HAQO, 403 μg/ml; peroxidase, 101 μg/ml; H$_2$O$_2$, 1500 μg/ml.   1) <1/3 sec, 2) 2 sec, 3) 3 sec, 4) 5 sec, 5) 10 sec, 6) 30 sec, 7) 90 sec.   (b) pH 6.9 (0.025 M phosphate buffer).   Concentration of 4HAQO, 389 μg/ml; peroxidase, 31 μg/ml; H$_2$O$_2$, 1500 μg/ml.   1) <1/3 sec, 2) 1 sec, 3) 1$\frac{1}{3}$ sec, 4) 2$\frac{2}{3}$ sec, 5) 3$\frac{2}{3}$ sec, 6) 5 sec, 7) 10 sec, 8) 30 sec, 9) 90 sec.   (c) pH 4.6 (0.02 M acetate buffer). Concentration of 4HAQO, 429 μg/ml; peroxidase, 105 μg/ml; H$_2$O$_2$, 1500 μg/ml.   1) 1 sec, 2) 2 sec, 3) 3 sec, 4) 5 sec, 5) 10 sec, 6) 15 sec, 7) 20 sec.

reached a maximum after 4 sec, and could no longer be seen after 1 min.   This again is consistent with the short lifetime of this compound.

Under acidic conditions (pH 4.6), the spectral change was different: That is, a broad absorption band centered at about 580 mμ appeared, and no transient band could be observed (Fig. 5c).   This suggests that the nitroso intermediate is unstable under acidic conditions.   However, the reaction mixture became very turbid under acidic conditions and the spectra after 5 sec were not very reliable.

Figure 6 shows the spectral changes at shorter wavelengths.   Usually after 4 sec almost all the 4HAQO was oxidized, although the rate of its oxidation largely depended on the enzyme concentration.   The final reaction products, however,

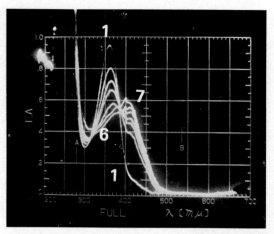

FIG. 6.   Changes in absorption spectra of 4HAQO in the ultraviolet and visible regions caused by enzymatic oxidation.   pH of the reaction mixture, 6.9 (0.025 M phosphate buffer).   Concentration of 4HAQO, 21 μg/ml; peroxidase, 39 μg/ml; H_2O_2, 1500 μg/ml. 1) 0 sec, 2) 1/3 sec, 3) 2/3 sec, 4) 1 sec, 5) 2 sec, 6) 4 sec, 7) 20 sec.   The small peak at 400 mμ is not a signal, but a noise originating from the light source (xenon lamp).

were quite different from those formed during alkaline oxidation, judging from the spectral changes.   This is ascribable to the pH of the reaction mixture, for it is well known that the condensation reaction of the nitroso compound to yield the azo compound proceeds best in an alkaline medium.   It should be mentioned here that the transient band at 456 mμ which was assigned to the free radical could not be observed during enzymatic oxidation.

A free radical could be detected in the enzymatic reaction by ESR measurement, even though no absorption band assignable to it was observed.   The ESR signals and their time courses are shown in Fig. 7, along with those produced during alkaline oxidation.   Unlike formation of the nitroso compound, formation of the free radical did not depend upon the pH value, and the same ESR signal was observed at pH 7.3 (Fig. 7) and at pH 4.6 (not indicated).   This suggests that the pathways for formation of the nitroso compound and the free radical are different. As reported previously (18), an ESR signal with 6 lines was obtained during alkaline oxidation.   During the enzymatic oxidation, however, the signal was a triplet, suggesting that the free radical produced during enzymatic oxidation is different from that produced during alkaline oxidation.

The structure of the free radical produced enzymatically could not be determined by examination of the hyperfine structure of the ESR signal because too little free radical was produced and its lifetime was too short.   However, a tentative assignment was made based on the mechanism of enzymatic oxidation and the features of the signal obtained in the following manner.   Peroxidative oxidation reactions often generate an –O· radical from a hydroxyl group (23), so it is probable that the hydrogen atom of the hydroxyl group of 4HAQO is transferred to the peroxidase-H_2O_2 complex (compound I) or compound II (see Discussion) to produce the radical

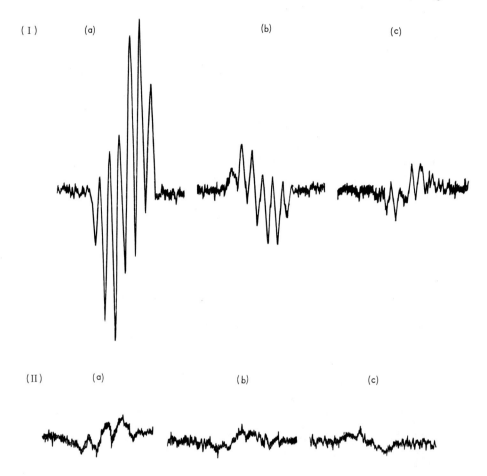

Fig. 7. ESR spectra of free radicals produced by alkaline (I) and enzymatic (II) oxidations of 4HAQO and time courses of their appearance. (I) Alkaline oxidation. pH of the reaction mixture, 12.5. Concentration of 4HAQO, 415 μg/ml. Times after start of reaction: (a) 60 sec, (b) 150 sec, (c) 260 sec. (II) Enzymatic oxidation. pH of the reaction mixture, 7.3 (0.025 M phosphate buffer). Concentration of 4HAQO, 410 μg/ml; peroxidase, 105 μg/ml; H_2O_2, 1500 μg/ml. Times after start of reaction: (a) 60 sec, (b) 210 sec, (c) 330 sec.

(I). The observed triplet signal with signals of equal intensity is reasonably explained in terms of the interaction of the unpaired electron on the oxygen atom with the neighboring nitrogen atom. Furthermore, the observed splitting of about 8 gauss is within the limits of those of other nitroxide radicals (4, 14).

The structure of the free radical produced in an alkaline medium has been determined to be (II) by analyzing the hyperfine structure of isotope-substituted 4-hydroxyaminoquinoline 1-oxide and by comparing the values of the spin densities obtained from the coupling constants with those calculated by the unrestricted SCF MO method (7).

However, the radical generated in an organic solvent was used for the analysis.

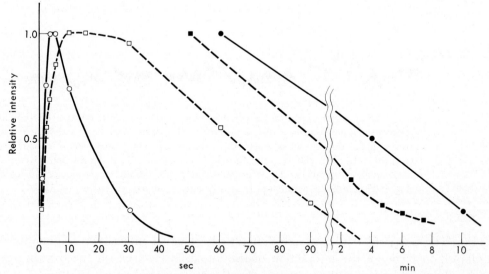

(I)   (II)   (III)

It is therefore questionable whether the same radical is produced in aqueous alkali. As stated above, almost all the 4HAQO is converted to its anionic species in alkaline medium, so that it is quite likely that the radical produced in an alkaline medium has structure (III).

Time Courses of Appearance of the Nitroso Intermediate and Free Radicals

It is very important to follow the time courses of appearance of the inter- mediates, since various transient species appear and disappear during the oxidative reactions. Figure 8 shows the decay curves of the nitroso intermediate and free radicals measured by their absorption and ESR spectra. It can be seen that the nitroso intermediate has a shorter life than the free radicals. Thus it is improbable that the nitroso intermediate is produced from the radicals. It can also be seen that

FIG. 8. Time courses of appearance of the nitroso intermediate and free radicals during alkaline and enzymatic oxidations of 4HAQO. The time courses of the appearance of the nitroso intermediate were estimated from the absorbance at 650 and 675 mμ in the alkaline and enzymatic oxidations, respectively. Corrections were made for shift of the base line when the reaction mixture became turbid. Time courses of the appearances of free radicals were calculated directly from the intensity of the ESR signal.
○———○, Abs. of nitroso compd. enz. oxid. (pH 7.3); □------□, Abs. of nitroso compd. alkaline oxid. (pH 12.5); ●———●, ESR of free radical enz. oxid. (pH 7.3); ■------■, ESR of free radical alkaline oxid. (pH 12.5)

the nitroso compound produced by the enzymatic oxidation is less stable than that produced during alkaline oxidation, while the radical produced during enzymatic oxidation is more stable than that formed during alkaline oxidation. The former observation indicates that 4-nitrosoquinoline 1-oxide is more stable in an alkaline medium. The latter is probably due to a marked difference in the reactivities of the two types of radicals. In fact, the radical produced in an alkaline medium dimerizes and condenses easily under these conditions.

Effect of Ascorbic Acid on the Alkaline and Enzymatic Oxidations of 4HAQO

In a previous paper it was reported that appropriate reducing agents, such as

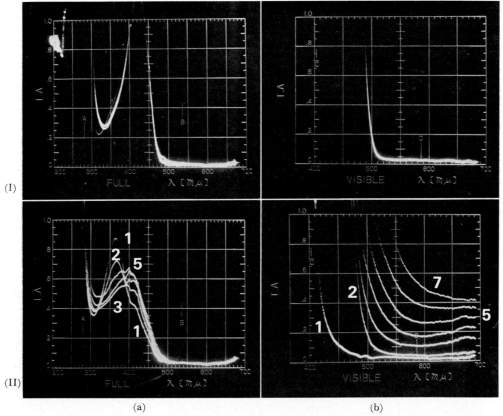

(a)   (b)

FIG. 9. Effect of ascorbic acid upon the spectral changes of 4HAQO during alkaline (I) and enzymatic (II) oxidation in the ultraviolet and visible (a) and visible (b) regions. (I) Alkaline oxidation. pH of the reaction mixture, 10.5 (0.02 M glycine-sodium hydroxide buffer). (a) Concentration of 4HAQO, 21 μg/ml; ascorbic acid, 100 μg/ml. (b) Concentration of 4HAQO, 415 μg/ml; ascorbic acid, 2010 μg/ml. The photographs show that no change in absorption spectra occurs in the presence of ascorbic acid. (II) Enzymatic oxidation. pH of the reaction mixture, 7.3 (0.025 M phosphate buffer) (a) Concentration of 4HAQO, 21 μg/ml; peroxidase, 42 μg/ml; H_2O_2, 1500 μg/ml; ascorbic acid, 100 μg/ml. 1) 1/3 sec, 2) 1 sec, 3) 5 sec, 4) 15 sec, 5) 30 sec. (b) Concentration of 4HAQO, 403 μg/ml; peroxidase, 101 μg/ml; H_2O_2, 1500 μg/ml; ascorbic acid, 1500 μg/ml. 1) <1/3 sec, 2) 1 sec, 3) 2 sec, 4) 3 sec, 5) 5 sec, 6) 10 sec, 7) 30 sec.

(a)   (b)

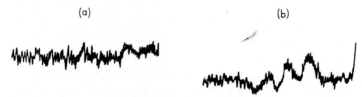

FIG. 10.   Effect of ascorbic acid upon free radical production during alkaline (a) and enzymatic (b) oxidations.   Conditions were the same as for (I) and (II) in Fig. 7, respectively, except for the presence of ascorbic acid (2010 μg/ml for (a) and 1760 μg/ml for (b)).   (a) and (b) are the signals 60 sec after the reactions started.

ascorbic acid, effectively protected 4HAQO from alkaline oxidation (8).   The present section is concerned with the effect of ascorbic acid upon formation of the nitroso intermediate and free radicals produced enzymatically and nonenzymatically. Figures 9 and 10 show that the effect of ascorbic acid upon the enzymatic oxidation is markedly different from its effect on alkaline oxidation.   Addition of ascorbic acid (about five times the amount of 4HAQO) completely inhibited the alkaline oxidation, as reported previously, and therefore no nitroso intermediate or free radical was detected.   On the other hand, ascorbic acid had no substantial effect upon enzymatic formation of the nitroso intermediate or free radical, although it seemed to cause a slight decrease in the reaction rate.   It is well known that ascorbic acid decomposes in an alkaline medium, yielding a proton and an electron, which may effectively prevent the anion of 4HAQO from further oxidation.   In the enzymatic oxidation the reaction mixture is neutral or acidic, so that ascorbic acid cannot act effectively as an antioxidant.   It should be noted that the signal and rate of production of the radical were the same in the presence and absence of ascorbic acid (Figs. 7 and 10).   Ascorbic acid can be oxidized by the peroxidase-H_2O_2 system to produce a radical with a doublet (23), but no such signal was detected, indicating that 4HAQO may be a better substrate of this enzyme system than ascorbic acid.

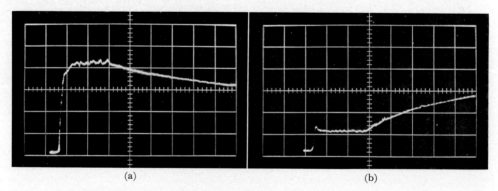

(a)   (b)

FIG. 11.   Time courses of the changes in absorbance at 355 mμ (a) and 410 mμ (b) in the initial stage of enzymatic oxidation of 4HAQO.   One division of the abscissa scale is 100 msec and one division of the ordinate scale is $\frac{1}{6}$ absorbance.   pH of the reaction mixture, 7.3 (0.025 M phosphate buffer).   Concentration of 4HAQO, 16 μg/ml; peroxidase, 40 μg/ml; H_2O_2, 1500 μg/ml.   (a) Change in absorbance at 355 mμ.   Light source, xenon lamp.   (b) Change in absorbance at 410 mμ.   Light source, tungsten lamp.

Time Courses of Absorbance Changes in the Initial Stage of Enzymatic Oxidation

Figure 11 shows the changes in absorbance at 355 and 410 mμ in the initial stage of the enzymatic oxidation.   It can be seen that the enzymatic oxidation starts about 250 msec after mixing.

Attempt to Detect Nitroso Intermediate during Reduction of 4NQO

4NQO is metabolized to 4HAQO *in vivo*, so it seemed desirable to demonstrate that the nitroso intermediate was formed in the reduction of 4NQO.   We tried to do this both chemically ($SnCl_2$–HCl) and enzymatically (C. L. Kluverig diaphorase-$NADH_2$ or $NADPH_2$), but did not succeed.   The overall rate of the reaction was very slow.   However, as 4-nitrosoquinoline 1-oxide is readily reduced to 4HAQO, an insufficient amount may accumulate to allow its detection directly with the present technique.   Therefore, the oxidative reactions were studied exclusively in the present work.

DISCUSSION

The present experiments clearly demonstrate that 4-nitrosoquinoline 1-oxide and free radicals are produced during oxidation of 4HAQO either enzymatically or nonenzymatically.   This is also indirect evidence for the participation of the nitroso compound in the reductive conversion of 4NQO to 4HAQO.

It is at present difficult to say whether 4-nitrosoquinoline 1-oxide is actually in-volved in 4NQO carcinogenesis since tests on its carcinogenicity are impossible be-cause it is so labile.   However, it is well known that nitroso compounds readily combine with primary amines to yield azo compounds.   Kosuge *et al.* (*11, 12*) found that one such azocompound was produced during alkaline oxidation of 4HAQO in the presence of aniline.   Similar reactions might be expected between 4-nitrosoquinoline 1-oxide and the amino groups of nucleic acids or proteins.   Ishi-zawa and Endo's suggestion (*6*) that the inactivation of phage DNA by 4HAQO may be brought about by the effective binding of 4-nitrosoquinoline 1-oxide with DNA is worth noting in this connection.

4HAQO itself is a more potent carcinogen than 4NQO (*3, 21*), and mammalian tissues may contain an enzyme system which catalyzes the oxidation of 4HAQO forming the nitroso compound and free radical.   It is then quite probable that the oxidative reaction of 4HAQO is essential for the carcinogenetic effect of 4NQO. This possibility has been discussed by Kawazoe and Araki (*9*).

If the general mechanism proposed for the peroxidative oxidation (*23*) is applied to the present system, the reaction scheme can be summarized in next page:

According to the scheme, the nitroso compound is the end product, which seems to be contradictory to the present data.   One explanation of this is that there is another pathway, such as a two-electron oxidation pathway, for oxidation of the present substrate.   Further studies are necessary on the mechanism of oxidation.

Next, the relationship between the two transient molecular species produced

Peroxidase   + H_2O_2 $\longrightarrow$ Compound - I   (1)

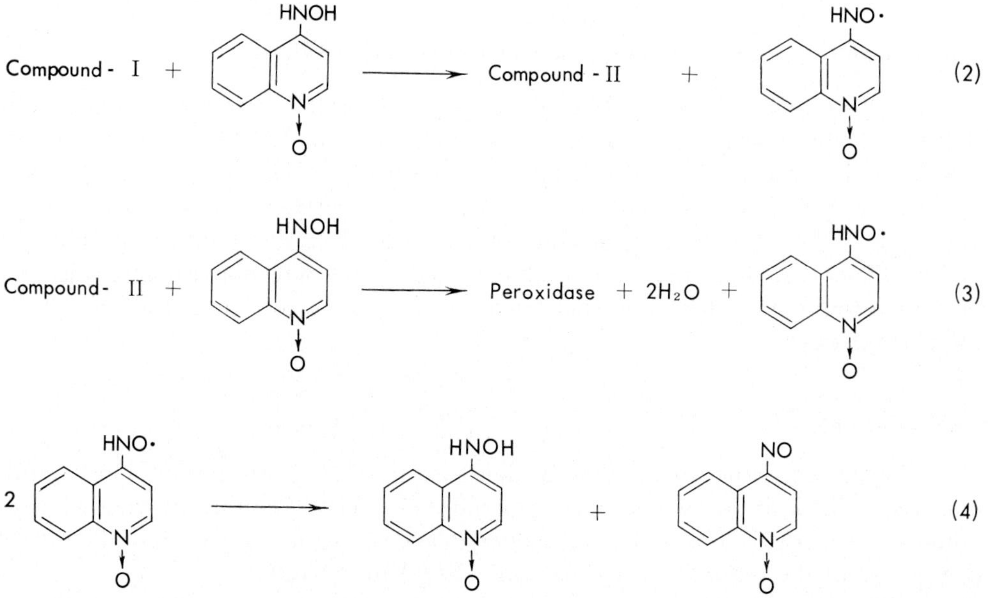

Compound - I   +   (4-HNOH quinoline N-oxide) $\longrightarrow$ Compound - II   +   (4-HNO· quinoline N-oxide)   (2)

Compound - II   +   (4-HNOH quinoline N-oxide) $\longrightarrow$ Peroxidase   + $2H_2O$ +   (4-HNO· quinoline N-oxide)   (3)

2 (4-HNO· quinoline N-oxide) $\longrightarrow$ (4-HNOH quinoline N-oxide)   +   (4-NO quinoline N-oxide)   (4)

during the oxidation of 4HAQO must be explained.   Our data show that the nitroso compound decays more rapidly than free radicals.   This implies that the nitroso compound is not formed from free radicals in the main pathway of the reaction.   In the enzymatic oxidation, however, it is possible that the nitroso compound is also produced from the free radical according to equation (4).   In fact, when the reaction mixture was allowed to stand for a long time, an absorption maximum reappeared at about 355 mμ and gradually increased in intensity.   A decrease in intensity of the band occurred at a longer wavelength.   This indicates that 4HAQO may be reproduced according to the reaction in equation (4).   The nitroso compound will also be generated.   However, we did not confirm this possibly because, as stated already, the reaction mixture became very turbid, and also possibly because an insufficient amount of nitroso compound accumulated through this pathway to allow its detection.   Furthermore all our other findings seem to be consistent with the existence of two different pathways for production of the nitroso compound and free radicals. The reductive conversion of the nitroso compound to two types of free radicals is very unlikely under the oxidative conditions in the present experiments.   Thus the oxidative process of 4HAQO can be summarized in next page:

Recently, Bartsch et al. (1, 2) found that the proximate carcinogen, N-hydroxy N-2-acetylaminofluorene, is oxidized enzymatically as well as chemically to yield a nitroxide radical which is converted to N-acetoxy-2-acetylaminofluorene and 2-nitrosofluorene with a dimeric molecule as an intermediate.   In their experiments

enz. ,enzymatic oxidation; non enz., non enzymatic oxidation

all the compounds were relatively stable, and so it was easy to test the carcinogenicities of the intermediates and to analyze the reaction mechanism.   In fact, both the intermediates were found to be carcinogenic to rats (*5, 15, 16*), thus establishing the participation of a free radical in carcinogenesis.   The mechanism of the present reaction differs in detail from that of N-hydroxy-N-2-acetylaminofluorene, but the participation of the nitroso compound and free radical in 4NQO and 4HAQO carcinogenesis may also be anticipated.

SUMMARY

The oxidative reaction of the proximate carcinogen, 4-hydroxyaminoquinoline 1-oxide, was investigated by spectroscopic and ESR measurements.   Using a rapid scan spectrophotometer it was possible to detect directly an unstable intermediate, which was 4-nitrosoquinoline 1-oxide.   The nitroso compound could be produced by enzymatic oxidation with horseradish peroxidase and hydrogen peroxide as well as by alkaline oxidation.   Enzymatic production of the nitroso compound is of great interest in connection with 4NQO and 4HAQO carcinogenesis.   The very short lifetime of the nitroso compound may imply its extreme reactivity with tissue components.   In addition to the nitroso compound, relatively stable free radicals could also be detected during the oxidative reactions.   The ESR spectrum of the free radical produced by enzymatic oxidation was different from that produced by alkaline oxidation, indicating that the two free radicals have different structures.   The time courses of appearance of the intermediates indicated that the nitroso compound decays more rapidly than the free radicals.   Alkaline oxidation of 4HAQO was inhibited by addition of ascorbic acid to the reaction mixture, but the enzymatic oxidation was not.   The nitroso compound could not be detected during reduction of 4NQO.

The authors thank Dr. Yutaka Kawazoe for suppling the purified 4HAQO hydrochloride and Dr. Waro Nakahara and Dr. Eiji Ochiai for their encouragement and interest throughout this work.

REFERENCES

1. Bartsch, H., and Hecker, E.   On the Metabolic Activation of the Carcinogen N-Hydroxy-N-2-acetylaminofluorene. III.   Oxidation with Horseradish Peroxidase to Yield 2-Nitrosofluorene and N-Acetoxy-N-2-acetylaminofluorene.   Biochim. Biophys. Acta, *237*: 567–578, 1971.

2. Bartsch, H., Traut, M., and Hecker, E.   On the Metabolic Activation of N-Hydroxy-N-2-acetylaminofluorene. II.   Simultaneous Formation of 2-Nitrosofluorene and N-Acetoxy-N-2-acetylaminofluorene from N-Hydroxy-N-2-acetylaminofluorene *via* a Free Radical Intermediate.   Biochim. Biophys. Acta, *237*: 556–566, 1971.

3. Endo, H., and Kume, F.   Comparative Studies on the Biological Actions of 4-Nitroquinoline 1-Oxide and Its Reduced Compound, 4-Hydroxyaminoquinoline 1-Oxide.   Gann, *54*: 443–453, 1963.

4. Forrester, A. R., Ogilvy, M.M., and Thomson, R.H. Mode of Action of Carcinogenic Amines.   Part I. Oxidation of N-Arylhydroxamic Acids.   J. Chem. Soc. (C), 1081–1083, 1970.

5. Hecker, E., Traut, M., and Hopp, M.   Über die Carcinogene Wirkung von 3-Amino-$\varDelta^{1,3,5(10)}$-oestratrienen und von 2-Nitrosofluoren.   Z. Krebsforsch., *71*: 81–88, 1968.

6. Ishizawa, M., and Endo, H.   On the Mode of Action of a Potent Carcinogen, 4-Hydroxylaminoquinoline 1-Oxide on Bacteriophage T4.   Biochem. Pharmacol., *16*: 637–646, 1967.

7. Kataoka, N., Imamura, A., Kawazoe, Y., Chihara, G., and Nagata, C.   The Structure of the Free Radical Produced from Carcinogenic 4-Hydroxyaminoquinoline 1-Oxide.   Bull. Chem. Soc. Japan, *40*: 62–68, 1967.

8. Kataoka, N., Shibata, S., Imamura, A., Kawazoe, Y., Chihara, G., and Nagata, C.   Oxidation Reaction of Carcinogenic 4-Hydroxyaminoquinoline 1-Oxide.   Chem. Pharm. Bull., Tokyo, *15*: 220–225, 1967.

9. Kawazoe, Y., and Araki, M.   *In*; Nakahara, W. (ed.), Chemical Tumor Problems, pp. 45–104, Japanese Society for the Promotion of Science, Tokyo, 1970.

10. Keussler, V. V., and Lüttke, W.   Spektroskopische Untersuchungen an Nitrosoverbindungen 3.   Mitteilung: Die Dissoziationsenergie der Nitrosodimeren.   Z. Electrochem., *63*: 614–623, 1959.

11. Kosuge, T., and Yokota, M.   Formation of 4-Nitrosoquinoline 1-Oxide and Synthesis of 4-Phenylazoquinoline 1-Oxide.   Yakugaku Zasshi, *85*: 69–71, 1965 (in Japanese).

12. Kosuge, T., Zenda, H., and Sawanishi, H.   Formation of Pyridazino [3,4-C: 5,6-C′] Biquinoline Compounds.   Chem. Pharm. Bull., Tokyo, *17*: 2389–2391, 1969.

13. Kosuge, T., Zenda, H., Yokota, M., Sawanishi, H., and Suzuki, Y.   Further Evidence for Formation of 4-Nitrosoquinoline 1-Oxide.   Chem. Pharm. Bull., Tokyo, *17*: 2181–2183, 1969.

14. Mackor, A., Wajer, Th. A. J. W., and de Boer, Th. J.   C-Nitroso Compounds.

Part I. The Formation of Nitroxides by Photolysis of Nitroso Compounds as Studied by Electron Spin Resonance.   Tetrahedron Letters, 2115–2123, 1966.

15.   Miller, E. C., McKechnie, D., Poirier, M. M., and Miller, J. A.   Inhibition of Amino Acid Incorporation *in vitro* by Metabolites of 2-Acetylaminofluorene and by Certain Nitroso Compounds.   Proc. Soc. Exptl. Biol. Med., *120*: 538–541, 1965.

16.   Miller, J. A., and Miller E. C.   *In*; Homburger, F. (ed.), Progress in Experimental Tumor Research, vol. 11, pp. 273–301, Karger, Basel, 1969.

17.   Nagata, C., Ioki, Y., Inomata, M., and Imamura, A.   Electron Spin Resonance Study on the Free Radicals Produced from Carcinogenic Aminonaphthols and N-Hydroxy-aminonaphthalenes.   Gann, *60*: 509–522, 1969.

18.   Nagata, C., Kataoka, N., Imamura, A., Kawazoe, Y., and Chihara, G.   Electron Spin Resonance Study on the Free Radicals Produced from 4-Hydroxyaminoquinoline 1-Oxide and Its Significance in Carcinogenesis.   Gann, *57*: 323–335, 1966.

19.   Nagata, C., Kodama, M., and Tagashira, Y.   Electron Spin Resonance Study on the Interaction between Chemical Carcinogens and Tissue Components. II. Free Radical Produced by Stirring Aromatic Hydrocarbons with Tissue Components such as Skin Homogenates or Proteins.   Gann, *58*: 493–504, 1967.

20.   Okabayashi, T., and Yoshimoto, A.   Reduction of 4-Nitroquinoline 1-Oxide by Microorganism.   Chem. Pharm. Bull., Tokyo, *10*: 1221–1226, 1962.

21.   Shirasu, Y.   Further Studies on Carcinogenic Action of 4-Hydroxy-aminoquinoline 1-Oxide.   Gann, *54*: 487–495, 1963.

22.   Sugimura, T., Okabe, K., and Endo, H.   The Metabolism of 4-Nitroquinoline 1-Oxide. I. Conversion of 4-Nitroquinoline 1-Oxide to 4-Aminoquinoline 1-Oxide by Rat Liver Enzyme.   Gann, *56*: 489–501, 1965.

23.   Yamazaki, I., Mason, H. S., and Piette, L.   Identification, by Electron Paramagnetic Resonance Spectroscopy, of Free Radicals Generated from Substrates by Peroxidase.   J. Biol. Chem., *235*: 2444–2449, 1960.

Discussion of Paper by Drs. Matsuyama and Nagata

DR. MAGEE: The interesting work of Dr. Nagata suggests that further work should be done on the carcinogenicity of C-nitroso compounds.

DR. WEISBURGER: Following the comment by Proffessor Magee on testing C-nitroso compounds for carcinogenicity it seems appropriate to recall that 2-nitrosofluorene was found to be carcinogenic by the Miller group in Wisconsin and by the Hecker group in Heidelberg. Of course, C-nitroso compounds can be metabolized further *in vivo*.

DR. PREUSSMANN: In one of your slides you compared C-nitroso and N-nitroso compounds. I think it should be stressed that the similarities between these two classes of compounds are rather formal ones. C-Nitroso compounds usually are highly reactive, and you have given a beautiful example of this. On the other hand, N-nitroso compounds like dimethylnitrosamine are not reacted chemically, at the nitroso groups. These latter compounds very probably require enzymatic activation *in vivo* to form chemically reactive forms.

DR. NAKAHARA: I might add that free radicals have not been considered seriously by many organic chemists, because it is difficult to get hold of them. Yet the free radical reaction does take place, and from the point of view of bioenergetics it cannot be disregarded in the truly proximate mechanism by which normal cells are altered into malignant ones.

DR. WEISBURGER: Professor Nakahara, pointing to the absence of studies of free radicals as carcinogens, offers a sound observation. In the United States efforts were made to detect free radicals in tobacco smoke with indecisive results. We need to consider the possibility that different mechanisms may operate in cancer induction in various target organs, reactive esters in one organ, carbonium ions in another and even free radicals in another organ.

Pancreatic Tumors in Rats Induced by 4-Nitroquinoline 1-Oxide Derivatives

Yuzo HAYASHI, Hitoshi FURUKAWA, and Toshiaki HASEGAWA

Shionogi Research Laboratory, Shionogi & Co., Ltd., Osaka, Japan

Since Nakahara and his colleagues succeeded in producing skin cancer in mice by painting the skin with 4-nitroquinoline 1-oxide (*24*), extensive studies have been made on the carcinogenic mechanism of this compound. Results indicate that 4-nitroquinoline 1-oxide is converted metabolically to 4-aminoquinoline 1-oxide *via* its 4-hydroxyamino derivative for exhibition of its carcinogenic activity. This conclusion is deduced from the following evidence: (1) 4-Hydroxyaminoquinoline 1-oxide itself was shown to be a potent carcinogen (*4, 36*); (2) 4-nitroquinoline 1-oxide can be converted to 4-hydroxyaminoquinoline 1-oxide (*25, 39, 40*) *in vivo* as well as *in vitro*; and (3) the carcinogenic activity of substituted 4-nitroquinoline 1-oxides appears to be parallel to their own redoxpotentials *in vitro* to give the corresponding derivatives of 4-hydroxyaminoquinoline 1-oxide (*14, 15*).

4-Nitroquinoline 1-oxide and 4-hydroxyaminoquinoline 1-oxide appear to be quite comparable (*3*) with regard to their carcinogenicity, as well as to some other biological activities such as mutagenicity in microorganisms, λ-phage induction in lysogenic *E. coli* and nuclear inclusion-body formation. For example, subcutaneous injection of either of these compounds into mice induces sarcomas *in loco* (*3, 4, 36*) and lung cancer (*19, 21*). However, the carcinogenic effects of these two compounds differ somewhat in organspecificity. For example, 4-nitroquinoline 1-oxide (*24, 42*) has a more specific carcinogenic effect on the epidermis or epidermoid tissue than 4-hydroxyaminoquinoline 1-oxide (*36*). Hozumi *et al.* (*12*) reported that 4-hydroxyaminoquinoline 1-oxide only induced skin cancer in mice when dimethylsulfoxide was used as the solvent. Mori (*20*) compared the effects of 4-hydroxyaminoquinoline 1-oxide and 4-nitroquinoline 1-oxide when given to mice by gastric instillation, and found that the former induced adenocarcinoma of the glandular stomach and duodenum, whereas the latter induced epidermoid cancer in the forestomach. Recently, Shirasu *et al.* (*31*) reported that intravenous injection of 4-hydroxyaminoquinoline 1-oxide induced cancer of the intestine, renal tubules and meninx.

Our own studies on the pathological effects of various quinoline derivatives in rats have shown that 4-hydroxyaminoquinoline 1-oxide strongly affects the exocrine acini of the pancreas resulting in a high incidence of adenoma or adenoma-like lesions (7).   We also noted a unique ability of a derivative of 4-hydroxyaminoquino-line 1-oxide, 6-diethylaminomethyl-4-hydroxyaminoquinoline 1-oxide, to cause either diabetes or islet cell adenomas in rats (5).   Details of these experiments are described in this paper.

Acute Effects of 4-Hydroxyaminoquinoline 1-Oxide on the Pancreas

While studying the acute toxicity of 4-hydroxyaminoquinoline 1-oxide in rats, it was found that intravenous injection of this compound in a dose greater than the LD_{50} (13.3±1.7 mg/kg, i.v.) invariably caused acinar necrosis of the pancreas and changes in various other tissues, such as disruption of the lymphatic tissues, epithelial degeneration of the gastrointestinal tract and necrosis of the proximal convoluted tubules of the kidney.

The severity of the pancreatic lesions varied with the dose and the time after injection.   When given a dose of 20 mg/kg rats showed gross evidence of pancreatic edema by 24 hr, and histological examination showed diffuse necrosis of the acinar cells.   After a dose of 10 mg/kg, the gross appearance of the pancreas was normal, but areas of necrosis of the acinar cells were observed histologically.   The remaining acinar cells underwent either shrinkage or various grades of cytoplasmic alteration, such as decrease of zymogen granules, vacuolation or loss of basophilia.   Electron microscopic examination of these cells revealed cisternal dilatation of the rough endoplasmic reticulum, development of lipiddroplets and various-sized autophagic vacuoles which contained amorphous material, membranous debris and, occasionally, well-preserved endoplasmic reticulum.   The degenerative changes occurred preferentially in the acinar cells, and the ductal epithelial cells appeared well preserved.   The islet cells occasionally displayed karyopycnosis after a dose of 20 mg/kg body wt. or more.   It should be mentioned that the selective damage of pancreatic acini by 4-hydroxyaminoquinoline 1-oxide was greater in dogs than in rats.

Pancreatic Tumors Induced by 4-Hydroxyaminoquinoline 1-Oxide

Effect of a single dose

Five-week-old Sprague-Dawley rats were used.   Thirty animals of each sex were injected intravenously with an acidic aqueous solution of 4-hydroxyamino-quinoline 1-oxide at a dose of 6, 9 or 13 mg/kg body wt.   Twenty-four rats which died from the toxic effects of the compound or from respiratory infection were excluded.   The other rats were killed 162 to 400 days after the injection.

The incidences of tumors in each group are shown in Table 1.   A remarkable finding was the high incidence of pancreatic tumors in groups receiving the carcinogen.   These tumors were round, multiple tumors of up to 7 mm in diameter, which were soft, and yellowish-grey.   Their incidence was significantly higher in males than

TABLE 1. Incidence of Tumors in Rats after a Single Intravenous Injection of 4-Hydroxyaminoquinoline 1-Oxide

Dose (mg/kg)	Sex	Number of rats		Number of rats with tumors						
		Initial	Effec- tive[a]	Pancreas		Intes- tinal carci- noma	Renal ade- noma	Breast		Other tumor
				Exo- crine tumor	Islet cell tumor			Carci- noma	Fibro- ade- noma	
0	♂	20	19	0	0	0	0	0	0	1[b]
6	♂	10	7	7	0	0	1	0	0	0
9	♂	10	6	6	0	2	0	0	0	0
13	♂	10	3	3	0	1	1	0	0	0
0	♀	15	14	0	0	0	0	0	2	0
6	♀	10	10	4	0	1	0	1	2	0
9	♀	10	7	4	0	3	1	0	0	1[c]
13	♀	10	2	1	1	0	1	0	0	1[d]

[a] Number of rats which survied more than 160 days.
[b] Pheochromocytoma of the adrenal.
[c] Leukemia.
[d] Pulmonary adenoma.

in females. Histologically, the tumors consisted of neatly arranged acini containing zymogen granules. The component cells were smaller than normal acinar cells, and arranged around a central lumen. The nuclei were located at the end of the cells distant from the central lumen. Mitotic figures were seen but were usually infrequent. Under an electron microscope, well-developed parallel arrays of rough endoplasmic reticulum were observed in the cytoplasm. Ductal structures were only seen in one tumor in which one area had a cystoadenoma-like appearance. The adjacent pancreatic tissue was compressed to form a false capsule, while true fibrous encapsulation was inconspicuous. There was no local invasion, spread to the mesentery, or distant metastasis. In contrast with the frequent occurrence of exocrine tumors, only one islet cell tumor was seen in a female rat, which had received 13 mg/kg body wt. of 4-hydroxyaminoquinoline 1-oxide.

Besides these discrete tumors, there were invariably minute foci of atypical acini, in which the cells were larger than normal acinar cells and had fewer zymogen granules. The nuclei were rather irregular in contour, with marginal condensation of chromatin, and contained distinct nucleoli. The cytoplasm showed intense basophilia. It was uncertain whether transition from atypical acini to tumors occurred.

Effect of repeated doses

Twenty 5-week-old male Sprague-Dawley rats were given 8 weekly intravenous injections of 4-hydroxyaminoquinoline 1-oxide in doses of 5 mg/kg body wt. Nine rats which died during this treatment were excluded. The other rats were killed between the 160th and 220th day after treatment. Pathological examination revealed the occurrence of 4 leukemias, 4 intestinal cancers and 1 breast cancer in these animals. Exocrine tumors of the pancreas were found in 7 animals, and an islet cell tumor in 1 animal.   The gross and histological features of these tumors were the same as those induced by a single dose of carcinogen.   Atypical acini were also noted in this group.

Islet Cell Tumor of the Pancreas Induced by 6-Diethylaminomethyl-4-hydroxyaminoquinoline 1-Oxide

To obtain a very watersoluble derivative of 4-hydroxyaminoquinoline 1-oxide, the 6-diethylaminomethyl derivative was synthesized.   In a preliminary test in rats, it was noted that a single intravenous injection of this compound in a dose of 80 mg/kg body wt. induced degenerative changes of the pancreatic islet cells, while the exocrine acinar cells appeared to be well preserved.   To confirm the tissue-selective carcinogenicity of this compound, the following experiment was carried out.

Four-week-old male Sprague-Dawley rats, 12 to a group, were given 8 weekly intravenous injections of 6-diethylaminomethyl-4-hydroxyaminoquinoline 1-oxide dihydrochloride in a dose of 10, 20 or 40 mg/kg body wt.   About 120 days after the last injection, 2 of the rats which had received 40 mg/kg body wt. exhibited growth retardation with polyuria and glycosuria; these animals were killed on the 211st day.   Histological examination revealed marked atrophy of the pancreatic islets and hydropic degeneration of the distal convoluted tubules of the kidney (osmotic nephrosis).   Another 4 rats in this group displaying the same symptoms were killed between the 250th and 340th day.   Histologically, atrophy of the pancreatic islets was seen in all rats, and osmotic nephrosis in 3 animals.   Glycosuria also developed in 1 rat after 10 mg/kg body wt. of carcinogen.

The other rats were killed for pathological examination on the 400th day.   The incidences of tumors in each group are shown in Table 2.   Exocrine tumors of the pancreas developed in 5 rats, while islet cell tumors developed in 20 of 34 rats.   The islet cell tumors were round or oval, measuring 2 to 8 mm in diameter, and were firm and varied in color from yellowish-white to brownish-red according to their

TABLE 2.   Incidences of Tumors and Diabetes in Rats after 8 Weekly Intravenous Injections of 6-Diethyl-aminomethyl-4-hydroxyaminoquinoline 1-Oxide

Dose per inject. (mg/kg)	Number of rats		Number of rats with tumors						Number of rats with	
	Initial	Effective[a]	Pancreas		Intestinal carcinoma	Pulmonary adenoma	Hemangioendothelioma	Other tumor	Glycosuria	Osmotic nephrosis
			Exocrine tumor	Islet cell tumor						
0	12	11	0	0	0	0	0	1[b]	0	0
10	12	11	1	6	0	0	0	1[b],2[e]	1	1
20	12	12	4	9	3	2	1	1[c],1[e]	0	0
40	12	11	0	5	2	1	2	1[c],1[d]	6	5

[a]   Number of rats which survived more than 200 days.
[b]   Pituitary adenoma.
[c]   Follicular adenoma of the thyroid.
[d]   Leukemia.
[e]   Ear duct cancer.

blood content. Histologically, they were circumscribed by a fibrous capsule. The tumor cells were cuboidal or polyhedral in shape and were arranged in short, anastomosed cords, single- or double-cell columns, or small clusters. The cytoplasm of most cells contained aldehyde-fuchsin positive granules, and β-granules were demonstrated by electron microscopy. The nuclei were round or oval and centrally located, and contained small nucleoli. The surrounding exocrine epithelium appeared to be compressed, although no local invasion or distant metastasis was detected.

It is interesting that 6-diethylaminomethyl-4-hydroxyaminoquinoline 1-oxide strongly affects the pancreatic islet cells, resulting in severe atrophy or a high incidence of tumors. 4-Hydroxyaminoquinoline 1-oxide itself has little affect on the islet cells, so the diethylaminomethyl group at C_6 may contribute to this tissue affinity. A similar situation has been shown for the diabetogenic activity of streptozotocin (27), 2-deoxy-2-(3-methyl-3-nitrosoureido)-D-glucopyranose, in which the glucose moiety of the molecules is considered to have a potential carrier function, facilitating transport across the β-cell membrane (28).

DISCUSSION

In longevity experiments (34, 43), it has been noted that the spontaneous occurrence of pancreatic tumors is extremely rare in rats. Therefore, the present experiments resulting in a high incidence of exocrine tumors or islet cell tumors following administration of 4-nitroquinoline 1-oxide derivatives appear to be significant. However, it is uncertain whether these tumors are true adenomas or hyperplastic nodules, since it was also shown that carcinogenic quinolines could produce degenerative changes in exocrine acinar cells or islet cells. Rowlatt (33) reported that, as with liver tumors, it is difficult to distinguish between hyperplastic nodules and autonomous neoplasms of the pancreas, although features such as the large size and small number of lesions, the presence of a capsule, and the absence of atrophy or postinflammatory changes elsewhere in the pancreas suggest that the lesion is an adenoma rather than a reactive hyperplastic nodule.

Recently we noted that a nucleolar alteration, characterized by segregation of the granular and fibrillar components into separate zones, developed in the exocrine acinar cells of the pancreas in rats following injection of 4-hydroxyaminoquinoline 1-oxide (8). The nucleolar alteration is known to occur in a series of *in vivo* and *in vitro* cell systems after treatment with various chemicals, including actinomycin D (30), acridine orange (29), 4-nitroquinoline 1-oxide (6, 9, 31) and aflatoxin B (41). These substances have the ability to form complexes (16, 23, 38) with DNA in some fashion and to interfere with DNA-mediated RNA synthesis. Reynolds et al. (6) discussed the possibility that nucleolar segregation could be used as a morphological marker for a special type of cell injury involving DNA. In recent biochemical studies, 4-hydroxyaminoquinoline 1-oxide was also found to form a complex with DNA. On the basis of these findings, it can be postulated that 4-hydroxyaminoquinoline 1-oxide, when injected into rats, reaches the pancreatic tissue and interacts with nuclear DNA.

Exocrine acini of the pancreas are known to be highly sensitive to certain chemicals that interfere with protein synthesis, cholesterol synthesis or nucleic acid metabolism. These include puromycin (*18*), ethionine (*11*), aminopentane carboxylic acid (*1*), triparanol (*13*) and actinomycin D (*32*). Injuries of the pancreatic islet cells result from administration of various diabetogenic agents (*28*), including alloxan, streptozotocin and dithizone. Experimental data on the induction of pancreatic tumors by chemicals have also been reported by several investigators. Exocrine adenomas or adenomatous growth of the pancreas could be induced in rats by long-term administration of 4'-fluoro-4-aminodiphenyl (*10*), N,N'-2,7-fluorenylenebisacetamide or N-2-fluorenylacetamide (*22*). Schoental *et al.* (*35*) reported the occurrence of adenocarcinomas of the islet cells and adenomas of the exocrine pancreas in rats after a single dose of pyrrolizidine alkaloids from *Amsinckia intermedia.* Rakieten *et al.* (*26*) found that combined administration of streptozotocin, a naturally occurring nitrosourea, with nicotinamide to rats is associated with a high incidence of pancreatic islet cell tumors. Druckrey *et al.* (*2*) reported the consistent induction of adenocarcinomas of the exocrine pancreas in guinea pigs by long-term administration of methylnitrosourea or methylnitrosourethane in the drinking water. All these data, together with the present findings, raise the possibility that the occurrence of pancreatic tumors in humans is, at least in part, due to environmental or occupational exposure to certain chemicals. Recently, Li *et al.* (*17*) published statistical data which suggest that occupational exposure of chemists increases their risk of incurring lymphoma or pancreatic cancer.

SUMMARY

Exocrine tumors as well as islet cell tumors of the pancreas were induced in rats by 4-nitroquinoline 1-oxide derivatives. Sixty 35-day-old Sprague-Dawley rats (30 of each sex) were given a single intravenous injection of 6, 9 or 13 mg/kg body wt. of 4-hydroxyaminoquinoline 1-oxide, which is a proximate carcinogen of 4-nitroquinoline 1-oxide. Within 7 days after the injection 14 rats died with edema and hemorrhage of the intestine, disruption of lymphatic tissues and degeneration of the exocrine acini of the pancreas. Between the 162nd and 400th day 35 rats were killed for pathological examination. Among these, 7 cases of intestinal cancer, 4 cases of renal adenoma and 1 case each of pulmonary adenoma and myelogenic leukemia were noted. In addition pancreatic tumors were found in 9 of 19 females and 16 of 16 males. These were round, multiple tumors, measuring up to 5 mm in diameter, and were characterized histologically by neatly arranged acini containing zymogen granules. Mitotic figures were infrequent and neither local invasion nor distant metastasis was detected.

In another series of experiments 36 male Sprague-Dawley rats were given weekly intravenous injections of 10, 20 or 40 mg/kg body wt. of 6-diethylaminomethyl-4-hydroxyaminoquinoline 1-oxide for 8 weeks. Six of the rats which received 40 mg/kg of carcinogen and 1 rat which received 10 mg/kg exhibited polyuria and glycosuria, and pathologically they showed severe atrophy of the pancreatic islets. On the 400th day the surviving rats were killed for pathological examination.

Among these, 5 cases of intestinal cancer, 3 cases of pulmonary adenoma and 3 cases of hemangioendothelioma were noted. Exocrine tumors of the pancreas appeared in 5 rats, while islet cell tumors occurred in 20 of 34 rats. The islet cell tumors were up to 8 mm in diameter and firm in consistency. The tumor cells were cuboidal or polyhedral and were arranged in anastomosed cords, single- or double-cell columns or small clusters. Examination by electron microscope showed that the majority of the cells had β-granules in the cytoplasm. It is considered that the diethylaminomethyl group of the molecule has a potential carrier function, bringing about contact with the islet cells.

The authors wish to express their sincere thanks to Dr. Eiji Ochiai, Emeritus Professor of University of Tokyo for his interest and encouragement throughout this study. Thanks are also due to Dr. Manabu Fujimoto, Shionogi Research Laboratory, for his valuable criticism and suggestions.

REFERENCES

1. Chenard, J., and Auger, C. Cytoplasmic Changes in Pancreatic Acinar Cells of the Rat Caused by One-Amino-Cyclopentane Carboxylic Acid (ACPC). Amer. J. Path., *52*: 825–840, 1968.
2. Druckrey, H., Ivankovic, S., Bücheler, J., Preussmann, R., und Thomas, C. Erzeugung von Magen- und Pankreas-Krebs beim Meerschweinchen durch Methylnitrosoharnstoff und -urethan. Z. Krebsforsch., *72*: 167–182, 1968.
3. Endo, H., and Kume, F. Comparative Studies on the Biological Actions of 4-Nitroquinoline 1-Oxide and Its Reduced Compound, 4-Hydroxyaminoquinoline 1-Oxide. Gann, *54*: 443–453, 1963.
4. Endo, H., and Kume, F. Induction of Sarcoma in Rats by Subcutaneous Injection of 4-Hydroxyaminoquinoline 1-Oxide. Naturwissenschaften, *50*: 525–526, 1963.
5. Hayashi, Y., Furukawa, H., and Hasegawa, T. Unpublished.
6. Hayashi, Y., and Hasegawa, T. Nucleolar Alterations of Alveolar Epithelial Cells in Rats Following a Single Injection of 4-Nitroquinoline 1-Oxide. Gann, *61*: 347–352, 1970.
7. Hayashi, Y., and Hasegawa, T. Experimental Pancreatic Tumor in Rats after Intravenous Injection of 4-Hydroxyaminoquinoline 1-Oxide. Gann, *62*: 329–330, 1971.
8. Hayashi, Y., and Hasegawa, T. Unpublished.
9. Hayashi, Y., Hasegawa, T., and Toyoshima, K. Nucleolar Alterations of Peripheral Nerve Cells in Rats Following Administration of 4-Hydroxyaminoquinoline 1-Oxide. Experientia, *27*: 925–926, 1971.
10. Hendry, J. A., Matthews, J. J., Walpole, A. L., and Williams, M. H. C. Tumours Induced in Rats with 4'-Fluoro-aminobiphenyl. Nature, *175*: 1131–1132, 1955.
11. Herman, L., and Fitzgerald, P. J. The Degenerative Changes in Pancreatic Acinar Cells Caused by DL-Ethionine. J. Cell Biol., *12*: 277–296, 1962.
12. Hozumi, M. Induction of Skin Tumors in Mice by Painting with 4-Hydroxyaminoquinoline 1-Oxide. Gann, *60*: 161–165, 1969.
13. Hruban, Z., Swift, H., and Slesers, A. Effect of Triparanol and Diethanolamine on the Fine Structure of Hepatocytes and Pancreatic Acinar Cells. Lab. Invest., *14*: 1652–1672, 1965.

14. Kawazoe, Y., Araki, M., and Nakahara, W.   The Structure-Carcinogenicity Relationship among Derivatives of 4-Nitro- and 4-Hydroxyaminoquinoline 1-Oxides. Chem. Pharm. Bull., Tokyo, *17*: 544–549, 1969.

15. Kawazoe, Y., Tachibana, M., Aoki, K., and Nakahara, W.   The Structure-Carcinogenicity Relationship among Derivatives of 4-Nitro- and 4-Hydroxyaminoquinoline 1-Oxides.   Biochem. Pharm., *16*: 631–636, 1967.

16. Lerman, L. S.   Structural Considerations in the Interaction of DNA and Acridin. J. Mol. Biol., *3*: 18–30, 1961.

17. Li, F. P., Fraumeni, J. F., Mantel, N., and Miller, R. W.   Cancer Mortality among Chemists.   J. Natl. Cancer Inst., *43*: 1159–1164, 1969.

18. Longnecker, D. S., and Farber, E.   Acute Pancreatic Necrosis Induced by Puromycin.   Lab. Invest., *16*: 321–329, 1967.

19. Mori, K.   Preliminary Note on Adenocarcinoma of the Lung in Mice Induced with 4-Nitroquinoline N-Oxide.   Gann, *52*: 265–270, 1961.

20. Mori, K.   Carcinoma of the Glandular Stomach of Mice by 4-Nitroquinoline 1-Oxide or 4-Hydroxyaminoquinoline 1-Oxide.   Proc. Jap. Cancer Ass. 26th Gen. Mtg., Nagoya, p. 187, 1967 (in Japanese).

21. Mori, K., Kondo, M., Koibuchi, E., and Hashimoto, A.   Induction of Lung Cancer in Mice by Injection of 4-Hydroxyaminoquinoline 1-Oxide.   Gann, *58*: 105–106, 1967.

22. Morris, H. P., Wagner, B. P., Ray, F. P., Stewart, H. L., and Snell, K. C.   Comparative Carcinogenic Effects of N,N'-2,7-Fluorenylenebisacetamide by Intraperitoneal and Oral Routes of Administration to Rat with Particular Reference to Gastric Carcinoma.   J. Natl. Cancer Inst., *29*: 977–1011, 1962.

23. Müller, W.   Bindung von Actinomycinen und Actinomycin-Derivaten an Desoxyribonucleinsäure.   Naturwissenschaften, *49*: 156–157, 1962.

24. Nakahara, W., Fukuoka, F., and Sugimura, T.   Carcinogenic Action of 4-Nitroquinoline 1-Oxide.   Gann, *48*: 129–137, 1957.

25. Okabayashi, T., and Yoshimoto, A.   Reduction of 4-Nitroquinoline 1-Oxide by Microorganism.   Chem. Pharm. Bull., Tokyo, *10*: 1221–1226, 1962.

26. Rakieten, N., Gordon, B. S., Beaty, A., Cooney, D. A., Davis, R. D., and Schein, P. S. Pancreatic Islet Cell Tumors Produced by the Combined Action of Streptozotocin and Nicotinamide.   Proc. Soc. Exptl. Biol. Med., *137*: 280–283, 1971.

27. Rakieten, N., Rakieten, M. L., and Nadkarni, M. V. Studies on the Diabetogenic Action of Streptozotocin (NSC-37917).   Cancer Chemother. Rep., *29*: 91–98, 1963.

28. Rerup, C. C.   Diabetes Produced by Drug Damage to Insulin-Secreting Cells. Pharmcol. Rev., *22*: 484–517, 1970.

29. Reynolds, R. C., and Montgomery, P. O'B.   Nucleolar Pathology by Acridine Orange and Proflavine.   Amer. J. Path., *51*: 323–339, 1967.

30. Reynolds, R. C., Montgomery, P. O'B., and Hughes, B.   Nucleolar " Caps " Produced by Actinomycin D.   Cancer Res., *24*: 1269–1277, 1964.

31. Reynolds, R. C., Montgomery, P. O'B., and Karney, D. H. Nucleolar "Caps"— a Morphologic Entity Produced by the Carcinogen 4-Nitroquinoline N-Oxide.   Cancer Res., *23*: 535–538, 1963.

32. Rodriguez, T. G.   Ultrastructural Changes in the Mouse Exocrine Pancreas Induced by Prolonged Treatment with Actinomycin D.   J. Ultrastruct. Res., *19*: 116–129, 1967.

33. Rowlatt, U.   Spontaneous Epithelial Tumors of the Pancreas of Mammals.   Brit. J. Cancer, *21*: 82–107, 1967.

34. Rowlatt, U., and Roe, F. J. C. Epithelial Tumors of the Rat Pancreas. J. Natl. Cancer. Inst., *39*: 17–32, 1967.

35. Schoental, R., Fowler, M. E., and Coady, A. Islet Cell Tumors of the Pancreas Found in Rats Given Pyrrolizidine Alkaloids from *Amsinckia intermedia* Fisch and Mey and from *Heliotropium supinum* L. Cancer Res., *30*: 2127–2131, 1970.

36. Shirasu, Y., and Ohta, A. A Preliminary Note on the Carcinogenicity of 4-Hydroxyaminoquinoline 1-Oxide. Gann, *54*: 221–223, 1963.

37. Shirasu, Y., Mizutani, T., and Yamamoto, S. Carcinogenicity of 4-Hydroxyamino-quinoline 1-Oxide Injected in Mice and Rats. 10th Internat. Cancer Cong., Houston, U.S.A., Abstracts, pp. 20–21, 1970.

38. Sporn, M. B., Dingman, C. W., Phelps, H. L., and Wogen, G. N. Aflatoxin B_1; Binding to DNA *in vitro* and Alteration of RNA Metabolism *in vitro*. Science, *151*: 1539–1541, 1966.

39. Sugimura, T., Okabe, K., and Endo, H. The Metabolism of 4-Nitroquinoline 1-Oxide. I. Conversion of 4-Nitroquinoline 1-Oxide to 4-Aminoquinoline 1-Oxide by Rat Liver Enzyme. Gann, *56*: 489–501, 1965.

40. Sugimura, T., Okabe, K., and Nagao, M. The Metabolism of 4-Nitroquinoline 1-Oxide. III. An Enzyme Catalyzing the Conversion of 4-Nitroquinoline 1-Oxide to 4-Hydroxyaminoquinoline 1-Oxide in Rat Liver and Hepatomas. Cancer Res., *26*: 1717–1721, 1966.

41. Svoboda, D., Racela, A., and Higginson, J. Variations in Ultrastructural Nucleolar Changes in Hepatocarcinogenesis. Biochem. Pharm., *16*: 651–657, 1967.

42. Takayama, S. Skin Carcinogenesis with a Single Painting of 4-Nitroquinoline N-Oxide. Gann, *51*, 139–145, 1960.

43. Thompson, S. W., Huseby, R. A., Fox, M. A., Davis, C. L., and Hunt, R. D. Spontaneous Tumors in the Sprague-Dawley Rat. J. Natl. Cancer Inst., *27*: 1037–1057, 1961.

Discussion of Paper by Drs. Hayashi et al.

DR. HIGGINSON: Congratulations on an excellent paper.   Pancreatic carcinoma is now becoming of major significance in North America and in Western Europe. It is most satisfactory to have an experimental morphological model now available to study this phenomenon.   It is of interest that Dr. Hayashi also found that males were more susceptible than females as in the United States.

I would also like to emphasize that we should reconsider the I.V. route as possibly the best method of showing the potential carcinogenic range of a proximate carcinogen.   Thus in I.V. injection cells are exposed to a wide range of concentrations of the proximate carcinogen and the critical level may more likely be reached. In contrast, with long-term feeding it is possible that cells are exposed to a more constant level and the critical level never obtained.   The nitrosamines have shown the advantages also of I.V. testing.   I believe this deserves further discussion and may serve as morphological models more similar to those found in man.

DR. HAYASHI: Thank you very much for your comment.

DR. STICH: Are the pancreatic tumors transplantable?   Do the various tumors differ antigenically?

DR. HAYASHI: So far, I have not succeeded in transplantation.

DR. DAWE: I am interested in the frequency with which you observed the large-cell, atypical acinar lesion in the exocrine pancreas.   I ask this because the lesions appear similar to others that I have seen in the salivary glands of untreated, normal mice.   I have interpreted such lesions as foci of polyploid—probably tetraploid—cells that were not neoplastic or otherwise abnormal.

DR. HAYASHI: The atypical acini appeared in all rats given 4HAQO.   The pathological entity of such lesions is uncertain.   A type of transformed cell without the capability to divide rapidly might be a possibility.   Histologically, the atypical acini resemble the lesion of the pancreas in aged rats.   So, as another possibility, I would like to mention that 4HAQO can promote a senile change of the pancreas besides inducing tumors.

DR. PREUSSMANN: Is there a special reason why you kill your experimental animals after 400 days? Have you also results from experiments with longer exposure?

DR. HAYASHI: The Sprague-Dawley rats in our laboratory are shown to suffer from severe contracted kidney at the age of 1 year to 1.5 years.   This is the reason why I stopped the experiment on the 400th day.

EXPLANATION OF PHOTOS

FIG. 1.   An area of the pancreas from a rat 48 hr after injection of 10 mg/kg body wt. of 4-hydroxyamino-quinoline 1-oxide, showing focal necrosis of the exocrine acini (upper left).   Islet cells appear intact.   H-E. ×250.

FIG. 2.   An area of the pancreas from a rat 24 hr after injection of 80 mg/kg body wt. of 6-diethylamino-methyl-4-hydroxyaminoquinoline 1-oxide.   Islet cells exhibit nuclear pycnosis.   H-E.   ×160.

FIG. 3.   An exocrine tumor (5×4 mm) of the pancreas from a rat given 6 mg/kg body wt. of 4-hy-droxyaminoquinoline 1-oxide.

FIG. 4.   An area of the pancreatic tumor shown in Fig. 3.   Cells containing zymogen granules are arranged around central lumina.   H-E.   ×250.

FIG. 5.   An exocrine tumor (6×5 mm) of the pancreas from a rat given 9 mg/kg body wt. of 4-hydroxya-minoquinoline 1-oxide.   One area (left) has a cystoadenoma-like appearance.   H-E.

FIG. 6.   An area of the pancreatic tumor shown in Fig. 5, showing cystic spaces lined by cuboidal epithelial cells.   H-E.   ×250.

FIG. 7.   An area of the pancreas from a rat 400 days after injection of 9 mg/kg body wt. of 4-hydroxy-aminoquinoline 1-oxide, showing a focus of atypical acini.   The component cells are larger than normal acinar cells, and contain large, single nuclei or occasionally double nuclei.   The cytoplasm appears stongly basophilic.   H-E.   ×250.

FIG. 8.   An area of the pancreas from a rat after 8 weekly injections of 40 mg/kg body wt. of 6-diethyl-aminomethyl-4-hydroxyaminoquinoline 1-oxide, showing severe atrophy of a pancreatic islet.   H-E.   ×400.

FIG. 9.   An islet cell tumor (3×2 mm) of the pancreas from a rat after 8 weekly injections of 20 mg/kg body wt. of 6-diethylaminomethyl-4-hydroxyaminoquinoline 1-oxide.   The tumor tissue appears to be circumscribed by a thin fibrous capsule.

FIG. 10.   An area of the pancreatic islet cell tumor shown in Fig. 9.   The tumor cells are arranged in single- or double-cell columns.   H-E.   ×160.

FIG. 11.   An islet cell tumor (9×5 mm) of the pancreas from a rat after 8 weekly injections of 20 mg/kg body wt. of 6-diethylaminomethyl-4-hydroxyaminoquinoline 1-oxide.   The tumor tissue is surrounded by a thick fibrous capsule.

FIG. 12.   An area of the islet cell tumor shown in Fig. 11.   The tumor cells appear to be closely packed and are arranged in double-cell columns.   H-E.   ×160.

FIG. 13.   Electorn micrograph showing an area of a pancreatic islet cell tumor from a rat given 8 weekly injections of 20 mg/kg body wt. of 6-diethylaminomethyl-4-hydroxyaminoquinoline 1-oxide. β-Granules are seen in each of the tumor cells.   Uranyl acetate-lead citrate.   ×6000.

FIG. 14.   A portion of an exocrine acinar cell of the pancreas from a rat 2 hr after injection of 20 mg/kg body wt. of 4-hydroxyaminoquinoline 1-oxide.   The nucleolus is reduced in size.   The fibrous and granular components are separated into distinct zones.   Uranyl acetate-lead citrate.   ×80000.

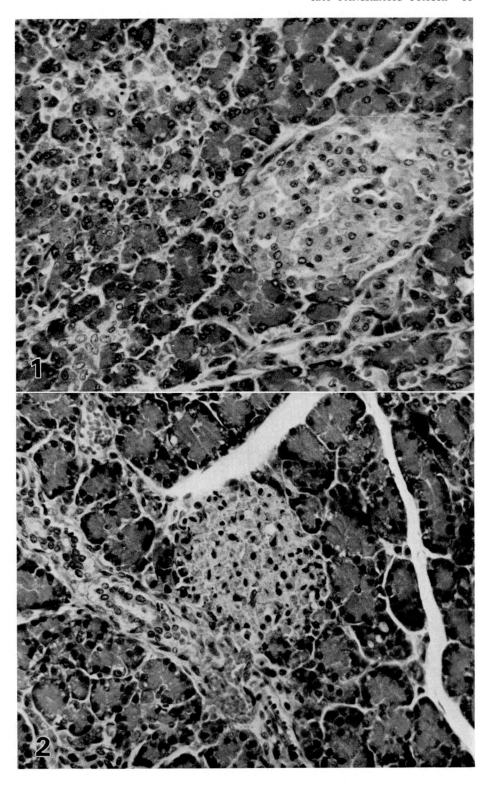

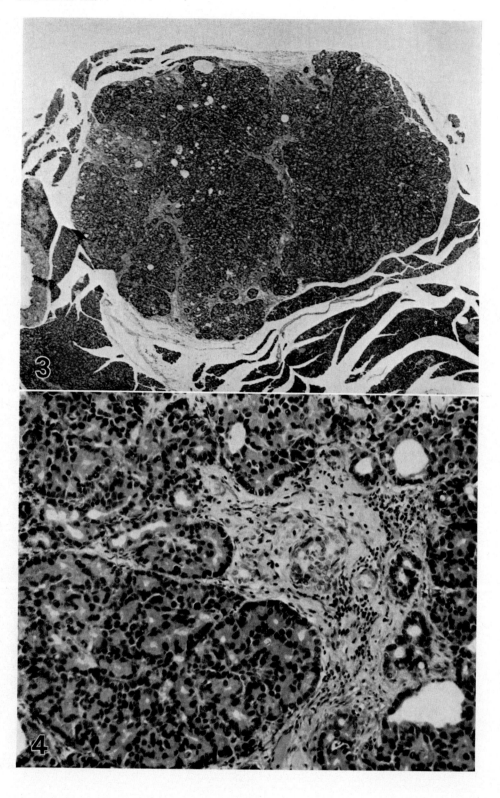

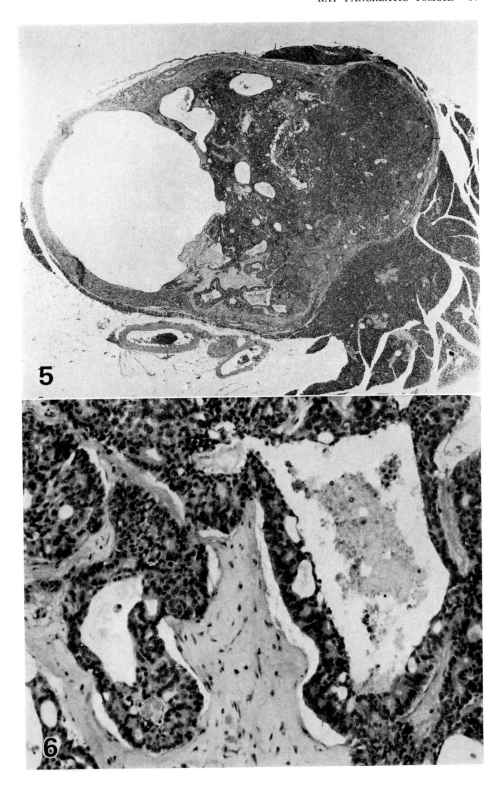

5

6

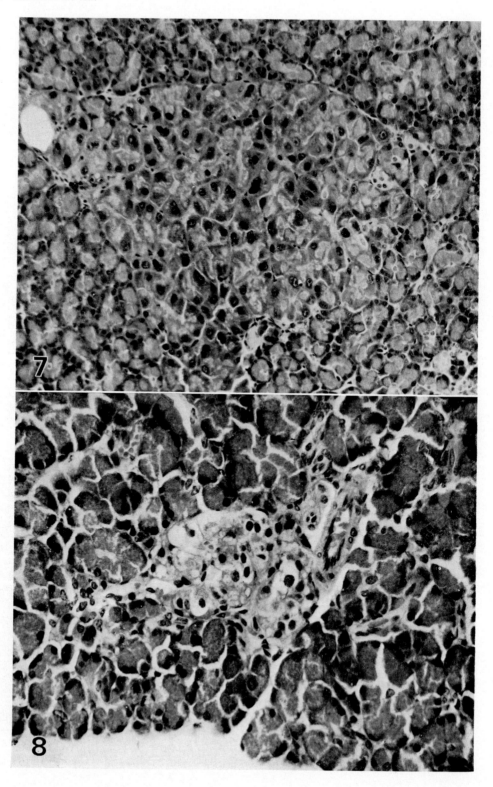

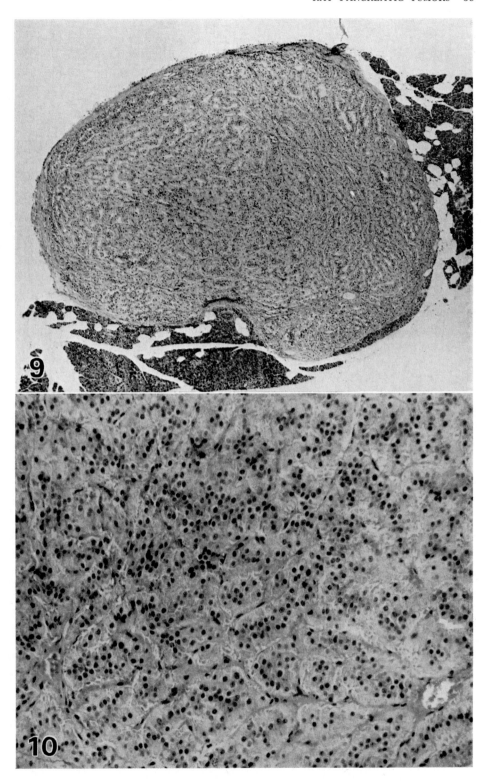

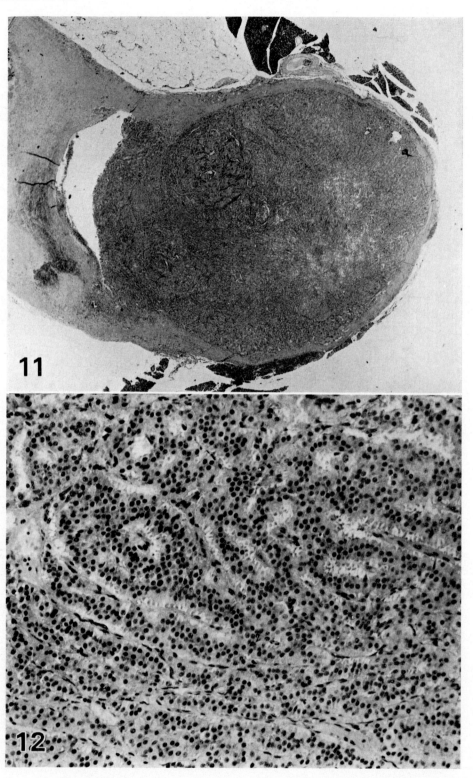

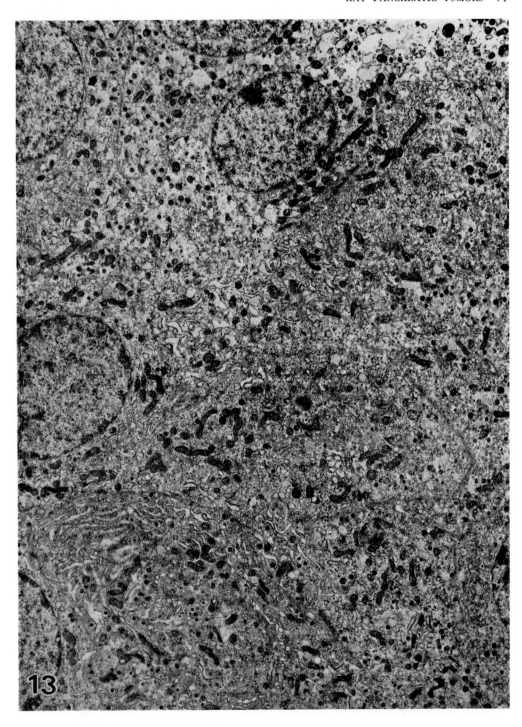

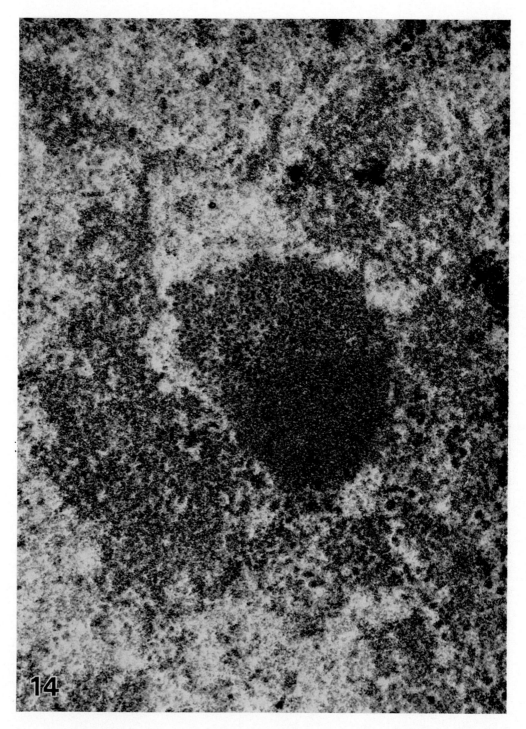

Organospecific Carcinogenesis in the Digestive Tract

H. DRUCKREY

Forschergruppe Praeventivmedizin am Max-Planck-Institut für Immunobiologie, Freiburg, West Germany

Epidemiological and statistical studies on the geographic pathology of cancer in general, and especially of tumors in the alimentary tract, reported by Stewart (*50*) and in the comprehensive work of Segi and his group (*47*), provided increasing evidence for the important role of exogenous factors in the causation of cancer. Beyond that, the observation of striking differences between the incidence of certain types of carcinomas even in neighboring places leads to the conclusion that the exogenous factors involved must be organospecific.

This conclusion is strongly supported by experimental results. In recent years a great number of new chemical carcinogens have been detected, specifically inducing malignant tumors in almost every organ of experimental animals with high accuracy and regularity as my colleagues and I have demonstrated (*14, 15*) as well as Preussmann *et al.* (*41*). In this paper the specific induction of carcinomas in three organs of the digestive tract, namely, in the esophagus, stomach, and colon, will be reported.

METHODS

The substances used were synthesized in our institute by R. Preussmann or obtained from commercial sources (Dr. Th. Schuchardt, München, West Germany) and characterized by adequate specifications for identity, purity, stability, and toxicity. Experimental animals in most cases were rats of our inbred BDstrains, described by Druckrey (*3*), or outbred guinea pigs. Standard diet was alternately altromin pellets and Latz-crackers. When the first clinical symptoms of tumor development occurred, the standard diet was replaced by a pap-like diet in order to keep the animals alive as long as possible. Oral administration of the respective carcinogens was made by means of the drinking water 5 days per week, and subcutaneous injections once a week. The dosages are indicated in mg/kg body wt., and, for

73

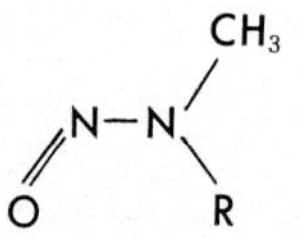

$$\underset{O}{\overset{}{\diagdown}} N - N \underset{R}{\overset{CH_3}{\diagup}}$$

examples:

R = butyl   -CH₂-CH₂-CH₂-CH₃

= amyl   -CH₂-CH₂-CH₂-CH₂-CH₃

= benzyl   -CH₂-phenyl

= phenylethyl   -CH₂-CH₂-phenyl

= acetic acid   -CH₂-COOH
(sarcosin)

FIG. 1. Methyl-alkyl-nitrosamines inducing carcinomas of the esophagus at any route of administration.

comparison, in percent of the LD_{50}. In inhalation experiments the rats were exposed to vapors in a 1-m³ closed box, and the concentration was calculated in ppm according to molecular weight (mMol = 22.4 ml gaseous substance). At autopsy every organ, including the brain and nervous system, was carefully inspected. Only carcinomas were evaluated, and the yield calculated as positive animals relative to the number of survivors at the time of first tumor appearance.

Esophagus

The conspicuous incidence of esophageal carcinomas observed in certain parts of Africa, Puerto Rico, Kasakhistan (USSR), Iran, China, and in the region of Nara (Japan) suggested that exogenous factors, probably in the diet, are responsible. As far as chemical carcinogens are considered, even though they are still unknown, a high specificity must be assumed.

The experimental induction of carcinomas in the esophagus in rats was first observed with N-nitroso-piperidine by Druckrey, Preussmann, Schmähl and Müller (*17a*). In systematic studies on relationships between chemical structure and carcinogenic effects of N-nitroso compounds it has been shown by Druckrey, Preussmann and Schmähl (1963) and Druckrey, Preussmann, Ivankovic and Schmähl (*15*) that almost all nonsymmetrical dialkylnitrosamines are specific carcinogens to the esophagus. Methyl-alkyl-nitrosamines, a few examples of which are formulated in Fig. 1, revealed the highest efficacy and specificity. In the first series of experiments the substances were given in the daily drinking water. All treated rats developed multiple squamous carcinomas exclusively in the esophagus. Figure 2 shows a few examples. Some compounds, like methyl-benzyl-nitrosamine, were effective already at a dosage of 0.25 mg/kg body wt.

The length of the induction period was between 200 and 600 days depending on dosage. The quantitative evaluation of the results, plotted in a probit net, yielded linear regressions of high characteristic ($s = \pm 15\%$) for all individual dosage groups and compounds tested.

In order to decide whether the carcinogenic effect is merely a local one or really specific, some methyl-alkyl-nitrosamines were tested for comparison by subcutaneous injections, once a week. No local sarcomas occurred, and carcinomas exclusively of the esophagus were observed as shown in Fig. 2(d). Intravenous injections yielded identical results. In a last series of experiments treatment by inhalation was used. Rats were exposed to methylbutylnitrosamine vapors at a concentration of 25 ppm in the air for 1 hr every week, and again carcinomas of the esophagus were observed by Druckrey, Landschütz and Preussmann (9), as shown in Fig. 2. This proves conclusively the high organospecificity of asymmetrical methyl-alkyl-nitrosamines. At the same time it demonstrates that cancer of the esophagus can be caused also by absorptive and not only by locally-acting carcinogens.

Our results, including more than 250 cases, have been confirmed by Weisburger, Mantel et al. (58a) and many others. With this, reliable models for any research on esophageal cancer are at hand. In this respect it deserves attention that N-nitroso-compounds can easily originate in the human environment by reaction of nitrous acid or nitrogen oxides with alkylamines or amides, as first indicated by Druckrey and Preussmann (12). In the meantime this problem was successfully studied, particularly by Sander, Schweinsberg and Menz (44a), as will be reported by J. Sander, S. Mirvish, and M. Ishidate.

In South Africa the use of the fruit of solanum incanum for curdling milk was suspected to be one factor, among others, responsible for the high incidence of esophageal cancer in certain populations of Bantus. The presence of several nitrosamines has been demonstrated, and dimethylnitrosamine identified in analytical studies of Du Plessis, Nunn and Roach (20). The fruit, kindly supplied by W. A. Roach from South Africa and constituting 20% of the diet of 80 rats, was tested for carcinogenicity at our institute by J. Gimmy. No malignant tumors were observed after more than 2 years. The negative result, however, cannot be considered as evidence because many dialkylnitrosamines are volatile and probably evaporated on the transport from Africa to Germany. Since I know of several examples in which the volatility (and instability) of nitrosamines was disregarded, I wanted to mention this potentiality.

In regard to the causation of cancer by environmental carcinogens, an important problem is whether or not a temporary, limited exposure is sufficient, and at what period of prenatal or postnatal development does the target organ become sensitive to organospecific carcinogens. This has been studied in rats using methyl-butyl-nitrosamine in a single subcutaneous injection of 30 mg/kg body wt. In trans-placental experiments no carcinomas of the esophagus occurred in the offspring. However, when given at one of the first days after birth, a number of cases were observed even at this low dose. Three examples are shown in Fig. 2g–i.

The results of our experiments present conclusive evidence for the view that nitrosamines are " indirect " carcinogens and need metabolic activation in order to form an alkylating intermediate, as first demonstrated by Dutton and Heath (20a)

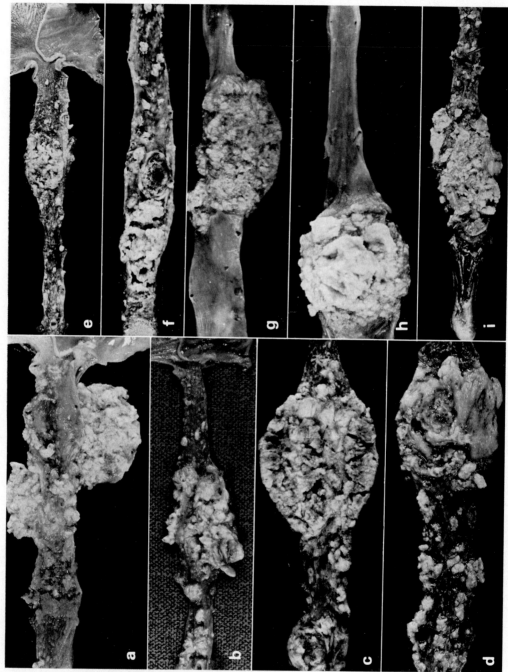

Fig. 2.   Specific induction of squamous carcinomas of the esophagus in BDrats by non symmetrical methyl-alkyl-nitrosamines.   (a) Methyl-benzyl-NA, oral doses daily of 0.25 mg/kg.
Death after 567 days.   (b) *idem*, 1 mg/kg.   Death after 273 days.   (c) Methyl-amyl-NA, oral
doses daily of 3 mg/kg.   Death after 254 days.   (d) *idem*, subcutaneous injections 10 mg/kg
once/week.   Death after 289 days.   (e) and (f) Methyl-butyl-NA, inhalation, 25 ppm 1 hr/week.
Death after 243 and 254 days, respectively.   (g)–(i) Methyl-butyl-NA, single subcutaneous
doses of 30 mg/kg to 10-day-old sibling rats.   Death after 478, 527 and 538 days, respectively.

with dimethylnitrosamine as an example. This compound, however, never produced cancer of the esophagus. Therefore, the organospecific effect of methyl-alkyl- (and of some cyclic)nitrosamines must be attributed to the presence of one longer alkyl group. This suggested that the first step of metabolic activation might be an enzymatic α-hydroxylation (Druckrey, Preussmann, Schmähl, and Müller, *17a*), which is supported by systematic studies by McMahon (1966). Hydroxylation of the α-CH_2 group necessarily leads to an asymmetrical carbon atom. This possibility, so far neglected in literature, may be one explanation for specific effects of methyl-alkyl-(and cyclic) nitrosamines, not observed with the dimethyl compound.

Furthermore, the molecular structure of dialkylnitrosamines is coplanar and, accordingly, *cis* and *trans* isomers are possible, as indicated by Rao and Bhaskar (*41a*). The grade of binding between N-N is considerably higher than that of a single bond, and rotation about this axis has a very high barrier of 23 kcal. The two potential boundary structures are formulated in Fig. 3. The dipole-moment of dimethylnitrosamine is 3.98 Debye, and the nitroso-oxygen has a pronounced nucleophilic reactivity. If hydroxylation occurs in *cis* position to the oxygen, a hydrogen bridge will be formed, probably leading to spontaneous dealkylation by concerted reaction as formulated in Fig. 3. These views are supported by calculations of the electronic structures of nitrosamines and their hydroxylated derivatives, recently published by Nagata and Imamura (*36*). Hydroxylation in *trans* position would lead to other pathways.

Even though the organotropism to the esophagus cannot be explained at present, it seemed necessary to mention at least the possibility of different and specific biochemical mechanisms. In any case, whatever mechanism may be proposed in the future, it must be consistent with the different specificity of carcinogenic nitrosamines, well established in animal experiments.

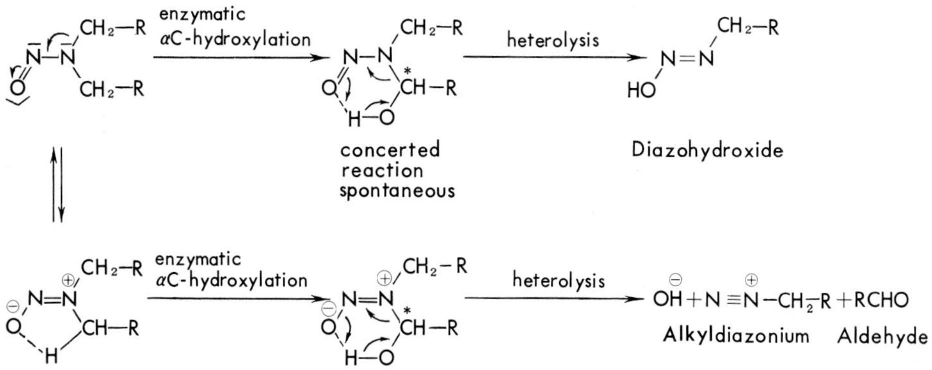

FIG. 3. Dialkylnitrosamines, molecular structure, enzymatic α-hydroxylation and subsequent dealkylation by concerted reaction, yielding alkyldiazohydroxide and -diazonium, respectively, as " proximate " alkylating carcinogen.

Stomach

As in carcinoma of the esophagus, epidemiological studies on stomach cancer revealed considerable geographic differences. The incidence is high in Chile,

Poland, Iceland, and, particularly, in Japan, as reported by Wynder, Kmet, Dungal and Segi (*61*) and by Segi, Kurihara and Matsuyama (*47*). In Japan the mortality from gastric carcinomas amounts to 50% of all cancer fatalities in males and is about seven times higher than that in the United States. The old theory of Konjetzny (*26, 27*), according to which the carcinomas originate " on the soil of chronic gastritis," cannot be considered as satisfying because it gives no explanation as to the etiology of this particular type of gastritis. Although a positive statistical correlation exists, Imai, Kubo and Watanabe (*24*) reported epidemiological evidence that environmental carcinogens are a major cause of human gastric carcinomas. This view is supported by the fact that a decreasing incidence is observed in many countries, probably due to improvements of food hygiene. Already in 1959, Sato, Fukuyama and Suzuki (*45*) directed attention to the high intake of salted foods in several places in Japan as a potential factor. However, at that time no decision was possible. With regard to the vital importance of this problem the development of experimental models became urgent.

The induction of squamous carcinomas of the forestomach in rats by 4-nitrostilbene, as reported by Druckrey, Schmähl and Mecke (*18*), probably was the first successful attempt. The dosage was 40 mg% in the diet, and all 11 treated rats died from this cancer after 400–500 days. Since 4-aminostilbene in comparative experiments did not induce cancer of the forestomach, the nitro group apparently is essential. I wanted to mention this old observation because of the parallelism to the carcinogenicity of 4-nitroquinoline N-oxide, discovered by Nakahara and Fukuoka (*37*), and because I feel that aromatic nitro compounds deserve special attention. This the more, as Mori, Ohta, Murakami *et al.* (*35*) succeeded in the production of mucosal and adenocarcinomas of the stomach of mice with 4-hydroxyaminoquinoline N-oxide hydrochloride.

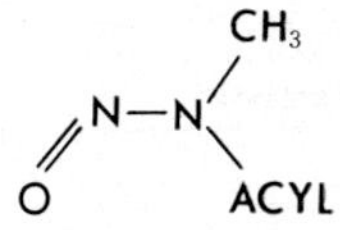

methyl-nitroso-

ACYL=CO-CH$_3$	-acetamide
=CO-CH$_2$-CH$_3$	-propionamide
=CO-O-C$_2$H$_5$	-urethane
=CO-NH$_2$	-urea
=CO-NH-CO-CH$_3$	-acetyl-urea
=CO-NH-CO-NH$_2$	-biuret
=C(NH)-NH-NO$_2$	-nitro-guanidine

Fig. 4.   Methyl-acyl-nitrosamides inducing carcinomas of the stomach after oral administration.

Decisive progress resulted from systematic studies with methyl-acyl-nitros-amides. The formulas of some compounds are compiled in Fig. 4. In contrast to dialkylnitrosamines, which need an enzymatic activation, the nitrosamides are unstable and, accordingly, direct-acting carcinogens. Methylnitrosourethane (MNUT) and -urea (MNU), given in the drinking water to rats, regularly induced multiple and large carcinomas of the forestomach, as shown by Schoental (45a) and by Druckrey, Preussmann, Schmähl and Müller (17b). In experiments with MNUT in hamsters the simultaneous occurrence of carcinomas of the esophagus was observed by Herrold (22). The simple carboxamides methylnitroso-acetamide and -propionamide (unpublished results) proved to be highly effective, and produced cancer of the forestomach already at a dosage of 1 mg/kg, as shown in Fig. 5.

In order to find a model for the induction of adenocarcinomas, we used guinea

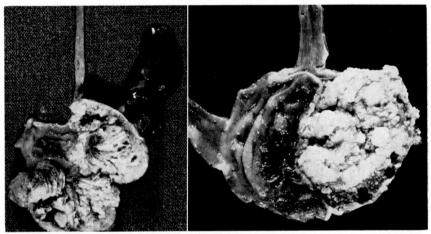

Fig. 5. Carcinomas of the forestomach of rats, induced by methylnitroso-carboxylamides in the daily drinking water. Left: acetamide, 1 mg/kg; death after 524 days. Right: pro-pionylamide, 1 mg/kg; death after 624 days.

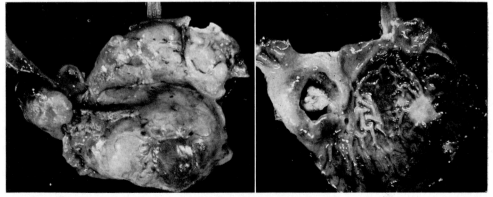

Fig. 6. Gastric carcinomas of guinea pigs, induced by left: methyl-nitrosourea, 1.5 mg/kg 5 times/week; death after 875 days. Right: methyl-nitrosourethane 2 mg/kg 5 times/week; death after 642 days.

pigs (6), since their whole stomach is glandular, like that of men. MNUT and MNU, were given at a dosage of 2.5 mg/kg body wt. in the drinking water 5 times per week with several interruptions because of severe toxic symptoms. In total, 64 animals survived for more than 1 year. After 450 to 1,000 days gastric carcinomas were observed in 16 animals of both experiments, 13 of them after treatment with MNUT which, accordingly, is particularly suitable for this purpose. Most tumors were localized in the pyloric region. Figure 6 shows the gross appearance of two gastric carcinomas, strikingly resembling human stomach cancer. The same applies to the histology, recently described by Bücheler and Thomas (2). To our surprise, 16 other guinea pigs had carcinomas of the pancreas with metastases in the liver and lungs, and 13 carcinomas were observed in the experiment with MNUT.

Although nitrosamides generally are considered to be direct-acting carcinogens, other conspicuous differences between the effects of MNUT and MNU were observed by Druckrey, Preussmann, Ivankovic and Schmähl (15). By intravenous injection in rats, MNUT [special precautionary measures are necessary in handling MNUT, as indicated by Druckrey and Preussmann (11)] was extremely toxic, and induced exclusively carcinomas of the lungs, whereas MNU proved to be a specific carcinogen for the brain, and did not produce any lung tumors. Accordingly, it seemed necessary to look for differences between the biochemical mechanisms involved. The breakdown of MNUT is considerably enhanced by thiol compounds, as shown by Schoental (45b), and the formation of the thio-half-acetal as an intermediate was demonstrated by Schoental and Rive (46). In contrast, we found the heterolysis of MNU is not affected by cysteine, probably because the carbonyl group is much less reactive. Furthermore, MNUT is liquid whereas MNU is crystalline. This indicates the existence of a hydrogen bridge to the nitroso-oxygen, which may also occur in MNUT after reaction with thiols. Under this assumption the probable biochemical mechanisms of action of MNUT and MNU are formulated in Fig. 7, in which a breakdown by concerted reaction is proposed, directly yielding methyl-diazohydroxide (or diazotate) as a " proximate " alkylating carcinogen.

A new area in stomach cancer research was opened by the admirable work by Sugimura and Fujimura (52), demonstrating the specific production of carcinomas

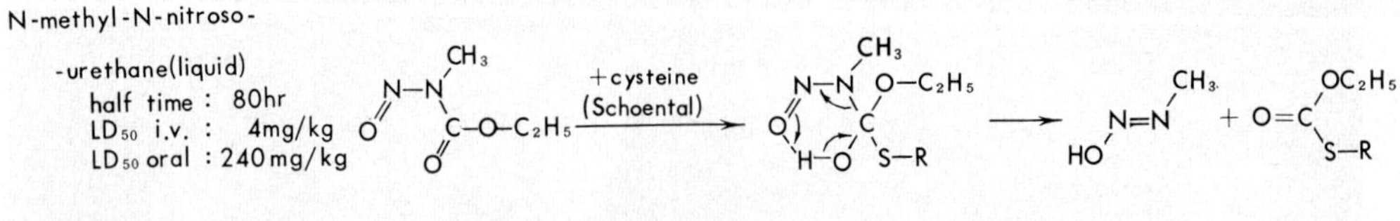

FIG. 7. Differences between structure, reactivity and breakdown of methylnitrosourethane and -urea, both yielding methyldiazohydroxide as the " proximate " alkylating carcinogen.

in the glandular stomach of rats by N-methylnitroso-N-nitroguanidine (MNNG), if the substance is given at low dosages in the drinking water. The experiment was successfully repeated by Sugimura, Fujimura, Kogure, Baba *et al.* (*54*) and by Sugimura, Fujimura and Baba (*53*). The highest yield of adenocarcinomas was observed when the treatment was discontinued after 7 months, as reported by Fujimura, Kogure, Sugimura and Takayama (*21*). The results were confirmed in the United States by Bralow, Gruenstein, Meranze, Bonakdapur and Shimkin (*1*). Recently, stomach cancer in dogs was produced for the first time in experiments by Sugimura, Tanaka, Kawachi *et al.* (*57*). Papers by Sugimura, Hirono, Takayama, and by Narisawa in our program will certainly report on new and stimulating results with MNNG.

From the chemical standpoint, MNNG is a guanidide of nitric acid or, in general terms, a N'-acylated methylnitrosoguanidine. In this connection it seemed of interest that some carcinomas of the glandular stomach of rats have been observed by Stewart, Snell *et al.* (*51*) in experiments with 2,7-bis-(acetylamido)-fluorene, but not with the monofunctional compound. For such reasons we became interested in N'-acylated derivatives of methylnitrosourea (MNU), and particularly in N-methyl-nitroso-N'-acetyl-urea (AcMNU) and -N'-carbamoylurea=biuret (MNBU). Both compounds were synthesized by R. Preussmann at our institute. The chemical structures and some relevant data are presented in Fig. 8 comparing to MNU and MNNG.

AcMNU is rather unstable, but its solubility in water of 15 g% is remarkably high. The substance was given to rats in the drinking water 5 days per week. Two dosage groups were given 4 and 2 mg/kg respectively, corresponding to 1.6 and 0.8% of acute LD_{50}. After 330 days the treatment was discontinued. In the first group 8 out of 10 rats died between the 412th and 567th day with extended and partly perforated tumors of the glandular stomach. Histologically, adenocarcinomas were observed in 6 cases, and polymorphous sarcomas in 2 cases. Four of these rats had additional neurogenic tumors, 2 had gliomas of the brain and 2 had malignant neurinomas of the PNS (peripheric nervous system). The lower dosage of 2

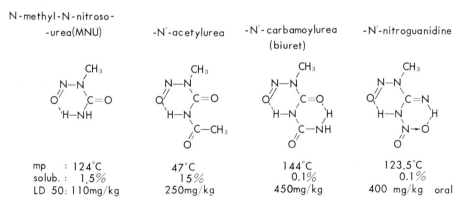

FIG. 8. Methylnitrosourea (MNU) and some of its N'-acyl derivatives, inducing stomach carcinomas in rats and (MNU) guinea pigs if given at low dosages in the drinking water.

mg/kg, however, produced exclusively adenocarcinomas of the glandular stomach in all 13 treated rats, and the medium induction time was 500 days as already reported by Druckrey, Ivankovic and Preussmann (*7*). The example in Fig. 9a demonstrates the similarity to human stomach cancer.

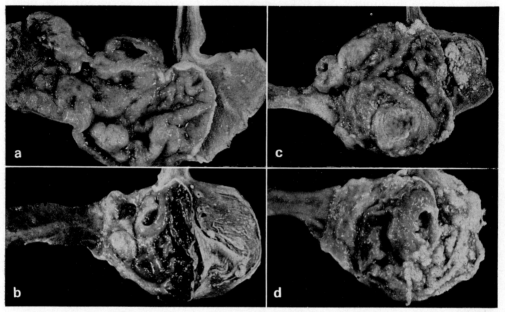

Fig. 9. Adenocarcinomas of the glandular stomach of rats, induced by acetyl-methylnitro-sourea, 2 mg/kg, 5 times/week. (a) in the drinking water, death after 465 days. (b)–(d) in milk, death after 381, 408 and 408 days, respectively.

The results support the observation by Fujimura, Kogure, Sugimura and Takayama (*21*), in experiments with MNNG, that the specific induction of gastric carcinomas can be obtained most effectively by using a low dosage for a limited period. Under such conditions AcMNU apparently is a reliable model substance. Since the nonacetylated MNU by oral administration to rats produces mainly cancer of the forestomach (besides brain tumors), the striking organotropism of AcMNU to the glandular stomach probably must be attributed to the acylation of the second N atom, which is considered an interesting parallelism to the similar effect of MNNG.

Hirayama (*23*) suggested that the low intake of milk may be responsible for the high incidence of gastric carcinomas in Japan. For this reason we felt obliged to use our model to study the problem of whether or not the induction of stomach cancer can be prevented by a large intake of milk. A group of 25 rats was treated with AcMNU given in milk instead of water, using again the dosage of 2 mg/kg. The duration of the treatment was extended to 408 days, 78 days longer than in the foregoing experiments, in order to secure possible negative outcome. During this period 3 rats died from pneumonia. All the remaining 22 rats without exception died within the following 200 days with large adenocarcinomas of the glandular stomach, as shown in Fig. 9b, c, d. Simultaneous carcinomas of the forestomach were observed in 8 of these rats, and additional brain tumors in 6 cases, probably due to the prolonged exposure. Metastases of the adenocarcinomas were found in the lungs of 2 rats (unpublished results, experiments with T. Tan).

The quantitative evaluation of the cumulative incidence of the gastric carcinomas depending on the individual induction time is presented in Fig. 10 for both experiments. AcMNU was given in water and in milk. The graph demonstrates the high accuracy of the obtained results, reflecting even small differences in exposure time. Accordingly, AcMNU is considered as the most suitable substance for the specific induction of gastric adenocarcinomas.

In the next experiment we used methyl-nitrosobiuret (MNBU), another N′-acylated derivative of MNU. It is relatively stable and less toxic than AcMNU. The chemical structure and some relevant data are presented in Fig. 8. The substance was given in the drinking water 5 days per week for 1 year to 2 groups at dosages of 10 and 5 mg/kg (2.2 and 1.1% of LD_{50}). In the first group only 4 out of 16 rats developed gastric cancer, and the others died with malignant tumors of the brain and PNS. The low dosage, however, produced large carcinomas exclusively of the glandular stomach in 7 out of 10 rats. The gross appearance is shown in Fig. 11. In contrast to the outcome of these chronic experiments, the application of a single high dose by stomach tube induced mainly squamous carcinomas of the

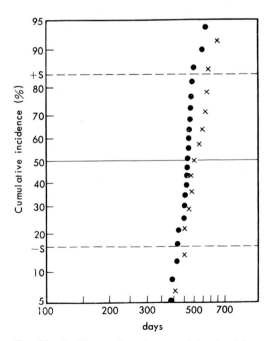

Fig. 10. Incidence of carcinomas of the glandular stomach, induced by acetyl-methylnitrosourea, 2 mg/kg body wt. 5 times / week in BDrats. ×, in the drinking water, stopped after 330 days and 468 mg/kg; ●, in milk, stopped after 408 days and 560 mg/kg. Crdinate, cumulative incidence, %. Abscissa, time of death (2.5-fold elongated).

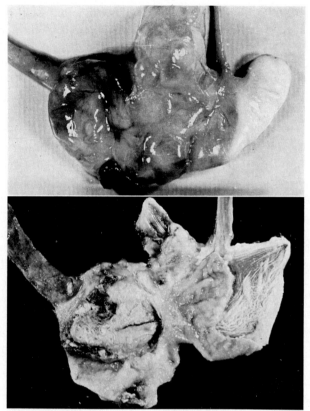

Fig. 11.   Adenocarcinoma of the glandular stomach of a rat, induced by methylnitrosobiuret, 5 mg/kg, 5 times / week in the drinking water.   Death after 500 days.

forestomach, and only a few adenocarcinomas, as recently reported by Druckrey, Landschütz, Preussmann and Ivankovic (*10*).

In order to study whether or not the N′-acetyl group alone is responsible for the carcinogenicity to the glandular stomach, we tested N′-acetyl-ethylnitrosourea (AcENU) for comparison.   The dosages were 6 and 2 mg/kg (1.5 and 0.5% LD_{50}), given in the drinking water 5 times per week to a total of 38 rats.   In total, the following tumor cases were observed: 3 carcinomas of the forestomach, 4 adenocarcinomas of the glandular stomach, 4 of the duodenum, 6 of the cecum or colon, 13 of the mammary glands, 2 malignant tumors of the nervous system and 12 leukemias. The results obtained after the low dosage are included in Table 1.   Accordingly, AcENU, in contrast to AcMNU, exerts its carcinogenic effect also on other parts of the alimentary tract, in a manner similar to that observed in experiments with MNNG by Sugimura, Fujimura and Baba (*53*).

Since the carcinogenic effect apparently is modified by the alkyl group, the homologous series of alkyl-nitrosoureas from ethyl- to *n*-pentyl-, synthesized by R. Preussmann, was tested for carcinogenicity by oral administration in BD rats by J. Stekar and T. Tan (unpublished).   A synopsis of the obtained results is presented in Table 1 with special consideration of carcinomas in the digestive tract.   The

TABLE 1. Carcinogenesis in the Digestive Tract, Induced by Alkyl-nitrosourea Compounds in Rats. Administration in Drinking Water (Milk) 5 Times/Week, Discontinued after About 1 Year

Alkyl nitrosourea	LD_{50} mg/kg	Dosage mg/kg	Rats number	Malignant tumors					
				Eso-phagus	Stomach		Duo-denum	Colons rectum	Other sites
					Fore	Gland			
Acetyl-methyl-	250	2	35	—	8	35	—	—	6 brain
Methyl-biuret	450	5	10	—	7	—	—	—	1 brain
Ethyl-	300	2	20	—	—	1	1	—	7 neurog. 10 leukemias
Acetyl-ethyl-	550	2	20	—	1	2	2	6	2 neurog., 7 mamma 5 leukemias
n-Propyl-	530	8	45	—	3	7	10	4	2 neurog., 3 lungs 4 leukem. 6 mamma
n-Butyl-	400	20	60	1	10	8	1	1	20 leukemias 17 mamma, 3 neurog.
n-Pentyl-	560	20	24	7	7	—	—	2	1 neurogen. 5 mamma, 2 kidney

differences between the effects of the various compounds are clearly recognizable. Ethyl-nitrosourea (2 mg/kg) had very little effect on the alimentary tract, and produced mainly leukemias and tumors of the nervous system. The result was practically identical to that after intravenous injections, as reported by Druckrey, Preussmann, Ivankovic and Schmähl (*15*). With *n*-propyl-nitrosourea (8 mg/kg), however, carcinomas in various parts of the digestive tract were obtained. The high incidence of 10 adenocarcinomas of the duodenum, apparently characteristic for the effect of this compound, is surprising. Most of these tumors were multiple, large, and highly invasive, as shown in Fig. 12a. The *n*-butylhomologue at a dosage of 20 mg/kg produced mainly leukemias in 20 out of 60 rats, and breast cancer in 17 female rats, but also carcinomas in the upper digestive tract, 10 cases in the forestomach and 8 in the glandular stomach (Fig. 12b). The results are similar to those reported by Odashima (*40*), Yokoro, Imamura *et al.* (*63*) and Narisawa, Sato *et al.* (*39*). Pentyl-nitrosourea, which has not been studied so far, was given to 24 rats at a dosage of 20 mg/kg. The principal result was the occurrence of squamous carcinomas of the esophagus (Fig. 12c) in 7 rats, whereas only 1 case occurred in the 190 animals treated with other alkyl-nitrosourea compounds.

Considering the results of all these experiments together, alkyl-nitrosoureas such as MNNG are carcinogenic to various parts of the digestive tract, when given by the oral route. Since all these compounds are relatively unstable, and no enzymatic activation process is needed for the formation of the corresponding alkyldiazonium, a direct carcinogenic effect may be assumed. However, the significant differences observed between the individual compounds (Table 1) suggest the possibility of different mechanisms of action. Since physical properties such as the degree of stability and solubility are particularly different between MNNG and Ac MNU, these properties cannot play important roles, although both substances at low dosage are the most selective inducers of gastric carcinomas. The common factor is that they are methyl compounds and acylated at the second N atom. Ac-

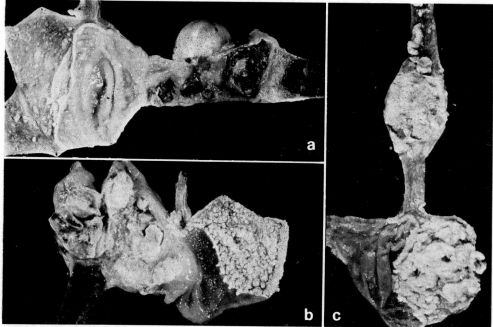

FIG. 12.   Carcinomas of the digestive tract, induced by alkylnitrosourea compounds, given in the drinking water of rats 5 times / week.   (a) Adenocarcinoma of the duodenum, n-propyl-NU, 16 mg/kg for 30 weeks.   Death after 281 days.   (b) Adenocarcinoma of the glandular stomach and hyperkeratosis of the forestomach, n-butyl-NU, 20 mg/kg for 37 weeks.   Death after 300 days.   (c) Squamous carcinomas of the esophagus and forestomach, n-pentyl-NU, 20 mg/kg.   Death after 457 days.

cordingly, studies on the systematic variations of these two groups may contribute to a better understanding of the mechanisms involved.

The induction period for adenocarcinomas of the glandular stomach was generally long, between 380 and 600 days in rats, and rather independent of the dosage, whereas that of squamous carcinomas of the forestomach was considerably shorter in experiments with high doses.   The striking prevalence of tumors of the forestomach and the low incidence in the glandular stomach particularly after a single high dose, however, are probably due to the high sensitivity of the glandular mucosa to the cytotoxic effects of the alkylating substances.   As already demonstrated by Takayama, Saito, Fujimura and Sugimura (58), MNNG given in the drinking water produces within a few weeks degenerative processes and increasing degrees of erosion of the mucosa, particularly in the antral part of the stomach. On the grounds of similar observations with AcMNU, Druckrey, Ivankovic and Preussmann (7) came to the conclusion that stomach cancer at least in these experiments does not originate " on the soil of chronic gastritis or ulcus " as proposed by Konjetzny (21), but that the reverse explanation is probable, namely that the chronic gastritis and erosions develop on the soil of carcinogenically injured mucosa, and should be considered pre- or " paracancerous " lesions.

The carcinogenicity of a great number of N-nitroso compounds opened new aspects in the potential etiology of human cancer, since they may easily originate from alkyl-amines or -amides in the presence of nitrous acid or -oxides, widespread in the human environment, as first indicated by me and co-workers (*11, 19*).   In recent years the formation of nitrosamines and nitrosamides in the stomach and their carcinogenic effect were demonstrated in numerous examples by Sander (*43*), Sander, Bürkle, Flohe and Aeikens (*44*), Ivankovic and Preussmann (*25*), Montesano and Magee (*34*), and Mirvish (*33*).   The potential importance of nitrosamines as environmental carcinogens is discussed by Lijinsky and Epstein (*29*).   Zaldivar (*64*) directed attention to the exceedingly high incidence of gastric and esophagus cancer in certain parts of Chile where the drinking water has a high nitrate content due to the widespread use of nitrate fertilizers.   Even though more systematic studies are needed for a proper judgement, this is an important example of widespread carcinogens in the human environment, the knowledge of which may contribute to active cancer prevention measures.

Colon and Rectum

The incidence of cancer of the colon and rectum, like that of other organs, shows striking differences in various countries, as reported by Segi, Kurihara and Matsuyama (*47*).   It is particularly high in the United States, where colonic cancer was responsible for more than 41,000 fatalities in 1964, according to Wynder and Shigematsu (*62*).   Although exogenous factors probably play an important role, as discussed by these authors and by Stewart (*50*) on the basis of experimental results obtained with bracken, cycasin and 4-aminodiphenyl compounds, the etiology is still unknown.

The induction of intestinal neoplasms in rats with glycoside cycasin and aglycone methylazoxymethanol (MAM) was first reported by Laqueur (*28*).   When the chemical formula of the aglycone became known (personal communication of H. L. Stewart, 1962), revealing a striking similarity to that of dimethylnitrosamine, I became interested in systematic studies on the potential carcinogenicity of symmetric dialkylhydrazines, azo- and azoxyalkanes.   First experiments with the ethyl compounds, given to rats by subcutaneous injections, revealed a high carcinogenicity, inducing tumors in certain remote organs [Druckrey, Preussmann *et al.* (*16*)] but no local sarcomas at the site of injections.   This gave evidence that the substances should be considered " indirect " carcinogens.   Further support came from transplacental experiments.   Hydrazo-, azo- and azoxy-ethane, when given to pregnant rats as a single dose by any route of administration after the 11th day of gestation, induced malignant tumors of the nervous system in almost all offspring as reported by Druckrey, Ivankovic, Preussmann *et al.* (*8*).

For biochemical reasons it was assumed that these compounds enzymatically become α-hydroxylated and subsequently dealkylated by concerted reaction, eventually yielding alkyldiazonium as alkylating intermediates in a manner similar to that observed in experiments with dialkylnitrosamines.   The probable reaction mechanism is formulated in Fig. 13.   The oxidative dealkylation of one alkyl group by incubation with the microsomal fraction of rat liver and the formation of the

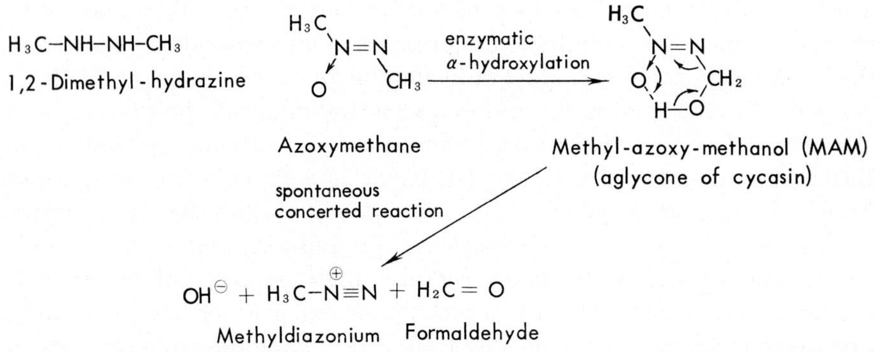

$$H_3C-NH-NH-CH_3$$

1,2-Dimethyl-hydrazine

FIG. 13.   Probable mechanism of carcinogenic action of 1,2-dimethylhydrazine and azoxy-methane by α-hydroxylation and subsequent dealkylation by concerted reaction, yielding methyldiazonium as the " proximate " alkylating carcinogen.

aldehyde have been demonstrated by Preussmann *et al.* (*41*), and the alkylation of RNA and DNA with MAM *in vivo* has been reported by Shank and Magee (*48*). Since the relevant step of metabolic activation is an enzymatic one, the possibility of organospecific effects was assumed.   In the following chapter the specific induction of colon and rectum carcinomas by hydrazo- and azoxymethane compounds will be reported.

1,2-Dimethylhydrazine-2HCl (melting point 168°C, commercially available from Dr. Th. Schuchardt, München, West Germany) was dissolved in water, and the solution neutralized by sodium carbonate of pH 6.   In order to inactivate metal ions, which would lead to rapid dehydrogenation, a few mg of ethylene-di-aminotetracetate (EDTA) were added.   The doses were calculated to the free base (factor 0.45).   The acute LD_{50} in rats was 215 mg/kg after subcutaneous injection and 100 mg/kg after oral administration.   This striking difference indicates that the liver is involved in metabolic toxification.

In chronic experiments of Druckrey, Preussmann, Matzkies and Ivankovic (*17*) 2 groups of 13 rats each received weekly subcutaneous injections of 21 and 7 mg/kg, respectively, of 1,2-dimethylhydrazine (DMH).   After 3 months, the rats treated with the higher dosage exhibited severe diarrhea and icterus.   Therefore the treatment was discontinued.   In the following months, prolapse of the tumorous rectum was observed in some cases.   All 13 rats in this group died with malignant intestinal cancer.   Autopsy revealed multiple and partly large tumors of the colon in 10 rats and of the rectum in 8.   Additional tumors of smaller size were observed in the duodenum of 7 rats, the small intestine of 4, and the liver of 2.   The medium induction time was 184 ± 24 days and the total dose 517 mg/kg.

The treatment with the lower dosage of 7 mg (3% of the LD_{50}) per week was discontinued after 263 days.   In this group all rats later died with intestinal cancer exclusively.   Multiple carcinomas of the colon were observed in 12 and of the rectum in 6 rats.   The gross appearance of these neoplasms is depicted in Fig. 14a.   Only 2 rats had cancer of the duodenum in addition.   The medium induction time was 333 ± 59 days, almost twice that observed in the foregoing experiment.   The dependency of the induction time upon dosage is presented in Fig. 15.   The results,

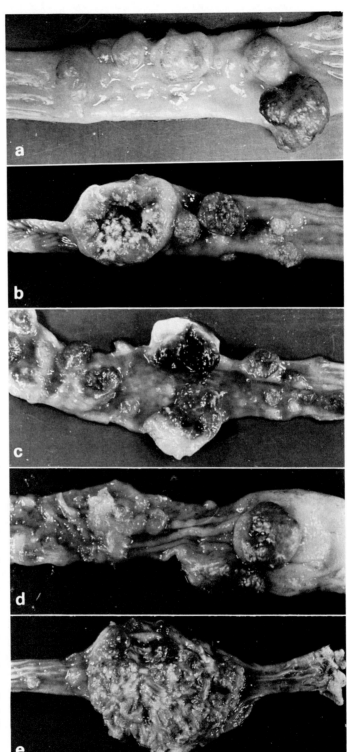

FIG. 14.   Specific induction of adenocarcinomas of the colon and rectum of rats (anus to the right side).

(a) 1,2-Dimethylhydrazine, subcutaneous injections of 7 mg/kg weekly for 37 weeks.   Death after 402 days.

(b) *idem*, 21 mg/kg, once/week, by stomach tube for 11 weeks. Death after 220 days.

(c) Azoxymethane, subcutaneous injections of 6 mg/kg, once/week, for 46 weeks. Death after 380 days.

(d) *idem*, a single subcutaneous injection of 12 mg/kg to a newborn rat at the age of 3 days.   Death after 377 days.

(e) *idem*.   Death after 402 days.

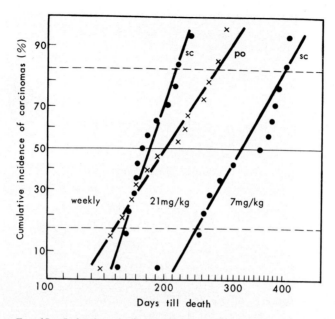

Fig. 15. Induction of colonic and rectal carcinomas in rats by 1,2-dimethylhydrazine, 7 and 21 mg/kg, respectively, once/week (abscissa fivef-old elongated). ●, subcutaneous injections; ×, stomach tube, stopped after 12 doses.

compiled in Table 2, demonstrate that 1,2-dimethylhydrazine is a resorptive and specific carcinogen for colonic and rectal mucosa.

Histological examination, performed by C. Thomas of the Institute of Pathology in Freiburg, revealed adenocarcinomas in all cases, mostly associated with polyps in all stages of progressing malignancy, and a striking resemblance to human colonic and rectal carcinomas.

In the meantime, our results were confirmed in experiments on mice by Wiebecke, Löhrs, Gimmy and Eder (59), and on rats by Wittig, Wildner and Ziebarth (60). In one group of rats in their experiments, the rectum was closed by colostomy. Nevertheless rectal carcinomas were observed in more than 50% of the treated rats, indicating a hematogenous action. This is in agreement with observations by Löhrs, Wiebecke and Eder (31), according to which cytotoxic effects occurred in the regeneration zone of the intestinal crypts already a few weeks after subcutaneous injection of DMH.

The most active organ in oxidative dealkylation is the liver. Therefore comparative experiments were performed by Druckrey, Preussmann et al. (17) by oral administration of DMH. Fourteen rats received 21 mg/kg once a week by stomach tube. This high dosage was badly tolerated, and the treatment had to be discontinued already after 78 days and a total dose of 252 mg/kg. One rat died from pneumonia. All 13 remaining rats died with multiple colonic carcinomas, the gross appearance of which is shown in Fig. 14b. In addition, 4 of these rats had carcinomas of the rectum, 3 had carcinomas of the duodenum, and 1 had a large adenosarcoma of the left kidney. The results are included in both Fig. 15 and Table 2.

In 6 rats monstrous cystic degeneration of the liver was observed, but no liver cancer. The medium induction time of 206 ± 48 days was rather short, which indicates that a short period of treatment is enough for regular production of colonic cancer.

The low dosage of 3 mg/kg in the drinking water 5 days per week surprisingly did not produce intestinal cancer, but very malignant hemangioendotheliomas of the liver instead with multiple metastases in the lungs. This indicates metabolic activation in the liver, already shown in experiments *in vitro*, and explains the relatively high toxicity after oral administration. The carcinogenic intermediate apparently is very short living. In order to induce intestinal cancer by the oral route, DMH must be given at a dosage high enough to surpass the activation capacity of the relevant enzymes of the liver which are damaged by the hepatotoxicity of DMH.

In order to determine whether the surprising organospecific effect to the colonic mucosa is due to the hydrazine structure or to the methyl groups, azoxymethane (AOM) was tested for comparison. The synthesis by oxidation of DMH is rather difficult, and yields only a small amount of AOM (azoxymethane is commercially obtainable from Dr. Th. Schuchardt, München, West Germany). AOM is a liquid substance (boiling point 98°C), stable, and soluble in water at all proportions. The acute LD_{50} was 27 mg/kg and independent of the route of administration.

Chronic experiments were performed by subcutaneous injections in BD rats once a week at 3 dosages of 12 (pilot group), 6, and 2 mg/kg. The highest dosage proved to be very toxic, and only 3 rats survived for more than 6 months. All 3 rats died with rectal carcinomas; medium induction time was 235 days. After 6 mg/kg was given to 16 rats, all animals developed multiple tumors of the large bowel, often simultaneously at different sites. Cancer of the colon was observed in 13 rats and of the rectum in 11 rats. Gross appearance, depicted in Fig. 14c, and histology were identical to those found in experiments with DMH. One rat had

TABLE 2. Induction of Colonic and Rectal Adenocarcinomas in Rats by 1, 2-Dimethylhydrazine, Azoxymethane, 1-Methyl-2-butylhydrazine and Methylazoxybutane

Substance	Route	Dosage p. week mg/kg	Medium induct. time days	Rats with multiple intestinal carcinomas				Additional
				Number	Intest.	Colon	Rectum	
Symmetric	sc	7*	333	13/13	2	16	6	0
dimethyl-hydrazine	sc	21	184	13/13	11	10	8	2 liver
	oral	21*	206	13/14	3	13	4	1 kidney
Azoxymethane	sc	2	500	7/16	0	6	1	8 liver
	sc	6	380	16/16	1	13	11	1 liver
	sc	12	235	3/3	0	0	3	0
Symmetric	sc	25	420	4/15	1	1	3	2 olfact.
methyl-butyl-hydrazine	oral	25	400	3/14	0	0	3	9 olfact.
Methyl-azoxy-butane	sc	30	500	11/17	1	10	0	5 skin
				total:	19	69	39	

* Treatment discontinued after 11 to 36 weeks.

hepatic carcinomas additionally.   The medium time till death was 380 days.   The lower dosage of 2 mg/kg was also effective.   Seven out of 16 treated rats died after about 500 days with colonic and rectal carcinomas.   Eight rats had malignant hemangioendotheliomas of the liver with multiple metastases in the lungs, as observed after a low oral dose of DMH.   The results, reported by Druckrey, Preussmann, Matzkies, and Ivankovic (17) and in detail by Druckrey (4) are compiled in Table 2.

In order to collect more information on the relationships between chemical structure and organospecific carcinogenicity, a great number of other hydrazo-, azo- and azoxyalkanes were systematically tested in experiments on rats.   Some results have been reported already by Preussmann, Druckrey, Ivankovic and Hodenberg (41) and by Druckrey (4).   Intestinal cancer was induced exclusively by such derivatives, in which one of the two alkyl groups was methyl.   A few examples are included in Table 2.   However, additional tumors of certain other organs, particularly neuroblastomas of the olfactory bulbs, were observed.   In contrast to the methane homologues, hydrazo-, azo- and azoxy-ethane, though multipotent carcinogens, never induced colonic or rectal carcinomas.   The striking differences in organotropy between the methyl and ethyl derivatives suggest that different and apparently highly specific processes are involved in the oxidative dealkylation of these two groups of related compounds.   In this respect it deserves attention that alpha hydroxylation of the ethyl group necessarily produces an asymmetrical C atom, which may be responsible for certain specific effects not observed with the methyl homologues.   On the other hand, the correspondence of the results obtained with both DMH and AOM indicates that the organotropic carcinogenicity for the colon and rectum is attributable to the methyl groups.   These, however, must be placed in the symmetrical 1,2 position, since the asymmetrical 1,1-dimethyl-hydrazine is only a very weak carcinogen, and dimethylnitrosamine, in spite of its chemical similarity to AOM, did not produce intestinal carcinomas.

After these studies of chemical and biochemical aspects, the mechanism of the organotropism to the colon remained unknown.   In order to find out whether or not the compounds might be activated directly by the colonic mucosa or the intestinal flora, we tested azoxymethane by rectal instillation, in cooperation with J. Gimmy (not yet published).   Since resorptive effects had to be avoided, low dosages of 0.06 and 0.2 mg per rat, once a week, were used on 2 groups of 25 rats each.   After 2 years the outcome was negative.   After 830 days and a total dose of more than 10 mg, corresponding to 40 mg/kg, cancer of the colon was observed in 3 rats.   On the other hand, methylnitroso-nitroguanidine by rectal administration to rats did produce a high yield of carcinomas of the colon and rectum within a few months, as recently reported by Narisawa, Sato et al. (39).   According to these results, which agree with the observations by Wittig, Wildner and Ziebarth (60) in experiments on rats with colostomy, the action of AOM in the colon is resorptive and hematogenous.

The induction of cancer was generally regarded as the result of chronic exposure. In systematic, quantitative experiments with various carcinogens, however, it has been demonstrated by Druckrey (3) that carcinogenesis is an accelerated process, progressing to the square or even higher power of time and, accordingly, can be started by a single high dose. The question of whether or not the latter is possible in the induction of intestinal cancer remained. A single subcutaneous injection of DMH, 200 mg/kg, was given to 10 rats. After 260 to 410 days 3 rats died with multiple carcinomas of the colon and 6 with nephroblastomas. Corresponding experiments were performed with azoxymethane, using different routes of administration. Twenty rats received a single dose of 16 or 30 mg/kg by stomach tube. Within 300 to 600 days almost all animals developed tumors. At autopsy, 8 rats had carcinomas of the colon and rectum and 8 others nephroblastomas. In addition, most rats of this group showed monstrous cystic degeneration of the liver. A single subcutaneous injection of 20 mg/kg produced intestinal cancer in 6 out of 20 rats and nephroblastomas in 12 rats. These kidney tumors, frequently observed in experiments with single doses of N-nitroso compounds, appeared earlier and grew faster than the intestinal carcinomas, so that most rats died before the manifestation of the latter could be expected.

The efficacy of a single dose permitted systematic studies on the problem of which periods of pre- or postnatal development the intestinal mucosa becomes susceptible to carcinogens. In transplacental experiments on rats on the 15th day of gestation, DMH and AOM, even at the highest tolerated dose, were neither teratogenic nor carcinogenic to the fetus. Only when a single dose was given to rats on the last day of pregnancy did some of the offspring later die with malignant tumors of the nervous system or nephroblastomas. No intestinal tumors were observed. On the other hand, methylazoxymethanol-glycoside (cycasin) did produce intestinal and neurogenic cancer in the offspring as demonstrated by Spatz and Laqueur (49). Hence α-hydroxylation seems to be the essential step in metabolic activation, as formulated in Fig. 13. The enzyme system for the activation of DMH and AOM apparently begins to occur only during the perinatal period of development. Since the corresponding ethyl compounds proved to be highly carcinogenic to the fetus already on the 15th day of gestation as reported by me and co-workers (8), this gives additional evidence of the existence of differences between the enzymatic activation of the methyl and ethyl compounds.

In postnatal experiments a single subcutaneous injection of AOM in doses ranging from 4 to 20 mg/kg was given to rats of the ages of 1, 3, 10, 30 and 60 days. The results are compiled in Table 3. The induction of intestinal cancer was already possible in newborn rats. After treatment at the ages of 1 or 3 days, 40 out of 148 rats died with multiple carcinomas of the colon and rectum. Gross appearance, depicted in Fig. 14d and e, and histology were identical to those observed in experiments with adult rats. The highest incidence of almost 50% was obtained when rats of the age of 30 days were used. Accordingly, the susceptibility of the colonic mucosa to cancerous transformation seems to be especially high after weaning, and decreases with increasing age. The age dependency of the susceptibility of the individual organs to carcinogens deserves serious attention. It is most striking in the nervous system, which proved to be extremely susceptible during fetal and neonatal development, as demonstrated by me and co-workers (6) in systematic studies with hydrazo-, azo-, and azoxy-ethane. This was also recognizable in the experiments with azoxymethane, although this carcinogen, in contrast to the ethane compounds, has no neurotropic properties. Nevertheless, malignant tumors of the brain and nervous system were observed in 20 out of 92 rats treated on the first day after birth. In the older age groups the incidence of neurogenic tumors decreased sharply. Only 1 neurogenic tumor was found among 86 rats treated at the age of 60 days. The third tumor type, nephroblastoma, occurred in all groups, and an age-dependent susceptibility of the kidney was not recognizable. If all malignant tumors observed after treatment at the first day are summarized, the incidence was 72%. From this it follows that the metabolic activation capacity of azoxymethane is already almost complete in newborn rats. The dose-response relationships are indicated at the bottom of Table 3.

TABLE 3. Colon Carcinomas, Nephroblastomas and Neurogenic Neoplasms Induced by a Single Subcutaneous Injection of Azoxymethane in BDrats of Various Ages. Relationships between Dose and Tumor Incidence

Age at treatment Days	Number of rats type of tumor			
	Colon carcinoma	Nephro- blastoma	Neuro- blastoma	Negative
1	21	25	20	26
3	19	21	4	12
10	9	13	3	9
30	24	4	3	18
60	36	13	1	36
adult	6	12	0	6

	single dose			
	4	6	12	20 mg/kg
yield:	18	31	60	84 percent

DISCUSSION

The problem of organospecific effects undoubtedly is of fundamental importance in pharmacology. As one approach, it was proposed to use such substances which represent an inactive " transport form " and become effective only after metabolic activation. This applies to various groups of "indirect" carcinogens. Therefore, a great number of such compounds have been tested in systematic studies mainly on rats, and striking organospecific effects have been observed. Two examples are reported in this paper. The first is the specific induction of carcinomas of the esophagus by nonsymmetrical dialkylnitrosamines, and the second the induction of adenocarcinomas of the colon and rectum by 1,2-dimethylhydrazine or azoxymethane.

Among the nitrosamines those derivatives were the most effective in which one alkyl group was methyl, and the other n-butyl, amyl, benzyl or phenylethyl. The organotropism to the esophagus proved to be completely independent of the route of administration, whether oral, parenteral or by inhalation. In contrast to this, esophageal cancer was never observed in experiments with dimethylnitrosamine.

Since diethylnitrosamine and higher homologues did produce a limited incidence, the presence of the -CH$_2$R group seems to be crucial. In this respect it deserves attention that enzymatic α-hydroxylation, which probably is the first and decisive step in metabolic activation, leads to an asymmetric C atom in this group. The induction of carcinomas of the esophagus was possible already in the first days after birth, but not in transplacental experiments. This indicates that the relevant enzyme system occurs only during the perinatal period of development.

The specific induction of colonic and rectal adenocarcinomas was observed exclusively with symmetrical dialkylhydrazines and azoxyalkanes in which at least one alkyl group was methyl. However, the best results were obtained with 1,2-dimethylhydrazine and azoxymethane, especially by subcutaneous injection of high weekly doses for a limited period. Even a single dose was effective, inducing multiple carcinomas of the colon and rectum as also observed after treatment of newborn, suckling and weaned rats. In transplacental experiments, however, both substances were neither teratogenic nor carcinogenic. In contrast to the methane compounds, hydrazo-, azo-, and azoxy-ethane, though multipotent carcinogens, never produced intestinal cancer, but proved to be highly teratogenic and carcinogenic to rat fetuses in early stages of development.

These striking differences between the actions of the methyl and ethyl compounds demonstrate that the enzymes involved in the metabolic activation cannot be identical or nonspecific, but must be different. The observation of distinct and characteristic organotropism in systematic studies with various types of " indirect " carcinogens suggests that the so-called mixed-functional drug-metabolizing enzymes are in fact a group of specific hydroxylases. Furthermore, the " proximate " carcinogens resulting from metabolic activation apparently are very short-lived intermediates, because cancer was induced exclusively in the respective target organs, and, in transplacental experiments, there was no transmission of the activated product from the maternal organism to the fetus. Accordingly, the relevant step of activation occurs in the target organ itself. This indicates that organospecific enzymes are involved.

Even though no explanation can be given at present of such organospecific mechanisms, the use of " indirect " carcinogens, particularly in transplacental and neonatal experiments, offers a new tool for studies of organospecific enzymes and their formation in the course of ontogenic development.

The third example presented in this paper is the specific induction of adenocarcinomas of the glandular stomach in rats, especially by N'-acetyl-methylnitrosourea by oral administration. In contrast to the forementioned substances it is a " direct " -acting carcinogen which does not need enzymatic activation. More surprising is the specific effect on the glandular mucosa of the stomach, first observed by Sugimura and Fujimura (52) in experiments with N'-nitro-methylnitrosoguanidine. The common factor in both substances is the acylated second N atom. This indicates that deacylating enzymes of the mucosa may play a role, since methylnitrosourea did produce gastric carcinomas in guinea pigs, which have no forestomach. The induction time for adenocarcinomas was very long in both guinea pigs and rats, whereas that for cancer of the forestomach was significantly shorter, especially if high doses were used.   Accordingly, the induction of carcinomas of the glandular stomach in rats suggests that a specific mechanism is involved.

In contrast to the specific effect of the methyl compound, N'-acetyl-ethyl-nitrosourea did not produce gastric adenocarcinomas in rats.   Therefore, the methyl group also seems to be essential.   Comparative studies with n-propyl-, butyl- and pentyl-nitrosourea led to different results, and the localization of the tumors observed was dependent on the nature of the alkyl group.   It is of interest that the effects even of " direct " -acting carcinogens can be modified by variation of alkyl groups.

The " ultimate " carcinogen of all groups of substances tested in these experiments probably is the corresponding alkyldiazohydroxide or -diazonium, as formulated in Figs. 3, 8 and 13.   Accordingly they belong to the greater class of alkylating carcinogens.   There is sufficient evidence of the alkylation of nucleic acids. The interactions with nitroso compounds will be discussed in the papers of P. D. Lawley and of P. N. Magee at this symposium.   The fact that the " ultimate " alkylating intermediate, namely methyldiazonium, probably is identical in the three groups of carcinogens leads to the conclusion that the different organospecific effects are attributable either to the structure of the original molecule or to its enzymatic activation.

The purpose of this paper was to demonstrate that organospecific induction of carcinomas in three parts of the digestive tract, the esophagus, the glandular stomach, and the colon and rectum, is in fact possible with high regularity and accuracy. Each organotropic effect was characteristic for one type of well-defined substance, producing cancer exclusively in one of these three organs and never in the other two. Some compounds which have been found suitable for the induction of cancer in the various parts of the digestive tract of rats are listed in Table 4 together with data on dosage, median induction time and yield.

Progress in every field of cancer research, be it morphogenesis, biochemistry, immunology, virology or chemotherapy, largely depends upon the availability of reliable experimental models for all types of malignant tumors.   Their specific induction naturally can be expected from chemical carcinogens.   Therefore, sys-

TABLE 4.   Selective Induction of Carcinomas in Special Parts of the Digestive Tract of Rats.   Examples of Methods.   Administration in Drinking Water 5 Times/Week, and Subcutaneous Injections Once/Week for 20 Weeks.

Target organ	Substance	Dosage		t_{50} days	Yield %	Other organs
		Appl.	mg/kg			
Tongue	diazoacetic-ethylester	drink	5	575	50	forestomach
Esophagus	methyl-butyl-nitrosamine	any	1	250	95	none
	methyl-phenylethyl-nitrosamine	any	1	230	95	none
Forestomach	methyl-nitroso-urethane	drink	5	330	90	none
Gland. stomach	N'-acetyl-methylnitrosourea	drink	2	500	90	brain
	N-methyl-N-nitroso-biuret	drink	5	500	70	brain
Duodenum	n-propyl-nitroso-urea	drink	16	350	25	forestomach
Colon, rectum	1, 2-dimethyl-hydrazine	s. c.	10	300	95	duodenum
	azoxy-methane	s. c.	6	300	95	duodenum

tematic studies in chemical carcinogenesis, including relationships between chemical structure and action, to which Japanese scientists have contributed so much, are regarded as fundamental in experimental cancer research. Beyond that the results of such studies will provide a basis for the prevention of cancer, which lastly is the most reasonable and most effective way to overcome this dreadful disease.

SUMMARY

Organospecific carcinogenesis in three parts of the digestive tract, namely the esophagus, glandular stomach, and colon mainly of rats is reported. Nonsymmetrical methyl-alkylnitrosamines proved to be selective and very potent carcinogens for the esophagus by any route of administration. Esophageal carcinoma induction was possible already soon after birth; this was not the case in transplacental experiments.

Adenocarcinomas of the glandular stomach were first observed in experiments with methylnitrosourethane and -urea in guinea pigs. Stimulated by the results of Sugimura and Fujimura (52) with N'-nitro-N-methylnitrosoguanidine, N'-acetyl-N-methylnitrosourea was tested in rats. At low dosages of 2 mg/kg in drinking water or milk for a limited period it produced gastric adenocarcinomas in all of 35 rats so treated. This specific effect was not obtained with the corresponding ethyl compound. Propyl-, butyl- and pentyl-nitrosourea by oral administration produced cancer in various parts of the digestive tract, the brain, and the breast and leukemias, each substance in a characteristic pattern, dependent on the nature of the alkyl group.

Symmetrical 1,2-dimethylhydrazine and azoxymethane proved to be specific inducers of intestinal cancer. After subcutaneous injections of 7 and 5 mg/kg, once a week for a few months, almost all treated rats later died with multiple adenocarcinomas of the colon and rectum. The induction of colonic cancer was also possible by single dose of azoxymethane in newborn rats, but not in transplacental experiments.

Relationships between chemical structure and organospecific carcinogenicity, and the probable reaction mechanisms are discussed. The quantitive evaluation of the results revealed high accuracy. Therefore the three groups of substances provide reliable models for the regular and specific induction of carcinomas of the esophagus, the glandular stomach, and the colon and rectum.

I would like to mention the names of my co-workers, S. Ivankovic, R. Preussmann, J. Stekar, C. Landschütz, J. Gimmy, J. Bücheler, U. Griesbach, A. Lange and T. Tan. The author is indebted to the Deutsche Forschungsgemeinschaft for generous support.

REFERENCES

1. Bralow, S. P. Gruenstein, M., Meranze, D. R., Bonakdapur, A., and Shimkin, M. B. Adenocarcinoma of Glandular Stomach and Duodenum in Wistar Rats Ingesting N-Methyl-N'-nitro-N-nitrosoguanidine, Histopathology and Associated Secretory Changes. Cancer Res., *30*: 1215–1222, 1970.

2. Bücheler, J., and Thomas, C. Experimentell Erzeugte Drüsenmagentumoren bei Meerschweinchen und Ratte. Beitr. Path., *142*: 194–209, 1971.

3. Druckrey, H. Quantitative Aspects in Chemical Carcinogenesis, *In*; Truhaut, R. (ed.), Potential Carcinogenic Hazards from Drugs, UICC Monograph Series, *7*: 60–77, Springer, Berlin, New York, 1967.

4. Druckrey, H. Production of Colonic Carcinomas by 1,2-Dialkylhydrazines and Azoxyalkanes, *In*; Burdette, W. J. (ed.), Carcinoma of the Colon and Antecedent Epithelium, pp. 267–279, Thomas, Springfield, 1970.

5. Druckrey, H. Genotypes and Phenotypes of Ten Inbred Strains of BD-rats. Arznei-mittelforsch., *21*: 1274–1278, 1971.

6. Druckrey, H., Ivankovic, S., Bücheler, J., Preussmann, R., und Thomas, C. Erzeugung von Magen- und Pankreas-Krebs beim Meerschweinchen durch Methylnit-roso-harnstoff und -urethan. Z. Krebsforsch., *71*: 167–182, 1968.

7. Druckrey, H., Ivankovic, S., und Preussmann, R. Selektive Erzeugung von Car-cinomen des Drüsenmagens bei Ratten durch orale Gabe von N-Methyl-N-nitroso-N'-acetylharnstoff (AcMNH). Z. Krebsforsch., *75*: 23–33, 1970.

8. Druckrey, H., Ivankovic, S., Preussmann, R., Landschütz, C., Stekar, J., Brunner, U., and Schagen, B. Transplacental Induction of Neurogenic Malignomas by 1,2-Diethyl-hydrazine, Azo-, and Azoxy-ethane in Rats. Experientia, *24*: 561–562, 1968.

9. Druckrey, H., Landschütz, C., und Preussmann, R. Oesophagus-Carcinome nach Inhalation von Methyl-butylnitrosamin (MBNA) an Ratten. Z. Krebsforsch., *71*: 135–139, 1968.

10. Druckrey, H., Landschütz, C., Preussmann, R., und Ivankovic, S. Erzeugung von Magenkrebs und Neurogenen Malignomen durch orale Gabe von Methyl-nitroso-biuret (MNB) an Ratten. Z. Krebsforsch., *75*: 229–239, 1971.

11. Druckrey, H. und Preussmann, R. Zur Entstehung carcinogener Nitrosamine am Beispiel des Tabakrauchs. Naturwissenschaften, *49*: 498–499, 1962.

12. Druckrey, H. and Preussmann, R. N-Nitroso-N-methylurethane, a Potent Car-cinogen. Nature, *195*: 1111, 1962.

13. Druckrey, H., Preussmann, R., Blum, G., Ivankovic, S., und Afkham, J. Erzeugung von Karzinomen der Speiseröhre durch unsymmetrische Nitrosamine. Naturwis-senschaften, *50*: 100–101, 1963.

14. Druckrey, H., Preussmann, R., and Ivankovic, S. N-Nitroso Compounds in Or-ganotropic and Transplacental Carcinogenesis. Ann. New York Acad. Sci., *163*: 676–696, 1969.

15. Druckrey, H., Preussmann, R., Ivankovic, S., und Schmähl, D. Organotrope Carcinogene Wirkungen bei 65 Verschiedenen N-Nitroso-Verbindungen an BD-Ratten. Z. Krebsforsch., *69*: 103–201, 1967.

16. Druckrey, H., Preussmann, R., Ivankovic, S., Schmidt, C. H., So, B. T., und Thomas, C. Carcinogene Wirkung von Azoäthan und Azoxyäthan an Ratten. Z. Krebs-forsch., *67*: 31–45, 1965.

17. Druckrey, H., Preussmann, R., Matzkies, F., und Ivankovic, S. Selektive Erzeugung von Darmkrebs bei Ratten durch 1,2-Dimethyl-hydrazin. Naturwissenschaften, *54*: 285–286, 1967.

17a. Druckrey, H., Preussmann, R., Schmähl, D., und Müller, M. Chemische Konstitu-tion und carcinogene Wirkung bei Nitrosaminen. Naturwissenschaften, *48*: 134–135, 1961.

17b. Druckrey, H., Preussmann, R., Schmähl, D., und Müller, M. Erzeugung von Ma-genkrebs durch Nitrosamide an Ratten. Naturwissenschaften, *48*: 165, 1961.

18. Druckrey, H., Schmähl, D., und Mecke, R., Jr. Erzeugung von Magenkrebs an Ratten durch 4-Nitrostilben. Naturwissenschaften, *42*: 128, 1955.

19. Druckrey, H., Steinhoff, D., Beuthner, H., Schneider, H., und Klärner, P. Prüfung von Nitrit auf Chronisch-toxische Wirkung an Ratten. Arzneimittelforschung, *13*: 320–323, 1963.

20. Du Plessis, L. S., Nunn, J. R., and Roach, W. A. Carcinogen in a Transkeian Bantu Food Additive. Nature, *222*: 1198–1199, 1969.

20a. Dutton, A. H. and Heath, D. F. Demethylation of Dimethylnitrosamine in Rats and Mice. Nature, *178*: 644, 1956.

21. Fujimura, S., Kogure, K., Sugimura, T., and Takayama, S. The Effect of Limited Administration of N-Methyl-N'-nitro-N-nitrosoguanidine on the Induction of Stomach Cancer in Rats. Cancer Res., *30*: 842–848, 1970.

22. Herrold, K. M. Epidermoid Carcinomas of Esophagus and Forestomach Induced in Syrian Hamsters by N-Nitroso-N-methylurethane. J. Natl. Cancer Inst., *37*: 389, 1966.

23. Hirayama, R. The Epidemiology of Cancer of the Stomach in Japan with Special Reference to the Role of Diet. *In*; UICC Monograph Series, *10*: 37–48, Springer, Berlin, Heidelberg and New York, 1967.

24. Imai, T., Kubo, T. and Watanabe, H. Chronic Gastritis in Japanese with Reference to High Incidence of Gastric Carcinoma. J. Natl. Cancer Inst., *47*: 179–195, 1971.

25. Ivankovic, S., und Preussmann, R. Transplacentare Erzeugung Maligner Tumoren nach oraler Gabe von Äthylharnstoff und Nitrit an Ratten. Naturwissenschaften, *57*: 460, 1970.

26. Konjetzny, G. E. Über die Beziehungen der Chronischen Gastritis mit Ihren Folgeerscheinungen und des Chronischen Magenulcus zur Entwicklung des Magenkrebses. Beitr. Klin. Chir., *85*: 455–519, 1913.

27. Konjetzny, G. E. Der Magenkrebs. F. Enke Verlag, Stuttgart, 1938.

28. Laqueur, G. L. The Induction of Intestinal Neoplasms in Rats with the Glycoside Cycasin and Its Aglycone. Virchows Arch. Path. Anat., *340*: 151–163, 1965.

29. Lijinsky, W., and Epstein, S. Nitrosamines as Environmental Carcinogens. Nature, *225*: 21–23, 1970.

30. Lijinsky, W., Loo, J., and Ross, A. E. Mechanism of Alkylation of Nucleic Acids by Nitrosodimethylamine. Nature, *218*: 1174–1175, 1968.

31. Löhrs, U., Wiebecke, B., und Eder, M. Morphologische und Autoradiographische Untersuchung der Darmschleimhautveränderungen nach Einmaliger Injektion von 1,2-Dimethyl-hydrazin. Z. Ges. Exp. Med., *151*: 297–307, 1969.

32. Mirvish, S. S. Kinetics of Dimethylamine Nitrosation in Relation to Nitrosamine Carcinogenesis. J. Natl. Cancer Inst., *44*: 633–639, 1970.

33. Mirvish, S. S. Kinetics of Nitrosamide Formation from Alkylureas, N-Alkylurethans, and Alkylguanidines: Possible Implications for the Etiology of Human Gastric Cancer. J. Natl. Cancer Inst., *46*: 1183–1193, 1971.

34. Montesano, R., and Magee, P. N. Evidence of Formation of N-Methyl-N-nitrosourea in Rats Given N-Methylurea and Sodium Nitrite. Int. J. Cancer, *7*: 249–255, 1971.

35. Mori, K., Ohta, A., Murakami, T., Tamura, M., and Kondo, M. Carcinoma of the Glandular Stomach of Mice Induced by 4-Hydroxyaminoquinoline-1-oxide Hydrochloride. Gann, *60*: 151–154, 1969.

36. Nagata, C., and Imamura, A. Electronic Structures and Mechanism of Carcinogenicity for Alkylnitrosamines. Gann, *61*: 169–176, 1970.

37. Nakahara, W., and Fukuoka, F.   Study of Carcinogenic Mechanism Based on Experiments with 4-Nitroquinoline-N-oxide.   Gann, *50*: 1–15, 1959.

38. Nakahara, W., Fukuoka, F., and Sugimura, T.   Carcinogenic Action of 4-Nitroquinoline-N-oxide.   Gann, *48*, 129–137, 1948.

39. Narisawa, T., Sato, T., Hayakawa, M., Sakuma, A., and Nakano, H.   Carcinoma of the Colon and Rectum of Rats by Rectal Infusion of N-Methyl-N'-nitro-N-nitrosoguanidine.   Gann, *62*: 231–234, 1971.

40. Odashima, S.   Leukemogenesis of N-Nitrosobutylurea in the Rat.   I.   Effect of Various Concentrations in the Drinking Water to Female Donryu Rats.   Gann, *61*: 245–253, 1970.

41. Preussmann, R., Druckrey, H., Ivankovic, S., and v. Hodenberg, A.   Chemical Structure and Carcinogenicity of Aliphatic Hydrazo-, Azo-, and Azoxy-compounds and Triazenes, Potential *in vivo* Alkylating Agents.   Ann. New York Acad. Sci., *163*: 697–716, 1969.

41a. Rao, C. N. R., and Bhaskar, K. R.   Spectroscopy of the Nitroso-Group.   *In*; Feuer, H. (ed.), The Chemistry of the Nitro- and Nitroso-Groups, p. 155, Interscience Publish., New York, 1969.

42. Saito, T., Inokuchi, K., Takayama, S., and Sugimura, T.   Sequential Morphological Changes in N-Methyl-N'-nitro-N-Nitrosoguanidine Carcinogenesis in the Glandular Stomach of Rats.   J. Natl. Cancer Inst., *44*: 769–783, 1970.

43. Sander, J.   Induktion maligner Tumoren bei Ratten durch orale Gabe von N,N'-Dimethylharnstoff und Nitrit.   Arzneimittelforsch., *20*: 418–419, 1970.

44. Sander, J., Bürkle, G., Flohe, L., und Aeikens, B.   Untersuchungen *in vitro* über die Möglichkeit einer Bildung Cancerogener Nitrosamide im Magen.   Arzneimittelforsch., *21*: 411–414, 1971.

44a. Sander, J., Schweinsberg, F., und Menz, H. P.   Untersuchungen über die Entstehung cancerogener Nitrosamine im Magen.   Zschr. Physiol. Chem., *349*: 1691–1697, 1968.

45. Sato, T., Fukuyama, T., and Suzuki, T.   Studies of the Causation of Gastric Cancer.   2.   The Relation between Gastric Cancer Mortality Rate and Salted Food Intake in Several Places in Japan.   Bull. Inst. Publ. Health. Japan, *8*: 187–198, 1959.

45a. Schoental, R.   Carcinogenic action of diazomethane and of Nitroso-N-methylurethane.   Nature, *188*: 420–421, 1960.

45b. Schoental, R.   Interaction of the Carcinogenic N-Methyl-nitrosourethane with Sulphydryl Groups.   Nature, *192*: 670, 1961.

46. Schoental T., and Rive, D. J.   Interaction of N-Alkyl-N-nitroso-urethanes with Thiols.   Biochem. J., *97*: 466–474, 1965.

47. Segi, M., Kurihara, M., and Matsuyama, T.   Cancer Mortality for Selected Sites in 24 Countries.   No. 5. Dept. Publ. Health, Tohoku University, Sendai, Japan, 1969.

48. Shank, R. C., and Magee, P. N.   Similarities between the Biochemical Actions of Cycasin and Dimethylnitrosamine.   Biochem. J., *105*: 521–527, 1967.

49. Spatz, M., and Laqueur, G. L.   Transplacental Induction of Tumours in Sprague-Dawley Rats with Crude Cycad Material.   J. Natl. Cancer Inst., *38*: 233–239, 1967.

50. Stewart, H. L.   Site Variation of Alimentary Tract Cancer in Man and Experimental Animals as Indicators of Diverse Etiology.   Proc. 9. Intern. Cancer Cong. UICC Monogr. Ser. *9*: 15, Springer- Verlag, Berlin, Heidelberg, New York, 1967.

51. Stewart, H. L., Snell, K. C., Morvis, H. P., Wagner, B. P., and Ray, F. E.   Car-

cinoma of the Glandular Stomach of Rats Ingesting N,N'-2,7-Fluorenylenebisace-tamide. Natl. Cancer Inst. Monogr., *5*: 105–139, 1961.

52. Sugimura, T., and Fujimura, S. Tumour Production in Glandular Stomach of Rat by N-Methyl-N'-nitro-N-nitrosoguanidine. Nature, *216*: 943–944, 1967.

53. Sugimura, T., Fujimura, S., and Baba, T. Tumor Production in the Glandular Stomach and Alimentary Tract of the Rat by N-Methyl-N'-nitro-N-nitrosoguanidine. Cancer Res., *30*: 455–465, 1970.

54. Sugimura, T., Fujimura, S., Kogure, K., Baba, T., Saito, T., Nagao, M., Hosoi, H., Shimosato, Y., and Yokoshima, T. Production of Adenocarcinomas in Glandular Stomach of Experimental Animals by N-Methyl-N'-nitro-N-nitrosoguanidine. Gann Monograph, *8*: 157–196, 1969.

55. Sugimura, T., Fujimura, S., Nagao, M., Yokoshima, T., and Hasegawa, M. Reaction of N-Methyl-N'-nitro-N-nitrosoguanidine with Protein. Biochim. Biophys. Acta, *170*: 427–429, 1968.

56. Sugimura, T., Kawachi, T., Kogure, K., Tanaka, N., Kazama, S., and Koyama, Y. A Novel Method for Detecting Intestinal Metaplasia of the Stomach with TES Tape. Gann, *62*: 237–238, 1971.

57. Sugimura, T., Tanaka, N., Kawachi, T., Kogure, K., Fujimura, S., and Shimosato, Y. Production of Stomach Cancer in Dogs by N-Methyl-N'-nitro-N-nitrosoguanidine. Gann, *62*: 67, 1971.

58. Takayama, S., Saito, T., Fujimura, S., and Sugimura, T. Histological Findings of Gastric Tumors Induced by N-Methyl-N'-nitro-N-nitrosoguanidine in Rats. Gann Monograph, *8*: 197–208, 1969.

58a. Weisburger, J. H., Weisburger, E. K., Mantel, N., Hadidian, Z., and Fredrickson, T. New Carcinogenic Nitrosamines in Rats. Naturwissenschaften, *53*: 508, 1966.

59. Wiebecke, B., Löhrs, U., Gimmy, J., und Eder, M. Erzeugung von Darmtumoren bei Mäusen durch 1,2-Dimethylhydrazin. Z. Ges. Exp. Med., *149*: 277–278, 1969.

60. Wittig, G., Wildner, G. P., und Ziebarth, D. Der Einfluss der Ingesta auf die Kanzerisierung des Rattendarmes durch Dimethylhydrazin. Arch. Geschwulst-forsch., *37*: 105–115, 1971.

61. Wynder, E. L., Kmet, J., Dungal, N., and Segi, M. An Epidemiological Investigation of Gastric Cancer. Cancer, *16*: 1461–1496, 1963.

62. Wynder, E. L., and Shigematsu, T. Environmental Factors of Cancer of the Colon and Rectum. Cancer, *20*: 1520, 1967.

63. Yokoro, K., Imamura, N., Takizawa, S., Nishihara, H., and Nishihara, E. Leukemogenic and Mammary Tumorigenic Effects of N-Nitrosobutylurea in Mice and Rats. Gann, *61*: 287–289, 1970.

64. Zaldivar, R. Geographic Pathology of Oral, Esophageal, Gastric, and Intestinal Cancer in Chile. Z. Krebsforsch., *75*: 1–13, 1970.

Discussion of Paper by Dr. Druckrey

DR. MAGEE: You have shown that 1,2-dimethylhydrazine is powerfully carcinogenic for the colon and in earlier studies that 1,1-dimethylhydrazine was not carcinogenic.   What about monomethylhydrazine?

Dr. Andrew Hanks in my laboratory has shown that 1,2-dimethylhydrazine
does methylate nucleic acids in the body.

DR. DRUCKREY: Monomethylhydrazine was practically not carcinogenic.   Only
sporadic tumors were observed after oral, subcutaneous or intravenous administration.   Alkylation of nucleic acids was first reported by Shank and Magee (1967),
using methylazoxymethanol.

DR. HEIDELBERGER: You have very elegantly demonstrated exquisite organ specificity of these carcinogens.   What is your working hypothesis to explain this organ
specificity?

DR. DRUCKREY: All our experimental results with dialkylnitrosamines, hydrazo-,
azo-, and azoxyalkanes indicate that the first step of activation is enzymatic α-
hydroxylation.   Furthermore, striking differences between the organotropic carcinogenicity of related compounds, particularly between methyl and ethyl derivatives strongly suggest that highly specific hydroxylases are involved in the metabolic
activation of these " indirect " carcinogens.

DR. HIGGINSON: I would like to ask Professor Druckrey to comment on the importance of a latent period in determing organ specificity.   Thus DEN will kill rats with
liver carcinoma, but careful examination will show minute carcinomata of the
esophagus.   In other words specificity here is essentially a factor of a latent period
which presumably represents the speed of metabolism of the compound by the two
organs.   Is it possible that with other nitrosamines the high mortality from one
cancer will obscure the occurrence of tumors in other organs?   Thus, organ specificity
may be essentially a relative rather than an absolute phenomenon.

DR. DRUCKREY: In our experiments, diethylnitrosamine produced liver cancer exclusively at a daily dosage of more than 0.6 mg/kg.   At lower dosage also carcinomas of the esophagus were observed and at the lowest dosage of less than 0.1
mg/kg carcinomas and neuroblastomas in the ethmobubinalia of rats.   On the other

hand, there are in fact examples for the importance of the time factor in organo-specific carcinogenesis.

Induction of Stomach Cancer by N-Methyl-N'-nitro-N-nitrosoguanidine : Experiments on Dogs as Clinical Models and the Metabolism of This Carcinogen

Takashi SUGIMURA, Takashi KAWACHI, Kikuko KOGURE, Minako NAGAO, Noritake TANAKA, Shinji FUJIMURA, Shozo TAKAYAMA, Yukio SHIMOSATO, Masatoshi NOGUCHI, Noriyuki KUWABARA, and Tatsuya YAMADA

National Cancer Center Research Institute, Tokyo, Japan [*T.S., T.K., K.K., M.N., N.T., S.F., Y.S.*] ; *Cancer Institute, Japanese Foundation for Cancer Research, Tokyo, Japan* [*S.T., N.K.*] ; *National Cancer Center Hospital, Tokyo, Japan* [*M.N., T.Y.*]

The problem of stomach cancer is of national interest in Japan. Our work on the production of stomach cancer by the administration of N-methyl-N'-nitro-N-nitrosoguanidine (MNNG) to experimental animals has two purposes. The first is to use animals as models for studies of the carcinogenic processes involved in the development of stomach cancer in human beings. To this end, we studied carcinogenesis in the stomach of dogs. The second purpose of this work is to study the metabolism of MNNG in relation to its peculiar feature of interaction with biological substances. Studies on this kind of biological interaction of a carcinogen with biological materials should be useful in elucidating the actions of naturally occurring carcinogens.

MNNG has been used as a potent mutagen in microbiology and its carcinogenicity was reported by Druckrey, Schoental and by us in 1966 (*1, 12, 21*).

The development of many adenocarcinomas in the glandular stomach of rats and hamsters after the administration of MNNG solution as drinking water has been well documented (*3, 11, 17–19*), and there are also reports of its effects on dogs (*14, 19, 22*).

Induction of Stomach Cancer in Rats and Hamsters upon Administration of MNNG

Figure 1 shows a gastric adenocarcinoma in the glandular stomach of a rat which had received MNNG solution (83 μg/ml) for 7 months, and which was killed 8 months later. It is interesting that in this single stomach, we found two different types of adenocarcinoma. One was a differentiated type of adenocarcinoma and the other a signet ring cell-type carcinoma. Figure 2 shows metastases of these two types of tumor. A metastasis of the differentiated type of adenocarcinoma developed in the liver (Fig. 2A), while a metastasis of the signet ring cell type of carcinoma (diffuse-type adenocarcinoma) developed in a lymph node (Fig. 2B).

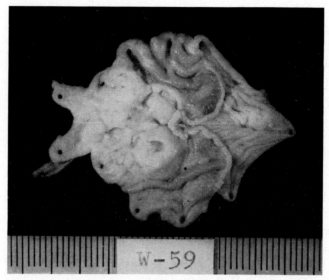

Fig. 1.   Gross appearance of cancer in the glandular stomach of a rat.   A gastric carcinoma developed in the glandular stomach of a rat which had received 83 μg/ml of MNNG for 7 months.   The animal was killed 8 months later.   This tumor was composed of two different types of adenocarcinoma: a differentiated type and a signet ring cell type.

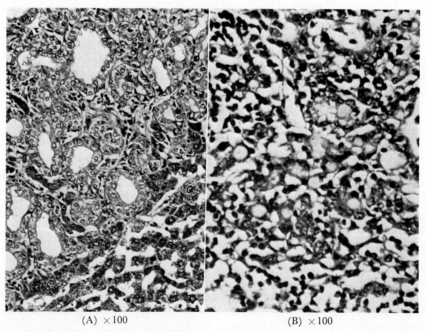

(A) ×100   (B) ×100

Fig. 2.   Histological appearance of the metastatic foci of the stomach cancer shown in Fig. 1. (A) Metastasis of the differentiated type of adenocarcinoma in the liver.   (B) Metastasis of the signet ring cell type of adenocarcinoma in a local lymph node.

Figure 3 shows an anaplastic adenocarcinoma in the glandular stomach of a hamster which was killed 6 months after the administration of 50 μg/ml of MNNG

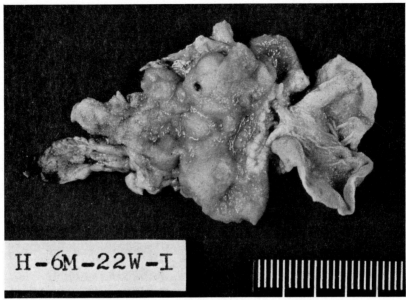

FIG. 3. Gross appearance of cancer in the glandular stomach of a hamster. An anaplastic adenocarcinoma developed in the glandular stomach of a hamster after administration of MNNG for 6 months. The animal was killed 6 months later.

for 6 months. Under optimum experimental conditions, about two-thirds of the rats which received MNNG developed adenocarcinomas in the glandular stomach.

Induction of Stomach Cancer in Dogs by the Administration of MNNG

Dogs also developed gastric carcinomas upon the administration of MNNG solution as drinking water. Dogs have a fairly large stomach and its histological structure resembles that of man. It was easy to carry out radiographic and endoscopic examinations on dogs after MNNG administration to follow the process of development of gastric cancer. Figure 4 shows an X-ray photograph of the stomach of a dog taken 7 months after the administration of the MNNG solution (83 μg/ml) for 15 months. Radiography was performed by the double-contrast method after introducing a suspension of barium sulfate and air through a gastric tube into the stomach of animals under anaesthesia. Irregularly shaped deposits of barium in the cardiac portion are suggestive evidence of cancer growth. Figure 5 is a photograph of the stomach of the same dog. He was killed 2 months after the radiography shown in Fig. 4. As was expected by the radiologists at the hospital of the National Cancer Center, a cancerous growth with ulcerations was found in the posterior wall of the cardiac portion of the stomach. Histologically, it was classified as an adenocarcinoma that had invaded the wall almost to the serosa. Other adenocarcinomas were found in the antral portion of the stomach, and some of them were quite anaplastic. Figure 6 is a photograph taken by endoscopy of the stomach of a dog that had been treated with MNNG for 15 months. The endoscopist in our hospital suspected that this abnormal change found in the antral region was the focus of a

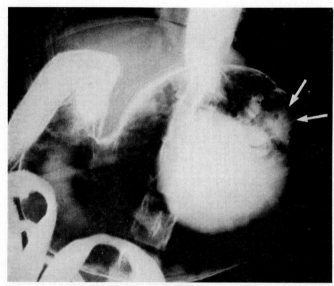

FIG. 4.   A double-contrast X-ray photograph of the stomach of a dog.   This dog had received MNNG for 15 months.   The radiograph was taken 7 months after stopping the administration of MNNG.   Barium deposit in the cardiac portion indicates cancerous growth.

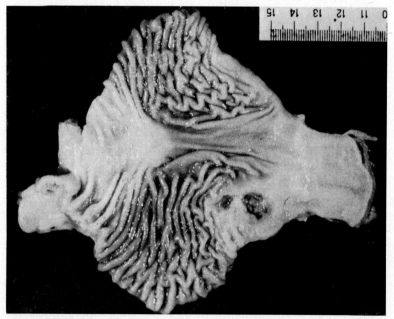

FIG. 5.   Gross appearance of the stomach of a dog.   This animal was killed 2 months after taking the radiograph shown in Fig. 4.   An adenocarcinoma with ulcerations was found in the posterior wall of the cardiac portion of the stomach.

carcinoma.   Figure 7 shows the histological appearance of a specimen taken by biopsy from a similar focus in the antral region of the stomach of a dog that had been treated with MNNG for 15 months.   A surgical pathologist diagnosed this as an

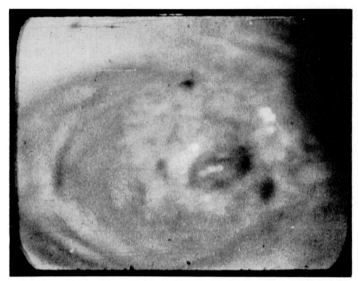

FIG. 6.   A photograph of the stomach of a dog taken by endoscopy. This dog received MNNG for 15 months, and this photograph was taken 14 months after stopping the administration of MNNG.   Cancerous change was observed in the antral region of the stomach.

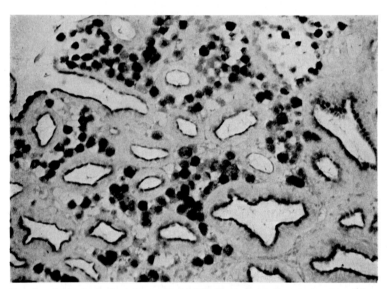

FIG. 7.   A histological specimen obtained by biopsy from the antral region of the stomach shown in Fig. 6.   The specimen was stained with PAS-Alcian blue.   A signet ring cell-type carcinoma was found in the mucosa only.

early gastric adenocarcinoma also, even though the carcinoma was still localized in the mucosal layer and had not penetrated into the submucosal layer yet.   The specimen showed structural and cellular atypia.

Seven dogs have so far been autopsied, and all of them had gastric carcinomas in the cardiac and/or antral region of the stomach.   Other dogs, which have cancerous foci and are still alive, are being followed up.   This technique for diagnosing early stomach cancer has just been developed over the past decade, primarily in Japan, by clinical pathologists, radiologists and endoscopists.   However, it should be mentioned that there is little information on the process of growth from incipient stomach cancer to big tumors.   There are still many questions that remain unanswered. For instance, *how long can one keep a patient with early stomach cancer under observation before the decision to operate is made? Or how fast and how frequently does early stomach cancer develop into an advanced carcinoma?*   At this point, we feel that experiments on dogs should provide precise information for understanding the development of stomach cancer in human beings.

Interaction of MNNG with Biological Materials

There are many reports that MNNG causes methylation of nucleic acids *in vitro* and *in vivo* (5–7, 15, 20).   MNNG can modify proteins by transferring its nitro-amidino moiety to either the ε-amino group of lysine or the sulfhydryl group of cysteine (6, 8–10, 13, 20).   Figure 8 shows the nitroamidination of lysine in a pep-

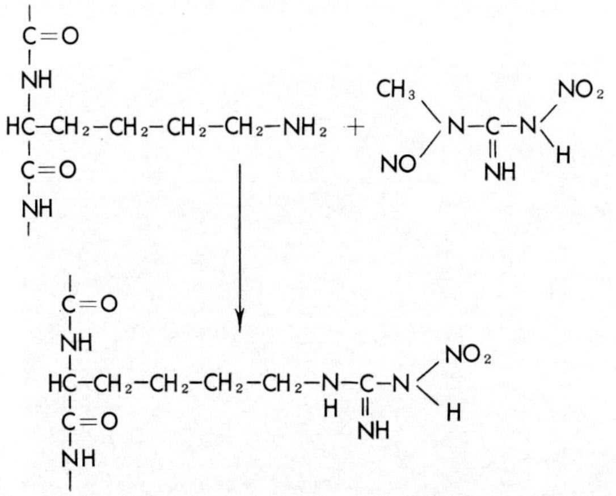

FIG. 8.   Conversion of the lysine residue of a protein to a nitrohomoarginine residue by nitroamidination with MNNG.

tide.   In this reaction, the lysine residue is converted to a nitrohomoarginine residue. Consequently, after treatment with MNNG, the characters of proteins may change. To test this, horse cytochrome *c* was incubated with MNNG, labeled at the guanidino carbon at a neutral pH at room temperature.   The modified cytochrome *c* was separated by column chromatography on IRC-120.   Cytochrome *c* with a certain number of nitroamidino residues was purified.   Modified cytochrome *c* did not act as an electron acceptor in the presence of mitochondrial NADH-cytochrome *c* oxidoreductase, as shown in Fig. 9 (9).   Figure 10 shows the electrofocusing of native cytochrome *c* and cytochrome *c* modified with MNNG.   The upper band is native cytochrome *c* and the lower band is cytochrome *c* with three nitrohomoarginine residues.   Modified cytochrome *c* clearly had a different isoelectric point.

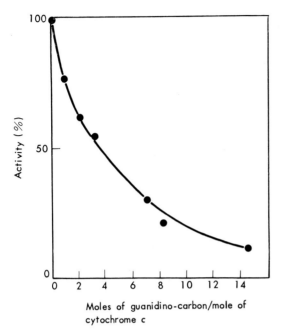

FIG. 9. Rate of enzymatic reduction of MNNG-modified cytochrome c. The reaction mixture contained in 0.5 ml: 25 μmoles of phosphate buffer (pH 7.4), 0.5 μmole of KCN, 24 nmoles of native or modified cytochrome c, 2 μmoles of NADH and 1.8 μg of mitochondrial protein. The increase of absorbance was measured at 550 nm.

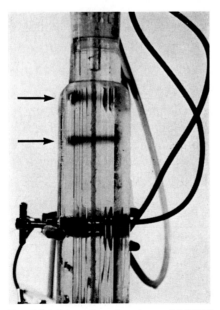

FIG. 10. Separation of native and MNNG-modified cytochrome c by electrofocusing. Apparatus, LKB 8100–10; pH range, 7–10; conditions, 4°C, 72 hr.

TABLE 1. Paper Chromatography of Hydrolyzed Histone from [Guanidino-^{14}C] MNNG-Treated Cells

Solvent system	Rf value	
Number	Authentic L-nitro-homoarginine	Radioactive product isolated from histone
1	0.13	0.13
2	0.30	0.30
3	0.03	0.04
4	0.71	0.70

Solvent system: 1, n-Butanol-methyl ethyl ketone-water-conc. NH$_4$OH (25:15:7:3, by vol.); 2, n-butanol-formic acid-water (75:15:15, by vol.); 3, n-butanol-ethanol-water (5:1:4, by vol.); 4, 10% citrate saturated phenol (under NH$_3$ vapor).

Ascites tumor cells were incubated with MNNG labeled at the guanidino carbon. Then the histone was isolated from the cells and digested with papain and leucine amino peptidase. From the resulting acid-soluble fraction, a single radioactive peak was obtained on paper chromatography. The Rf-values of this radioactive amino acid in three different solvent systems coincided with those of the authentic L-nitrohomoarginine, as shown in Table 1 (*10*). This indicates that the nitroamidination of lysine in histone actually occurred in intact cells which were exposed to MNNG.

Next, rats were given [^{14}C-guanidino] MNNG through a gastric tube, and histone was extracted from their stomachs. Radioactive nitrohomoarginine was also detected in this histone preparation. Thus, it is certain that MNNG modified protein both *in vivo* and *in vitro*.

The experiments with cytochrome c and histone are simply models, proving that protein is modified by MNNG; but the results suggest that some proteins, which play a more crucial role in carcinogenesis, may also be modified by MNNG.

Overall Metabolism of MNNG in vivo

When radioactive MNNG was administered orally to rats, the radioactivity was quickly excreted in the urine. As shown in Table 2, about 90% of the radioactivity was excreted in the urine within 24 hr after the administration of MNNG, labeled at either the methyl or guanidino carbon. Furthermore it should be emphasized that most of the radioactivity in the urine was excreted within the first 9 hr after its administration. After the administration of MNNG, labeled at either the methyl

TABLE 2. Excretion of Radioactivity in the Urine, Feces and Expired Air

	[Guanidino-^{14}C] MNNG (% of total radioactivity)	[Me-^{14}C] MNNG (% of total radioactivity)
Urine	93.3	87.1
Feces	0.2	0.2
Expired air	3.7	9.7

Rats, weighing about 250 g each, were given 2 μCi of [guanidino-^{14}C] MNNG or [Me-^{14}C] MNNG by stomach tube. Radioactivity excreted within 24 hr after MNNG administration was measured.

or guanidino carbon, all the radioactivity in the urine was extracted with ethyl ether. It was found to exist almost exclusively as N-methyl-N'-nitro-guanidine (MNG), as identified with a radiochromatoscanner. This suggests that there may be a metabolic pathway for conversion of MNNG to the denitroso derivative (4).

In vitro Conversion of MNNG to MNG in the Presence of Tissue Extract

MNNG is fairly stable under neutral conditions and its concentration in solution was easily determined from the absorption at 402 nm. MNG has no absorption at 402 nm. Consequently, the conversion of MNNG to MNG could be determined quantitatively by measuring the decrease in optical absorption at 402 nm. Table 3 shows the conversions of MNNG to MNG, using extracts of rat stomach, liver and kidney tissues. As control proteins, bovine albumin and cytochrome c were incubated with MNNG, but they did not cause any conversion of MNNG to MNG.

TABLE 3. Conversion of MNNG to MNG by Tissue Extracts

	(nmole/min/mg prot.)
Stomach	6.83
Liver	41.40
Kidney	20.90
Bovine albumin	0.48
Horse cytochrome c	1.80

Tissues were homogenized with 9 volumes of 0.1 M potassium phosphate buffer (pH 7.5). Homogenates were centrifuged at $105,000 \times g$ for 60 min, and supernatants were used as tissue extracts. The reaction mixture contained in 2.0 ml : 10 μmoles of MNNG, 50 μmoles of phosphate buffer (pH 7.5) and 0.2 ml of tissue extract.

TABLE 4. Partial Purification of " Active Protein " from Rat Liver

	Protein (mg)	Activity (nmole of MNG/min)	Specific activity (nmole/min/mg prot.)
Supernatant	1462	16740	11.4
$(NH_4)_2SO_4$ fractionation 50–70%	351	4392	12.5
Sephadex G-100	38.5	1672	43.4
DEAE-cellulose	14.0	1030	73.6

A protein(s) with activity to convert MNNG to MNG was partially purified from rat liver, using ammonium sulfate fractionation, gel filtration on Sephadex and DEAE-cellulose column chromatography, as shown in Table 4. About an 8-fold purification was achieved with a yield of 7%. The activity was not lost on dialysis, but was lost on boiling the preparation. The reaction had an optimum pH around 7.2. Apparently this protein behaves like an " enzyme." The partially purified " enzyme " was incubated with MNNG labeled at the guanidino carbon, and the mixture was passed through a Sephadex G-25 column. As shown in Fig. 11, the protein was eluted in the void volume. Then a radioactive, low molecular

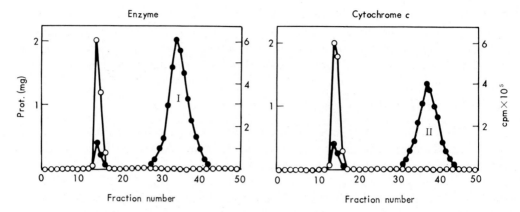

Fig. 11. Gelfiltration on a Sephadex G-25 column of a partially purified "enzyme" or cytochrome c with [guanidino-^{14}C] MNNG. Reaction mixture (0.6 ml), containing 3 μmoles, 50 μCi of MNNG and 4 mg of protein in 0.1 M phosphate buffer (pH 7.5), was incubated at room temperature for 60 min in the dark. The column size was 1 × 40 cm. The column was eluted at 4°C with 0.01 M phosphate buffer (pH 7.0). The fraction size was 1 ml. The reaction products (I and II) were subjected to paper chromatography, using n-butanol-acetic acid-water (4: 1: 2, by vol.) as a solvent.

○———○, Protein (mg); ●———●, cpm × 10^5

	λ_{max}	Rf	expected substance
I	267 nm	0.67	MNG
II	278	0.82	MNNG

weight compound was eluted in a single peak. This peak had no absorption at 402 nm but had an absorption maximum at 267 nm and an Rf value of 0.67 on paper chromatography, using n-butanol-acetic acid-water (4: 1: 2, by vol.) as a solvent. These properties coincided with those of MNG. Contrary to this, when MNNG labeled at the guanidino carbon was incubated with cytochrome c and then treated in the same way as the protein, cytochrome c was eluted in the void volume and the radioactive, low molecular weight compound was eluted as a single peak. But it showed the absorption and Rf values characteristic of unchanged MNNG. Upon taking a stoichiometric measurement of the reaction of the partially purified "enzyme," the formation of the denitroso compound exactly accounted for the decomposition of MNNG. All these results suggest the presence of "enzymatic activity" to produce MNG from MNNG.

DNA Damage by MNNG and Its Repair

Figure 12 shows a quick method for detecting possible damage of nucleic acids by MNNG that might be subject to repair. The central well in an agar plate contained 150 μg of MNNG. *Escherichia coli*, a wild strain, was spread over the surface of the dish on the left, while a mutant lacking DNA polymerase (pol A$_1$) was spread over the dish on the right, as described by Slater, Anderson and Rosenkrantz (16). DNA polymerase I is known to be involved in the process of repair of damaged DNA. It is clear that the inhibiting zone is much wider in the dish with the mutant than in

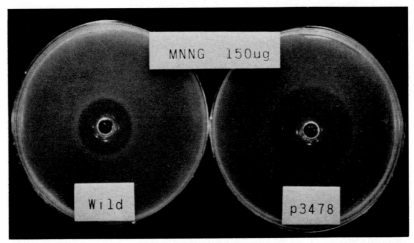

FIG. 12. Effects of MNNG on *Escherichia coli*, wild type, and a mutant lacking DNA polymerase. Effect of MNNG on the growth of *E. coli*, wild strain [W3110 (T⁻)], and its DNA polymerase-deficient mutant [P3478 (T⁻, pol A₁)]. Exponentially growing *E. coli* cells were suspended in 3 ml of soft (0.75%) agar and then spread on the surface of a hard (1.5%) agar plate (30 ml). The bottom of the center well was sealed with 80 μl of melted agar and then 50 μl of aqueous MNNG solution (3 mg/ml) was introduced. Plates were incubated at 37°C for 16 hr.

that with the wild strain. This clearly indicates that MNNG caused some damage to DNA that is repairable by the *E. coli* cells.

SUMMARY

As shown in Fig. 13, when MNNG is administered *in vivo*, it is quickly converted to the denitroso derivative because the stomach, liver and intestine actively convert MNNG to MNG, and biologically inert MNG is rapidly excreted in the urine. Thus, only the stomach can be affected by this carcinogen. This may explain the specific production of stomach cancer by MNNG. Our experiments showed that MNNG modifies protein as well as nucleic acid. At present it is uncertain which of these reactions is the cause of its carcinogenic activity.

One important feature of our studies on stomach carcinogenesis is the application of this technique to dogs, since these animals can be used as models for studies on the clinical course of early stomach cancer on a scientific and experimental basis.

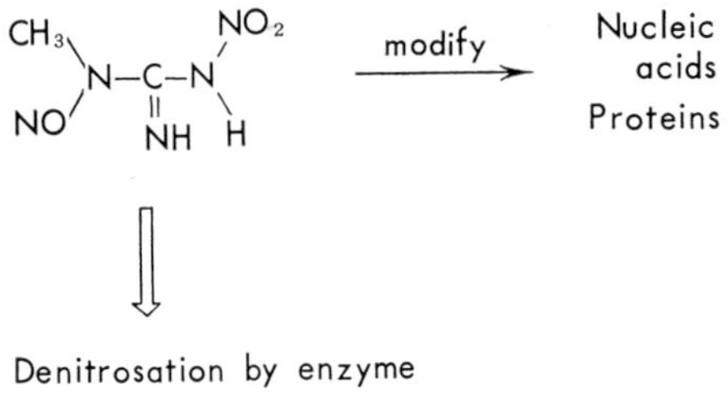

Denitrosation by enzyme

FIG. 13. Fate of MNNG *in vivo*.

This work was supported by grants from the Ministry of Health, the Ministry of Education, the Naito Foundation and the Society for the Promotion of Cancer Research.

REFERENCES

1. Drukrey, H., Preussmann, R., Ivankovic, S., So, B. T., Schmidt, C. H., und Bücheler, J. Zur Erzeugung Subcutaner Sarkome an Ratten. Carcinogene Wirkung von Hydrazodicarbonsäure-bis-(methyl-nitrosamid), N-Nitroso-N-*n*-butyl-harnstoff, N-Methyl-N-nitroso-nitroguanidin und N-Nitroso-imidazolidon. Z. Krebsforsch., *68*: 87–102, 1966.

2. Fujimura, S., Kogure, K., Oboshi, S., and Sugimura, T. Production of Tumors in Glandular Stomach of Hamsters by N-Methyl-N′-nitro-N-nitrosoguanidine. Cancer Res., *30*: 1444–1448, 1970.

3. Fujimura, S., Kogure, K., Sugimura, T., and Takayama, S. The Effect of Limited Administration of N-Methyl-N′-nitro-N-nitrosoguanidine on the Induction of Stomach Cancer in Rats. Cancer Res., *30*: 842–848, 1970.

4. Kawachi, T., Kogure, K., Kamijo, Y., and Sugimura, T. The Metabolism of N-Methyl-N′-nitro-N-nitrosoguanidine in Rats. Biochim. Biophys. Acta, *222*: 409–415, 1970.

5. Lawley, P. D. Methylation of DNA by N-Methyl-N-nitrosourethane and N-Methyl-N-nitroso-N′-nitroguanidine. Nature, *218*: 580–581, 1968.

6. Lawley, P. D., and Thatcher, C. J. Methylation of Deoxyribonucleic Acid in Cultured Mammalian Cells by N-Methyl-N′-nitro-N-nitrosoguanidine. Biochem. J., *116*: 693–707, 1970.

7. McCalla, D. R. Reaction of N-Methyl-N′-nitro-N-nitrosoguanidine and N-Methyl-N-nitroso-*p*-toluenesulfonamide with DNA in Vitro. Biochim. Biophys. Acta, *155*: 114–120, 1968.

8. McCalla, D. R., and Reuvers, A. Reaction of N-Methyl-N′-nitro-N-nitrosoguanidine with Protein: Formation of Nitroguanido Derivatives. Canad. J. Biochem., *46*: 1411–1415, 1968.

9. Nagao, M., Hosoi, H., and Sugimura, T. Modification of Cytochrome *c* with N-Methyl-N′-nitro-N-nitrosoguanidine. Biochim. Biophys. Acta, *237*: 369–377, 1971.

10. Nagao, M., Yokoshima, T., Hosoi, H., and Sugimura, T. Interaction of N-Methyl-N′-nitro-N-nitrosoguanidine with Ascites Hepatoma Cells *in vitro*. Biochim. Biophys. Acta, *192*: 191–199, 1969.

11. Saito, T., Inokuchi, K., Takayama, S., and Sugimura, T. Sequential Morphological Changes in N-Methyl-N′-nitro-N-nitrosoguanidine Carcinogenesis in the Glandular Stomach of Rats. J. Natl. Cancer Inst., *44*: 769–783, 1970.

12. Schoental, R. Carcinogenic Activity of N-Methyl-N-nitroso-N′-nitroguanidine. Nature, *209*: 726–727, 1966.

13. Schulz, U., and McCalla, D. R. Reaction of Cysteine with N-Methyl-N-nitroso-*p*-toluenesulfonamide and N-Methyl-N′-nitro-N-nitrosoguanidine. Canad. J. Chem., *47*: 2021–2027, 1969.

14. Shimosato, Y., Tanaka, N., Kogure, K., Fujimura, S., Kawachi, T., and Sugimura, T. Histopathology of Tumors of Canine Alimentary Tract Produced by N-Methyl-N′-nitro-N-nitrosoguanidine, with Particular Reference to Gastric Carcinomas. J. Natl. Cancer Inst., *47*: 1053–1070, 1971.

15.   Singer, B., Fraenkel-Conrat, H., Greenberg, J., and Michelson, A. M.   Reaction of Nitrosoguanidine (N-Methyl-N'-nitro-N-nitrosoguanidine) with Tobacco Mosaic Virus and Its RNA.   Science, *160*: 1235–1237, 1968.

16.   Slater, E. E., Anderson, M. D., and Rosenkranz, H. S.   Rapid Detection of Mutagens and Carcinogens.   Cancer Res., *31*: 970–973, 1971.

17.   Sugimura, T., and Fujimura, S.   Tumor Production in Glandular Stomach of Rat by N-Methyl-N'-nitro-N-nitrosoguanidine.   Nature, *216*: 943–944, 1967.

18.   Sugimura, T., Fujimura, S., and Baba, T.   Tumor Production in the Glandular Stomach and Alimentary Tract of the Rat by N-Methyl-N'-nitro-N-nitrosoguanidine. Cancer Res., *30*: 455–465, 1970.

19.   Sugimura, T., Fujimura, S., Kogure, K., Baba, T., Saito, T., Nagao, M., Hosoi, H., Shimosato, Y., and Yokoshima, T.   Production of Adenocarcinomas in Glandular Stomach of Experimental Animals by N-Methyl-N'-nitro-N-nitrosoguanidine. Gann Monograph, *8*: 157–196, 1969.

20.   Sugimura, T., Fujimura, S., Nagao, M., Yokoshima, T., and Hasegawa, S.   Reaction of N-Methyl-N'-nitro-N-nitrosoguanidine with Protein.   Biochim. Biophys. Acta, *170*: 427–429, 1968.

21.   Sugimura, T., Nagao, M., and Okada, Y.   Carcinogenic Action of N-Methyl-N'-nitro-N-nitrosoguanidine.   Nature, *210*: 962–963, 1966.

22.   Sugimura, T., Tanaka, N., Kawachi, T., Kogure, K., Fujimura, S., and Shimosato, Y.   Production of Stomach Cancer in Dogs by N-Methyl-N'-nitro-N-nitrosoguanidine.   Gann, *62*: 67–68, 1971.

Discussion of Paper by Drs. Sugimura et al.

DR. TAKAHASHI: In our laboratory, we are studying gastric carcinogenesis induced by MNNG, combined with various surfactants, in the drinking water of rats.   In our experimental groups, we obtained some undifferentiated adenocarcinomas as well as many well-differentiated adenocarcinomas.   Furthermore, these spread directly into the omentum, the liver and the pancreas.   Lymphatic invasion and metastasis into the intestinal lymph nodes were observed.   Meanwhile, in the control group, we observed neither lymphatic invasion nor metastasis.   The increase in the incidence of anaplastic adenocarcinoma is considered to be due to surfactants used as vehicles for MNNG.

DR. DRUCKREY: Did you test ethylnitroso-N'-nitroguanidine for comparison? Do you think that the deacylation of MNNG, the splitting off of the nitrogroup, may play a role in the specific effect on the glandular stomach?

DR. SUGIMURA: We have done experiments using the ethyl derivative.   The incidence of tumors and patterns of tumor distribution are about the same as in the experiment using MNNG.   I do not think there is a reaction to denitrate.

DR. PREUSSMANN: You demonstrated very convincingly an enzymatic denitrosation of MNNG.   Have you any results that indicate whether similar effects are also possible with other N-nitroso compounds, for example, with dimethylnitrosamine or other nitrosamines?

DR. SUGIMURA: We intend to study the effects of denitrosation on other nitroso compounds.

DR. MAGEE: Would you please comment on the significance of the reaction of the guanidino moiety of MNNG with proteins, since this moiety does not occur in any other nitroso carcinogens?

DR. SUGIMURA: I am not saying this particular nitroamidination for modifying protein is the only important one.   Rather, I want to emphasize that the modification of protein in general should be reevaluated.

DR. WEISBURGER: In addition to the biochemical reactions of MNNG, the alkylation of nucleic acid with the methyl residue and the transfer of the remainder of the molecule to protein lysine end groups, a similar situation has been reported for 1-(2-chloroethyl)-3-cyclohexyl-1-nitrosourea (CCNU), a drug used in cancer chemotherapy, which is also carcinogenic in rodents.   Thus, Cheng, Fujimura, Grunberger, and Weinstein (Cancer Research, *32*: 22–27, 1972) demonstrated that nucleic acids were modified by alkylation from the chloroethyl or better the ethylene group, whereas proteins underwent cyclohexylcarbamoylation.   Prejean, Griswold, Casey, Peckham, Weisburger, Weisburger, and Wood (Proceedings Am Assn Cancer Research, *13*: 112, 1972) presented a preliminary report on the carcinogenicity of CCNU.

Induction of Stomach Cancer by a Single Dose of N-Methyl-N'-nitro-N-nitrosoguanidine through a Stomach Tube

Iwao Hirono and Chiken Shibuya

Department of Pathology, Gifu University School of Medicine, Gifu, Japan

Induction of carcinoma in the glandular stomach of rodents had been difficult, but recently Sugimura and his co-workers (*3–5*) succeeded in inducing a high incidence of adenocarcinomas in the glandular stomach of rats by administrating N-methyl-N'-nitro-N-nitrosoguanidine (MNNG) in the drinking water. On the other hand, Schoental (*2*) reported that tumors were induced exclusively in the forestomach after forced administration of MNNG through a stomach tube.

To elucidate the factors causing this difference in the locations of tumors in the stomach, we studied the development of gastric tumors in rats after a single dose of MNNG, suspended in various vehicles and administered through a stomach tube. After injecting the suspensions of MNNG, the emptying time of the stomach was determined, since this was thought to be a possible factor involved in the induction of gastric tumors. The results obtained are reported below and compared with those reported by previous workers.

MATERIALS AND METHODS

Chemicals

The MNNG used was purchased from Daiichi Pure Chemicals Co., Ltd., Tokyo, Japan. This compound is only slightly soluble in saline or olive oil, so it was ground in a mortar before use. Even so, it did not dissolve completely. So it was administered to the rats in suspension in the strict sense of the word.

Animals

Two-month-old ACI rats of both sexes were used. All animals were maintained on diet CE-2 from the Central Laboratory of Experimental Animals, Tokyo, Japan, and water. Both food and water were withheld from the night before to about 7 hr after administration of MNNG.

Experiment with MNNG suspensions in saline

Thirty-six rats were divided into 3 groups of 12 animals each (Table 1). Groups I and II received a single intragastric dose of 250 mg MNNG/kg body weight through a stomach tube. MNNG was given as suspensions in 1.0 ml (Group I) or 4.0 ml (Group II) of physiological saline per rat. Group III was given a single dose of 50 mg MNNG/kg body weight, suspended in 4.0 ml of saline.

Experiment with MNNG suspended in olive oil

Twenty-two rats were divided into 2 groups of 11 animals each. Animals were given a single intragastric dose of 250 mg MNNG/kg body weight through a stomach tube, suspended in 1.0 ml (Group IV) or 4.0 ml (Group V) of olive oil. The control group of 6 rats received no treatment. All the animals were autopsied when they died, or when they became moribund and then were killed. All organs were fixed with 10% formalin, sectioned, and stained with hymatoxylin and eosin. Histological diagnoses of lesions with marked atypical epithelial growth in the glandular stomach were based on the criteria of Stewart (*1*). Experiments were terminated 480 days after the administration of MNNG.

Emptying time of the stomach after MNNG administration

Rats were starved overnight and then given an MNNG suspension through a stomach tube, as described above. One to 3 rats were sacrificed 2, 4 and 10 hr after the administration of the MNNG suspensions; and the fluid content in the stomach was determined. Rats were examined in the same way after a single dose of saline, olive oil or 30% aqueous ethanol without MNNG.

RESULTS

Experiment with MNNG suspended in physiological saline

A few animals died of acute toxicity or pneumonia after the administration of the MNNG suspensions, but most animals survived for more than 300 days (Table 1). In the surviving animals, most tumors were found in the stomach. These tumors

TABLE 1. Incidence of Tumors Induced by a Single Dose of N-Methyl-N'-nitro-N-nitrosoguanidine (MNNG)

Experimental group	Dose of MNNG (mg per kg body wt.)	Vehicle	Number of rats used	Number of rats surviving beyond 300 days	Number of rats with tumors	Incidence of tumors (%)	Number of rats with gastric tumors	Incidence of gastric tumors (%)
I	250	1.0 ml of saline	12	11	5	45.4	5	45.4
II	250	4.0 ml of saline	12	11	6	54.5	4	36.3
III	50	4.0 ml of saline	12	10	1	10.0	1	10.0
IV	250	1.0 ml of olive oil	11	9	6	66.6	6	66.6
V	250	4.0 ml of olive oil	11	10	7	70.0	7	70.0

TABLE 2. Summary of Sites and Types of Tumors Induced by a Single Dose of N-Methyl-N′-nitro-N-nitrosoguanidine

Tumor site and type		Number of rats with tumors				
		Group I	Group II	Group III	Group IV	Group V
Forestomach :	Papilloma	4	2	1	4	2
	Squamous cell carcinoma		1			2
	Sarcoma					1
Glandular stomach :	Adenoma		1		2	3
	Adenocarcinoma		1		1	1
	Leiomyoma		1			
	Sarcoma	1				1
Duodenum :	Adenoma					1
Jejunum :	Adenoma					1
	Adenocarcinoma		2			

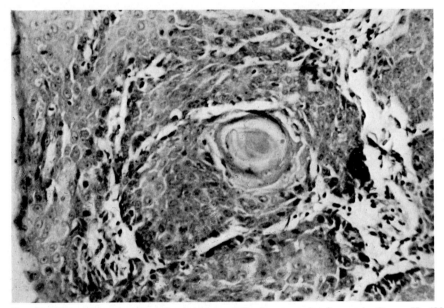

Fig. 1. Keratotic squamous cell carcinoma of the forestomach of a rat in Group II, 480 days after a single dose of MNNG. ×280.

varied from miliary plaque-like lesions to nodules the size of a fingertip.   Among the gastric tumors in rats in Group I there were 4 papillomas of the forestomach and one sarcoma of the glandular stomach, as shown in Table 2.   Among the tumors induced in Group II, there were 2 papillomas, one squamous cell carcinoma (Fig. 1) of the forestomach, and 1 case each of adenoma, adenocarcinoma (Figs. 2 and 3) and leiomyoma of the glandular stomach.   Histologically, signet ring cell carcinoma was observed in part of the adenocarcinoma.   The tumor cells infiltrated all of the layers of the stomach wall, invading the gastric serosa (Fig. 4).   In Group II, adenocarcinomas were found in the jejunum (Fig. 5).   The incidences of gastric tumors in rats surviving for more than 300 days after intragastric administration of MNNG

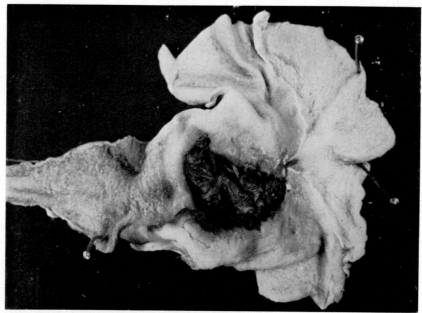

FIG. 2.   An ulcerated tumor of the glandular stomach of a rat in Group II, 368 days after a single dose of MNNG.

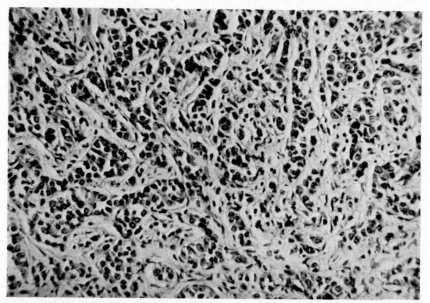

FIG. 3.   Histological appearance of the tumor of the glandular stomach shown in Fig. 2. Adenocarcinoma.   ×280.

were 45.4% in Group I and 36.3% in Group II. Thus, on administration of 250 mg MNNG/kg body weight, no significant difference was noted in the incidence of tumors, when carcinogens in different volumes were given.   In Group III, which received a single intragastric dose of 50 mg MNNG/kg body weight through a

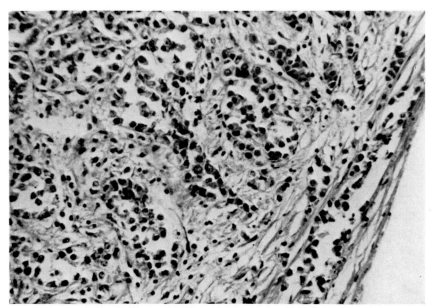

FIG. 4.   Another part of the tumor shown in Fig. 3.   Tumor cells show that atypical glandular structures infiltrate all layers of the stomach wall and invade the gastric serosa.   ×280.

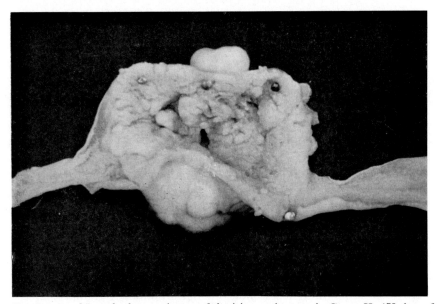

FIG. 5.   An ulcerated adenocarcinoma of the jejunum in a rat in Group II, 475 days after administration of MNNG.

stomach tube, only 1 out of 10 animals developed a gastric tumor.   Table 3 gives a comparison of the incidences of tumors in the forestomach and glandular stomach. Six of 9 rats with gastric tumors in Groups I and II had tumors in the forestomach only, two had tumors in the glandular stomach only, and one had tumors in both the forestomach and glandular stomach.

TABLE 3.　Sites in the Stomach of Tumors Induced by a Single Dose of N-Methyl-N'-nitro-N-nitrosoguanidine

Experimental group	Animal numbers	Forestomach	Glandular stomach
I	1		+
	2	+	
	3	+	
	4	+	
	5	+	
II	1	+	
	2		+
	3	+	+
	4	+	
III	1	+	
IV	1		+
	2	+	
	3	+	+
	4		+
	5	+	
	6	+	
V	1	+	+
	2	+	
	3		+
	4	+	+
	5		+
	6	+	
	7	+	+

Total, 23; forestomach, 12; glandular stomach, 6; both forestomach and glandular stomach, 5.

Experiment with MNNG suspended in olive oil

Most animals survived for more than 300 days after treatment with MNNG in olive oil in the same way as those treated with MNNG in saline (Table 1).　The incidences of gastric tumors were 66.6% in Group IV and 70.0% in Group V.　Thus, there was no significant difference in the incidences of gastric tumors after the administration of 1.0 ml and 4.0 ml of MNNG suspension, as was true also with the administration of MNNG in different volumes of physiological saline.　However, the incidence of tumors in Groups IV and V (MNNG in olive oil) seemed to be higher than in Group I and II (MNNG in saline).　The incidences of tumors in the forestomach and the glandular stomach were similar, *i.e.*, 5 out of the 13 rats with gastric tumors had tumors in the forestomach, 4 had tumors in the glandular stomach and the remaining 4 had tumors in both the forestomach and the glandular stomach, as shown in Table 3.　The histological types of tumors were similar to those in Groups I and II (Figs. 6 and 7, and Table 2).　A case of adenocarcinoma of the glandular stomach in Group IV was of an undifferentiated type with metastases in the lymph nodes of the mesentery (Figs. 8, 9 and 10).　In Group V, 1 rat with a duodenal adenoma and one with a jejunal adenoma were found.　Furthermore, proliferative changes of the intrahepatic bile duct and degenerative, cystic dilation of the proli-

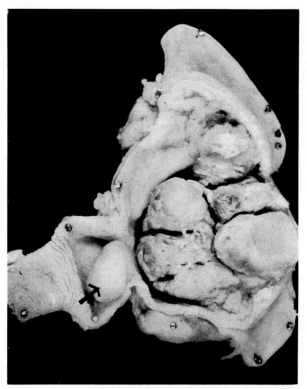

FIG. 6. Sarcoma of the glandular stomach and adenomatous polyp (arrow) of the duodenum of a rat in Group V, 480 days after administration of MNNG.

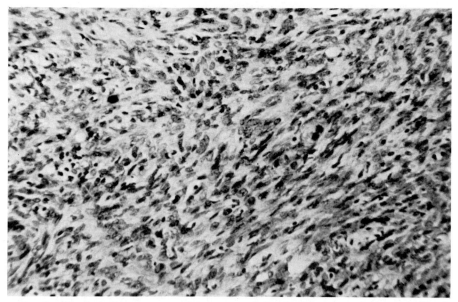

FIG. 7. Histological appearance of the tumor of the glandular stomach shown in Fig. 6. Spindle cell fibrosarcoma. ×280.

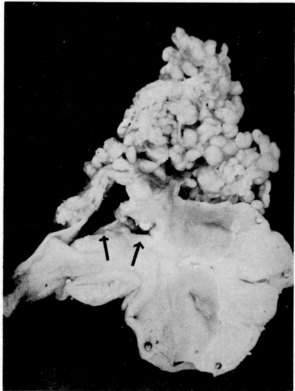

FIG. 8. An ulcerated tumor of the glandular stomach and its metastasis in the lymph nodes of the mesentery in Group IV, 470 days after treatment.

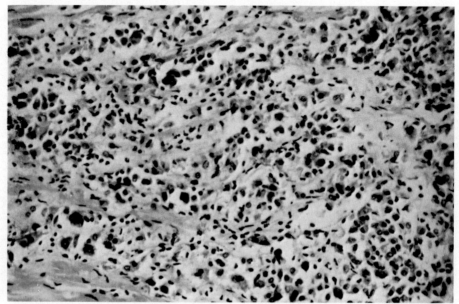

FIG. 9. Histological appearance of the tumor of the glandular stomach shown in Fig. 8. Undifferentiated adenocarcinoma. ×280.

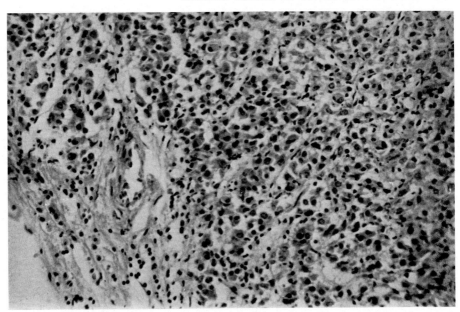

FIG. 10. Histological appearance of the metastasis in the lymph nodes of the tumor shown in Fig. 8. ×280.

TABLE 4. Emptying Time of Stomach after Administration of Suspensions of N-Methyl-N'-nitro-N-nitrosoguanidine in Saline or Olive Oil

Suspension		Time after administration		
Dose of MNNG (mg/kg b. w.)	Vehicle	2 hr (%)	4 hr (%)	10 hr (%)
	4.0 ml of saline alone	Empty		
250	1.0 ml of saline	90[a]	90	90
250	4.0 ml of saline	80	80	80
50	4.0 ml of saline	80	80	10–20
	4.0 ml of olive oil alone	20–30	Nearly empty	
250	1.0 ml of olive oil	90	90	90
250	4.0 ml of olive oil	90	90	90
	1.0 ml of 30% ethanol alone	Nearly empty	Empty	
100	1.0 ml of 30% ethanol	100	Nearly empty	Nearly empty
50	1.0 ml of 30% ethanol	100	Nearly empty	Empty

[a] Fluid content as a percentage of the volume of suspension introduced into the stomach.

ferated bile ducts were frequently encountered in animals in Groups IV and V. One of the 16 animals in the control group had a cecal adenoma.

Emptying time of the stomach after MNNG administration

The stomach was emptied quite rapidly after the introduction of physiological saline or olive oil into the stomach through a stomach tube (Table 4). However, most of the suspensions of 250 mg MNNG/kg body wt. in saline or olive oil still remained in the stomach after 10 hr. The emptying time was shorter after the administration of a suspension of 50 mg MNNG/kg body wt. in saline than with a suspension of 250 mg MNNG/kg body wt.   The stomach was emptied completely within 4 hr after administration of 1.0 ml of 30% ethanol.   The emptying time was also shorter after administration of the MNNG suspension in ethanol, as shown in Table 4.

DISCUSSION

In the present work, tumors were induced not only in the forestomach, but also in the glandular stomach by a single dose of MNNG through a stomach tube. Schoental (2) reported that tumors were induced only in the forestomach when suspensions of 50–100 mg MNNG/kg body wt. in 30% ethanol were given to young rats through a stomach tube 3 to 5 times at intervals of several months. In the present study, tumors of the glandular stomach were only induced in rats which received 250 mg MNNG/kg body wt.   Therefore, the cause of the restricted site of occurrence of gastric tumors, i.e., the forestomach, in Schoental's experiment may be due to the small dose of MNNG that she used.

We determined the emptying time of the stomach after administration of MNNG suspensions by measuring the volume of fluid remaining in the stomach, not the amount of MNNG remaining.   Nevertheless, we found that the emptying time was much shorter (less than 4 hr) with MNNG suspensions in 30% ethanol than with suspensions in saline or olive oil.   Thus, another cause for the difference in the localization of tumors in the stomach in Schoental's work and our own may be due to a difference in the emptying times of the stomach after MNNG administration. However, the significance of the emptying time in carcinogenesis of the stomach is still uncertain.

Sugimura et al. (3–5) reported that gastric tumors developed exclusively in the pyloric region of the glandular stomach, when rats were given 33 to 167 μg/ml of MNNG in their drinking water.   They hypothesized that because the animals were taking the carcinogen in the drinking water ad libitum the solution might be translocated directly to the pyloric region of the glandular stomach where MNNG exerted its carcinogenic action.   However, it is difficult to explain the discrepancy between their observations and ours.

Six (26%) of the 23 animals with gastric tumors in our work had tumors of the glandular stomach only.   So it may be possible to produce tumors of the glandular stomach only by some modification of the administration technique, even with the administration of a single dose of MNNG through a stomach tube.

SUMMARY

The incidence and location of tumors in the stomach induced by a single dose of N-methyl-N'-nitro-N-nitrosoguanidine through a stomach tube were studied in inbred ACI strain rats.   Animals were divided into 5 groups: Groups I and II received single intragastric doses of 250 mg N-methyl-N'-nitro-N-nitrosoguanidine/kg body wt. as suspensions in 1.0 and 4.0 ml, respectively, of physiological saline; Group III received 50 mg/kg as a suspension in 4.0 ml of saline; Groups IV and V received 250 mg/kg as suspensions in 1.0 and 4.0 ml, respectively, of olive oil. Both food and water were withheld from the night before to about 7 hr after the carcinogen was administered. Experiments were terminated 480 days after the treatment.

The incidences of gastric tumors in rats surviving for over 300 days after treatment were 45.4% in Group I, 36.3% in Group II, 10.0% in Group III, 66.6% in Group IV and 70.0% in Group V. These tumors were induced not only in the forestomach, but also in the glandular stomach; and 6 out of the 23 rats with gastric tumors had tumors only in the glandular stomach. Histologically, the tumors induced were, in the order of decreasing frequency: papillomas, adenomas, adenocarcinomas, squamous cell carcinomas and a sarcoma. The incidence of gastric tumors induced by a single dose of 250 mg/kg body wt. of N-methyl-N'-nitro-N-nitrosoguanidine was almost the same, whether the carcinogen was given as a 1.0 ml or 4.0 ml suspension, whether given in saline or olive oil. However, it seemed to be higher in groups receiving suspensions in olive oil than in those receiving suspensions in saline.

This study was supported by a grant-in-aid for scientific research from the Ministry of Education and Cancer Research Subsidy, 1970–71, from the Japanese Ministry of Health and Welfare.

REFERENCES

1. Hare, W. V., Stewart, H. L., Bennett, J. G., and Lorenz, E. Tumors of the Glandular Stomach Induced in Rats by Intramural Injection of 20-Methylcholanthrene. J. Natl. Cancer Inst., *12*: 1019–1055, 1952.
2. Schoental, R. Carcinogenic Activity of N-Methyl-N-nitroso-N'-nitroguanidine. Nature, *209*: 726–727, 1966.
3. Sugimura, T., and Fujimura, S. Tumour Production in Glandular Stomach of Rat by N-Methyl-N'-nitro-N-nitrosoguanidine. Nature, *216*: 943–944, 1967.
4. Sugimura, T., Fujimura, S., and Baba, T. Tumor Production in the Glandular Stomach and Alimentary Tract of the Rat by N-Methyl-N'-nitro-N-nitrosoguanidine. Cancer Res., *30*: 455–465, 1970.
5. Sugimura, T., Fujimura, S., Kogure, K., Baba, T., Saito, T., Nagao, M., Hosoi, H., Shimosato, Y., and Yokoshima, T. Production of Adenocarcinomas in Glandular Stomach of Experimental Animals by N-Methyl-N'-nitro-N-nitrosoguanidine. Gann Monograph, *8*: 157–196, 1969.

Discussion of Paper by Drs. Hirono and Shibuya

DR. HIGGINSON: Is there any evidence that the adenocarcinomas of the glandular stomach show histological differentiation into diffuse and intestinal types similar to those seen in man? In man, the existence of these two types has been regarded as an index of two different etiologies.   The latter is found most frequently in countries with a high incidence of cancer and occurs more and more infrequently in countries with a decrease in gastric carcinoma.   Accordingly, researchers should clarify the various types of adenocarcinomas produced in order to see if the same phenomenon does occur.

DR. SUGIMURA: As you pointed out Dr. Sugano and his group proposed the intestinal type and diffuse type of adenocarcinomas in human beings.   According to our research, roughly 80% were tumors of the intestinal type.   Only a few cases of intestinal metaplasia occurred when MNNG was used.   So I am not sure yet whether intestinalization can really be correlated causatively with the intestinal type of adenocarcinoma.

DR. MAGEE: You have clearly shown the importance of the vehicle in determining the incidence of tumors of the glandular stomach with MNNG.   Have you tried similar experiments using other carcinogenic nitrosamides, such as nitrosomethylurea or nitrosomethylurethan?

DR. HIRONO: I have not yet tried them.

Carcinogenesis in Newborn and Suckling Rats Induced by N-Methyl-N'-nitro-N-nitrosoguanidine

Shozo Takayama, Noriyuki Kuwabara, Nobuo Nemoto, and Yoko Azama

Cancer Institute, Japanese Foundation for Cancer Research, Tokyo, Japan

N-Methyl-N'-nitro-N-nitrosoguanidine (MNNG) has been known to be a powerful mutagenic substance since the report of Mandell and Greenberg (5). The carcinogenicity of MNNG given to rats parenterally was described by Schoental (6), Druckrey *et al.* (2), and Sugimura *et al.* (10). Subsequently, MNNG solution given as drinking water was found to produce high incidences of adenocarcinomas in the glandular stomach of rats (1, 7–9), hamsters (3), and dogs (9). The induction of gastric tumors after a single dose of MNNG administered through a stomach tube was studied in an inbred strain of ACI rats (4). MNNG induced skin cancer locally when applied to the skin of noninbred ICR mice (11).

This paper reports studies on the carcinogenic action of a single dose of N-methyl-N'-nitro-N-nitrosoguanidine (MNNG) in newborn and suckling rats.

Induction of Various Tumors in Newborn and Suckling Rats

In this experiment, male and female (ACI ♂ × Sprague-Dawley ♀)F$_1$ rats were used. The parental line of ACI rats was originally obtained from the National Cancer Institute, Bethesda; and the animals have been bred in our laboratory since 1966 by brother to sister mating. Sprague-Dawley rats were obtained from a commercial animal supply source in Tokyo.

Animals were treated with MNNG either within 24 hr after birth or 7 days after birth.

MNNG was a commercial preparation supplied by the Aldrich Chemical Company, Milwaukee. It was dissolved in saline immediately before use.

Group 1: Forty-five rats were injected subcutaneously in the dorsal region on the day of birth with 2 μg per rat of MNNG in 0.2 ml of saline.

Group 2: Forty-eight rats were treated the same as those in Group 1, except that the dose was 10 μg per rat.

Group 3:   Sixty-one rats were treated the same as those in Group 1, except that the dose was 100 μg per rat.

Group 4:   Fifty-five rats were injected intraperitoneally on the seventh day after birth with 600 μg of MNNG in 0.2 ml of saline.

Group 5:   Thirty untreated rats were used as controls.

Experiment with Newborn Rats

In this experiment, 86 of the 154 rats that received a single subcutaneous injection of MNNG within 24 hr after birth died within one month after the injection. The cause of death was acute toxicity due to MNNG and cannibalism by the mother.

The main pathological findings with respect to tumors are shown in Table 1. In all, 46 rats were still alive 12 months later.   As shown in this table, most of the tumors in these animals were found in the small intestine, especially in Group 3.

A fibrosarcoma (Fig. 1) and a myosarcoma were found about midway along the small intestine.   These tumor masses were quite large, being 2.5–3.0 cm in diameter.   A hemangioma was found in the spleen of a male rat killed after 18 months (Fig. 2).   The tumor, projecting from the surface of the spleen, appeared as a red

TABLE 1.   Neoplastic Lesions Induced by a Single Dose of MNNG

Site	Histological findings	Experimental group			
		1	2	3	4
Stomach	Forestomach papilloma				+
	Squamous cell carcinoma				+
	Adenocarcinoma				+
	Fibrosarcoma				+
	Hemangiosarcoma			+	
Small intestine	Adenocarcinoma			++	+++
	Fibrosarcoma			+	++
	Myosarcoma			+	
Liver	Adenoma			+	
	Liver cell carcinoma				+
Spleen	Hemangioma			+	
Peritoneal cavity	Neurinoma				++
	Teratoma				+
	Fibrosarcoma			+	+++
Kidney	Wilms' tumor				+
Uterus	Myosarcoma			+	
Ovary	Granulosa cell tumor	+	+	+	++
	Myosarcoma				+
Heart	Sarcoma				+
Lung	Adenocarcinoma			+	
Breast	Adenocarcinoma				+
Skin					+
Subcutis	Fibrosarcoma	+		+	

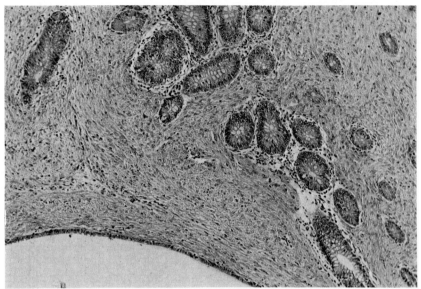

FIG. 1.   Fibrosarcoma of the small intestine.   The tumor involves the whole layer of the small intestine.   Hematoxylin and Eosin.   ×120.

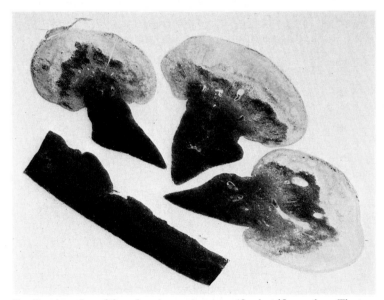

FIG. 2.   A section of the spleen in a male rat sacrificed at 18 months.   The tumor is projecting from the surface of the spleen.   ×5.

nodule the size of the tip of a small finger.   Granulosa cell tumors were found in the ovaries of 3 female rats.

Experiment with Suckling Rats

Table 2 shows that 38 rats survived for more than 12 months.   Thus, the survival of suckling rats was significantly less than that of newborn rats.   The relation between age at treatment and subsequent tumor development appeared to be different in newborn and suckling rats.   The incidence of tumors was higher in rats treated 7 days after birth than in those treated at birth (Table 3).

TABLE 2.   Number of Rats Surviving over 12 Months

Group	Number of rats injected at birth	Number and sex of rats at weaning		Number of rats surviving over 12 months	
1	45	15	♂ 8 / ♀ 7	10	♂ 4 / ♀ 6
2	48	22	♂ 9 / ♀ 13	12	♂ 6 / ♀ 6
3	61	31	♂ 16 / ♀ 15	24	♂ 12 / ♀ 12
4	55	46	♂ 20 / ♀ 26	38	♂ 19 / ♀ 19
Control	30	29	♂ 12 / ♀ 17	26	♂ 11 / ♀ 15

TABLE 3.   Tumor Incidence Caused by Single Injections of MNNG into Newborn and Suckling Rats

Group	Number of tumors	%
1	2/10	20.0
2	1/12	8.3
3	12/24	50.0
4	24/38	63.2
Control	0/26	0

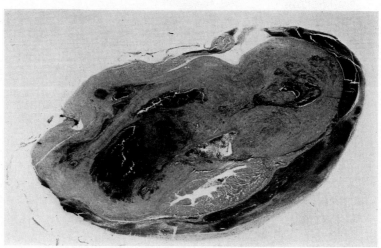

FIG. 3.   A section of the heart in a male rat sacrificed at 18 months.   The heart was replaced by tumor tissue.   ×5.

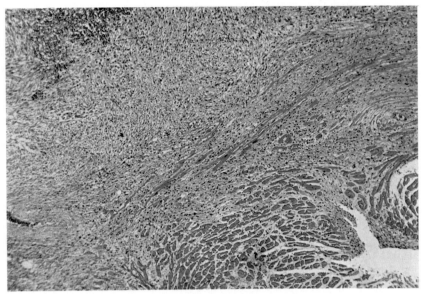

FIG. 4. Histological picture of the heart tumor shown in Fig. 3. Hematoxylin and eosin. ×120.

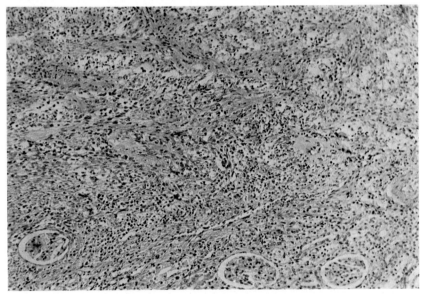

FIG. 5. Histological picture of a Wilms' tumor. Hematoxylin and eosin. ×120.

The locations, numbers and histological types of induced tumors are shown in Table 1. As shown in this table, intraperitoneal injections of MNNG into suckling rats induced mainly gastrointestinal tumors and tumors apparently originating in the peritoneal membrane. Among the 38 surviving rats, 24 had some type of tumor and 10 of them had gastrointestinal tumors.

Of the 6 rats with tumors in the peritoneum, 2 had nerve sheath tumors of

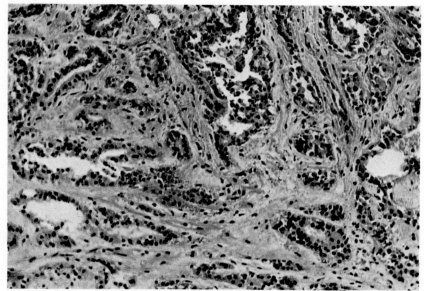

FIG. 6. Histological picture of mammary adenocarcinoma. Hematoxylin and Eosin. ×180.

the parietal peritoneum, 1 had a teratoid tumor, and 3 had fibrosarcomas. A tumor of the heart was observed in 1 male rat which was killed after 18 months. This tumor was diagnosed as a rhabdomyosarcoma (Figs. 3 and 4). In addition to the above neoplasms, a few other tumors were found at the autopsy, namely, a Wilms' tumor (Fig. 5), a liver cell carcinoma, two granulosa cell tumors, a sweat gland adenocarcinoma, and a mammary adenocarcinoma (Fig. 6). Another common finding in male rats treated with MNNG at birth or 7 days after birth was small testes. In sections, the germinal epithelium appeared atrophic and few or no spermatozoa were present in the epididymis. Endometrial changes were seen in only one female treated with MNNG at birth. No consistent changes were found in the adrenal glands or thyroid.

Incorporation of Labeled MNNG into the Lipid-free, Acid-insoluble Fraction of Various Organs

The possible relationship between the incorporation of labeled MNNG into lipid-free, acid-insoluble material obtained from various organs and tumor development by MNNG was investigated.

The same strains of rats were used as in the previous experiment. Preparations of MNNG labeled with carbon-14 either in the methyl group or in the guanidino group were obtained from Daiichi Pure Chemical Co., Ltd., Tokyo.

Newborn rats were injected subcutaneously with 2 μCi of labeled MNNG. Suckling rats were injected intraperitoneally with 2 μCi of labeled MNNG. The animals were killed at intervals by decapitation.

Various organs were homogenized with 4 or 9 volumes of distilled water in a Teflon homogenizer. Two aliquots of each homogenate were spread over paper disks and washed three times with cold 5% trichloroacetic acid and twice with cold

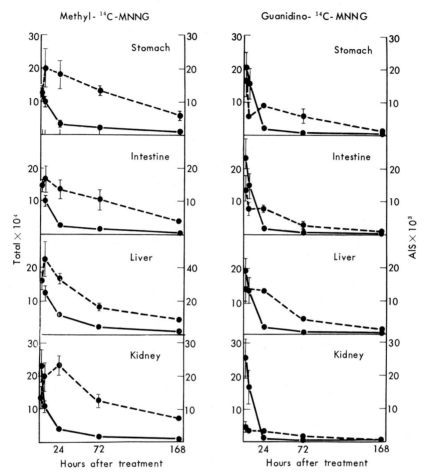

FIG. 7.   Incorporation of ^{14}C-labeled MNNG in stomach, intestine, liver and kidney.
●————●, cpm/g total; ●------●, cpm/g AIS.

ethanol.   Then the paper was dried and its radioactivity was determined in a toluene scintillator (toluene, 1,000 ml; PPO, 5 g; POPOP, 100 mg), using a Packard liquid scintillation counter.   The incorporation of radioactivity into various organs was measured at intervals after the injection of labeled MNNG into newborn rats.

The incorporation of radioactive MNNG into the stomach, intestine, liver and kidney reached a maximum within the first 6 hr after injection and then decreased, rapidly at first and then more slowly.   After 7 days the radioactivity in these organs was very low (Fig. 7).

Figure 8 shows the radioactivity of acid-insoluble, lipid-free material from various organs of newborn rats.   In this experiment, the rats were given either methyl-labeled MNNG (results shown in the figure as black lines) or guanidino-labeled MNNG (results shown as oblique lines).   As shown in Fig. 8, 2 hr after the injection of methyl-labeled MNNG, the levels of radioactivity in the liver, subcutis, and spleen were much higher than in other organs. However, when guanidino-labeled MNNG was used, the subcutis showed the highest level of incorporation. Seven days after administration of methyl-labeled MNNG, the liver retained the highest level of radioactivity followed by the subcutis, heart, kidney, and mesen-

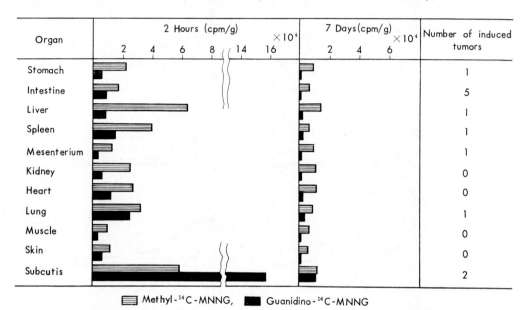

FIG. 8   Radioactivity of acid-insoluble lipid-free material from various organs of newborn rats after administration of ^{14}C-labeled MNNG.

Organ	2 Hours (cpm/g) ×10⁴	7 Days (cpm/g) ×10⁴	Number of induced tumors
Stomach			4
Intestine			6
Liver			1
Spleen			0
Mesenterium			6
Kidney			1
Heart			1
Lung			0
Muscle			0
Skin			2

☰ Methyl-^{14}C-MNNG,   ■ Guanidino-^{14}C-MNNG

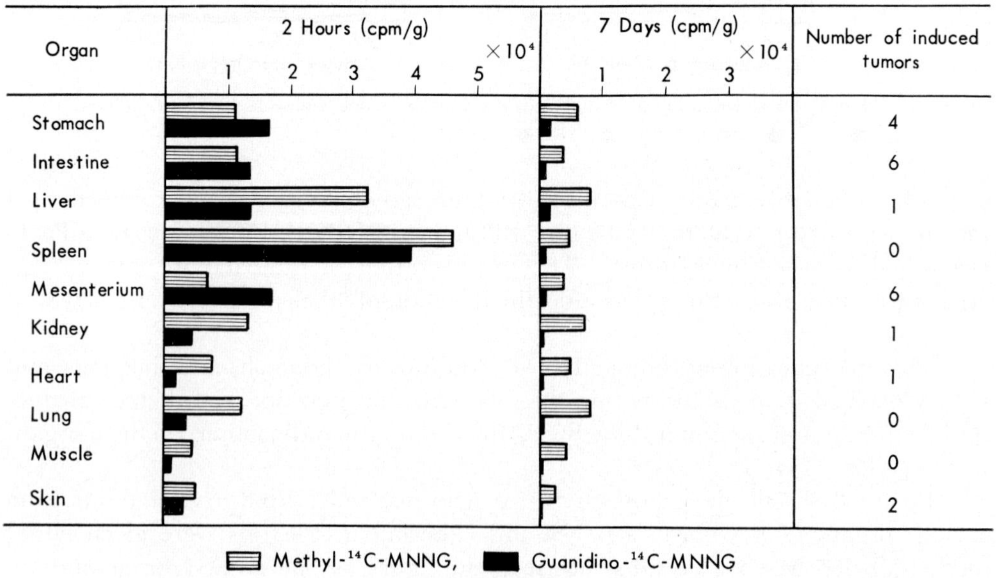

FIG. 9.   Radioactivity of acid-insoluble lipid-free material from various organs of suckling rats after administration of ^{14}C-labeled MNNG.

terium. With guanidino-labeled MNNG, the subcutis retained a much higher level than other organs.

Figure 9 shows the results of a similar experiment in which the labeled compound was administered 7 days after birth. As indicated in Fig. 9, with methyl-labeled MNNG, the spleen and liver retained the highest radioactivity; and this was almost double that in the stomach and intestine. Seven days after the injection, the liver and lungs showed the highest level of incorporation, followed by the kidney and stomach. Incorporation of guanidino-labeled MNNG into the liver, stomach and mesenterium was higher than that into other organs.

However, from this biochemical study we could not find any close relationship between the level of incorporation of labeled MNNG and its metabolites into various organs and the site of carcinogenic action of MNNG.

SUMMARY

The incidence of tumors produced by MNNG was lower in newborn and suckling rats than in adults.

The rats treated with MNNG at birth or during the suckling period developed mesenchymal tumors in various organs, while when adult rats receive MNNG they rarely develop mesenchymal tumors. This may depend on the functional and structural immaturity of the tissues of the test animals at the time of the administration of MNNG, since at birth, tissues in general are still in a labile state. In a biochemical study, no correlation was found between the carcinogenic action of MNNG and the level of its incorporation into acid-insoluble, lipid-free material in various organs.

This investigation was supported by grants-in-aid for scientific research from the Ministry of Education and Ministry of Health and Welfare, Japan.

REFERENCES

1. Bralow, S. P., Gruenstein, M., and Meranze, D. R. Adenocarcinoma of Glandular Stomach and Duodenum in Wistar Rats Ingesting N-Methyl-N'-nitro-N-nitrosoguanidine, Histopathology and Associated Secretory Changes. Cancer Res., *30*: 1215–1222, 1970.
2. Druckrey, H., Preussmann, R., und Ivankovic, S. Zur Erzeugung subcutaner Sarcome an Ratten. Carcinogene Wirkung von Hydrazodicarbonsäure-bis-(methyl-nitrosamid), N-Nitroso-N-n-butyl-harnstoff, N-Methyl-N-nitroso-nitroguanidine und N-nitroso-imidazolidon. Z. Krebsforsch., *68*: 87–102, 1966.
3. Fujimura, S., Kogure, K., and Oboshi, S. Production of Tumors in Glandular Stomach of Hamsters by N-Methyl-N'-nitro-N-nitrosoguanidine. Cancer Res., *30*: 1444–1448, 1970.
4. Hirono, I., and Shibuya, C. Induction of Gastric Cancer by a Single Administration of N-Methyl-N'-nitro-N-nitrosoguanidine. Proc. Japan. Cancer Assoc., *30*: 29, 1971.
5. Mandell, J. D., and Greenberg, J. A New Chemical Mutagen for Bacteria 1-

Methyl-3-nitro-1-nitrosoguanidine.   Biochem. Biophys. Res. Commun., *3*: 577–577, 1960.

6. Schoental, R.   Carcinogenic Activity of N-Methyl-N-nitroso-N'-nitroguanidine. Nature, *209*: 726–727, 1966.

7. Sugimura, T., and Fujimura, S.   Tumour Production in Glandular Stomach of Rat by N-Methyl-N'-nitro-N-nitrosoguanidine.   Nature, *216*: 943–944, 1967.

8. Sugimura, T., Fujimura, S., and Baba, T.   Tumor Production in the Glandular Stomach and Alimentary Tract of the Rat by N-Methyl-N'-nitro-N-nitrosoguanidine. Cancer Res., *30*: 455–465, 1970.

9. Sugimura, T., Fujimura, S., and Kogure, K.   Production of Adenocarcinomas in Glandular Stomach of Experimental Animals by N-Methyl-N'-nitro-N-nitrosoguanidine.   Gann Monograph, *8*: 157–196, 1969.

10. Sugimura, T., Nagao, M., and Okada, Y.   Carcinogenic Action of N-Methyl-N'-nitro-N-nitrosoguanidine.   Nature, *210*: 962–963, 1966.

11. Takayama, S., Kuwabara, N., Azama, Y., and Sugimura, T.   Skin Tumors in Mice Painted with N-Methyl-N'-nitro-N-nitrosoguanidine and N-Ethyl-N'-nitro-N-nitrosoguanidine.   J. Natl. Cancer Inst., *46*: 973–980, 1971.

Discussion of Paper by Drs. Takayama et al.

Dr. Druckrey: In your experiments with newborn rats, did you observe brain tumors?

Dr. Takayama: We did not examine the newborn rats for brain tumors.   But we intend to do it the next time.

Dr. Mirvish: A possible reason for the induction by MNNG of mesenchymal tumors in newborn but not in adult rats could be that the stomach of an adult rat removes MNNG and does not allow it to reach other tissues.   This removal could be by acid-catalyzed or (as we have heard from Dr. Sugimura) enzyme-catalyzed denitrosation.   Both processes could be deficient in the newborn rat stomach, due to a lack of HCl and/or the denitrosating enzyme.

Dr. Odashima: In addition to age specificity, we should also consider strain specificity, because in our experiment using adult Donryu rats we got more mesenchymal tumors of the gastrointestinal tract than of epithelial origins.

Dr. Takayama: I think so too, but this afternoon Professor Druckrey presented his findings on the carcinogenicity of azoxymethanol.   He also found many cases of neuroblastomas when the carcinogen was administered at the newborn stage. This may depend on the functional and structural immaturity of the tissues at the time of the administration of carcinogens.

Dr. Magee: Do you know how long MNNG persists in the animal body as the unchanged molecule, either in the newborn or adult or both?

Dr. Takayama: I have no idea.   Do you have any idea about it, Dr. Sugimura?

Dr. Sugimura: Concerning your question, I would like to mention the importance of investigating the enzyme activity that catalyzes the denitrosation reaction in newborn or suckling animals.   Meanwhile, Dr. Bralow indicated the resistance of some particular strain of rat to MNNG.   Enzyme activity should be investigated in the strain of rats which Dr. Bralow used.

DR. WEISBURGER: Was there a dose response with the very small amounts of MNNG administered once as 2, 10, and 100 μg doses?

DR. TAKAYAMA: I would like to investigate this aspect in more detail in the near future.

DR. SANDERS: Concerning Dr. Weisburger's question about the dose response curves for tumor induction by MNNG, I can state that, when tested with cells in culture, MNNG has a unique form of dose response curve.   It is more toxic to cells in the S phase than to cells in the rest of the cycle.   Moreover, damage to cells not in the S phase is more readily repaired than damage to cells in the S phase.   I cannot say whether similar considerations will apply to the whole animal.

Tumors of the Colon and Rectum Induced by N-Methyl-N'-nitro-N-nitrosoguanidine

Tomio Narisawa, Hiroshi Nakano, Masaru Hayakawa, Tadayoshi Sato, and Akira Sakuma

Department of Surgery, Akita University School of Medicine, Akita, Japan [T.N.]; Department of Surgery, Tohoku University School of Medicine, Sendai, Japan [H.N., M.H., T.S., A.S.]

1) A high incidence of colo-rectal cancer was induced experimentally by a simple new method. Three groups of female Donryu rats were injected with N-methyl-N'-nitro-N-nitrosoguanidine as a carcinogen. Animals in Groups I and II received daily injections of 0.5 ml of 0.25% aqueous solution of the carcinogen in the lumen of the colon and rectum through the anal orifice for 28 to 32 days and 7 days, respectively. Animals in Group III received 0.3 ml of the solution daily for 41 days.

2) Colo-rectal tumors were found in 20 of the 26 rats autopsied 40 to 60 weeks after the beginning of the series of injections, that is, in 77% of the cases. In all, 69 colo-rectal tumors were found in these rats as either single or multiple tumors. All the tumors were polyps and polypoid tumors. The tumors were all located in the segment from the left colonic flexure to the rectum. No tumors were found in other organs.

3) A microscopic examination showed that there were 14 hyperplastic polyps, 35 atypical adenomatous polyps, 7 suspected cancers and 13 cancers. Atypical adenomatous polyps seemed to become malignant. The tumors were very similar to human colo-rectal tumors. The incidences of tumors and the malignant changes were the same in all groups.

4) When injected into the lumen of the large intestine, the carcinogen apparently interacted with the mucosa of the large intestine by direct contact.

5) The dosages of N-methyl-N'-nitro-N-nitrosoguanidine used seemed suitable and did not have any significant toxic effect on the animals other than their carcinogenic effect.

The purpose of the present study was to develop a simple method for selective induction of experimental cancer in the large intestine. N-Methyl-N'-nitro-N-nitrosoguanidine was used as a carcinogen and infused into the lumen of the colon and rectum of rats through the anal orifice. Using this technique, a high incidence of colo-rectal cancers and atypical adenomatous polyps were produced (*9*).

MATERIALS AND METHODS

Female Donryu rats, approximately 7 weeks old, initially weighing about 120 g, were used. N-Methyl-N'-nitro-N-nitrosoguanidine was used as a 0.25% aqueous solution. For its injection, each rat was lightly anesthetized by ether inhalation. Then, an 8 cm long metal tube connected with a syringe was inserted into the lumen of the large intestine through the anal orifice and the carcinogen solution was injected.

The experimental animals were divided into 4 groups (Table 1). Animals in

TABLE 1. Experimental Design

Group	Method of colo-rectal infusion	Number of examined rats
I	0.25% MNNG aqueous solution 0.5 ml daily for 28–32 days	29
II	0.25% MNNG aqueous solution 0.5 ml daily for 7 days	7
III	0.25% MNNG aqueous solution 0.3 ml daily for 41 days	16
IV (control)	aqua 0.5 ml daily for 28 days	6

Groups I and II received 0.5 ml of the carcinogenic solution daily for 28 to 32 days and 7 days, respectively. Animals in Group III received 0.3 ml of the carcinogen solution daily for 41 days. The control animals in Group IV were infused with 0.5 ml of aqua daily for 28 days. The total dosage of carcinogen infused per animal was 35 to 40 mg in Group I, 8.75 mg in Group II, and 30.75 mg in Group III. The animals had free access to Oriental MF chow and water.

To confirm the adequacy of this experimental procedure, 0.5 ml of Methylene Blue solution in place of the carcinogen solution was infused into the colon and rectum of laparotomized rats. Subsequent examination of these animals showed that the tip of the inserted tube had reached the left colonic flexure, and that the

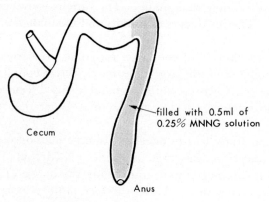

Cecum

filled with 0.5ml of
0.25% MNNG solution

Anus

FIG. 1. Method of experiment.

segment from the left colonic flexure to the rectum was well stained with Methylene Blue.   Thus, the carcinogen seemed to come in contact with the mucous membrane in the region shown in Fig. 1.

A total of 58 rats, which died or were sacrificed within 60 weeks after the beginning of carcinogen administration, were examined macroscopically and microscopically.   After macroscopic examination, the large intestine and other organs were excised and fixed in a 10% formalin solution.   Then, sections were prepared for microscopic study.

To test the toxicity of N-methyl-N'-nitro-N-nitrosoguanidine injected into the large intestine, the body weight of experimental animals was also examined.

RESULTS

Gross findings

The incidence of colo-rectal tumors in the experimental animals that were infused with the carcinogen solution was extremely high (Fig. 2).   Tumors were

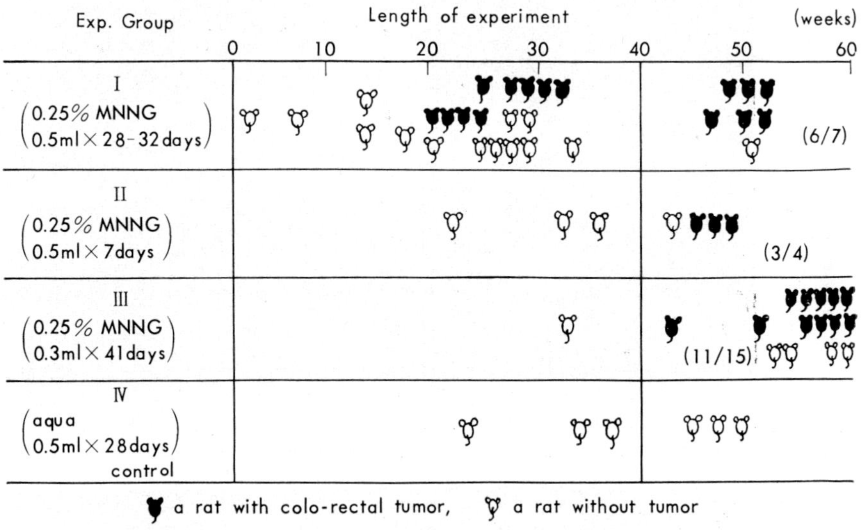

Fig. 2.   Tumor incidence in rats and length of experiment (weeks).

found in 29 of the 47 rats which died or were sacrificed between 20 and 60 weeks after the beginning of the experiment.   Moreover, 20 of the 26 rats, which died or were sacrificed after between 40 and 60 weeks, had colo-rectal tumors (incidence, 77%).   The incidence of tumors in the 3 groups were similar.   The first tumor was found in a rat in Group I sacrificed after 20 weeks.

The tumor-bearing animals had one or more tumors in the colon and/or rectum (Figs. 3–6).   Thus, fourteen rats had a single tumor, six had 2, two had 3, two had 4, one had 5, three had 6, and one had 7 multiple tumors.   In all, 69 colo-rectal tumors were observed in these 29 rats.   All the tumors protruded, *i.e.*, they were pedunculated polyps, sessile polyps, or polypoid tumors with an ulceration at the center.

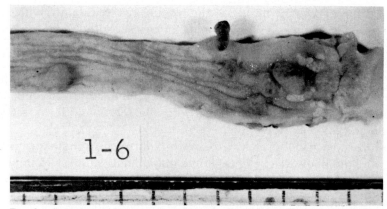

FIG. 3. Six tumors in the colon and rectum of a rat sacrificed 50 weeks after the beginning of the experiment.

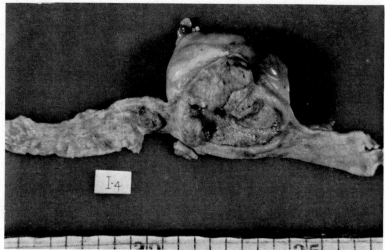

FIG. 4. Two tumors with craters in the colon. The large one measures $3.8 \times 3.8 \times 3.0$ cm. This rat died from colonic obstruction after 50 weeks.

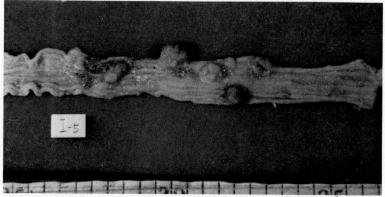

FIG. 5. Six tumors in the colon of a rat sacrificed after 50 weeks. Many types of tumors are present.

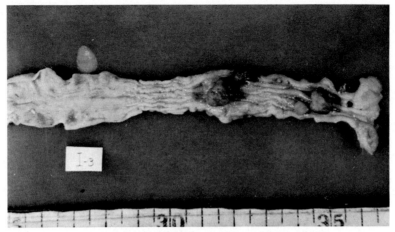

FIG. 6. Six tumors in the colon and rectum of a rat sacrificed after 50 weeks.

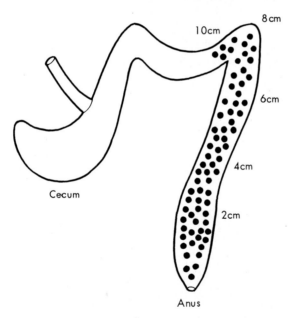

FIG. 7. Distribution of 69 tumors.

The smallest tumor was 0.2×0.1 cm, and the largest was $3.8 \times 3.8 \times 3.0$ cm (Fig. 4). The tumors were all located in the region from the left colonic flexure to the rectum, as shown in Fig. 7. No tumor was observed in the upper large intestine, and no tumors developed in other organs. No tumors were found in the 6 control rats in Group IV.

Microscopic findings

Four types of tumors were distinguished microscopically, *i.e.*, hyperplastic polyps, atypical adenomatous polyps (Fig. 8), suspected carcinomas, and carcinomas

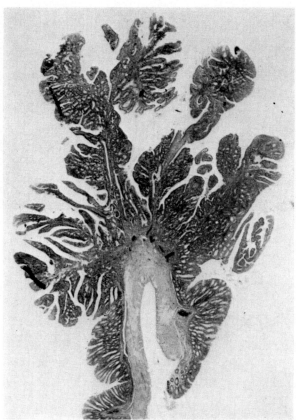

FIG. 8. Section of one of the tumors seen in Fig. 5. Atypical adenomatous cells of the polyp infiltrate the submucosa.

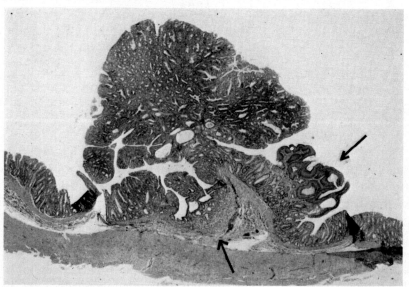

FIG. 9. Section of the tumor adjacent to the anus in Fig. 3. This appears to be a polyp with a short peduncle. Squamous cell metaplasia is found (right arrow).

(Figs. 9–13).   Of all the 69 tumors, 14 were hyperplastic polyps, 35 were atypical adenomatous polyps, 7 were suspected carcinomas, and 13 were adenocarcinomas. It was observed in some atypical adenomatous polyps that tumor growth extended into the submucosa.

On the other hand, in some of the carcinomas, tumor invasion extended into the proper muscle layer and/or the serosa.   Some tumors had a cancer focus with an

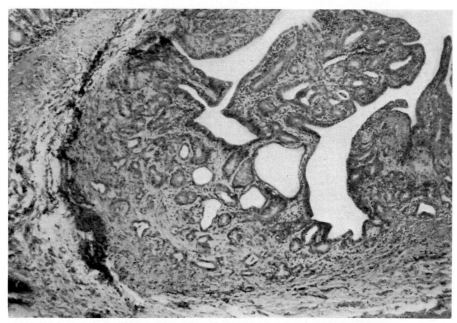

Fig. 10.   Microscopic appearance of the part indicated by an arrow (left) in Fig. 9.   Adenocarcinoma cells infiltrate into the submucosa.   The cancer focus is enclosed in an atypical adenomatous lesion.   The muscularis mucosa is seen in left upper corner.

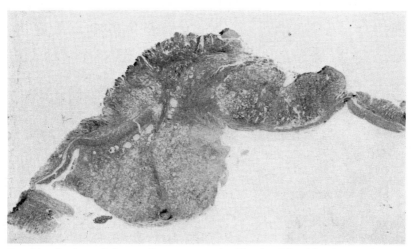

Fig. 11.   Section of the small tumor seen in Fig. 4.   Mucoid adenocarcinoma cells are seen infiltrating the serosa.

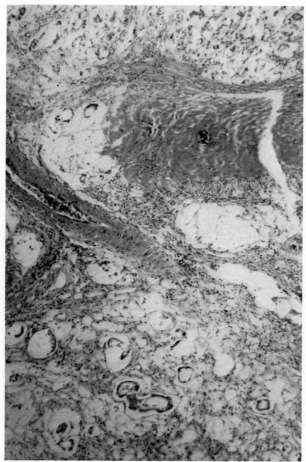

FIG. 12. Higher magnification of a part of the section in Fig. 11. The proper muscle layer is present in the center.

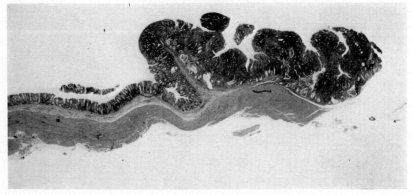

FIG. 13. Section of the tumor adjacent to the anus in Fig. 6. The tumor has a dish-like form, and adenocarcinoma cells infiltrate the submucosa.

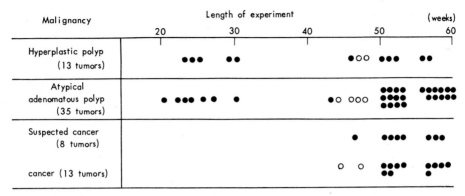

FIG. 14.   Malignancy of tumors and length of experiment (weeks).   ●, a tumor in the rat of Groups I and III;   ○, a tumor in the rat of Group II.

atypical adenomatous lesion, and the cancer focus was enclosed in an atypical adenomatous lesion.   These tumors were identified as adenocarcinomas.   However, no metastasis of lymph nodes was observed.   Microscopically too, no neoplastic lesions were found in the areas of the large intestine which appeared normal macroscopically.

The relationship between the experimental period and tumor malignancy is shown in Fig. 14.   The first atypical adenomatous polyp was found in a rat sacrificed 20 weeks after the beginning of the experiment, and the first adenocarcinoma was found in a rat sacrificed after 44 weeks.

Toxicity of N-methyl-N'-nitro-N-nitrosoguanidine
The toxic effect of the carcinogen judged by its effect on body weight was examined as follows.   Male Donryu rats, weighing about 130 g initially, were divided

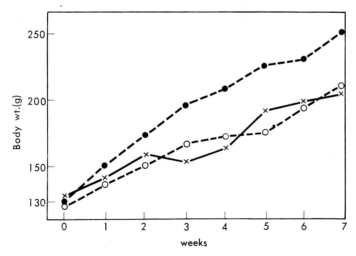

FIG. 15.   Mean body weight and length of experiment (weeks). D_1, 0.25% MNNG 0.5 ml × 28 days;   E, aqua 0.5 ml × 28 days;   ●------●, F (4 rats, nontreated);   ○------○, E (9 rats);   ×——×, D_1 (17 rats).

into three groups. Group D_1, 17 rats, received 0.5 ml of 0.25% N-methyl-N'-nitro-N-nitrosoguanidine solution daily for 28 days; Group E, 9 rats, received 0.5 ml aqua daily for 28 days, and Group F, 4 rats, was not treated. The mean body weight of the rats in each group was recorded weekly for 7 weeks (Fig. 15). Groups D_1 and E gained less weight than the untreated Group F for 4 weeks, but later weight gains in these 3 groups were similar. Therefore, the doses of N-methyl-N'-nitro-N-nitrosoguanidine used in the present experiment did not seem to cause significant toxicity.

DISCUSSION

Experimental stomach cancer can now be produced easily by oral administration of the potent carcinogen, N-methyl-N'-nitro-N-nitrosoguanidine (11–14). On the other hand, it had been very difficult to produce experimental colo-rectal cancer (1, 5, 6–8, 10), although Druckrey and his co-workers reported a high incidence of colo-rectal cancer with subcutaneous injection or oral administration of dimethylhydrazine and azoxymethane (2–4). However, these methods also caused development of carcinomas in other organs.

In the present study, a simple new method was developed for the selective induction of experimental cancer in the large intestine in rats. The four requirements of the method decided beforehand were: (1) cancer production with high incidence, (2) a simple technique, (3) induction of cancer in the colon and rectum only, and (4) the carcinogen should affect the glandular epithelia directly.

It was confirmed that the solution infused filled the lumen from the left colonic flexure to the rectum, and the tumors developed were uniformly distributed in the same area. Therefore, the N-methyl-N'-nitro-N-nitrosoguanidine infused into the lumen of the colon and rectum seemed to interact with the mucosa of the large intestine by direct contact. Detailed data on the direct interaction of the carcinogen with the glandular epithelium of the stomach have been reported by Sugimura and his colleagues (12).

However, the exact amount of the carcinogen which came in contact with the mucous membrane is unknown, because it was observed that most of the infused solution was evacuated from the anus soon after its injection. The doses of carcinogen used in the present experiment did not seem to have any significant toxic effect on animals apart from its tumorigenic effect. There was a high incidence of tumors induced, and they appeared as early as 20 weeks after the beginning of the experiment. The first adenocarcinoma was found in a rat sacrificed after 44 weeks. Consequently, the doses of N-methyl-N'-nitro-N-nitrosoguanidine infused into the large intestine seemed suitable.

Microscopically, some of the adenocarcinomas appeared to be produced by a malignant change from atypical adenomatous tumors, because in these tumors the carcinoma focus was enclosed by an atypical adenomatous lesion. Furthermore, carcinomas appeared later during the experiment than atypical adenomatous tumors. Some adenocarcinomas infiltrated into the proper muscle layer and/or the serosa. However, no metastasis to lymph nodes was observed in any of these animals.   The tumors induced were generally similar both macroscopically and microscopically to human colo-rectal tumors.   In other experimental series, metastasis to lymph nodes and peritonitis carcinomatosa were observed in a rat with adenocarcinoma in the colon.   No transplantation experiments were carried out in the present study.

The present experimental method should be useful in future studies on the carcinogenesis and especially the histogenesis and growth pattern of colo-rectal cancer.

This study was supported in part by a grant-in-aid for scientific research from the Ministry of Education.

REFERENCES

1. Berenblum, I., Haran, N., and Rosin, A.   The Carcinogenic Action in the Mouse of 20-Methylcholanthrene by Rectal Administration.   Amer. J. Pathol., *32*: 579–589, 1956.
2. Druckrey, H.   Production of Colonic Carcinomas by 1,2-Dialkyl-hydrazines and Azoxyalkanes.   *In*; Burdette, W. J. (ed.), Carcinoma of the Colon and Antecedent Epithelium, pp. 267–279, Thomas, Illinois, 1970.
3. Druckrey, H.   Organospecific Carcinogenesis in the Digestive Tract.   *In*; Nakahara, W. (ed.), Topics in Chemical Carcinogenesis, pp. 73–104, Univ. of Tokyo Press, Tokyo, 1972.
4. Druckrey, H., Preussmann, R., Matzkeis, F., und Ivankovic, S.   Selektive Erzeugung von Darmkrebs bei Ratten durch 1,2-Dimethylhydrazin.   Naturwissenschaften, *54*: 285–286, 1967.
5. Druckrey, H., Steinhiff, D., Preussmann, R., und Ivankovic, S.   Erzeugung von Krebs durch eine Eimalige Dosis von Methylnitrosoharnstoff und Verschiedenen Dialkylnitrosoaminen an Ratten.   Z. Krebsforsch., *66*: 1–10, 1964.
6. Krebs, C.   Experimenteller Alkoholkrebs bei Weissen Mäusen.   Z. Immunitäts-forsch. Exptl. Therap., *50*: 203–218, 1928.
7. Laqueur, G. L.   The Induction of Intestinal Neoplasms in Rats with the Glycoside Cycasin and its Aglycone.   Virchows Arch. Pathol. Anat., *340*: 151–163, 1965.
8. Laurens, J., and Bacon, H. E.   Studies on Experimental Carcinogenesis in the Colon and Rectum of the Rat.   J. Natl. Cancer Inst., *12*: 1237–1243, 1952.
9. Narisawa, T., Sato, T., Hayakawa, M., Sakuma, A., and Nakano, H.   Carcinoma of the Colon and Rectum of Rats by Rectal Infusion of N-Methyl-N'-nitro-N-nitrosoguanidine.   Gann, *62*: 231–234, 1971.
10. Schauer, A., Völlnagel, Th., und Wildanger, F.   Cancerizierung des Rattendarmes durch 1, 2-Dimethylhydrazin.   Z. Ges. Exp. Med., *150*: 87–93, 1969.
11. Sugimura, T., and Fujimura, S.   Tumor Production in Glandular Stomach of Rat by N-Methyl-N'-nitro-N-nitrosoguanidine.   Nature, *216*: 943–944, 1967.
12. Sugimura, T., Fujimura, S., Kogure, K., Baba, T., Saito, T., Nagao, M., Hosoi, H., and Shimosato, Y.   Production of Adenocarcinomas in Glandular Stomach of Experimental Animals by N-Methyl-N'-nitro-N-nitrosoguanidine.   Gann Monograph, *8*: 157–196, 1969.
13. Sugimura, T., Kawachi, T., Kogure, K., Tanaka, N., Fujimura, S., and Nagao, M.   Induction of Stomach Cancer by N-Methyl-N'-nitro-N-nitrosoguanidine.   *In*;

Nakahara, W. (ed.), Topics in Chemical Carcinogenesis, pp. 105–120, Univ. of Tokyo Press, Tokyo, 1972.

14.   Takayama, S., Saito, T., Fujimura, S., and Sugimura, T.   Histological Findings of Gastric Tumors Induced by N-Methyl-N'-nitro-N-nitrosoguanidine in Rats.   Gann Monograph, *8*: 197–208, 1969.

Discussion of Paper by Drs. Narisawa et al.

DR. SATO: I would like to add a few preliminary data obtained in a series of experiments which are being carried out in my laboratory, modifying Dr. Narisawa's
method.

The animals used were from the ACI strain of rats, inbred, male and female,
weighing about 100–120 g, obtained from the Fuji Animal Farm, Tokyo.   The
MNNG was dissolved in deionized water at a concentration of 2 mg/ml just before
administration.   In preparing the insertion tube, the end of a polyethylene tube
(No. 20, external diameter, 1.3 mm) was melted into globular form in order to avoid
intestine perforation, and then a hole was made in the globule with a needle.   Before the experiment, food was not given for 24 hr.   Under ether, anesthesia a
polyethylene tube was inserted about 15 cm into the colon through the anus, reaching the cecum of the rat, through which 1 ml of the solution containing 2 mg of
MNNG was administered twice a week.   The animals (41 rats) were divided into
four groups according to the total amount of MNNG administered, *i.e.*, 50 mg in
Group I, 30 mg in Group II, 20 mg in Group III, and 10 mg in Group IV.   The
animals were sacrificed when found moribund and then autopsied.   Tissues and
organs were fixed in a 10% formalin solution and stained with hematoxylin and
eosin.

Tumors of the colo-rectal area were found in 15 out of the 20 animals sacrificed
during the period from 7 to 13 months after the first administration of MNNG, as
shown in Table I.   Multiple tumors (3 to 10) were seen in each animal with tumors,

TABLE I.   Tumors of the Colon and Rectum in ACI Rats Caused by the Induction of N-Methyl-N'-nitro-
N-nitrosoguanidine (MNNG)

Amount of MNNG	Sex	Number of animals	
		Examined	With tumor(s)
50 mg	M	8[a]	7
	F	3[a]	3
30	M	3[a]	2
	F	2[a]	2
20	M	4[a]	1
	F	4[b]	0
10	M	5[b]	0
	F	6[b]	0

[a]   Sacrificed during the period from 7–13 months after the first administration of MNNG.

[b]   Animals still alive.

located in the left descendant colon and the rectum, the area within 10 cm from the anus. This was almost the same as seen in Dr. Narisawa's findings.   In most cases, pedunculated polyps were seen, except in 2 cases where the lesions were ulcerated. Metastasis was found in the regional lymph node in one case and widespread dissemination in the abdominal cavity was seen in another one.

According to our microscopic investigations, most of the tumors were adenocarcinomas of the well-differentiated type with moderate cellular and structural atypism, invading from the submucosa to the serosa through the muscle layers.   It is my impression that the tumors in the rats in this series of experiments were more malignant than those of the Donryu rats on which Dr. Narisawa reported.

DR. WEISBURGER: In the United States we have an intense interest in the induction of colo-rectal cancer by simple reliable techniques.   As part of our National Colon Cancer Program, we have a number of advisors, one of whom, Dr. Louis Miller of the University of Wisconsin, has suggested using the same technique that Dr. Narisawa and Dr. Sato have so successfully applied.

DR. SANDER: Did you do experiments with a single injection of the carcinogens too?
    Did you find a dosage effective in inducing single tumors in the colon?
    Are you able to predict in your model at what time in the experiment the different animals will develop tumors with security, so that you can start a therapeutic experiment?

DR. NARISAWA: A single injection experiment is under way right now.   Unfortunately for our purposes here, it is only in its 40th week and all of the animals are still alive.

DR. SATO: An experiment with a single application has not been tried yet.

DR. NARISAWA: We have not examined the model experiment of cancer chemotherapy or radiotherapy.

DR. HIGGINSON: Do you have any experience with testing the positivity to Gold's embryonal antigen in such tumors?

DR. HIRONO: In rats with a solitary tumor in the colon or rectum, was there any special site—prone to the development of tumors?

DR. NARISAWA: No correlation among tumor size, number of the tumors, and tumor localization was observed in our study.

Model Studies on the Etiology of Colon Cancer

John H. Weisburger*

Experimental Pathology Branch, National Cancer Institute, Bethesda, Maryland, U.S.A.

Contemporary Epidemiological and Other Evidence on Environmental Factors as Causes of Bowel Cancer

Segi and associates (*24*) have made significant contributions to the problem of the etiology of cancer and an understanding of causative factors in neoplastic disease by their studies of the geographic pathology of cancer at various sites. Specifically of interest in the context of the Princess Takamatsu Symposium and the subject of this paper are the findings that cancer of the colon and rectum exhibits sizable differences in incidence and in death rate as a function of geographic area. Thus, colon cancer ranks highest in Scotland in males and in Canada in females. Fortunately for the population in the host country to this symposium, Japan shows the lowest mortality rates due to colon cancer in males and females alike. Denmark has the highest incidence of cancer of the rectum, which some investigators believe may have different causative factors from that of the colon, and Chile has the lowest incidence. The incidence of cancer of the rectum is low in Japan, putting Japan somewhere in the middle between Chile and Denmark.

Further contributing factors in developing insight into elements in the environment responsible for neoplasia in the large bowel are studies on migrant populations (*8*, *26*). Of outstanding relevance are migrants from Japan, where, as noted above, the incidence of cancer of the lower intestinal tract is very low, to the United States where this type of cancer is among the highest. These studies demonstrate without question that genetics and related factors are of less importance than the environmental situation. In particular, diets consumed are key problems. The results of such investigations do, indeed, reveal that individuals of Japanese ancestry living in the United States, particularly second generation individuals, run the same risk of developing cancer of the colon as native-born Americans of different origins.

Parenthetically, it can be said that the situation for gastric cancer is just the reverse, gastric cancer being quite high in Japan and reasonably low in the United

---

* Present address: American Health Foundation, 2 East End Ave., New York, NY, 10021, U.S.A.

States (*2, 10*).   Migrants from Japan in the first generation have a lower rate than in Japan itself, but not yet as low as those individuals who have resided in the United States for their entire lives.   Furthermore, there is a small but perhaps meaningful difference between gastric cancer and colon cancer.   Individuals who migrate to the United States after having lived in the high gastric cancer incidence environment of Japan for the first 10 or 15 years and then spend the remainder of their lives in the United States do run almost the same risk of developing gastric cancer as if they had remained in Japan.   On the other hand, individuals who move from Japan to the United States after 15 years of age run the same risk of developing cancer of the bowel as if they had migrated earlier.   From these facts, the preliminary conclusion is drawn that cancer of the colon may relate to causative elements present in the environment throughout life, whereas gastric cancer may be developed as a result of exposure to an active agent early in life.

Thus, the question arises: What are the possible elements in the environment which lead to cancer of the colon in a population typical of the United States or the United Kingdom, particularly Scotland, which are absent or certainly present in much lower amounts in an environment such as that provided by Japan.   In a number of instances, cancer at various organ sites in man has been unambiguously connected to occupational exposure to specific chemicals, as for example, bladder cancer in dyestuff or rubber workers, lung cancer in uranium miners, and so on.   As a first approximation, it is probably true that the industrial environment and occupational hazards in Japan are not too different from those in the United States or in the United Kingdom.   Moreover, cancer of the colon is also quite low in the African environment, particularly among the native black population, in which instance an occupational contact is probably not involved (*1*).   All these factors taken together remove suspicion from occupational exposure as a causative element in colon cancer, although this need not necessarily be neglected in specific instances.   Certainly, prime consideration centers around dietary and nutritional elements, which are obviously different in regions of high and low colon cancer incidence.

Diets in low colon cancer regions typically are relatively poor in protein and fats of animal origin.   Moderate amounts of protein are derived from seafood which again contains low levels of fat.   Such diets are rich in carbohydrates and also vegetables and other ingredients, providing sizable amounts of bulk and high residue nutrients.

On the other hand, diets typical of western countries are rich in animal protein and animal fat (*34*).   They include other sources of lipids such as milk or vegetable fats, and because of the extensive milling and refining of the carbohydrate component, such foodstuffs provide relatively moderate bulk.   People in Denmark, where there is a high incidence of cancer of the colon, consume more meat than in neighboring Finland, where there is a low incidence of colon cancer and diets contain more milk proteins (*18*).

Furthermore, of possibly decisive interest in comparative studies are micronutrients, such as minerals and vitamins (*17, 23*).   Admittedly, insufficient relative values in various countries on these potentially rather important factors are available. More information in this area would be desirable.

This information then constitutes the overall background which needs to be studied intensively to gather insight into causative factors of colon cancer and possibly also cancer of the rectum. At the present time, only a beginning has been made into developing approaches to the understanding of the as yet unknown environmental agents responsible for cancer of the colon and rectum in man. Thus, the factors (1) high animal meat protein and (2) lack of bulk assume major significance.

Differences in diet in various populations have been associated with consequent variations of the intestinal bacterial flora. Recently, several studies along these lines, comparing populations with high, moderate, and low risk of colon cancer, have discovered an interesting relationship which deserves additional study (*1, 11, 12, 27*). Thus, populations in the high-risk groups appear to have a higher ratio of total anaerobic over aerobic bacterial flora. In fact, Japan had the lowest such ratio, 0.5, compared to 2.1 in western countries. Once specific differences in such bacterial systems are pinpointed, the question that will have to be asked is what these differences mean as regards the presence of select types of enzymes. As will be discussed below, the bacterial flora elaborates many different types of enzymes. It will be interesting to establish whether qualitative rather than quantitative differences exist in respect to such factors.

In a preliminary experiment in our laboratories, groups of rats excreted considerably more fecal material on a high residue natural diet than on a semi-synthetic low residue diet, as might be expected. On the other hand, two enzymes studied, namely, β-glucuronidase and azo-dye reductase, had rather similar specific activities, that is, units per mg of fecal material. Because of the large difference in weight of fecal material in rats on the two diets, the total units excreted per 24 hr were much higher in the fecal material from the animals on the high-residue chow. Further critical enzyme studies will be most useful.

Along these lines, it has been postulated that certain of the bile acids or related steroids might be metabolized by bacterial flora to materials which may be carcinogenic in the lower gut (*12*). This is an interesting avenue of approach. However, it is somewhat improbable and perhaps not rewarding to necessarily think in terms of a production of carcinogenic polynuclear aromatic hydrocarbons during this process, since it could well be that chemicals in the intermediate metabolic steps (*7, 13, 22*) are carcinogenic. Hydrocarbons would lead to enzyme induction in the gut, which, in turn, would stimulate detoxification of such molecules (*30*).

Another possibility, the production by bacterial flora of mycotoxins affecting the lower gut, should not be neglected. While at the present time no example is known of a colon-specific agent, it is not unlikely that such materials may be elaborated under the proper conditions.

Experimental Induction of Colo-rectal Cancer by Chemicals

2′,3-Dimethyl-4-aminobiphenyl

As a result of investigations in the area of structure-activity relationships with a number of aromatic amines, Walpole and his associates (*28, 29*) discovered that methyl-substituted 4-aminobiphenyls do yield cancer of the colon in rats in fair yields with a latent period of one year or less. The compound used most often in such studies, since the original discovery by Walpole, is 2',3-dimethyl-4-aminobiphenyl. A beginning has been made, but no detailed studies on the metabolism of this agent have been as yet undertaken.

It seems quite likely that this carcinogen would be metabolized in a manner similar to that of the parent 4-aminobiphenyl itself. In rats, this latter carcinogen undergoes acetylation and ring-hydroxylation, mostly at the 4' position, but also in a minor way at other ring positions. Significantly, hydroxylation on the nitrogen occurs, yielding N-hydroxy-4-acetylaminobiphenyl. It is the latter agent which most likely is an active carcinogenic intermediate (19).

It is quite probable that this key material is synthesized through conventional metabolic steps in the liver and excreted in the bile and also into the blood as a glucuronic acid conjugate (31). The metabolite entering the gut through the bile is hydrolyzed by bacterial β-glucuronidase provided by the bacterial flora when it reaches the lower part of the gut, along with the liberation of the free compound (Fig. 1). It is not known whether additional activation steps are required in the colon. For the liver, a sulfuric acid ester appears to be the active ultimate carcino-

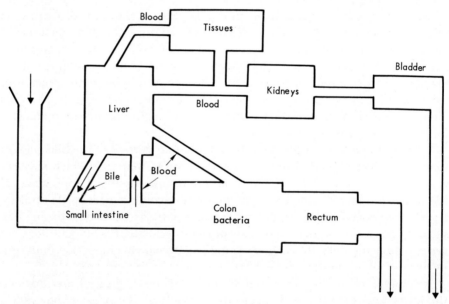

FIG. 1. A carcinogen after oral intake can pass through the gastrointestinal tract and affect the colon-rectal system directly, or after modification by enzymes from the intestinal mucosa, or even more often from the bacterial flora in the gut. It can also be absorbed, circulate, be metabolized by the liver, chiefly to more polar compounds, be excreted in the bile, reach the the lower portion of the tract where complexes such as glucuronides, sulfate esters and the like are hydrolyzed or bile acids are converted to metabolites again by the bacterial flora in the colon, which thus in either case assumes importance in leading to the active carcinogenic intermediates from procarcinogens. After parenteral administration, similar events occur once the material has reached the liver through the circulatory system. Specific metabolic reactions with certain carcinogens in portions of the gastrointestinal tract may also lead to the production of reactive intermediates, and thus accounting for select organotropic cancer induction.

gen (*3, 32*).   Secretion in the bile, documenting in part this overall pathway, has been adduced by Spjut and Noall (*25*), although the specific metabolites in the bile remain to be identified.

Cycasin

The carcinogenicity to the colon as well as liver and kidney of a natural product, cycasin, the β-glucoside of methylazoxymethanol, was discovered by serendipity in the studies of Laqueur and associates (*15*).   Cycasin, suspected to be a cause of amyotropic lateral sclerosis in man, when given chronically to rats in their diet, failed to induce this condition, but instead led to cancer, especially in the lower intestinal tract.   Laqueur demonstrated that the bacterial flora in the lower gut is uniquely involved in eliciting the carcinogenic intermediate methylazoxymethanol, because cycasin itself proves singularly inactive in germ-free animals.   On the other hand, injection or oral administration of the aglycone methylazoxymethanol, even in germ-free rats, yielded the same type of cancer as when cycasin was administered to conventional rats although not in the same yield.

1,2-Dimethylhydrazine and azoxymethane

Druckrey and associates (*5, 6*) developed another colon-specific carcinogen on the basis of the reports by Laqueur and associates about cycasin.   Thus, the powerful carcinogenicity to the bowel of 1,2-dimethylhydrazine was discovered.   This agent, as well as the closely related azoxymethane, induced a high incidence of cancer in the colon in the laboratory of Druckrey and associates, after a latent period of approximately 200 to 300 days, depending on the dosage.   It was discovered that if the compound is given orally, it also leads to cancer of the liver and kidney, given subcutaneously, as was the case in Druckrey's experiments, it yielded mainly cancers of the colon, some in the rectum, and depending on the dose, a few in the small intestine.   Mice and hamsters are also susceptible.

While specific studies on the metabolism of these agents have not yet been performed extensively, it seems possible that they are also metabolized in the liver by oxidation to methylazoxymethanol, which, in turn, is conjugated with glucuronic acid and excreted in the bile.   The glucuronide is split in the lower gut by enzymes provided by the bacterial flora (*31*).   Alternatively, the experiments of Wittig *et al.* (*33*) can be interpreted in terms of a colon-specific oxidation system giving the active carcinogenic intermediate in the mucosal cells.   More recently, Gennaro has obtained leads in the same direction by ingenious surgical transplant experiments (personal communication; Diseases Colon Rectum, in press).   Recently, Pegg and Hawks (*20*) demonstrated that there was increased tRNA methylation in the lower gut after an injection of 1,2-dimethylhydrazine.

Experimental Study of Dietary Factors in Colon Cancer Induction with 1,2-Dimethylhydrazine or with Azoxymethane

We have utilized these newly discovered colon-specific carcinogens to study the possible modifications of their action as a function of diet, modeled after some para-

TABLE 1.   Composition of Diets

Diet[a]	Casein	Fat[b]	Carbohydrate[c]
Basal	18%	5%	74.5%
Basal+1.4% trytophan	18	5	73.1
High fat	18	30	49.5
High protein	27	5	65.5
High protein+high fat	27	30	40.5

[a]   Includes H. M. W. salt mixture with added zinc carbonate, 2%, and vitamin mixture with vitamins at twice the necessary level, 0.5%.

[b]   Fat: corn oil, 5%; additional fat, Crisco.

[c]   Carbohydrate: starch, 0.5%; and remainder, Cerelose.

TABLE 2.   Survival of Male Rats Injected with 1, 2-Dimethylhydrazine

Diet	Weeks						
	0	10	14	18	22	26	30
	Number of rats						
Basal	24	22	22	22	19	10	4
Basal+tryptophan	18	18	18	18	18	11	6
High fat	18	17	15	8	2	0	
High protein	24	22	22	19	14	8	3
High protein+fat	24	23	17	8	0		

0.2 mM/kg DMH twice/week for 16 weeks, once/week for 10 more weeks.

meters drawn from epidemiology.   The diets used are shown in Table 1.   A basal diet included 18% casein and 5% fat.   Others contained high casein (27%), high fat (30% saturated fat), or high protein and high fat, the balance being carbohydrate added as cerelose (glucose).   The diets were fortified with adequate amounts of minerals, including additional zinc carbonate and vitamins at twice the normal level.   Male and female weanling Fischer strain rats (a highly inbred strain) were injected with 0.2 mM of 1,2-dimethylhydrazine or azoxymethane (12 mg/kg and 14.8 mg/kg, respectively).   Dimethylhydrazine was injected for 16 weeks (twice per week initially; in later tests, once per week), then once per week for 10 weeks, followed by a further holding period of 6 to 8 weeks without treatment on the various diets.   Azoxymethane was injected once a week for 12 weeks followed by a 12-week holding period.   A number of these experiments are still under way.   The present report, therefore, is a preliminary statement on findings to date.

In male rats, the regimen initially selected of two subcutaneous doses a week for 16 weeks led to a sizable mortality rate in the animals on the high fat or on the high fat plus high protein diet (Table 2).   Animals on high protein diet alone or the basal diet survived for the duration of the experiment.   Thus, it would appear that the high fat level is responsible for the increased toxicity at the dosage used.   Female rats were somewhat more tolerant to this regimen of carcinogen administration, although some mortality was seen also on the high fat diet (Table 3).   In this series of experiments extending over a period of approximately 30 weeks, gross tumors were seen in all diet groups in both male and female rats.   They were mainly in the

TABLE 3. Survival of Female Rats Injected with 1, 2-Dimethylhydrazine

Diet	Weeks						
	0	10	14	18	22	26	30
	Number of rats						
Basal	23	23	23	23	23	22	19
Basal+tryptophan	17	17	17	17	17	17	13
High fat	18	18	18	17	12	5	3
High protein	23	23	23	21	20	19	14
High protein+fat	24	24	24	22	21	15	12

0.2 mm/kg DMH s.c. twice/week for 16 weeks, once/week for 10 more weeks.

TABLE 4. Survival of Male Rats Injected with Azoxymethane

Diet	Weeks						
	0	10	12	14	18	22	24
	Number of rats						
Basal	20	17	16	14	13	8	6
Basal+tryptophan	25	24	22	20	17	12	7
High fat	25	20	17	12	8	6	6
High protein	20	18	18	18	15	15	11
High protein+fat	25	21	13	7	5	5	4

0.2 mm/kg AOM once/week for 12 weeks.

colon, although some lesions were also observed in the small intestine, particularly in animals on the high protein diet. In addition, some rats had kidney and liver lesions. Males exhibited pronounced atrophy of the testes.

Of interest is the finding that in male and female rats, an injection of dimethyl-hydrazine induced a high incidence of tumors of the external ear duct, irrespective of diet. This lesion was not apparent under the conditions utilized by Druckrey and associates in BD strain rats. However, the finding of ear duct tumors is of interest insofar as an entirely different type of colon carcinogen, Walpole's 3-methyl-4-aminobiphenyl derivatives, under some conditions and as a function of structure of the specific agent used, also induced ear duct tumors, in addition to tumors in the lower intestinal tract (28). Rats injected with azoxymethane for 12 weeks and killed 12 weeks later, making a total experimental period of 24 weeks, also exhibited a high incidence of ear duct tumors.

With azoxymethane also, animals on the diets containing 30% fat were affected adversely by the toxic effect of the compound, and relatively few animals lived into the cancer period (Table 4). The survivors on all diets exhibited a high yield of cancer in the colon, cecum and also in the small intestine. With the high level of carcinogens used, no influence of dietary regimen could be seen as regards the localization of the tumors.

The significant finding was made that the diet would affect the survival of the animals. The mechanism of toxicity of these agents as a function of diet deserves additional elaboration. It appears that animals on a high protein diet resist the toxic action most readily; those on an average protein level are intermediate, and those on a high fat level survived least well.

These range finding studies need additional refinement in order to meaningfully attack the problem of factors operating in human colon cancer formation.

DISCUSSION

The preliminary results obtained in our laboratories in inducing colon cancer with 1,2-dimethylhydrazine and azoxymethane in an inbred strain of rat confirm that this type of agent, indeed, does generate a high yield of these tumors. In addition, and not obvious under some conditions (5), we observed tumors of the ear duct. It may be recalled that in Walpole's hands with entirely different types of compounds in the 4-aminobiphenyl series, ear duct and colon cancers seemed to go hand in hand also. The significance of this connection is obscure at the present time, but certainly deserves further exploration.

The key additional finding was that diets high in fat exaggerated the toxic effect of azoxymethane and 1,2-dimethylhydrazine. In the absence of detailed data on the metabolic fate of these agents, it is difficult to offer a rational mechanistic explanation of this finding at the present time.

While detailed histologic evaluation of our material remains to be done, the overall impression is gained that tumor induction in the intestinal tract appears to be independent of the diet fed. However, lesions were seen in the pancreas on the basal diet containing 1.4% supplementary tryptophan. It could well be that with high dose levels of the carcinogens minor differences controlled by the type of diet would be obliterated. Therefore, further studies are necessary with lower dosages.

Several efforts were made to transplant the colon cancers obtained in this series with the highly inbred Fischer strain rat. No growth has been observed up until now, after subcutaneous or intraperitoneal transplantation in untreated and even radiation-pretreated rats. A transplantable intestinal cancer would be useful to further biochemical, kinetic and immunological studies, especially to develop studies on carcino-embryonic antigens. This area also deserves further intense attention.

COMMENT

How do these model studies in rodents bear on present concepts on the etiology of colon cancer in man? As was discussed in the introduction, migrant and other epidemiologic studies do attribute cancer at this site to environmental factors, most likely of a dietary nature, and within that group probably naturally occurring chemicals rather than synthetic ones.

Thus, the key question is the nature of those chemicals. Are they exogenous, and if so, of animal or vegetable origin? Do they arise from further metabolism in the liver, excretion in the bile of a complex, and resolution by bacterial enzymes in the gut which are obviously involved? Are they bacterial metabolites of the bile acids or steroids? Does the bacterial flora itself produce a mycotoxin under some conditions? Is the effect one of a primary carcinogen potentiated possibly by other factors, such as, irritation (*33*) from hard stools typical of western man and paralleling the potentiation of urinary, bladder and renal carcinogenesis by stones?

In some areas mineral elements have been suspected of playing a role, a possibility not to be neglected, considering that a number of key enzymes concerned with the cell cycle, DNA synthesis, or DNA repair are highly dependent on and involve specific metal ions.

The example of familial polyposis, a genetically controlled disorder which almost always tends to eventuate in colon cancer, may be a useful model for further study. It may well be that the high turnover rate of cells in the intestinal tract implies a certain risk of miscoding during DNA synthesis, or the operation of other elements during the mitotic cycle (*16*). Thus, it is conceivable that in a normal individual such tissues as the intestinal tract are also characterized by highly developed repair mechanisms capable of controlling and eliminating misfits of the cell duplication cycle.

Viewed from this perspective familial polyposis may be akin to *Xeroderma pigmentosum*, characterized by the absence of or faulty repair mechanisms. In fact, in such a model it could be visualized that colon cancer, in general, may be the consequence not of a primary carcinogen affecting DNA, but rather of an agent preventing the efficient operation of repair mechanisms. This speculative concept would regard colon cancer as the outcome of chronic deficiencies in certain essential nutritive elements. Experimental effort along those lines would also concern itself with the maintenance or, indeed, increase of repair systems, for example, by assuring a more than adequate supply of inorganic ions and of select vitamins like A and E, which at the same time would be relevant to a proper operation, not only of repair systems, but of the process of differentiation of epithelial tissues, such as the intestinal tract (*16*).

Unfortunately, at this time, there is no good experimental model with a high incidence of " spontaneous " colon cancer in which such delicate, intangible variables could be investigated more readily. It will be necessary, therefore, to utilize the known chemical colon carcinogens and tailor their action in a more delicate and refined way than used heretofore to be in a position to delve into some of the questions raised.

In addition to this type of experimental and laboratory approach, a great deal can be learned from a thorough and deliberate study of changing dietary conditions in countries like Japan and Finland, which heretofore have exhibited a relatively low incidence of colon cancer. However, because of alterations in personal dietary habits, there is now an increase in the rate of colon cancer development. Detailed clinical evaluation of such contemporary changes may provide insight into the key factors which then can be subjected to tests in experimental situations. Hopefully, these endeavors will soon reveal the key factors responsible for cancer of the colon, so that appropriate preventive measures can be recommended.

This is particularly important for the host country of this symposium, Japan. Indeed, Japan is an ideal country to implement experimental laboratory findings in preventive medicine with respect to cancer. Japan is a country where many types of cancer, so common in the western world, like cancer of the colon, breast, and prostate, are quite low. The major problem in Japan is cancer of the glandular stomach and cancer of the liver. These two types have exhibited appreciable decreases in the last few decades in the United States of America, and similar trends are in evidence in continental Europe and even, perhaps, in Japan.

The exact underlying causes for this decrease are not yet fully explained. It might seem reasonable to attribute this desirable decline to better and more balanced nutrients and possibly improved methods of preserving foodstuffs by refrigeration, antioxidants, and the like, which would avoid the production and presence of mycotoxins like aflatoxin. Also relevant may be the decreasing use of preservatives such as nitrite, which when present might lead to the formation of most hazardous and carcinogenic nitrosamines and nitrosoureas (9, 14, 21), a subject discussed by a number of speakers at this conference. Thus, if deliberate or unplanned modifications of the environment in Japan can lower the carcinogenic risks for the stomach and liver, without simultaneously increasing the chances for carcinogenesis in other organs, Japan will be an enviable country with a low prevalence of cancers of all types. That this situation should exist in Japan would be most appropriate inasmuch as the entire field of chemical carcinogenesis, on which rational prevention is based, originated in large measure in Japan with the discoveries of Yamagiwa and Ichikawa earlier in this century.

SUMMARY

Comparative studies on various types of cancer indicate that they often exhibit variations in incidence as a function of the country or area of residence. Thus, the factors related to local customs can be analyzed to gain insight into causative agents involved specifically with the disease by a combination of epidemiologic approaches and laboratory studies. In the case of colon cancer, epidemiological studies have shown that the incidence of this type of cancer is high in some western countries, like the United States of America and the United Kingdom, lower on the European continent, considerably lower in Japan and the Far East, generally, and very low in Africa.

Experimental colon cancer model studies were performed, simulating different dietary conditions, mainly by varying the protein and fat content of the diet. The animals were Fischer strain rats injected s.c. with either of the colon carcinogens, 1,2-dimethylhydrazine or azoxymethane, at 0.2 mm/kg twice a week for 16 weeks, then once a week for 10 more weeks. Observation of the rats for 6 weeks longer indicated that over all the high fat (30%) or the high fat, high protein (27%) diet led to higher mortality and shorter survival, compared with standard fat (5%) and high protein (27%) or the control diet (18% protein, 5% fat). Those animals living for more than 24 weeks on all diets showed colon tumors, some cancer in the small intestine, and/or cancer in the external ear duct. Male and female rats responded similarly, but females appeared to survive somewhat longer on the high fat diets. There was intestinal bleeding in the rats which died early and marked anemia in all cases. Depression of the hematocrit was less in females. Experiments with lower dose levels of the carcinogen are presently under way to specifically assess dietary factors involved in colon cancer development utilizing azoxymethane and 1,2-dimethylhydrazine.

REFERENCES

1. Burkitt, D. P.   Epidemiology of Cancer of the Colon and Rectum.   Cancer, *28*: 3–13, 1971.
2. Cutler, S. J.   Trends in Cancers of the Digestive Tract.   Surgery, *65*: 740–752, 1969.
3. DeBaun, J. R., Miller, E. C., and Miller, J. A.   N-Hydroxy-2-acetylaminofluorene Sulfotransferase: Its Probable Role in Carcinogenesis and in Protein-(methion-S-yl) Binding in Rat Liver.   Cancer Res., *30*: 577–595, 1970.
4. De Luca, L., Schumacher, M., and Nelson, D. P.   Localization of the Retinol-dependent Fucose-glycopeptide in the Goblet Cell of the Rat Small Intestine.   J. Biol. Chem., *246*: 5762–5765, 1971.
5. Druckrey, H.   Production of Colonic Carcinomas by 1,2-Dialkylhydrazines and Azoxyalkanes.   *In*; Burdette, W. J. (ed.), Carcinoma of the Colon and Antecedent Epithelium, pp. 267–279, Charles C. Thomas, Springfield, Illionis, 1970.
6. Druckrey, H.   Organospecific Carcinogenesis in the Digestive Tract.   *In*; Nakahar, W. (ed.), Topics in Chemical Carcinogenesis, p. 73, Univ. of Tokyo Press, Tokyo, 1972.
7. Eyssen, H., Sacquet, E., Evrard, E., and Van den Bosch, J.   Effect of Neomycin on Cholesterol Levels and Bile Acid Excretion in Germfree and Conventional Rats. Life Sci., *7*: 1155–1162, 1968.
8. Haenszel, W., and Correa, P.   Cancer of the Colon and Rectum and Adenomatous Polyps.   A Review of Epidemiologic Findings.   Cancer, *28*: 14–24, 1971.
9. Hawksworth, G., and Hill, M. J.   The Formation of Nitrosamines by Human Intestinal Bacteria.   Biochem. J., *122*: 28–29 1971.
10. Higginson, J.   Etiology of Gastrointestinal Cancer in Man.   Natl. Cancer Inst. Monograph, *25*: 191–198, 1967.
11. Hill, M. J., and Aries, V. C.   Faecal Steroid Composition and Its Relationship to Cancer of the Large Bowel.   J. Path., *104*: 129–139, 1971.
12. Hill, M. J., Drasar, B. S., Aries, V., Crowther, J. S., Hawksworth, G., and Williams, R. E. O.   Bacteria and Aetiology of Cancer of Large Bowel.   Lancet, *1*: 95–100, 1971.
13. Jänne, O. A., Laatikainen, T. J., and Vihko, R. K.   Effect of Reduction of the Intestinal Microflora on the Excretion of Neutral Steroids in Human Faeces and Urine.   Europ. J. Biochem., *20*: 120–123, 1971.
14. Klubes, P., and Jondorf, W. R.   Dimethylnitrosamine Formation from Sodium Nitrite and Dimethylamine by Bacterial Flora of Rat Intestine.   Res. Commun. Chem. Path. Pharm., *2*: 24–34, 1971.
15. Laqueur, G. L.   Contribution of Intestinal Macroflora and Microflora to Carcinogenesis.   *In*; Burdette, W. J. (ed.), Carcinoma of the Colon and Antecedent Epithelium, pp. 305–313, Charles C. Thomas, Springfield, Illinois, 1970.
16. Lipkin, M.   Proliferation and Differentiation of Normal and Neoplastic Cells in the Colon of Man.   Cancer, *28*: 38–40, 1971.
17. Marjanen, H.   Possible Causal Relationship between the Easily Soluble Amount

of Manganese on Arable Mineral Soil and Susceptibility to Cancer in Finland. Ann. Agric. Fenniae, *8*: 326–334, 1969.

18. Miettinen, J. K.   University of Helsinki, Personal communication.

19. Miller, J. A., Wyatt, C. S., Miller, E. C., and Hartmann, H. A.   The N-Hydroxylation of 4-Acetylaminobiphenyl by the Rat and Dog and the Strong Carcinogenicity of N-Hydroxy-4-acetylaminobiphenyl in the Rat.   Cancer Res., *21*: 1465–1473, 1961.

20. Pegg, A. E., and Hawks, A.   Increased Transfer Ribonucleic Acid Methylase Activity in Tumours Induced in the Mouse Colon by the Administration of 1,2-Dimethylhydrazine.   Biochem. J., *122*: 121–123, 1971.

21. Sander, J., Bürkle, G., Flohe, L., und Aeikens, B.   Untersuchungen *in vitro* über die Möglichkeit einer Bildung cancerogener Nitrosamide im Magen.   Arzneim.-forsch., *21*: 411–414, 1971.

22. Schiff, L., Carey, J. B., Jr., and Dietschy, J.   Bile Salt Metabolism, Charles C. Thomas, Springfield, Illinois, 1969.

23. Schroeder, H. A.   Losses of Vitamins and Trace Minerals Resulting from Processing and Preservation of Foods.   Amer. J. Clin. Nutr., *24*: 562–573, 1971.

24. Segi, M., Kurihara, M., and Matsuyama, T.   Cancer Mortality for Selected Sites in 24 Countries.   No. 5, 1964–1965, Tohoku University School of Medicine, Sendai, Japan, 1969.

25. Spjut, H. J., and Noall, M. W.   Experimental Induction of Tumors of the Large Bowel of Rats.   Cancer, *28*: 29–37, 1971.

26. Stewart, H. L.   Geographic Pathology of Cancer of the Colon and Rectum.   Cancer, *28*: 25–28, 1971.

27. Walker, A. R. P.   Diet, Bowel Motility, Faeces Composition and Colonic Cancer.   S. Afr. Med. J., *45*: 377–379, 1971.

28. Walpole, A. L.   *In*; Bielka, H. (ed.), Berliner Symposion über Fragen der Carcinogenese, pp. 9–11, Akademie-Verlag, Berlin, 1960.

29. Walpole, A. L., and Williams, M. H. C.   Aromatic Amines as Carcinogens in Industry.   Brit. Med. Bull., *14*: 141–145, 1958.

30. Wattenberg, L. W.   Studies of Polycyclic Hydrocarbon Hydroxylases of the Intestine Possibly Related to Cancer.   Cancer, *28*: 99–102, 1971.

31. Weisburger, J. H.   Colon Carcinogens: Their Metabolism and Mode of Action.   Cancer, *28*: 60–70, 1971.

32. Weisburger, J. H., Yamamoto, R. S., Williams, G. M., Grantham, P. H., Matsushima, T., and Weisburger, E. K.   On the Sulfate Ester of N-Hydroxy-N-2-fluorenyl-acetamide as a Key Ultimate Hepatocarcinogen in the Rat.   Cancer Res., *32*: 491–500, 1972.

33. Wittig, G., Wildner, G. P., und Ziebarth, D.   Der Einfluss der Ingesta auf die Kanzerisierung des Rattendarms durch Dimethylhydrazin.   Arch. Geschwulstforsch., *37*: 105–115, 1971.

34. Wynder, E. L., Kajitani, T., Ishikawa, S., Dodo, H., and Takano, A.   Environmental Factors of Cancer of the Colon and Rectum.   Cancer, *23*: 1210–1220, 1969.

Discussion of Paper by Dr. Weisburger

DR. HEIDELBERGER: Did the various diets you used affect the cancer incidence? Has the St. Mary's group in London actually demonstrated the production of carcinogens by an altered intestinal flora? Dr. Burkitt said that they have.

DR. WEISBURGER: Dr. Heidelberger, as chairman this morning, I failed to point out that in the United States at meetings of the American Association for Cancer Research in the last few years we have refrained from smoking, because we believe that this habit is an important cause of cancer in man.   But, with your question you have opened the door, if I may use a legalistic term, for a statement I meant to make at the conclusion of my lecture.

We are here in Japan, where cancer of the colon is still low, cancer of the prostate is low, cancer of the breast in women is low.   May the situation remain that way.   In Japan the major problems now are stomach cancer and liver cancer. If the trends followed in the United States and other Western countries are repeated here, cancer in stomach and liver will go down with the advent of better foodstuffs, containing perhaps less mycotoxins or nitrite-generated nitrosamines, for example.   Then, if the Japanese people avoid acquiring some of our poor Western-style dietary habits, Japan may be a remarkable country because all of its main types of cancer will be low.   I wish my Japanese colleagues and hosts luck in bringing to fruition this particular scheme, making Japan a perfect example of rationally based preventive medicine.

With the concentrations of carcinogen we used, the tumor incidence was similar on various diets.   I am afraid we tried to go too fast.   We gave high levels of the carcinogen, about twice the doses employed by Professor Druckrey and associates (7 mg/kg) when they saw almost exclusively colo-rectal cancer.   We noted, as I mentioned, some tumors in the small intestine.   There was no effect of diet discernible in respect to colon cancer incidence, except, of course, those animals on high fat diets that died early and, thus, did not have enough time to develop colon cancer.   The whole problem must be investigated further with much lower levels of carcinogens.

I have been in touch with Drs. Hill, Drasar and Williams of the St. Mary's Hospital group in London.   I am not aware that they have as yet demonstrated the presence of a colon carcinogen.   They are now working on the identification of several metabolites of steroids and of bile acids which are produced by the intestinal flora.   Tests of the carcinogenic activity of any such agents will be most important.

DR. SANDERS: When considering the causation of colon cancer, it is perhaps pertinent to remember the cytological peculiarities of the epithelial lining.   Not only is there continuous renewal of the epithelium from ileum cells in the crypts, and thus continuous cell division, but the cells differentiate as they move up the villi, so that there is continuous differentiation as well.   Thus, any agent that affects differentiation, *i.e.*, the pattern of expression of the genome, might be expected to have a high probability of acting at this site.

DR. WEISBURGER: Dr. Sanders, you are absolutely right.   In fact, Dr. Lipkin at Cornell University and New York Hospital has demonstrated that, whereas DNA synthesis, *i.e.*, thymidine incorporation, occurs in normal colon epithelial tissue only in the stem cells, in patients with colon cancer, DNA synthesis occurs all the way up on the crypts and there is less differentiation.   Dr. Lipkin is just now beginning a study of familial polyposis which is, as you know, a condition in which patients, genetically so disposed, develop polyps in the intestinal tract at a very early age. Later such polyps almost invariably end up as colon cancer.

I suggested that this condition might be perfectly analogous with colon epithelium to cases of *Xeroderma pigmentosum* in which deficient DNA repair systems have been pinpointed as the key defect.   This is why I am so interested in this morning's discussion, because it is directly related to what we mentioned just now, regarding my current concept and understanding of the problem of colon cancer in terms of faulty DNA repair.   Of course, these notions now need experimental exploration.

DR. HIGGINSON: Do you feel that your results should refer to colon, or colon and rectum? If so, can the animal model be used as a model for rectal carcinoma as well as colon carcinoma?

There is a different epidemiology for rectum and colon carcinoma.   A high incidence of colon and rectum carcinomas tends to show a similarity of patterns. However, while a very high incidence of colon cancer does not seem to occur in the absence of rectal carcinoma, the converse is even less true.

If colonic carcinoma is due to endogenous carcinogens, how would Dr. Weisburger explain the relatively different epidemiological patterns, *e.g.*, the normal frequency of rectal carcinoma in Japan and the low incidence of colonic carcinoma? Is this due to the fact that the human rectum is usually empty? Why have most epidemiological studies failed to show a correlation with constipation?

DR. WEISBURGER: Dr. Higginson, you raise many important questions.   I think all of us tend to oversimplify in our enthusiasm.   The metabolism studies I presented need still to be elaborated on and details refined.   We have done some preliminary work in examining some typical bacterial enzymes in the gut, such as β-glucuronidase, as a function of diet.   For example, with a natural diet high in residue (a commercial animal chow) and with a semisynthetic diet low in residue, I was quite amazed that the specific activity, units of enzyme per gram of fecal matter in rats, was quite similar.   Of course, the animals on the low residue diet put out much less fecal material and it had much less cecal content so the total amount of enzyme activity was much lower. β-Glucuronidase may be a poor model even though it is essential for liberating active carcinogen metabolites from conjugates.   We need to go into bacterial enzymes which metabolize steroids, bile acids, fats, or proteins, for example, to see if differences occur.

You will recall that the recent studies of Hill, Drasar *et al.* in London did seem to show quite a dramatic difference in the ratio of anaerobic to aerobic bacterial metabolic systems.   It could just be that some such system needs to be taken into account, even though one has doubts about the importance of the operation of aerobic reactions in the gut.   Of course, they isolated bacteria which in their test tubes are definitely aerobic.   But I wonder, under conditions of actual realistic use, whether or not these aerobic bacteria actually have a chance to operate.   Thus, the key question behind gut microflora is which metabolic enzyme systems are relevant to our question.   This is something we must investigate further.

Now lastly, I believe you asked me to elaborate on animal models and rectal cancer, that is, the problem of rectal versus colonic cancer.   As I mentioned, in animal models, irrespective of which agents you use, cancer develops at various sites all along the intestinal tract.   Indeed, the interesting and important studies of Drs. Narisawa and Sato we heard about this afternoon, where the agent MNNG is introduced intrarectally, seem to indicate to me at least that the colon mucosa down to the rectum is similarly sensitive all along.   Tumors were seen everywhere.   Thus, if you have distinct localization, it would suggest that one has a specific metabolism at certain points.   Frankly, with the system I proposed here, where we attribute operational significance to hydrolytic enzymes which split methylazoxymethanol glucuronide or an aminobiphenyl metabolite, it is clear that these enzymes exist way up in the cecum.   If this is true, we should not get cancers in the lower bowel, and yet we do.   That is why I say, we all tend to oversimplify.   We need to do much more.   I think we are at the beginning of an exciting series of experiments, and the contributions I have heard here this afternoon will help a great deal in focusing on this area.

Dr. Higginson, I think I should have said colon, mostly because as I understand it from discussions with my friends in Bethesda, who are versed in epidemiology, rectal cancer actually has a similar incidence here in Japan as in America or other Western countries, except for minor differences.   Therefore, some individuals in Bethesda, as well as my colleague Dr. Wynder in New York, visualize a different etiology for cancer in the colon in contrast to rectum.   However, in our experimental models, and also in others, as Dr. Druckrey so beautifully demonstrated this morning, we have not been able to distinguish this difference so far.   The chemical carcinogens used yield polyps and cancer in the colon as well as in the rectum.

Dr. Lawley: The mention of the possible importance of DNA " repair " leads to a discussion of the existence of several different mechanisms, some of which are more " error-prone " than others.   Further, different " lesions " may stimulate different repair mechanisms, *cf.*, the report by Dr. Stich.   Another factor may be differentiation, *e.g.*, Hahn has reported that some differentiated tissues do not repair, unless cell division is stimulated.   The interpretation of the effects of repair inhibition may, therefore, be complex, *e.g.*, inhibition of an " error-prone " mechanism could decrease mutagenesis and possibly inhibit tumor initiation.

DR. WEISBURGER: Dr. Lawley, I must say your points are certainly well taken. It is a novel idea to introduce the notion of repair in studies on induction mechanisms in colon cancer and cancer, in general.   Extensive experimental development is required, and I hope you will help.

DR. HEIDELBERGER: I agree with Dr. Lawley about the complexing of the DNA repair systems.   Just to illustrate this, human cells can repair DNA damage by excising thymine dimers following UV irradiation, whereas rodent cells repair DNA without excising thymine dimers.

DR. WEISBURGER: I agree, but this is, as I said before, where I have high hopes for Dr. Lipkin's project in collaboration with us.   We are studying critical enzymes in cases of familial polyposis not only in freshly collected human tissue samples, but also in cells from such patients grown *in vitro*.   Thus, we should be able to look specifically for these repair systems, or their decrease or absence, which we visualize to prevail under these conditions.

Rat Bladder Tumors Induced
by N-Butyl-N-(4-hydroxybutyl)nitrosamine

Nobuyuki Ito, Yoshio Hiasa, Keiji Toyoshima,* Eigoro Okajima,**
Yoshiyuki Kamamoto, Sachio Makiura, Yoshiteru Yokota,
Seiichi Sugihara, and Kinuko Matayoshi

First Department of Pathology, Nara Medical University, Nara, Japan

N-Butyl-N-(4-hydroxybutyl)nitrosamine is known as a potent carcinogen of the urinary bladder in rats and mice (*1, 2, 19, 32*).   This paper reports *in vivo* studies on the sensitivities of different strains of rats to N-butyl-N-(4-hydroxybutyl)nitrosamine and the effects of differences in doses and administration periods on bladder tumors induced by this carcinogen.   The effects on tumor growth of unilateral ureter ligation and treatment with another carcinogen before or after administration of N-butyl-N-(4-hydroxybutyl)nitrosamine were also studied.   Furthermore, the biological characteristics of cells of urinary bladder tumors in rats indued by N-butyl-N-(4-hydroxybutyl)nitrosamine were investigated *in vitro*.

Gross Findings on Bladder Tumors

N-Butyl-N-(4-hydroxybutyl)nitrosamine has been observed to induce tumors in various strains of rats and these developed only in the urinary bladder (*19, 30–32*). In the present work, in a very few cases, macroscopically detectable papillary tumors developed in the kidney, in the renal pelvis.   Many animals showed thickening of the urinary bladder wall, usually with vascular dilatation of the wall.   The large hypertrophic serosa of the bladder had an irregular surface and small miliary tumors were frequently seen on it.   Metastatic growth into the mesenteric or para-aortic lymph nodes was occasionally observed in rats which survived for long periods after treatment with carcinogens.   In the mucosa of the urinary bladder, white hyperplastic patches and papillomatous and hemorrhagic changes due to development of papillomatous tumors were usually seen after treatment with N-butyl-N-(4-hydroxybutyl)nitrosamine. Some urinary bladder tumors showed infiltrative growth into the bladder wall.

---

* Present address: Clinical Research Laboratory, Nara National Hospital, Nara, Japan
** Present address: Department of Urology, Nara Medical University, Nara, Japan

Microscopic Findings on Bladder Tumors

The normal distended bladder has a mucosal epithelium, 1 to 3 cells thick (Fig. 1). After carcinogenic treatment, there is a diffuse increase in cells, and nuclear irregularities are seen (Fig. 2). The focal changes of the bladder epithelium in rats treated with N-butyl-N-(4-hydroxybutyl)nitrosamine were of the following 3 kinds (*32*).

Hyperplasia—Thickening of the bladder epithelium (Fig. 3). This change was strictly localized and there was little stromal connective tissue. Nuclear irregularities and mitotic figures were rare.

Papilloma—Extensive epithelial proliferation, with a tendency to form papillomas (Fig. 4). Cellular irregularities were slight and a few mitotic figures were noticed in proliferative areas of the bladder epithelium.

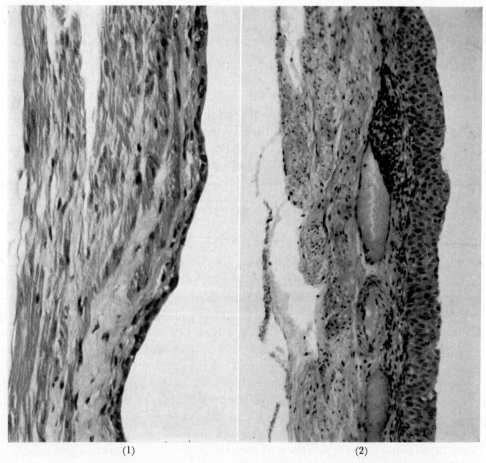

(1)   (2)

FIG. 1. Normal bladder epithelium. The epithelium is 1 to 3 cells thick. ×200.
FIG. 2. The bladder mucosal epithelium after carcinogen treatment shows a diffuse increase in cell number. ×100.

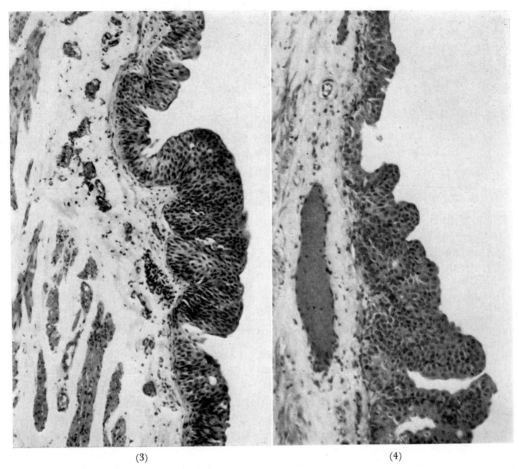

(3)   (4)

FIG. 3.   Focal hyperplasia of the bladder epithelium.   Nuclear irregularities and mitotic figures are rare.   ×100.

FIG. 4.   Extensive papillary proliferation of bladder epithelium.   A few mitotic figures are noticed in the proliferative area.   ×100.

Cancer—The tumors were usually transitional cell carcinomas (Fig. 5).   Squamous cell metaplasia and mitotic figures were frequent (Figs. 6 and 7).   Cystic degeneration, hemorrhage, and inflammatory changes in the stromal tissues were also noticed. Metastatic lesions had the same histological appearance as the primary areas of carcinoma (Fig. 8).   Papillomas and cancers resembled other chemically induced tumors (*10, 11, 14, 16, 17, 23, 24*) and also human bladder tumors (*20, 47, 48*).

Tumor Incidence

1)   Effect of the administration period of N-butyl-N-(4-hydroxybutyl)nitrosamine
   Male Wistar strain rats (Fuji Animal Farm, Tokyo), weighing an average of 150–160 g, were used.   Animals were given water containing 0.05% N-butyl-N-

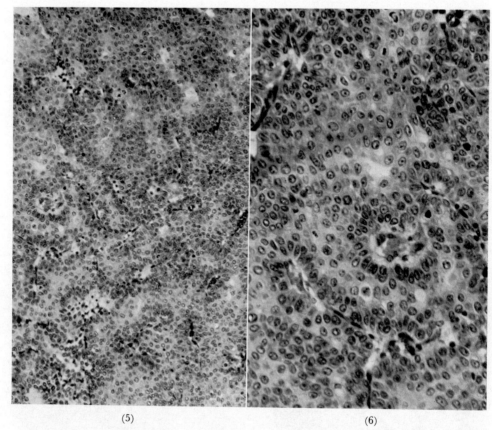

(5)   (6)

Fig. 5.   Transitional cell carcinoma of the bladder in a rat induced by N-butyl-N-(4-hydroxy-butyl)nitrosamine.   ×100.

Fig. 6.   Higher magnification of a transitional cell carcinoma of the bladder.   Many mitotic figures are seen.   ×200.

(4-hydroxybutyl)nitrosamine for 2, 4, 6, 8 or 12 weeks and then water without the carcinogen for 38, 36, 34, 32 or 28 weeks, respectively.   The histological changes in the urinary bladder after these periods of carcinogen administration are summarized in Table 1.

TABLE 1.   The Incidence of Tumors in Male Wistar Strain Rats Treated with 0.05% N-Butyl-N-(4-hydroxybutyl)nitrosamine (BBN) for Different Periods

Duration (weeks)		Number of rats	Body weight (g)		Changes in urinary bladder (%)		
with BBN	without BBN		Initial	Final	Hyperplasia	Papilloma	Cancer
2	38	18	167.6	504.4	12 (66.7)	6 (33.3)	0
4	36	11	162.7	526.4	11 (100.0)	8 (72.7)	2 (18.2)
6	34	17	166.8	469.6	16 (94.1)	15 (88.2)	11 (64.7)
8	32	10	166.3	452.0	10 (100.0)	9 (90.0)	9 (90.0)
12	28	9	166.5	386.2	9 (100.0)	9 (100.0)	9 (100.0)
0	38	5	167.6	425.8	0	0	0

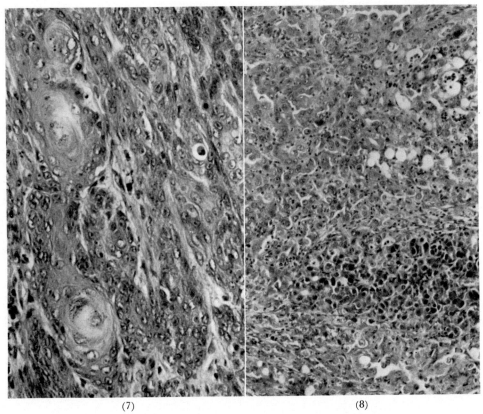

(7) (8)

Fig. 7. Squamous cell metaplasia observed in a bladder tumor. ×200.
Fig. 8. Metastatic lesion in a para-pancreatic lymph node. ×100.

After administering the carcinogen for 2 weeks and then carcinogen-free water for 38 weeks, 12 of the 18 rats (66.7%) developed hyperplasias of the urinary bladder epithelium. Six of the 18 rats (33.3%) developed papillomas, but none developed cancer. After administering the carcinogen for 4 weeks and then normal water for 36 weeks, all 11 rats developed hyperplasia of the urinary bladder epithelium. Eight of the 11 rats (72.7%) developed papillomas and 2 rats (18.2%) developed cancer of the bladder. After administering the carcinogen for 6 weeks, followed by carcinogen-free water for 34 weeks, 16 of the 17 rats (94.1%) developed hyperplasias, 15 rats (88.2%) developed papillomas, and 11 rats (64.7%) developed cancer. After administration of the carcinogen for 8 weeks and then normal water for 32 weeks, all 10 rats developed hyperplasia of the bladder epithelium, and 9 rats had papillomas and cancer of the bladder. After administration of the carcinogen for 12 weeks and then normal water for 28 weeks, all the animals developed hyperplasias, papillomas or cancers.

These results showed that histological changes of the urinary bladder epithelium in rats increase in frequency and extent as the period of N-butyl-N-(4-hydroxybutyl)nitrosamine administration increases. There was a large difference in the incidences of bladder cancer in the groups treated with carcinogen for 4 and 8 weeks. Previously, Ito *et al.* (*32*) observed differences in the incidence of cancer after the administration of the carcinogen for periods of up to 12 weeks, but in this previous work the observation period was only 20 weeks. It would be interesting to examine the difference in the pattern of incidence of cancer found with observation periods of 20 and 40 weeks.

2) *Effect of the dose*

Male Wistar strain rats were given 0.1% N-butyl-N-(4-hydroxybutyl)nitrosamine for 2 and 4 weeks and then normal water for 38 and 36 weeks, respectively, or 0.01% carcinogen for 20 and 40 weeks and then normal water for 20 and 0 weeks, respectively. Thus, the total intake of carcinogens in the two groups at each dose level was the same. The effects of these different doses on the incidences of tumors are shown in Table 2.

TABLE 2. Effects of the Differences in Doses of N-Butyl-N- (4-hydroxybutyl) nitrosamine (BBN) on the Incidence of Tumors in Male Wistar Strain Rats

Conc. of BBN in water (%)	Duration (weeks) with BBN	Duration (weeks) without BBN	Number of rats	Body weight(g) Initial	Body weight(g) Final	Hyperplasia	Changes in urinary bladder(%) Papilloma	Cancer
0.1	2	38	10	176.5	487.2	9 (90.0)	4 (40.0)	0
0.1	4	36	12	183.3	571.1	12 (100.0)	11 (91.7)	4 (33.3)
0.01	20	20	7	171.9	438.3	7 (100.0)	7 (100.0)	7 (100.0)
0.01	40	0	10	175.0	444.0	10 (100.0)	10 (100.0)	10 (100.0)

In the group receiving drinking water containing 0.1% N-butyl-N-(4-hydroxybutyl)nitrosamine for 2 weeks and then normal drinking water for 38 weeks, no bladder cancer was seen. In the group receiving water containing 0.1% carcinogen for 4 weeks and then normal water for 36 weeks, 4 of the 12 rats (33.3%) developed bladder cancer. However, in the groups receiving water containing 0.01% carcinogen for 20 or 40 weeks and then carcinogen-free water for 20 or 0 weeks, all animals developed cancer. These results suggest that continuous stimulation of the urinary bladder epithelium by the carcinogen is necessary for development of urinary bladder tumors in rats.

3) *Susceptibilities of different strains*

A significant difference was found in the induction of urinary bladder cancer in different strains of rats after the administration of water containing 0.05% N-butyl-N-(4-hydroxybutyl)nitrosamine for 8 weeks, and then normal water for 32 weeks. All the male ACI/NC rats (Fuji Animal Farm, Tokyo) tested developed bladder cancer, while 86% of the Wistar strain, 50% of the BDIX/N strain (originally from Prof. H. Druckrey, Freiburg, Germany), 40% of the Sprague-Dawley (JCL, Tokyo) and none of the Lewis strain (Fuji Animal Farm) rats tested developed cancer. Usually, in rats treated with N-butyl-N-(4-hydroxybutyl)nitrosamine, cancer only developed in the bladder (*29, 32*), but one case of transitional cell carcinoma of the

TABLE 3.   Strain Differences in the Incidence of Urinary Bladder Tumors in Male Rats Treated with 0.05% N-Butyl-N-(4-hydroxybutyl)nitrosamine (BBN) for 8 Weeks[a]

Strain	Number of rats	Changes in urinary bladder (%)			Change in kidney
		Hyperplasia	Papilloma	Cancer	
ACI/NC	6	6 (100.0)	6 (100.0)	6 (100.0)	0
Wistar	14	14 (100.0)	13 (92.3)	12 (85.7)	1[b]
BDIX/N	10	10 (100.0)	9 (90.0)	5 (50.0)	0
Sprague-Dawley	10	10 (100.0)	6 (60.0)	4 (40.0)	1[c]
Lewis	9	9 (100.0)	3 (33.3)	0	0

[a]   Examined after 40 weeks.
[b]   Transitional cell carcinoma in renal pelvis.
[c]   Nephroblastoma in renal cortex.

renal pelvis was seen in a Wistar strain rat and one case of nephroblastoma of the renal cortex was found in a Sprague-Dawley strain rat.

These results show that different strains of rats vary in susceptibility to the induction of bladder cancer by N-butyl-N-(4-hydroxybutyl)nitrosamine. Strain differences in carcinogenesis induced by ethionine were observed by Farber (25). It is known that β-glucuronidase activities in the liver, kidney and bladder differ in the ACI/NC, Wistar, BDIX, Sprague-Dawley and Lewis strains (30). However, no relationship between β-glucuronidase activity and the incidence of bladder tumors was observed. The factors causing the difference in the incidences of tumors in different strains require further study.

Effect of Unilateral Ureter Ligation

The middle or lower part of the left ureter of male Wistar strain rats was ligatured with cotton thread (33). Then, these animals and normal rats were given drinking water containing 0.025% N-butyl-N-(4-hydroxybutyl)nitrosamine for a period of 20 weeks. The incidences of bladder tumors in these animals are summarized in Table 4.

Cancers developed not only in the urinary bladder, but also in the renal pelvis and ureter. In the group with ligatured ureters that received the carcinogen, cancer developed in the renal pelvis in 9 of the 24 rats (37.5%), in the ureter in 5 rats (20.8%) and in the bladder in 23 rats (95.8%). However, no cases of cancer of the renal pelvis or ureter were seen in the group of normal rats receiving the carcinogen, although 11 of the 15 rats (73.3%) developed bladder cancer.

The carcinomas in the 3 different regions were all transitional cell carcinomas. These results show that stagnation of urine, containing an active carcinogen, in the renal pelvis, ureter and bladder may be important in the induction of tumors in the urinary system.

Studies on Implanted Urinary Bladders

The upper one-third of the urinary bladder of Wistar strain rats was resected

TABLE 4. Effect of the Ligation of the Left Ureter on the Development of Urinary System Tumors in Male Wistar Strain Rats Treated with 0.025% N-Butyl-N-(4-hydroxybutyl) nitrosamine (BBN) for 20 Weeks

Ureter ligation	BBN	Number of rats	Renal pelvis			Ureter			Urinary bladder		
			Hyperp.	Papill.	Cancer	Hyperp.	Papill.	Cancer	Hyperp.	Papill	Cancer
+	+	24	15 (62.5)	11 (45.8)	9 (37.5)	10 (41.7)	9 (37.5)	5 (20.8)	24 (100.0)	24 (100.0)	23 (95.8)
−	+	15	0	0	0	0	0	0	15 (100.0)	14 (93.3)	11 (73.3)
+	−	12	0	0	0	0	0	0	0	0	0
−	−	6	0	0	0	0	0	0	0	0	0

a) Hyperp., Hyperplasia; Papill., Papilloma.

TABLE 5. Changes in the Urinary Bladder and Implanted Bladder in the Wistar Strain Rats Treated with N-Butyl-N-(4-hydroxybutyl) nitrosamine (BBN)

Group	Sex[a]	Number of rats	Body weight (g)		Urinary bladder(%)			Implanted bladder		
			Initial	Final	Hyperplasia	Papilloma	Cancer	Hyperplasia	Papilloma	Cancer
BBN	M.	10	225.3	478.7	10 (100.0)	10 (100.0)	9 (90.0)	0	0	0
	F.	13	142.3	264.2	12 (92.3)	11 (84.5)	5 (38.5)	0	0	0
no BBN	M.	4	223.3	469.0	0	0	0	0	0	0
	F.	5	131.4	266.0	0	0	0	0	0	0

a) Male rats were given 0.01% BBN for 20 weeks and then normal water for 20 weeks and female rats were given 0.025% BBN for 20 weeks.

surgically. The resected region was then immediately implanted subcutaneously into the right side of the back. Starting 4 weeks later, these animals were given water containing 0.01% N-butyl-N-(4-hydroxybutyl)nitrosamine for 20 to 40 weeks (*29*). As seen in Table 5, no tumor developed in the implanted bladder after treatment with N-butyl-N-(4-hydroxybutyl)nitrosamine, but 90% of the rats developed transitional cell carcinomas in their functional bladder. Histologically, the mucosa area of the implanted bladder was 1 to 3 cells thick, while the muscular layer showed degenerative changes but no tumor was seen.

McDonald *et al.* (*37, 43*) showed that in dogs urinary constituents have a role in the production of bladder tumors induced by β-naphthylamine. If the carcinogen responsible for the development of bladder tumors induced by N-butyl-N-(4-hydroxybutyl)nitrosamine is carried in the blood, tumors should develop in the epithelium of the implanted bladder which has an intact blood supply. Thus, these results, together with the direct evidence obtained in the present work, indicate that bladder carcinogenesis induced by N-butyl-N-(4-hydroxybutyl)nitrosamine results from a urogenous stimulus.

Effect of N-Nitrosopiperidine

Male Wistar strain rats were divided into 5 groups. Animals were given water containing 0.05% N-butyl-N-(4-hydroxybutyl)nitrosamine for 8 weeks and/or were fed on a basal diet, containing 0.05% N-nitrosopiperidine for 4 weeks, following the schedule of carcinogen administration shown in Fig. 9. Cancer developed in the urinary bladder of 7 out of 9 rats (77.8%) in Group 1, while 30.0% and 45.5% of the animals in Groups 2 and 4, respectively, developed bladder cancer. The incidences of papillomas in Groups 2 and 4 were also lower than in Group 1. The

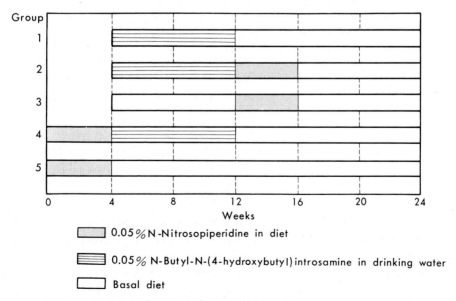

FIG. 9. Summary of schedule of carcinogen administration.

TABLE 6. Effects of Pre- or Posttreatment with 0.05% N-Nitrosopiperidine (NNP) on Rats Treated with 0.05% N-Butyl-N-(4-hydroxybutyl)nitrosamine (BBN)

Group[a]	Number of rats	Changes in urinary bladder(%)		
		Hyperplasia	Papilloma	Cancer
1 (BBN)	9	9 (100.0)	8 (88.9)	7 (77.8)
2 (BBN→NNP)	10	10 (100.0)	7 (70.0)	3 (30.0)
3 (NNP)	14	7 (50.0)	0	0
4 (NNP→BBN)	11	10 (90.9)	8 (72.7)	5 (45.5)
5 (NNP)	7	5 (71.4)	0	0

[a] For schedule of carcinogen administration, see Fig. 9.

results show that N-nitrosopiperidine inhibits bladder tumorigenesis in rats.   Two other chemical carcinogens were previously found to act antagonistically in rats (*28*), but the reason for this is not yet understood.

Changes in Long Term Survival after Administration of the Carcinogen

Male Wistar strain rats were given water containing 0.05% N-butyl-N-(4-hydroxybutyl) nitrosamine for 4 weeks and then normal water for 16, 36 or 56 weeks. Findings in these animals are summarized in Table 7.   The incidence of cancer of the bladder increased with an increase in the observation period.   Hyperplasia was found in 54.6% of the animals examined after 20 weeks and in 100% after 40 weeks, while after 60 weeks, the incidence had decreased.   The incidence of papillomas of the bladder showed the same pattern.   These results suggest that 2 types of hyperplastic precursor lesions may occur, namely, reversible and irreversible.   However, the change to papillomas is probably irreversible and later papillomas may change to cancers.

TABLE 7. Effect of Period after Administration of 0.05% N-Butyl-N-(4-hydroxybutyl)nitrosamine (BBN) on Bladder Changes in Male Wistar Strain Rats

Duration(weeks)		Observation period (weeks)	Number of rats	Body weight(g)		Changes in urinary bladder(%)		
with BBN	without BBN			Initial	Final	Hyperplasia	Papilloma	Cancer
4	16	20	11	160.2	430.9	6 (54.6)	1 (9.1)	0
4	36	40	11	162.7	526.4	11 (100.0)	8 (72.7)	2 (18.2)
4	56	60	11	172.0	510.8	9 (81.8)	7 (63.6)	4 (36.4)

In vitro Observations on Cells of Bladder Tumors

Cells of urinary bladder tumors (transitional cell carcinomas) induced in both a Wistar strain and a BDIX strain rat by N-butyl-N-(4-hydroxybutyl)nitrosamine and cells of a hyperplastic lesion of the urinary bladder epithelium in a BDIX strain rat treated with N-butyl-N-(4-hydroxybutyl)nitrosamine were cultured.   The methods used for tissue culture were as described previously (*46*).   Three cell lines were established: NBT-II (derived from the transitional cell carcinoma in the blad-

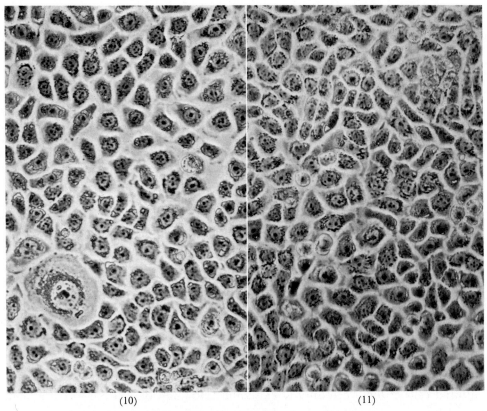

(10)   (11)

Fig. 10.   Phase-contrast micrograph of NBT-II cells.   ×100.
Fig. 11.   Phase-contrast micrograph of NBT-H cells.   ×100.

der of the Wistar rat), NBT-IV (derived from the transitional cell carcinoma in the bladder of the BDIX rat) and NBT-H (derived from the hyperplastic lesion of the bladder in the BDIX rat).

Under a phase-contrast microscope, cultures of these cell lines appeared as mosaic sheets of epithelium cells (Figs. 10 and 11).   Most cells were mononucleate, while a few had 2 or more nuclei.   Mitotic figures were seen.   There were no remarkable differences between the 3 cell lines.

The results obtained after the inoculation of the cultured cells into Wistar and BDIX strain rats are summarized in Table 8.   With NBT-II and -IV, the tumor developing at the site of the subcutaneous inoculation usually showed cystic changes, while with an intraperitoneal inoculation, disseminated tumors developed in the peritoneal cavity along with the formation of hemorrhagic ascites.   Microscopically, squamous cell carcinomas were observed with transitional cell carcinomas in some areas.   However, with NBT-H, no tumor formation was observed with either the subcutaneous or intraperitoneal inoculation.

The growth rates of culture cells in the 90th generation of NBT-II, 42nd generation of NBT-IV and 23rd generation of NBT-H were measured.   The results are shown in Fig. 12.   The cell numbers increased remarkably.   The growth rates of the

TABLE 8.   Transplantability of Cultured Urinary Bladder Tumor Cells

Cell line	Generation in culture	Culture days	Number of inoc. cells ($\times 10^6$)	Rat	Sex and number of rats	Site of inoc.	Number of rats with inoc. tumor	Av. observed survival in days[a]
NBT-II	70	675	1.3	Wistar(S)	M ; 3 F ; 2	I. P.	5	1	79
	74	713	2.5	„ (S)	M ; 4 F ; 3	I. P.	7	2	16
	94	805	2.5	„ (S)	F ; 3	I. P.	3	0	over 400
	96	813	10	„ (A)	F ; 4	I. P.	4	0	196
	108	873	3.0	„ (A)	M ; 1 F ; 1	I. P.	2	0	84
	108	873	3.0	„ (S)	M ; 1	S. C.	1	0	84
	108	873	1.0	„ (S)	M ; 1	S. C.	1	1	84
NBT-IV	5	135	2.5	BDIX(S)	M ; 2 F ; 3	S. C.	5	0	274
	10	195	0.8	„ (S)	M ; 2	S. C.	2	0	206
	12	204	5.0	„ (S)	M ; 3 F ; 2	S. C.	5	2	205
	19	328	2.5	„ (S)	M ; 3	I. P.	3	2	171
	38	461	1.3	„ (S)	M ; 2 F ; 5	I. P.	7	3	77
	43	479	1.0	„ (S)	M ; 1 F ; 2	I. P.	3	1	84
	43	479	3.0	„ (S)	F ; 1	S. C.	1	0	84
NBT-H	10	189	2.5	BDIX(S)	M ; 2 F ; 3	S. C.	5	0	220
	11	194	10	„ (S)	M ; 3 F ; 3	I. P.	6	0	214
	27	427	4.5	„ (A)	F ; 4	I. P.	4	0	188
	46	475	3.0	„ (S)	M ; 2 F ; 2	I. P.	4	0	106

(S), suckling ;   (A), adult ;   I. P., intraperitoneal ;   S. C., subcutaneous.
[a]   Survival period after inoculation.

cultured cells of the 3 cell lines were similar, although that of NBT-H was slightly lower than those of the others.   The chromosome numbers were examined in the 93rd generation of NBT-II, the 47th generation of NBT-IV and the 24th generation of NBT-H.   The cells examined showed a narrow range of chromosome numbers (Fig. 13).

DISCUSSION

Druckrey et al. (19) first reported that when N-butyl-N-(4-hydroxybutyl)-nitrosamine was given continuously in the drinking water for about 40 weeks, carcinomas of the squamous epithelium of the urinary bladder were selectively induced in all the BDIX strain rats tested.   Ito et al. (32) confirmed these results on the carcinogenic effect of N-butyl-N-(4-hydroxybutyl)nitrosamine on the urinary bladder of rats.   Histologically, the tumors, papillomas and carcinomas induced by N-butyl-N-(4-hydroxybutyl)nitrosamine were very similar to those produced after the administration of other chemical carcinogens (3–9, 12, 15, 18, 21, 22, 26, 27, 36, 38, 40–42, 44, 49, 50).

Before our work, there were few reports on the histogenesis of bladder tumors in rats treated with N-butyl-N-(4-hydroxybutyl)nitrosamine.   We observed diffuse growth of epithelial cells in the bladder of rats surviving for a long time after the administration of the carcinogen.   However, the hyperplastic changes of the bladder epithelium were of two types, reversible and irreversible.   Development of papil-

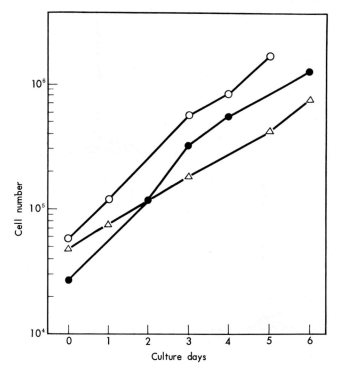

FIG. 12.   Growth rates of the 3 cell lines in Eagle's MEM with 20% calf serum.
○———○, NBT-IV (42nd generation); ●———●, NBT-II (90th generation); △———△,
NBT-H (23rd generation)

lomas and cancers were irreversible changes.   A diagram of the histogenesis of urinary bladder tumors induced with N-butyl-N-(4-hydroxybutyl)nitrosamine, based on the present work, is shown in Fig. 14.

In recent studies on the metabolism of N-butyl-N-(4-hydroxybutyl) nitrosamine in rats, Suzuki and Okada (45) did not find N-butyl-N-(4-hydroxybutyl)nitrosamine, as such, in the urine, but instead they identified N-butyl-N-(4-butyric acid) nitrosamine and a glucuronide type of compound in the urine.   These results suggest that a proximate derivative of N-butyl-N-(4-hydroxybutyl)nitrosamine may have a potent carcinogenic action on rat bladder.   The results of the ligation of one ureter show that, whereas the transitional epithelium of the renal pelvis, ureter and bladder seems to be susceptible to the carcinogenic action of N-butyl-N-(4-hydroxybutyl)nitrosamine, the renal parenchyma seems to be resistant.

We isolated 3 lines of cells from the bladder tumors induced by N-butyl-N-(4-hydroxybutyl)nitrosamine.   There are few previous reports on the biological characteristics of cultured bladder cells (13, 34, 35, 39).   Our 3 cell lines derived from urinary bladder tumors should be useful in studies on the biochemistry, biology and ultrastructure of these cells.

The interaction of other chemical carcinogens with N-butyl-N-(4-hydroxybutyl)nitrosamine, the fate of the latter, and the histological analysis of the cancer cells *in vivo* and *in vitro* require further study.

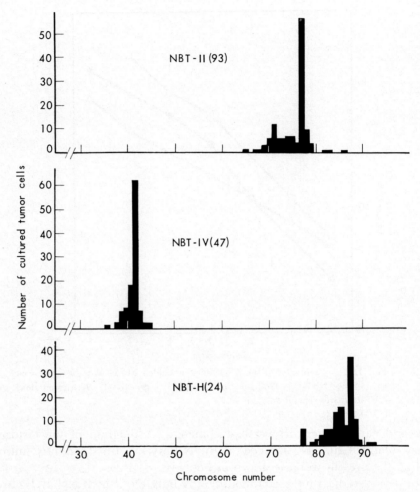

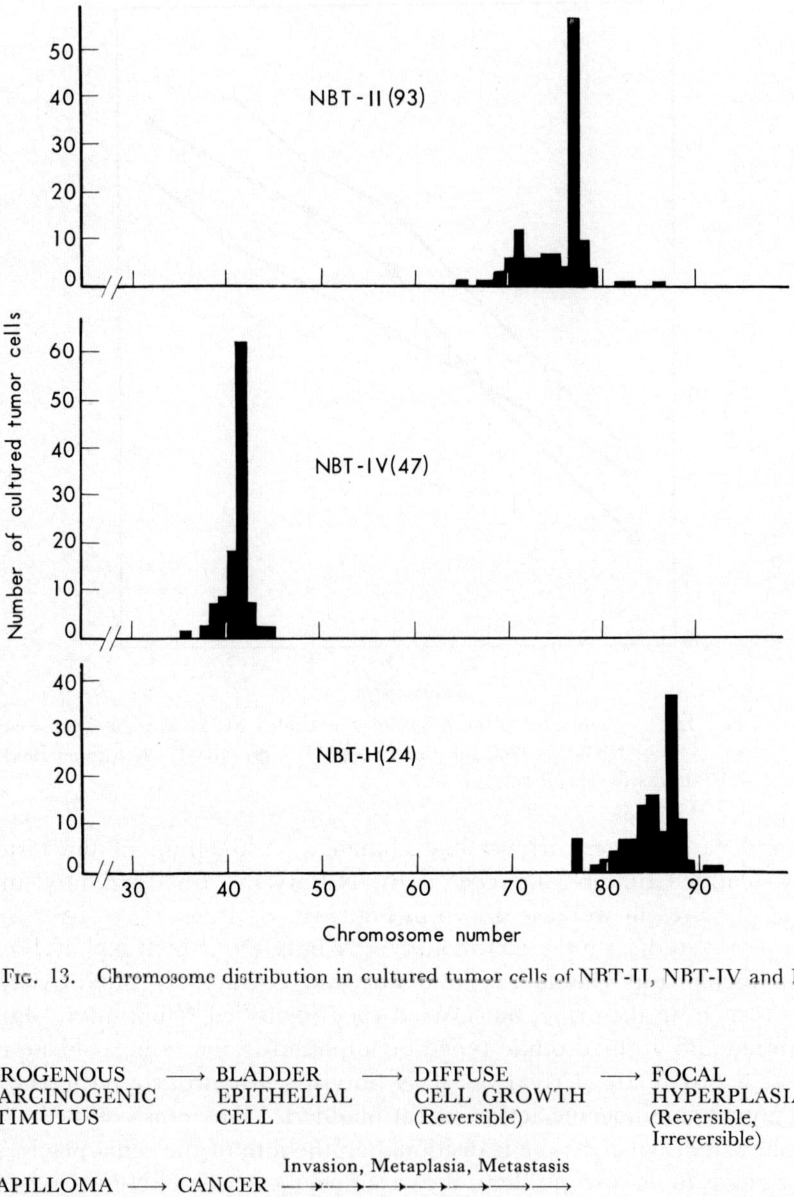

Fig. 13.   Chromosome distribution in cultured tumor cells of NBT-II, NBT-IV and NBT-H.

UROGENOUS	→	BLADDER	→	DIFFUSE	→	FOCAL	→
CARCINOGENIC		EPITHELIAL		CELL GROWTH		HYPERPLASIA	
STIMULUS		CELL		(Reversible)		(Reversible,	
						Irreversible)	

Invasion, Metaplasia, Metastasis

PAPILLOMA → CANCER ⟶⟶⟶⟶⟶⟶⟶
(Irreversible)

Fig. 14.   Histogenesis of urinary bladder cancer induced by N-butyl-N-(4-hydroxybutyl) nitrosamine.

SUMMARY

N-Butyl-N-(4-hydroxybutyl)nitrosamine is known to be a potent carcinogen, capable of selectively inducing urinary bladder tumors in rats and mice. The present work was on the histogenesis and biological characteristics of bladder tumors in rats. The incidences of urinary bladder tumors in rats were influenced by the administration period and dosage of the carcinogen, the strain of rats and the observation period after treatment with the carcinogens. Ligation of one ureter promoted bladder tumorigenesis in rats treated with N-butyl-N-(4-hydroxybutyl) nitrosamine, while pre- or posttreatment with N-nitrosopiperidine inhibited it. Experiments on an implanted bladder showed that a urogenous stimulus had a direct tumorigenic action on the bladder mucosa. Two cell lines derived from bladder cancers and one cell line derived from a hyperplastic lesion were established in tissue culture. The biological specificities of these cells were investigated.

This work was supported in part by a grant-in-aid for scientific research from the Japanese Ministry of Education, a grant from the Tokyo Biochemical Research Foundation and a grant from the Nara Anti-Cancer Association, which we gratefully wish to acknowledge.

REFERENCES

1. Akagi, G., Akagi, A., and Kimura, M. Tumor of Urinary Bladder Induced by N-Butyl-N-butanol(4)nitrosamine (BBN) in Mice and Rats. Proc. Japan Cancer Assoc., 29th Ann. Meeting, p. 65, 1970.

2. Akagi, G., Akagi, A., and Kimura, M. Changes of DNA Content during Urinary Bladder Carcinogenesis in Rats. Proc. Japan Cancer Assoc., 30th Ann. Meeting, p. 2, 1971.

3. Allen, M. J., Boyland, E., Duked, C. E., Herning, E. S., and Watson, J. G. A. Cancer of the Urinary Bladder Induced in Mice with Metabolites of Aromatic Amines and Tryptophan. Brit. J. Cancer, 11: 212–228, 1957.

4. Armstrong, E. C., and Bonser, G. M. Epithelial Tumors of the Urinary Bladder in Mice Induced by 2-Acetylaminofluorene. J. Path. Bact., 56: 507–512, 1944.

5. Battifora, H. A., Eisenstein, R., Sky-Peck, H. H., and McDonald, J. H. Electron Microscopy and Tritiated Thymidine in Gradation of Malignancy of Human Bladder Carcinomas. J. Urol., 93: 217–223, 1965.

6. Bonser, G. M. The Experimental Induction of Cancer of the Bladder. Acta Unio Intern. Contra Cancrum, 18: 538–544, 1962.

7. Bonser, G. M., Boyland, E., Busby, E. R., Clayson, D. B., Grover, P. L., and Jull, J. W. A Further Study of Bladder Implantation in the Mouse as a Means of Detecting Carcinogenic Activity: Use of Crushed Paraffin Wax or Stearic Acid as the Vehicle. Brit. J. Cancer, 17: 127–136, 1963.

8. Bonser, G. M., Bradshaw, L., Clayson, D. B., and Jull, J. W. A Further Study on the Carcinogenic Properties of ortho Hydroxy-amines and Related Compounds by Bladder Implantation in the Mouse. Brit. J. Cancer, 10: 539–546, 1956.

9. Boyland, E., Busby, E. R., Dukes, C. E., Grover, P. L., and Manson, D. Further Experiments on Implantation of Materials into the Urinary Bladder of Mice. Brit. J. Cancer, 18: 575–581, 1964.

10. Boyland, E., Dukes, C. E., and Grober, P. L. Carcinogenicity of 2-Naphthylhydroxylamine and 2-Naphthylamine. Brit. J. Cancer, 17: 79–84, 1963.

11. Boyland, E., Harris, J., and Horning, E. S. The Induction of Carcinoma of the Bladder in Rats with Acetamidofluorene. Brit. J. Cancer, 8: 647–654, 1954.

12. Boyland, E., Kinder, C. H., and Manson, D. The Biochemistry of Aromatic

Amines 8 Synthesis and Detection of Di-(2-amino-1-naphthyl)hydrogen phosphate, a Metabolite of 2-Naphthylamine in Dogs. Biochem. J., *75*: 175–179, 1961.

13. Bregman, R. U., and Bregman, E. T. Tissue Culture of Benign and Malignant Human Genitourinary Tumors. J. Urol., *86*: 642–649, 1961.

14. Bryan, G. T., Brown, R. R., and Price, J. M. Incidence of Mouse Bladder Tumors Following Implantation of Paraffin Pellets Containing Certain Tryptophan Metabolites. Cancer Res., *24*: 582–585, 1964.

15. Clayson, D. B., Jull, J. W., and Bonser, G. M. The Testing of *ortho* Hydroxy-amines and Related Compounds by Bladder Implantation and a Discussion of Their Structural Requirements for Carcinogenic Activity. Brit. J. Cancer, *12*: 222–230, 1958.

16. Clayson, D. B., Pringle, J. A. S., and Bonser, G. M. The Carcinogenic Action of 2-Aminodiphenylene Oxide and 4-Aminodiphenyl on the Bladder and Liver of the $C_{57} \times IF$ Mouse. Brit. J. Cancer, *21*: 755–762, 1967.

17. Clayson, D. B., Pringle, J. A. S., and Bonser, G. M. 4-Ethylsulphonylnaphthalene-1-sulphonamide: A New Chemical for the Study of Bladder Cancer in the Mouse. Biochem. Pharmacol., *16*: 619–626, 1967.

18. Druckrey, H., Preussmann, R., Ivankovic, S., und Schmähl, D. Organotrope carcinogene Wirkungen bei 65 verschiedenen N-Nitroso-Verbindungen an BD-ratten. Z. Krebsforsch, *69*: 103–201, 1967.

19. Druckrey, H., Preussmann, R., Ivankovic, S., und Schmidt, C. H. Selektive Erzeugung von Blasenkrebs an Ratten durch Dibutyl- und N-Butyl-N-butanol (4) nitrosamin. Z. Krebsforsch., *66*: 280–290, 1964.

20. Dukes, C. E. Tumors of the Bladder, p. 105, E. & S. Livingstone, Edinburgh, 1959.

21. Dunning, W. F., Curtis, M. R., and Maun, M. E. The Effect of Added Dietary Tryptophane on the Occurrence of 2-Acetylaminofluorene-induced Liver and Bladder Cancer in Rats. Cancer Res., *10*: 454–459, 1950.

22. Ertürk, E., Cohen, S. M., and Bryan, G. T. Urinary Bladder Carcinogenicity of N-[4-(5-Nitro-2-furyl)-2-thiazolyl]formamide in Female Swiss Mice. Cancer Res., *30*: 1309–1311, 1970.

23. Ertürk, E., Cohen, S. M., Price, J. M., and Bryan, G. T. Pathogenesis, Histology, and Transplantability of Urinary Bladder Carcinomas Induced in Albino Rats by Oral Administration of N-[4-(5-Nitro-2-furyl)-2-thiazolyl]formamide. Cancer Res., *29*: 2219–2228, 1969.

24. Ertürk, E., Price, J. M., Morris, J. E., Cohen, S. M., Leith, R. S., Von Esch, A. M., and Crovetti, A. J. The Production of Carcinoma of the Urinary Bladder in Rats by Feeding N-[4-(5-Nitro-2-furyl)-2-thiazolyl]formamide. Cancer Res., *27*: 1998–2002, 1967.

25. Farber, E. Ethionine Carcinogenesis. Advan. Cancer Res., *7*: 383–474, 1963.

26. Goldblatt, M. W., Henson, A. F., and Somerville, A. R. Metabolism of Bladder Carcinogens. III. The Metabolic Path of 2-[8-^{14}C]Naphthylamine in Several Animal Species. Biochem. J., *77*: 511–516, 1960.

27. Irving, C. C., Gutmann, H. R., and Larson, D. M. Evaluation of the Carcinogenicity of Aminofluorenols by Implantation into the Bladder of the Mouse. Cancer Res., *23*: 1782–1791, 1963.

28. Ito, N., and Farber, E. Effects of Trypan Blue on Hepatocarcinogenesis in Rats Given Ethionine or N-2-Fluorenylacetamide. J. Natl. Cancer Inst., *37*: 775–785, 1966.

29. Ito, N., Hiasa, Y., Kamamoto, Y., Makiura, S., Sugihara, S., Marugami, M., and

Okajima, E.   Histopathological Analysis of Kidney Tumors in Rats Induced by Chemical Carcinogens. Gann, *62*: 435–444, 1971.

30. Ito, N., Hiasa, Y., Kamamoto, Y., Makiura, S., Yokota, Y., Sugihara, S., Matayoshi, K., and Okajima, E.   Various Factors on the Development of Urinary Bladder Tumors in Rats Induced by N-Butyl-N-(4-hydroxybutyl)nitrosamine. Proc. Japan. Cancer Assoc., 30th Ann. Meeting, p. 2, 1971.

31. Ito, N., Hiasa, Y., Tamai, A., Kamamoto, Y., Makiura, S., and Okajima, E.   Studies on the Developmental Conditions of the Urinary System Tumors in Rats Induced by N-Butyl-N-(4–hydroxybutyl)nitrosamine. Proc. Japan. Cancer Assoc., 28th Ann. Meeting, p. 61, 1969.

32. Ito, N., Hiasa, Y., Tamai, A., Okajima, E., and Kitamura, H.   Histogenesis of Urinary Bladder Tumors Induced by N-Butyl-N-(4-hydroxybutyl)nitrosamine in Rats. Gann, *60*: 401–410, 1969.

33. Ito, N., Makiura, S., Yokota, Y., Kamamoto, Y., Hiasa, Y., and Sugihara, S.   Effect of Unilateral Ureter Ligation on Development of Tumors in the Urinary System of Rats Treated with N-Butyl-N-(4-hydroxybutyl)nitrosamine. Gann, *62*: 359–365, 1971.

34. Kamamoto, Y., Matayoshi, K., Hiasa, Y., Makiura, S., Sugihara, S., Marugami, M., and Ito, N.   Comparison on Three Cell Lines of Urinary Bladder Tumor in Rats and Effects of Bleomycin (A$_2$). Proc. Japan. Cancer Assoc., 30th Ann. Meeting, p. 239, 1971.

35. Lavin, P., and Koss, L. G.   Studies of Experimental Bladder Carcinoma in Fischer 344 Female Rats.   II.   Characterization of 3 Cell Lines Derived from Induced Urinary Bladder Carcinomas. J. Natl. Cancer Inst., *46*: 597–614, 1971.

36. Magee, P. N., and Barnes, J. M.   Carcinogenic Nitroso Compounds. Advan. Cancer Res., *10*: 163–246, 1967.

37. McDonald, D. F., and Lund, R. R.   The Role of the Urine in Vesical Neoplasm.   I.   Experimental Confirmation of the Urogenous Theory of Pathogenesis. J. Urol., *71*: 560–570, 1954.

38. Melicow, M. M., Uson, A. C., and Prise, T. D.   Bladder Tumor Induction in Rats Fed 2-Acetamidofluorene (2-AAF) and a Pyridoxine Deficient Diet. J. Urol., *91*: 520–529, 1964.

39. Okajima, E.   Studies on the Incidence of Experimental Bladder Tumor by 20-Methylcholanthrene and 4-Nitroquinoline-N-oxide, and on the Cellular Characteristics of Its Tumor by Tissue Culture.   II.   The Study on the Tissue Culture of Experimental Bladder Tumor Induced by 20-Methylcholanthrene and 4-Nitroquinoline-N-oxide. J. Nara Med. Assoc., *15*: 21–58, 1964 (in Japanese).

40. Okajima, E., Hiramatsu, T., Motomiya, Y., Iriya, K., Ijuin, M., and Ito, N.   Effect of DL-Tryptophan on Tumorigenesis in the Bladder and Liver of Rats Treated with N-Nitrosodibutylamine. Gann, *62*: 163–169, 1971.

41. Oyasu, R., Miller, D. A., McDonald, J. H., and Hass, G. M.   Neoplasma of Rat Urinary Bladder and Liver.   Rats Fed 2-Acetylaminofluorene and Indole. Arch. Pathol., *75*: 184–190, 1963.

42. Rodomski, J. L., Brill, E., and Glass, E. M.   Induction of Bladder Tumors and Other Malignancies in Rats with 2-Methoxy-3-aminodibenzofuran. J. Natl. Cancer Inst., *39*: 1069–1080, 1967.

43. Scott, W. W., and Boyd, H. L.   A Study of Carcinogenic Effect of beta-Naphthylamine on the Normal and Substituted Isolated Sinmoid Loop Bladder of Dogs. J. Urol., *70*: 914–925, 1953.

44. Strombeck, J. P., and Ekman, B.   Effect of 2-Acetylaminofluorene in Inducing Tumors of the Bladder.   Acta Pathol. Microbiol. Scand., *26*: 480–495, 1949.
45. Suzuki, E., and Okada, M.   Metabolism of N-Butyl-N-(4-hydroxybutyl)nitrosamine in the Rat.   Proc. Japan. Cancer Assoc., 30th Ann. Meeting, p. 3, 1971.
46. Toyoshima, K., Ito, N., Hiasa, Y., Makiura, S., and Kamamoto, Y.   Tissue Culture of Urinary Bladder Tumor Induced in a Rat by N-Butyl-N-(4-hydroxybutyl)nitrosamine: Establishment of Cell Line, Nara Bladder Tumor II.   J. Natl. Cancer Inst., *47*: 979–986, 1971.
47. Veenema, R. J., Fingerhut, B., and Girgis, A. S.   Histochemistry: A Possible Guide to Therapy of Bladder Tumors.   J. Urol., *90*: 736–746, 1963.
48. Veenema, R. J., Fingerhut, B., and Lattimer, J. K.   Experimental Studies on the Biological Potential of Bladder Tumors.   J. Urol., *93*: 202–211, 1965.
49. Walpole, A. L., Williams, M. H. C., and Roberts, D. C.   Bladder Tumors Induced in Rats of Two Strains with 3:2′ Dimethyl-4-aminodiphenyl.   Brit. J. Cancer, *9*: 170–176, 1955.
50. Weisburger, J. H., Hadidian, Z., Fredrickson, T. N., and Weisburger, E. K.   Bladder Cancer, A Symposium, 45, Birmingham; Esculpius Publ. Co., 1966.

Discussion of Paper by Drs. Ito et al.

Dr. Okada: The selective induction of bladder cancer in rats using dibutylnitrosamine (DBN) and butyl(4-hydroxybutyl)nitrosamine (BBN) was reported in 1964
by Professor Druckrey and his co-workers.   In their paper, in which the biochemical
mechanism and the importance of the terminal hydroxylation for the organotropic
effect of the nitrosamine were discussed (Fig. I), they mentioned briefly about the
metabolism of DBN.

Now, I would like to present the preliminary results of our work on the metabolism of BBN in the rat after oral administration in large doses (Fig. II).   Five
hundred mg of BBN was given orally to a Wistar rat and 48-hr urine was collected.
The urine was acidified to pH 1 and extracted with chloroform or methylene
chloride.   In the organic layer (A), no BBN could be detected by thin-layer chro-

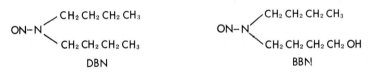

Fig. I.   Chemical structure of DBN and BBN.

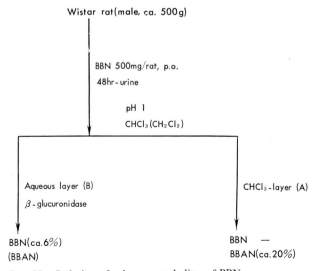

Fig. II.   Isolation of urinary metabolites of BBN.

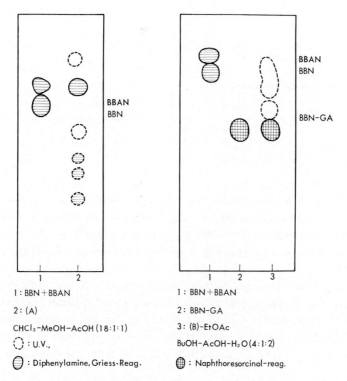

FIG. III. Thin-layer chromatography of urinary metabolities of BBN.

matography, while butyl(3-carboxypropyl)nitrosamine (BBAN) was obtained from (A) in about 20% of the dosage, whose identification will be mentioned later. On the other hand, the aqueous layer (B), in which no BBN or BBAN were detected by thin-layer chromatography, was hydrolyzed with beef liver β-glucuronidase to produce BBN in about 6% of the dosage.   The appearance of BBAN was also demonstrated by thin-layer chromatography after the enzymatic hydrolysis of (B).

Figure III shows the thin-layer chromatograms of (A) and (B) together with the authentic reference samples.   As seen in this chromatogram, no BBN was detected in (A).   Since the glucuronide in (B) was found to be easily extractable with ethyl acetate, the ethyl acetate extract of (B) was used here.   The principal metabolite in (B), giving positive tests for both nitroso group and glucuronic acid, was identified with the glucuronide of BBN (BBN-GA) which was prepared in a clear-cut manner that will be mentioned later on.

Figure IV indicates the preparation of BBAN from BBN.   The methyl ester of BBAN was also prepared.   BBAN isolated from rat urine as well as its methyl ester

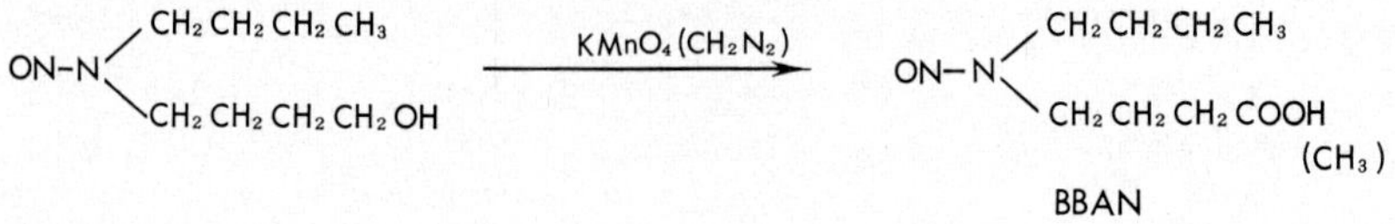

FIG. IV. Preparation of BBAN and its methyl ester from BBN.

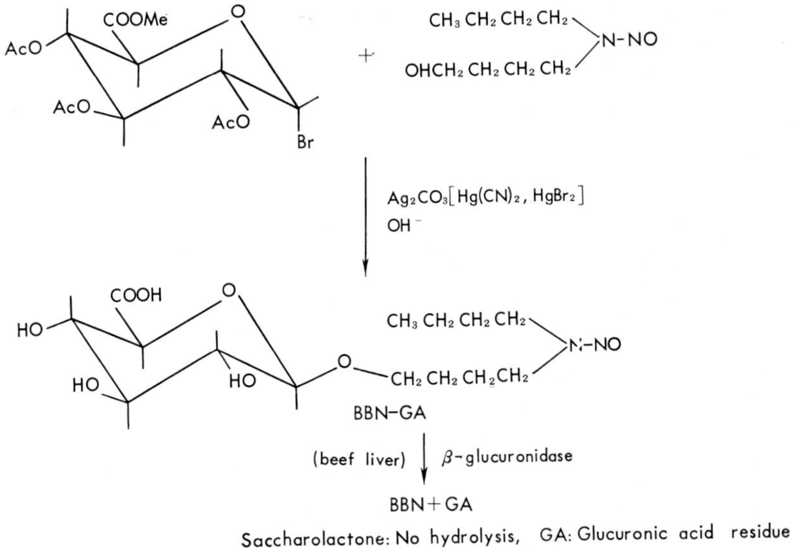

FIG. V. Synthesis of BBN-GA (β-D-glucosiduronate of BBN).

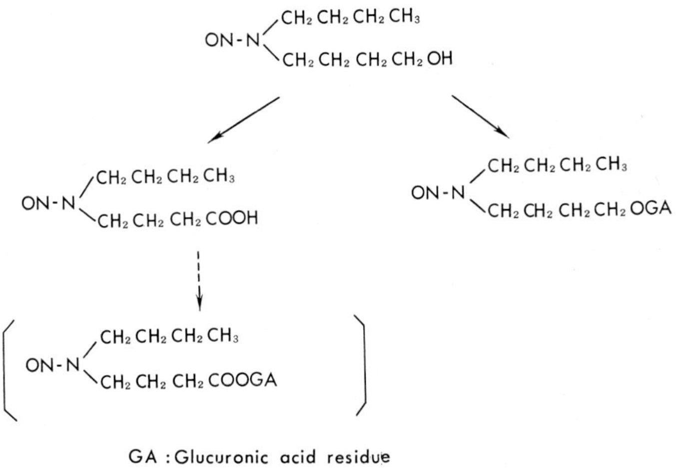

GA : Glucuronic acid residue

FIG. VI. Principal metabolic pathway of BBN in the rat.

was identical with the respective authentic specimen under the usual criteria, namely, thin-layer chromatography, infrared spectrum, NMR spectrum, and so on.

Figure V shows the preparation of BBN-GA. It was accomplished according to the usual method of glucuronide synthesis, as indicated. The synthetic BBN-GA was hydrolyzed by beef liver β-glucuronidase to afford BBN and glucuronic acid. The addition of saccharolactone, a specific β-glucuronidase inhibitor, to the incubation mixture prevented its complete hydrolysis.

In short, so far as a urinary metabolite having a nitroso group is concerned,

TABLE I.   Urinary Excretion of BBAN after Administration of BBN, BBAN and DBN to the Rat.

BBN	p.o.	*ca.* 20%	(4)
BBAN	p.o.	42–48%	(2)
DBN	p.o.	3– 8%	(3)
	s.c.	8–13%	(2)

BBN administered orally in the rat underwent mainly ω-oxidation to yield BBAN, while a part of the BBN was excreted in urine as the glucuronic acid conjugate.   No BBN was excreted intact in the urine (Fig. VI).

In view of the fact that a large quantity of BBAN was excreted in rat urine after oral administration of BBN, the urinary excretion of BBAN has been determined after administration of BBAN itself and DBN.   The preliminary results are shown in Table I.   About 45% of the orally administered BBAN was recovered unchanged from the urine.   While about 6% of the dosage was recovered as BBAN after oral administration of DBN, the subcutaneous injection of DBN resulted in the recovery of about 10% as BBAN.   This result seems to be interesting as well as significant in connection with the observations reported by Professor Druckrey and his co-workers about DBN, concerning the different frequencies of the production of bladder carcinomas between oral and subcutaneous administrations.

To determine the carcinogenic action of BBAN on rat urinary bladder as compared with that of BBN, an animal test is now under way in our laboratory.   Although the test is not yet finished, the preliminary result indicates definitely that BBAN is a more potent bladder carcinogen than BBN in the rat.   Thus, BBAN could be regarded as the so-called proximate form of BBN, as well as of DBN, the latter being metabolized through BBN to BBAN.

DR. SANDERS: Concerning the 3 established cell lines from bladder epithelium affected by BBN, are these cell lines in the strict sense—*i.e.*, capable of continuous propagation *in vitro* in cell strains, which will eventually undergo a " crisis " and fail to grow further *in vitro*?

Have you succeeded in establishing cell strains *in vitro* from a normal bladder?

In regard to your cell line NBT-H, which has hyperplastic bladder epithelium and which does not cause tumors when inoculated *in vivo*, is it affected in any way by further treatment with carcinogens *in vitro*?

DR. ITO: Already, all 3 cell lines are established.   However, we have never had any cell strains from a normal bladder.   About NBT-H, we have tried some treatment for inoculation, but we are still preparing the results.

DR. MAGEE: Dr. Marian Hicks, Middlessex Hospital Medical School, London, England, has induced bladder cancer in rats by 3 injections of N-nitrosomethylurea into the bladder lumen but failed to induce those tumors with a single similar injection.   What was the condition of the liver in the rats given nitrosopiperidine as well as BBN?   Will damage to the liver affect the metabolism of BBN?

DR. ITO: Very little liver damage was seen after treatment with N-nitrosopiperi-dine.   These findings were essentially the same as with NNP plus BBN.

DR. WEISBURGER: Are there any data about the production of BBAN in animals pretreated with nitrosopiperidine?

Did animals receiving nitrosopiperidine after BBN die of liver cancer? Could this account for the lower incidence of bladder cancer?

DR. ITO: I never tried pretreatment with nitrosopiperidine.   The animals were killed after only 5 months by carcinogenesis.   No liver cancer was observed.

DR. DAWE: I would simply like to comment that it is interesting that when you returned your cell line, derived from transitional cell carcinomas, back to sub-cutaneous tissue, the resulting tumors were squamous cell carcinomas.   This may very well reflect the different behavior of neoplastic epithelium when deprived of its usual stroma.   One wonders whether this change in morphologic expression is reversible or not.   It might be interesting to see how your cell lines behave when transplanted back into the bladder mucosa.

DR. ITO: We observed that squamous cell carcinomas were caused by inoculation into the intraperitoneal cavity and subcutaneous tissue of NBT-II and IV.   We never investigated whether the process was irreversible or not.

Influence of Disulfiram (Tetraethylthiuramdifulfide) on the Biological Actions of N-Nitrosamines

D. Schmähl and F. W. Krüger

The Institute of Experimental Toxicology and Chemotherapy, German Cancer Research Center, Heidelberg, West Germany

It is generally agreed that nitrosamines are not toxic themselves, but have to be metabolized to form a toxic and probably a carcinogenic intermediate. As was shown for dimethylnitrosamine (DMNA), the acute toxic effect is correlated with the formation of an alkylating agent (*4, 9, 15, 21*), which may be responsible for liver necrosis as well as for lung and liver hemorrhages, observed after the application of this compound. Reduction of this acute toxic effect has been recently reported by Fiume and co-workers (*4*) after an additional application of aminoacetonitrile, which also led to a reduced metabolism of DMNA, a decreased methylation of nucleic acids and a diminished incorporation of the ^{14}C activity into proteins.

Recently Scholler and his co-workers (*18*) described how the hepatotoxic effect of chloroform ($CHCl_3$) could be considerably reduced after an additional application of tetraethylthiuramdisulfide (disulfiram [DSF], Antabus®).

$$H_5\text{-}C_2 \diagdown \quad \overset{\text{S}}{\underset{}{\|}} \quad \diagup C_2H_5$$
$$\text{N-C-S-S-C-N}$$
$$H_5\text{-}C_2 \diagup \quad \underset{\text{S}}{\underset{}{\|}} \quad \diagdown C_2H_5$$

Antabus®, disulfiram.

Since it is known that chloroform as well as DMNA is not toxic *per se*, but has to be metabolized into a reactive intermediate, the aim of the study presented here was to investigate whether the toxicity of DMNA can be reduced by simultaneous application of DSF and whether this reduction is due to a diminished formation of an alkylating intermediate.

Since the amount of alkylating intermediates formed in the metabolism of higher nitrosamines (diethyl-, dipropyl- and dibutylnitrosamine) is comparatively small, we also investigated whether the toxic action of these compounds can be reduced.

Furthermore, it seemed to be relevant to investigate whether there is a correlation between the toxic and the carcinogenic activity of DMNA with reference to an additional treatment with DSF.

Toxicological and Biochemical Investigations

In these studies several hundred female Swiss and NMRI mice with an average weight of 20–25 g female and male Sprague-Dawley and BR 46 rats with an average weight of 250–350 g were used. Animals were maintained on an Altromin® pellet diet and unlimited water. DSF was applied orally through a stomach tube, suspended in a 4% starch solution, after the animals had been starved for 12 hr. DMNA was given in an aqueous solution, i.v., i.p. or orally. Animals that died were dissected and the livers examined histologically. The time of observation was limited to 10 days after treatment.

As can be seen in Fig. 1 and Table 1, a treatment 2 hr before the injection with 500 mg/kg DSF increased the LD_{50} to double its value in female NMRI mice as well

TABLE 1. Influence of Oral Disulfiram (DSF) Pretreatment (500 mg/kg) 2 hr before the Dimethylnitrosamine (DMNA) Application on DMNA Toxicity in Female Swiss Mice and Sprague-Dawley Rats

Species	DMNA mg/kg	DSF mg/kg	Number of animals survivors/died	LD_{50} mg/kg
Mouses	10 i. p.	—	6/0	
	14 ,,	—	9/3	
	16 ,,	—	2/10	15
	19 ,,	—	0/12	
	28 ,,	—	0/26	
	28 ,,	500 orally	7/13	27
Rat	45 orally	—	11/1	
	65 ,,	—	4/8	63
	75 ,,	—	0/12	
	100 ,,	500 orally	5/1	
	150 ,,	500 ,,	3/3	150
	200 ,,	500 ,,	2/4	
	250 ,,	500 ,,	0/6	
Rat	60 i. v.	—	4/2	
	80 ,,	—	0/6	
	110 ,,	—	0/6	63
	140 ,,	—	0/6	
	180 ,,	—	0/6	
	240 ,,	—	0/6	
	60 ,,	500 orally	6/0	
	80 ,,	500 ,,	6/0	
	110 ,,	500 ,,	4/2	130
	140 ,,	500 ,,	2/4	
	180 ,,	500 ,,	0/6	
	240 ,,	500 ,,	0/6	

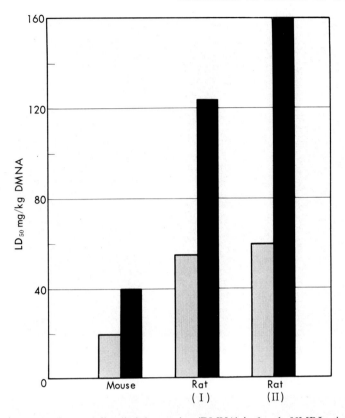

FIG. 1. LD_{50} of dimethylnitrosamine (DMNA) in female NMRI mice and male BR 46 rats without (empty columns) and with (hatched columns) disulfiram (DSF) pretreatment (500 mg/kg) 2 hr before DMNA application (DMNA i.p. in mice and i.v. (I) and orally (II) in rats).

as in male BR 46 rats. The LD_{50} of 15 mg/kg in Swiss mice and of 19 mg/kg in NMRI mice could be raised after oral pretreatment with 500 mg/kg DSF 2 hr before administering the intraperitoneal DMNA injection to 27 mg/kg and 40 mg/kg, respectively. Similar results were obtained in BR 46 and Sprague-Dawley rats. The LD_{50} in Sprague-Dawley rats of 63 mg/kg and in BR 46 rats of 55 mg/kg could be increased to 130 mg/kg and 124 mg/kg, respectively. This shows that at least in rats and mice the protective effect of DSF against DMNA poisoning is independent of strain, sex and method of application of DMNA. No difference was observed between i.v. or oral application. Therefore, unspecific adsorptive effects after both oral application of DSF and DMNA can be excluded.

Figures 2 and 3 demonstrate the protective effect of DSF in mice after histological examination of the liver. Every animal in a group of 20 received an i.p. dose of 20 mg/kg DMNA, which was lethal for the control group, whereas all animals in the experimental DSF group survived.

When DMNA was given in a dosage of, for example, 240 mg/kg to Sprague-Dawley rats, where the protective effect of the DSF pretreatment was no longer

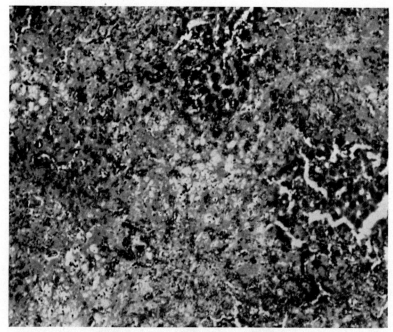

FIG. 2.   Necrosis of the liver of a mouse after i.p. application of 20 mg/kg dimethylnitrosamine. (1 : 125).

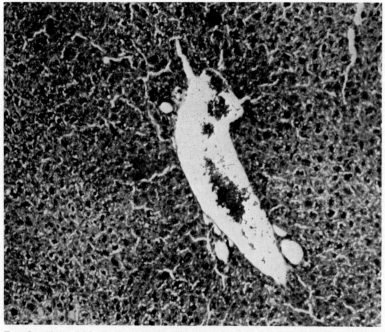

FIG. 3.   Normal histological picture of a mouse liver after i.p. application of 20 mg/kg dimethylnitrosamine (DMNA) and pretreatment with 500 mg/kg disulfiram 2 hr before the DMNA application.   (1 : 125).

effective, animals in both the experimental and the control group died 2–5 days after the application from liver necrosis and liver and lung hemorrhages without a significant difference in survival time. These symptoms agree with those well-known ones from the literature (*16*) that occur after DMNA poisoning in rats and mice.

Kinetic Studies

Table 2 illustrates the kinetics of the DMNA toxicity inhibition by DSF in NMRI mice. The upper part shows the protective effect of pre- (+) and post- (−) treatment with 500 mg/kg DSF, This dose, which was found to be effective in the experiments mentioned before, reduces the lethal dose of 48 mg/kg DMNA in mice to half. As can be seen from the table, only a pretreatment, given 2–4 hr before, had any effect on the acute toxicity of DMNA. The lower part of the table demonstrates the dose response of a DSF pretreatment 2 hr before the DMNA application, a time found to be most effective in the experiments listed in the upper part. It can be seen that dosages of DSF of less than 500 mg/kg were insufficient.

Even though a dose of 1,000 mg/kg is about twice as effective as a 500 mg/kg dose, a dose of 500 mg/kg DSF was applied in the following experiments to exclude any unpredictable side effects of the DSF treatment.

TABLE 2. Kinetic Studies: The Influence of Dosage and Timing of Disulfiram (DSF) Application on the Toxicity of 48 mg/kg Dimethylnitrosamine (DMNA) in Female NMRI Mice

DSF dosage (mg/kg)	Time of DSF treatment (hours)	Survivors (%)
500	+ 2	55
500	+ 4	45
500	+ 8	0
500	+12	0
500	+24	0
500	+48	0
500	− 2	0
500	− 4	0
50	+ 2	0
100	+ 2	0
200	+ 2	0
500	+ 2	45
1000	+ 2	70

Comparison of the Toxic and Methylating Action of DMNA

In order to investigate whether the inhibiting effect of DSF on DMNA poisoning is due to the methylating action of DMNA metabolites, the formation of ^{14}C-7-methylguanine in liver RNA was studied as a model system. Table 3 shows the influence of a 2 hr pretreatment with 500 mg/kg in Swiss mice on the formation of 7-methylguanine, after the intraperitoneal application of two different DMNA dosages and two different times of action.

TABLE 3.   Influence of Pretreatment 2 hr before the Injection with 500 mg/kg Disulfiram (DSF) on Labeling of Nucleic Acids and Methylation of Guanine in RNA after the Application of ^{14}C-Dimethylnitrosamine (DMNA)

Substances and dosages	Hours	Distribution of radioactivity and % of total counts			Spec. act.		Relative decrease of spec. act. 1=100%		Counts for 7-MG calculated from spec. act.	Relative decrease 7-MG 1=100%
		Guanine	7-MG	Adenine	RNA	DNA	RNA	DNA		
1) 1.5 mg/46μCi/kg DMNA-^{14}C i.v.	6	3.9	77.5	11.0	247	84			192.0	
2) 500 mg/kg DSF 1.5 mg/46μCi/kg DMNA-^{14}C	6	6.35	66.0	14.8	101	35	59	58.4	66.2	65.5
1) 1.5 mg/46μCi/kg DMNA-^{14}C i.p.	16	4.83	73.47	15.4	189	108			139.0	
2) 500 mg/kg DSF 1.5 mg/46μCi/kg DMNA-^{14}C	16	8.62	69.0	12.7	133	72	29.5	34	92.0	34.0
1) 10 mg/100μCi/kg DMNA-^{14}C i.v.	6	2.35	82.5	10.02	225	297			183	
2) 500 mg/kg DSF 10 mg/100μCi/kg DMNA-^{14}C	6	13.0	66.0	16.0	96	86	57.5	71	63.2	65.5
1) 10 mg/100μCi/kg DMNA-^{14}C i.p.	16	3.1	79.8	9.2	341	348			272.0	
2) 500 mg/kg DSF 10 mg/100μCi/kg DMNA-^{14}C	16	13.26	62.8	14.7	261	274	23	21	164.0	40.0

At this point, let's look at the data on Table 3.   The RNA was prepared by the modified method of Kidson, Kirby and Ralph (*10*), hydrolyzed with 1 N HCl at 100°C for 1 hr and then chromatographed on a Dowex column using a 1–2 N HCl gradient.   In order to achieve a real comparison of specific activities from the RNA of the experimental and control groups, 5 mg RNA were dissolved in 5 ml water and the UV-absorption at 260 nm was determined.   Slight differences in absorption were corrected by diluting a solution with a higher concentration until equal absorption of both solutions was obtained.

After the radioactivity of 1 ml was determined, the comparable amount of 7-methylguanine formed in the RNA was calculated by the following procedure. After chromatographic separation of nucleotides and bases, the radioactivity of an equal amount of each fraction was measured.   After background subtraction, the counts of all fractions were added.   One percent was chosen as the statistical error in counting, except in those samples with less than 100 counts per min.   By using the optical density and radioactive distribution pattern, the counts of the samples in the guanine as well as in the 7-methylguanine and the adenine region were added and related by percentages to the total amount of counts from all the samples.   The percentage obtained for 7-methylguanine was used to calculate the comparable amount of 7-methylguanine formed from the specific activity of the RNA.   For comparison of the experimental group with the controls, the amount of 7-methylguanine in the control groups was set at 100%.

TABLE 4.   Kinetic Studies: Influence of Different Times in Oral Pretreatment with 500 mg/kg Disulfiram (DSF) on Dimethylnitrosamine (DMNA) Poisoning in Comparison with the Toxicity of 48 mg/kg DMNA in Female NMRI Mice
(Biochemical investigations were done with animals killed 16 hr after the treatment.)

Substances and dosages	Distribution of radioactivity and % of total counts			Spec. act. imp./mg RNA	Relative decrease of spec. act. $1 = 100\%$ RNA	Counts for 7-MG calculated from spec. act.	Relative decrease of 7-MG $1 = 100\%$	% Sur-vivors
	Guanine	7-MG	Adenine					
1.5 mg/50 μCi/kg DMNA-^{14}C i. p.	8.47	68.89	12.93	153		105		0
2 hr pretreatment with 500 mg/kg DSF 1.5 mg/50 μCi/kg DMNA-^{14}C i.p.	24.90	41.85	19.27	95	38	40	62	55
4 hr pretreatment with 500 mg/kg DSF 1.5 mg/50 μCi/kg DMNA-^{14}C i.p.	24.61	47.0	16.7	105	31	49	54	45
24 hr pretreatment with 500 mg/kg DSF 1.5 mg/50 μCi/kg DMNA-^{14}C i.p.	17.4	57.05	13.61	150	8.5	85.5	19	0

As can be seen from Table 3, the specific activity of both RNA and DNA, as well as the formation of 7-methylguanine in RNA, is reduced when more DSF is added.   As indicated in the right-hand column, the inhibition of the formation of 7-methylguanine is higher 6 hr after the application of DMNA.   This is in contrast to the data obtained after 16 hr with both dosages.   This shows that the protective effect of DSF is most active during the first 6 hr and corresponds well with the toxicological data presented earlier.

This can be seen in more detail in Table 4, in which the protective effect of pretreatment with 500 mg/kg DSF on DMNA poisoning, given a constant dose of DMNA and a period of 16 hr, is illustrated.   In agreement with the kinetic studies on the toxic effect of DMNA, using a constant dose and different timing for the DSF application, the inhibition of guanine alkylation is most active 2 and 4 hr before the application of DMNA.   On the other hand, a pretreatment 24 hr before shows only a slightly reduced alkylation in comparison with the controls.   As can be seen in the left-hand part of Table 4, the additional application of DSF increases the biological incorporation of the ^{14}C activity of DMNA into the purine bases via the C_1-pool. Whether this is due to an increased synthesis of RNA or to a difference in metabolism of DMNA cannot be deduced from these data.   But, it is obvious from the above experiments that there is a clear correlation between the alkylating and the toxic action of DMNA.

According to the work of Stroemme (20), DSF is immediately reduced in vivo to form 2 molecules of dithiocarbamic acid and the alkylating agents readily react with the sulphhydryl groups.   Therefore, it seemed possible that the protective effect of DSF might be due to such a reaction.

So we investigated whether an equimolar amount of cysteine (250 mg/kg), applied in the same manner as DSF in rats and mice, has a similar protective effect against DMNA poisoning as a dose of 500 mg/kg DSF has.

We discovered that cysteine had no protective effect. It, therefore, seems more likely to assume a direct inhibition of DMNA metabolizing enzymes by DSF, as this has been reported for dopamine-β-oxydasis (6) and tryptophanpyrolasis (19). Barbituric acid derivatives are metabolized less by DSF, according to Giarman (5) and Graham (7). If the reduction of DMNA toxicity was due to an inhibition of metabolism, DSF would have no protective effect against nitrosomethylurea poisoning. This compound *in vivo* leads also to the formation of a methylcation, but needs no oxidative activation. The LD_{50} of nitrosomethylurea, determined to be 110 mg/kg in Swiss mice, was not influenced by the DSF pretreatment. This again shows that any protective effect on the part of the sulphhydryl groups can be excluded.

Other Nitrosamines

The next question we had to answer was whether DSF could diminish poisoning by higher alkylated nitrosamines, since the same pathway of oxidative activation was assumed for all dialkylnitrosamines (3).

Female NMRI mice and male Sprague-Dawley rats were used in these experiments. The substances tested were diethyl-, dipropyl-, dibutyl-, and methyl-

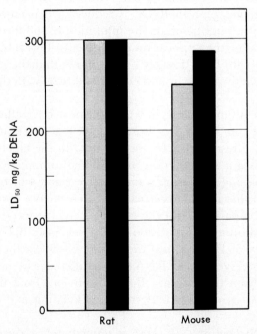

FIG. 4. The influence of a pretreatment given 2 hr before (500 mg/kg) with disulfiram (DSF) on toxicity of diethylnitrosamine (DENA) in male Sprague-Dawley rats (i.v.) and female NMRI mice (i.p.). Empty columns, without DSF pretreatment; hatched columns, with DSF pretreatment.

propylnitrosamine, which were applied intraperitoneally either in aqueous solution, or if not soluble enough in water, undiluted by a micro syringe.

Figure 4 shows the effect of DSF on acute diethylnitrosamine (DENA) poisoning in male Sprague-Dawley rats and female NMRI mice. It can be seen that the LD_{50} of this compound in mice was only slightly increased from 250 mg/kg to 290 mg/kg and the DSF had no effect whatsoever in rats. In these animals, a LD_{50} of 300 mg/kg was determined independently of the DSF pretreatment. This result is remarkable, because the symptoms and histology of acute DMNA and DENA toxicity differ very little, if at all.

Similar results were obtained when the protective effect of DSF (500 mg/kg) on poisoning with dipropyl- and dibutylnitrosamine was investigated. The DSF pretreatment did not reduce the LD_{50} of dipropylnitrosamine, determined in NMRI mice to be 420 mg/kg and in Sprague-Dawley rats to be 460 mg/kg, nor did it extend the life span of the animals. Since some of the animals died from the central symptoms 6–10 hr after the application of acutely toxic dosages of dipropylnitrosamine, the LD_{50} was divided into three portions, which were applied at 24 hr invervals. This prevented the central symptoms and induced a parenchymatous hepatotoxic death. The DSF pretreatment, however, did not prevent liver injury induced by dipropylnitrosamine in this way.

In the kinetic studies presented earlier, it was demonstrated that a dose of 1,000 mg/kg DSF was more efficient in protecting against DMNA poisoning. The influence of this dose on dipropylnitrosamine poisoning was investigated, but was found to be ineffective as well.

The LD_{50} of dibutylnitrosamine, determined to be 1,100 mg/kg in mice and 1,050 mg/kg in rats, could not be reduced by a pretreatment with 500 mg/kg of DSF 2 hr before the injections. Methyl-propylnitrosamine, an unsymmetrical dialkylnitrosamine, was investigated as described before. The LD_{50} of this compound was found to be 95 mg/kg in NMRI mice, which died 2–5 days after an intraperitoneal injection from liver necrosis. As described before for dialkylnitrosamines other than DMNA, pretreatment with 500 mg/kg DSF had no influence on a dose of 105 or 155 mg/kg methyl-propylnitrosamine. The only difference was that the life span of the DSF-treated animals was somewhat longer. The animals, however, only survived 24 hr more, which is not at all significant.

Investigations on the Effects of DSF Pretreatment on DMNA Carcinogenesis

Even though we agree with the papers presented by Heath (9) and Fiume *et al.* (4), that a definite correlation between the alkylation and toxicity of DMNA can be established, the existence of such a connection between alkylation and carcinogenicity has become doubtful during recent years [Krüger *et al.* (12), Den Engelse *et al.* (2), Lijinsky and Ross (14), Schoental (17)]. The significant reduction of alkylation by DMNA after pretreatment with DSF, therefore, seemed to be an excellent model to study, whether alkylation is correlated with carcinogenic action or not.

Carcinogenesis studies were carried out on 60 male Sprague-Dawley rats and

150 female NMRI mice, which were divided into three groups.   Two of these groups received DMNA orally; the other one was pretreated with 500 mg/kg DSF.   The last group received DSF only.   The substances were applied once every 5 days. Mice were treated with a single dose of 1.5 mg/kg and rats with a dose of 4.5 mg/kg DMNA in an aqueous solution, whereas DSF was applied in the usual manner (500 mg/kg 2 hr before the DMNA application, orally).   Each group of mice included 50 animals, whereas the rats were divided into two groups of 24 animals each. One group received DMNA with and one group without the DSF pretreatment. Twelve animals were treated with DSF alone.

These experiments, which were started on October, 1970, are still not quite finished (September, 1971).   Surprisingly, the death rate of the animals treated with DSF+DMNA was much higher than that of those treated with DMNA alone. On the day this report was written, 6 out of a group of 50 mice treated with DMNA +DSF were still alive.   Twenty-nine animals still survived in the DMNA series, and 44 in the group treated with DSF alone.   Five malignant tumors were observed in the combination group: 3 animals had ependymomas of the brain and 2 animals developed hemangioendotheliomas of the liver.   Only 2 mice from the group treated with DMNA showed malignant tumors of the liver.   These have not yet been examined histologically; but macroscopically, they appeared to be hemangioendotheliosarcomas.   No tumors were obtained in those animals treated only with DSF.

The experiments with rats showed the following results.   In the group of 24 animals treated with DSF+DMNA, 12 animals died.   The following tumors were observed in 7 rats: 1 ependymoma of the brain, 1 basalioma of the bulbus olfactorius, 1 squamous cell carcinoma, 1 tumor of the pars frontale, which has not yet been examined histologically, and 2 hepatocellular carcinomas of the liver.   In the group treated with DMNA, only 3 out of 24 animals developed malignant tumors and died. We obtained 1 cerebellum glioma, 1 estesio neuroepithelioma and 1 malignant tumor of the liver, which has not yet been examined histologically.   No animals died from the group treated with DSF alone.

These preliminary results presented here suggest that DSF pretreatment probably does not influence the carcinogenic action of DMNA.   In order to reduce the toxicity of the DSF+DMNA treatment, we have started experiments with other dosages, which are not yet finished.

DISCUSSION

The main result of the toxicological experiments was that the pretreatment with DSF in a dose of 500 mg/kg, given orally 2 hr before the intraperitoneal, intravenous or oral DMNA application, considerably reduced the acute toxic action of DMNA and the alkylation of RNA by this compound.   When alkylation was reduced to half after the DSF pretreatment, the LD_{50} was raised to double its value.   The reduction of DMNA toxicity is independent of strain and sex in both rats and mice. It was especially remarkable that DSF showed protective effects in DMNA but not in diethyl-, dipropyl-, dibutyl-, and methyl-propylnitrosamine toxicity.   These results suggest that DMNA and the other nitrosamines tested are metabolized by different enzyme systems, but they cannot answer the question of which enzymes are involved. This problem needs further investigation. It is very interesting, however, that the metabolism of chemically different compounds, such as chloroform and DMNA, are inhibited by DSF, whereas the toxicity of other nitrosamines, chemically very similar to DMNA, were unimpaired.

The results obtained from studying the protective action of DSF on DMNA carcinogenesis are interesting. Even though the protective action of DSF against DMNA toxicity could also be observed after animals were treated with DSF, as described above, for about 1 year, this pretreatment probably had no effect on DMNA carcinogenesis. These results are in agreement with those obtained by Alonso and Herranz (1), who found that chloramphenicol reduced the liver necrosis induced by DMNA, but discovered that the carcinogenic action was umimpaired. Similar results have been reported by Kipplinger and Kensler (11), who found that phenoxybenzamine inhibited the acute toxicity of CCl_4, but not its carcinogenic action. On the other hand, it was shown that acetanilide had a protective effect against the toxicity of 2-acetamino fluorene, as well as against the carcinogenic action of this compound (22), and the carcinogenic action of 4-dimethylaminoazobenzene was found to be reduced by the simultaneous application of chloramphenicol (13). Recently Hadjiolov (8) reported that the carcinogenic action of DMNA is inhibited by amino acetonitrile. Further investigation is needed to elucidate the problem of carcinogenesis inhibition by specific-acting chemicals.

We thank Mr. B. Eitel, Mr. E. Wolff, and Mrs. E. Kiausch for the financial support of our work.

REFERENCES

1. Alonso, A., und Herranz, G. Der Einfluß von Chloramphenicol auf die Leber-Cancerisierung durch Diäthylnitrosamin. Naturwissenschaften, 57: 249, 1970.
2. Den Engelse, L., Bentvelzen, P. A. J., and Emmelot, P. Studies on Lung Tumours. I. Methylation of Deoxyribonucleic Acids and Tumour Formation Following Administration of Dimethylnitrosamine to Mice. Chem. Biol. Interactions, 1: 395, 1969/70.
3. Druckrey, H., Preussmann, R., Ivankovic, S., und Schmähl, D. Organotrope carcinogene Wirkungen bei 65 verschiedenen N-Nitroso-Verbindungen an BD-Ratten. Z. Krebsforsch., 69: 103, 1967.
4. Fiume, L., Campadelli-Fiume, G., Magee, P. N., and Holsman, J. Cellular Injury and Carcinogenesis. Biochem. J., 120: 601, 1970.
5. Giarman, N. J., Flick, F. H., and White, J. M. Prolongation of Thiopental Anesthesia in the Mouse by Premedication with Tetraethylthiuram Disulfide (Antabuse). Science, 114: 35, 1951.
6. Goldstein, M. I. Inhibition of Norepinephrine Biosynthesis at the Dopamine-β-hydroxylation Stage. Pharmacol. Rev., 18: 77, 1966.
7. Graham, D. W., Carmichael, E. J., and Allmach, M. G. J. Pharm. Pharmacol., 3: 497, 1951.
8. Hadjiolov, D. The Inhibition of Dimethylnitrosamine Carcinogenesis in Rat Liver

by Aminoacetonitrile. Z. Krebsforsch., *76*: 91, 1971.

9. Heath, D. F. The Decomposition and Toxicity of Dialkylnitrosamines in Rats. Biochem. J., *85*: 72, 1962.

10. Kidson, C., Kirby, K. S., and Ralph, R. K. Isolation Characteristics of Rapidly Labelled RNA from Neutral Rat Liver. J. Mol. Biol., *7*: 312, 1963.

11. Kipplinger, G. F., and Kensler, C. J. Failure of Phenoxybenzamine to Prevent Formation of Hepatomas after Chronic Carbon Tetrachloride Administration. J. Natl. Cancer Inst., *30*: 837, 1963.

12. Krüger, F. W., Walker, G., and Wiessler, M. Carcinogenic Action of Dimethylnitrosamine in Trout Not Related to Methylation of Nucleic Acids and Protein *in vivo*. Experientia, *26*: 520, 1970.

13. Lacassagne, A., et Hurst, L. Action retardatrice du chloramphénicol sur le processusde cancérisation du foi du rat par le p-diméthylaminoazobenzene. Bull. Cancer, *54*: 405, 1967.

14. Lijinsky, W., and Ross, A. E. Alkylation of Rat Liver Nucleic Acids Not Related to Carcinogenesis of N-Nitrosamines. J. Natl. Cancer Inst., *42*: 1095, 1969.

15. Magee, P. N., and Hultin, T. Toxic Liver Injury and Carcinogenesis. Methylation of Proteins of Rat-Liver Slices by Dimethylnitrosamine. Biochem. J., *83*: 106, 1962.

16. Schmähl, D. Entstehung, Wachstum und Chemotherapie maligner Tumoren. Editio Cantor, Aulendorf, 1970.

17. Schoental, R. Lack of Correlation between Presence of 7-Methylguanine in Deoxyribonucleic Acid of Organs and the Localization of Tumors after a Single Carcinogenic Dose of N-Methyl-N-nitrosourethane. Biochem. J., *114*: 55, 1969.

18. Scholler, K. L., Müller, E., und Plehwe, U. Verstärkung und Unterdrückung der Toxizität von Chloroform für die Leber durch Pharmaka. Arzneim.-Forsch., *20*: 289, 1970.

19. Smith, A. A., and Wortis, S. B. Formation of Tryptophol in the Disulfiram-treated Rat. Biochim. Biophys. Acta, *40*: 569, 1960.

20. Stroemme, J. K. Metabolism of Disulfiram and Diethyldithiocarbamate in Rats with Demonstration of an *in vivo* Ethanol-induced Inhibition of the Glucuronic Acid Conjugation of the Thiol. Biochem. Pharmacol., *14*: 393, 1965.

21. Swann, P. F., and Magee, P. N. Nitrosamine-induced Carcinogenesis. The Alkylation of Nucleic Acids of the Rat by N-Methyl-N-nitrosourea, Dimethylnitrosamine, Dimethylsulphate and Methylmethanesulphonate. Biochem. J., *110*: 39, 1968.

22. Yamamoto, R. S., Glass, R. M., Frankel, H. H., Weisburger, E. K., and Weisburger, J. H. Inhibition of the Toxicity and Carcinogenicity of N-2-Fluorenylacetamide by Acetanilide. Toxicol. Appl. Pharmacol., *13*: 108, 1968.

Discussion of Paper by Drs. Schmähl and Krüger

DR. WEISBURGER: The data you showed with disulfiram remined me of the similar effect of SKF-525A as an inhibitor of microsomal enzymes. It shows an acute effect, but not a chronic action. In fact, chronic administration increases enzymes metabolizing drugs. Do you feel disulfiram acts likewise?

DR. KRÜGER: We have tested the protective effect of DSF after feeding it to animals for one year and have found the same inhibition of DMNA poisoning then as at the beginning of the experiments.

DR. SUGIMURA: Is there any experiment on *in vivo* inhibition of the DMNA metabolizing system by DSF?

DR. KRÜGER: No, we have not studied it yet.

DR. DRUCKREY: Can it be concluded from the presented results that different mechanisms are involved in the acute toxicity and carcinogenicity of dialkyl nitrosamines?

DR. KRÜGER: No, I think one cannot conclude this from this experiment definitely because so many animals in the group treated with DSF and DMNA died prematurely without developing tumors.

DR. MAGEE: What is the effect of disulfiram on microsomal hydroxylase enzymes? I was surprised to see that brain tumors appeared in the mice treated with DMNA and disulfiram.

DR. KRÜGER: Yes, the reduced metabolism of barbituric acid derivatives were reported by Giarman *et al.* (Science, *114*: 35, 1951) and Graham *et al.* (J. Pharm. Pharmacol., *3*: 497, 1951). The appearance of brain tumors may depend on the dosage used in this experiment.

New Aspects in Metabolism of Carcinogenic Nitrosamines

F. W. Krüger

The Institute of Experimental Toxicology and Chemotherapy, German Cancer Research Center, Heidelberg, West Germany

Since the discovery by Magee and Farber (*7*) that the *in vivo* application of the carcinogen dimethylnitrosamine led to the formation of 7-methylguanine in the nucleic acids of certain organs in rats, a correlation among the toxic, carcinogenic and alkylating actions of nitrosamines has been assumed. As a result of their investigations, Magee (*8*), Rose (*13*) and Druckrey (*1*) suggested the following general pathway for the conversion of nitrosamines into highly reactive alkylating agents. According to this proposed mechanism (Fig. 1), the initial step should be an enzymatic α-hydroxylation of one of the aliphatic chains, which is followed by its hydro lytic cleavage, and leads to the formation of the corresponding aldehyde and a monoalkylnitrosamine. From this last compound, after its rearrangement into the corresponding diazohydroxide, a diazoalkane is formed that then decomposes to the corresponding alkyl-cation by splitting off a nitrogen molecule.

Lijinsky and his co-workers have shown that the formation of 7-methylguanine *in vivo* after the application of both dimethylnitrosamine (DMNA) (*12*) and nitrosomethylurea (NMU) (personal communication) is a transmethylation and, therefore, does not involve the formation of diazomethane as an intermediate. Hence, the nature of the reactive intermediates in the formation of the alkyl-cation is not yet clear. But the formation of 7-ethylguanine after the application of diethylnitrosamine (DENA) (*9*) or nitrosoethylurea (NEU) (*11*), which can be thought of as an α-oxidized derivative of an N-nitroso compound, supports the assumption that α-oxidation of one of the alkyl chains leads to the transfer of the other.

However, with this exception, no 7-alkylguanine derivative other than 7-methylguanine could be detected in the genetic material after the application of various tritium-labeled cyclic nitrosamines, as was shown in comprehensive studies by Lee and Lijinsky (*4*), Lijinsky and Ross (*6*).

These results are in disagreement with the established theory of enzymatic nitrosamine activation. According to which, α-oxidation followed by hydrolytic cleavage

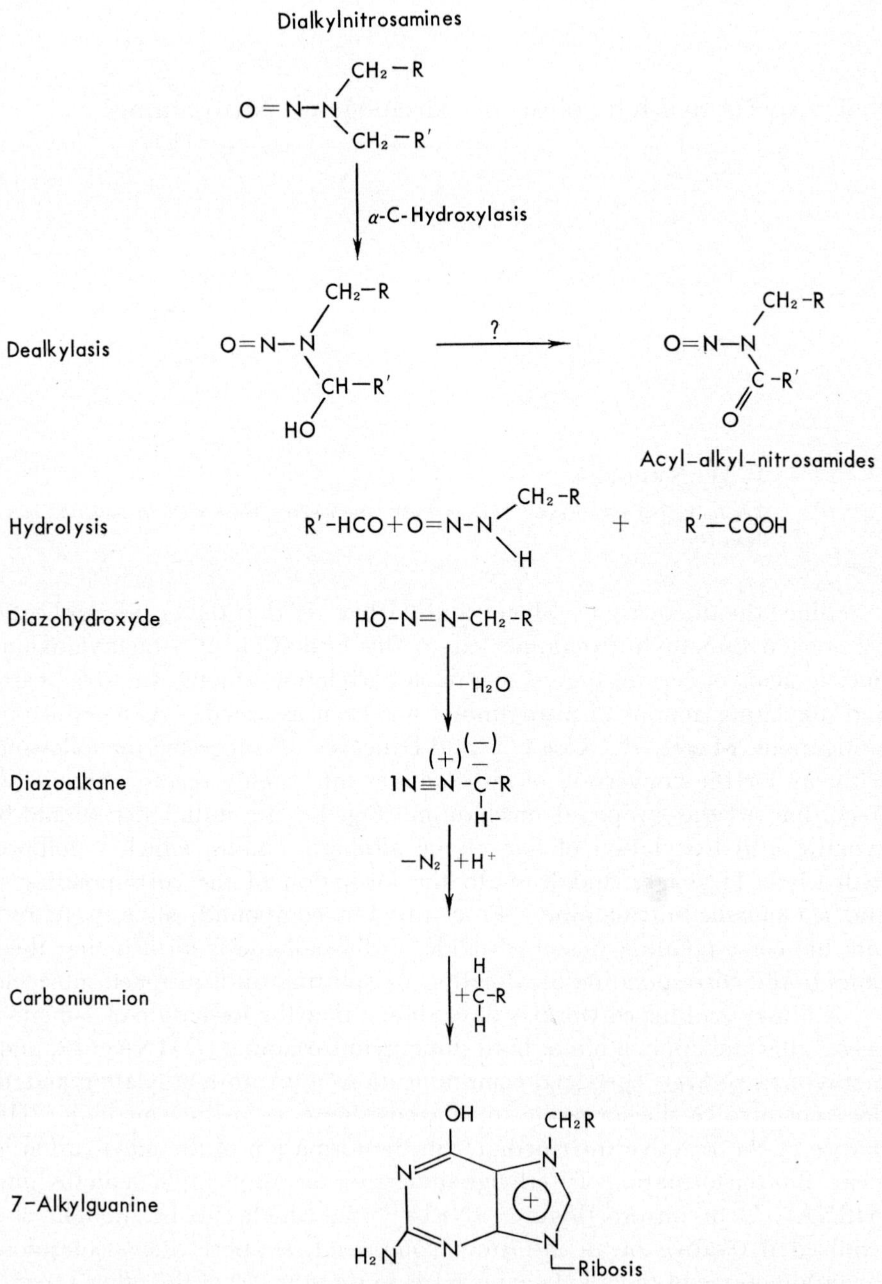

FIG. 1. Proposed mechanism for the alkylating intermediates from dialkylnitrosamines and dialkylnitrosamides.

of the heterocyclic ring system should finally lead to the transfer of the corresponding aldehyde or of carboxylic acid to the genetic material which should contain all the carbon atoms of the heterocyclic system (Fig. 2).

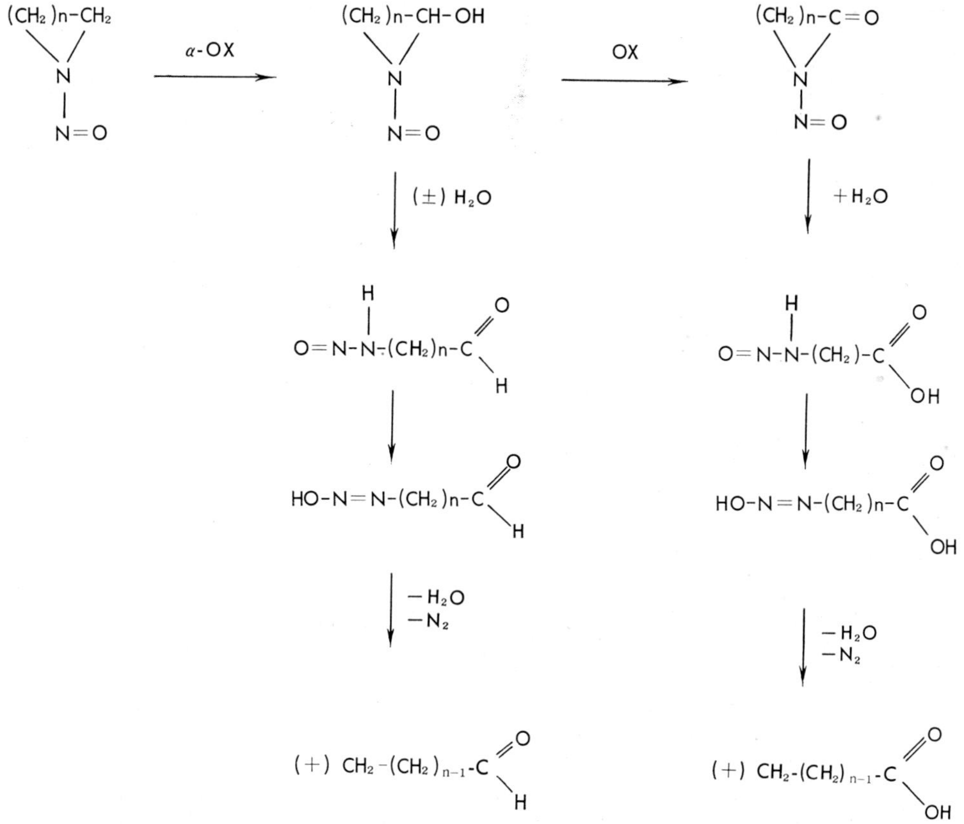

Fig. 2. Reactive products expected to be formed from cyclic nitrosamines after α-oxidation and the following steps (see Fig. 1).

Since it was shown by Magee and Lee (9) that methyl-butyl-nitrosamine had strong methylating properties, whereas 7-butylguanine could not be detected after the application of this compound, it seemed possible that cyclic and higher di-*n*-alkylnitrosamines are metabolically degraded to methyl-alkyl- or dimethylnitros-amines, which then react as methylating agents. If one adapts the established metabolic pathway of fatty acid degradation to nitrosamine metabolism, this seems to be theoretically possible (Fig. 3). Assuming that the first step would be an enzymatic dehydrogenation of the alkyl chain between the α- and the β-carbon, the subsequent addition of water to the double bond would lead to a β-hydroxylated product, since the inductive effect of a N-nitroso group would be qualitatively comparable with that of an activated carbonyl function.

As can be seen from Fig. 3, the final product would be a methyl-alkyl-nitros-amine or dimethylnitrosamine if both alkyl groups were degraded in the same way. According to this hypothetical mechanism, the formation of the methyl-nitroso compounds is due to the cleavage of the alkyl chain between the α- and the β-carbon. Therefore, the application of alkyl-nitrosamines, ^{14}C-labeled in the α-position, should lead to the formation of 7-methylguanine, whereas this reaction product should not be observed when the β-carbon is labeled.

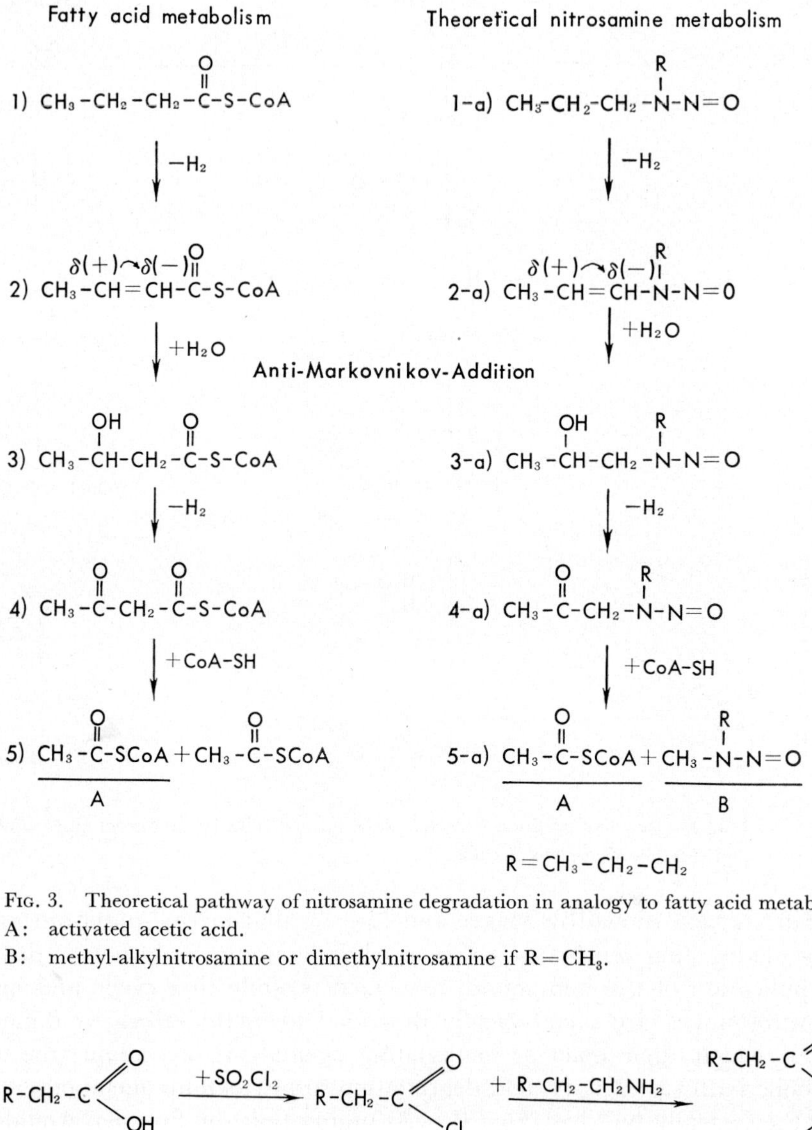

Fatty acid metabolism

Theoretical nitrosamine metabolism

1) $CH_3-CH_2-CH_2-\overset{\overset{\displaystyle O}{\|}}{C}-S-CoA$

1-a) $CH_3-CH_2-CH_2-\overset{\overset{\displaystyle R}{|}}{N}-N=O$

$\downarrow -H_2$

$\downarrow -H_2$

2) $CH_3-CH=CH-\overset{\overset{\displaystyle \delta(+)\frown\delta(-)}{\underset{\|}{O}}}{C}-S-CoA$

2-a) $CH_3-CH=CH-\overset{\overset{\displaystyle \delta(+)\frown\delta(-)}{\underset{|}{R}}}{N}-N=O$

$\downarrow +H_2O$

$\downarrow +H_2O$

Anti-Markovnikov-Addition

3) $CH_3-\overset{\overset{\displaystyle OH}{|}}{CH}-CH_2-\overset{\overset{\displaystyle O}{\|}}{C}-S-CoA$

3-a) $CH_3-\overset{\overset{\displaystyle OH}{|}}{CH}-CH_2-\overset{\overset{\displaystyle R}{|}}{N}-N=O$

$\downarrow -H_2$

$\downarrow -H_2$

4) $CH_3-\overset{\overset{\displaystyle O}{\|}}{C}-CH_2-\overset{\overset{\displaystyle O}{\|}}{C}-S-CoA$

4-a) $CH_3-\overset{\overset{\displaystyle O}{\|}}{C}-CH_2-\overset{\overset{\displaystyle R}{|}}{N}-N=O$

$\downarrow +CoA-SH$

$\downarrow +CoA-SH$

5) $\underline{CH_3-\overset{\overset{\displaystyle O}{\|}}{C}-SCoA+CH_3-\overset{\overset{\displaystyle O}{\|}}{C}-SCoA}$

5-a) $\underline{CH_3-\overset{\overset{\displaystyle O}{\|}}{C}-SCoA}+\underline{CH_3-\overset{\overset{\displaystyle R}{|}}{N}-N=O}$

A

A　　　　B

$R = CH_3-CH_2-CH_2$

FIG. 3.   Theoretical pathway of nitrosamine degradation in analogy to fatty acid metabolism.
A: activated acetic acid.
B: methyl-alkylnitrosamine or dimethylnitrosamine if $R=CH_3$.

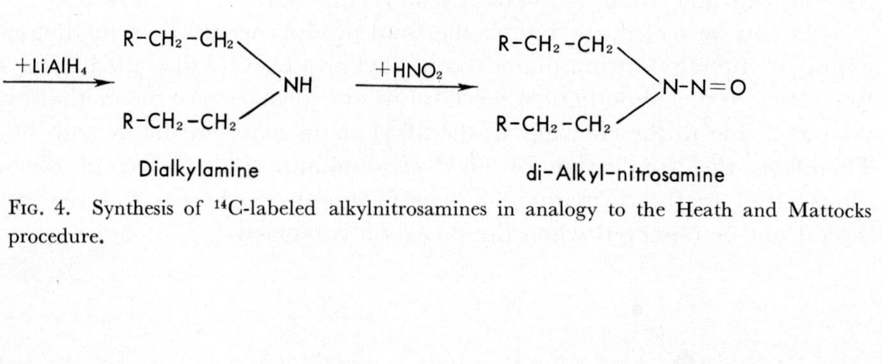

FIG. 4.   Synthesis of ^{14}C-labeled alkylnitrosamines in analogy to the Heath and Mattocks procedure.

Consequently, the alkylating properties of 1- and 2-¹⁴C-di-*n*-propylnitrosamine, respectively, and those of 1-¹⁴C-di-*n*-butylnitrosamine were investigated. They were synthesized from the appropriate carbonylic acids by the Heath and Mattocks procedure (2) (Fig. 4). 1-¹⁴C-Propionic or 1-¹⁴C-butyric acid were prepared by reacting the corresponding Grignard compounds with radioactive CO_2. The 2-¹⁴C-propionic acid was prepared from 1-¹⁴C-ethyl iodide and KCN, with sub-

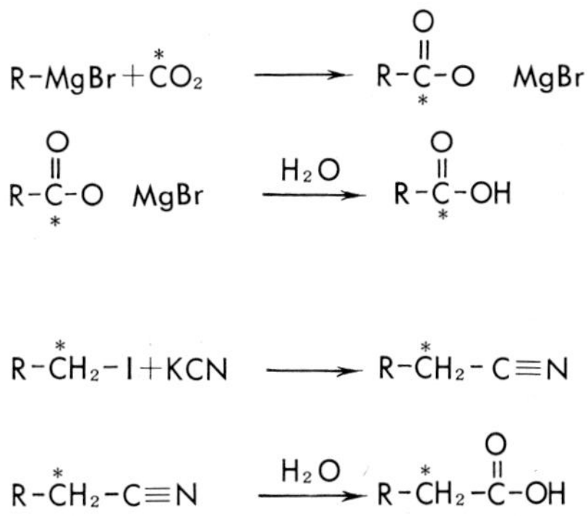

$$R-MgBr + \overset{*}{C}O_2 \longrightarrow R-\overset{O}{\underset{*}{C}}-O \ \ MgBr$$

$$R-\overset{O}{\underset{*}{C}}-O \ \ MgBr \xrightarrow{H_2O} R-\overset{O}{\underset{*}{C}}-OH$$

$$R-\overset{*}{C}H_2-I + KCN \longrightarrow R-\overset{*}{C}H_2-C\equiv N$$

$$R-\overset{*}{C}H_2-C\equiv N \xrightarrow{H_2O} R-\overset{*}{C}H_2-\overset{O}{C}-OH$$

Fig. 5.   Synthesis of 1- and 2-¹⁴C-labeled carbonic acids (Radio Chemical Centre, Amersham).

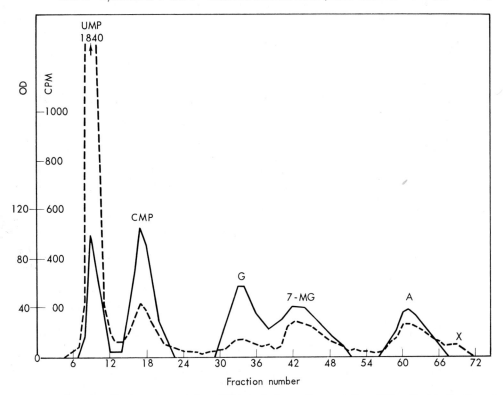

Fig. 6a.   Elution pattern of an RNA hydrolysate from rat liver 16 hr after application of 388 mg/2,000 μCi/kg 1-¹⁴C-di-*n*-propylnitrosamine, 50 mg RNA + 5 mg inactive 7-methylguanine added. CMP, cytidinemonophosphate; G, guanine; A, adenine; 7-MG, 7-methylguanine; UMP, uridinemonophosphate; ------, CPM; ———, optical density. Dowex 50WX2.

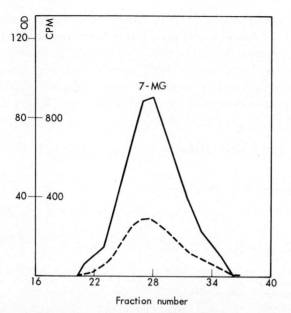

FIG. 6b. Rechromatography of fractions between adenine and guanine after application of 1-^{14}C-di-n-propylnitrosamine (compare with Fig. 6a), 100 mg RNA + 10 mg 7-methylguanine added. 7-MG, 7-methylguanine; --------, CPM/min; ———, optical density. Dowex 50WX2.

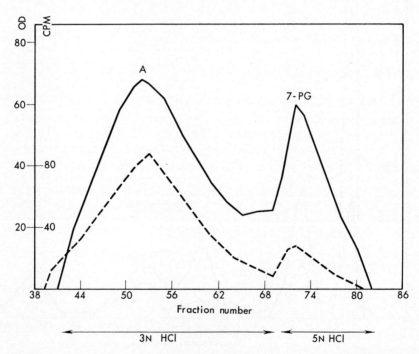

FIG. 6c. Rechromatography of fractions in the adenine region with after application of 1-^{14}C-di-n-propylnitrosamine (compare with Fig. 6a), 100 mg RNA + 10 mg inactive 7-propylguanine added. A, adenine; 7-PG, 7-propylguanine; --------, CPM/min; ———, optical density. Dowex 50 WX8.

sequent hydrolysis of the resulting nitrile (Fig. 5) by the Radio Chemical Centre, Amersham.   This synthesis of the carboxylic acids labeled in the 1-position excludes ^{14}C-methylalkyl or dimethylamine as impurities, and the subsequent steps leading to the corresponding labeled nitrosamines are carried out with inactive material. So, a contamination of the final products with ^{14}C-dimethyl- or ^{14}C-methyl-alkyl-nitrosamine is extremely unlikely.

In these experiments, male Sprague-Dawley rats with an average weight of 100–150 g were used.   The nitrosamines were applied undiluted intraperitoneally. The animals were killed 16 hr after the application.   The RNA from the liver was prepared by the modified Kidson procedure (*3*), as described by Swann and Magee (*10*), and was analyzed after acid hydrolysis by fractionation on the Dowex columns, using an increasing HCl gradient.   For the identification of unknown compounds, 7-methyl-, 7-propyl- or 7-butylguanine were added to the hydrolysates.   Proteins from the liver were purified as described by Magee and Hultin (*8*).   Following the application of 1- or 2-^{14}C-di-*n*-propylnitrosamine, the mesenteric fat tissues were removed, lyophilized, extracted with ether, and separated into neutral lipids and fatty acids, after hydrolysis with metanolic-aqueous potassium hydroxide.

Figure 6a shows the elution pattern of liver RNA after the application of 2,000

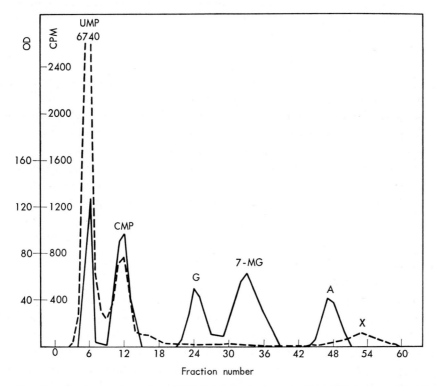

FIG. 7a. Elution pattern of an RNA hydrolysate from rat liver 16 hr after application of 400 mg/2,060 μCi/kg 2-^{14}C-di-*n*-propylnitrosamine. UMP, uridinemonophosphate; CMP, cytidinemonophosphate; G, guanine; 7-MG, 7-methylguanine; A, adenine; X, 7-propyl-guanine?; --------, CPM/min; ———, optical density. Dowex 50 WX2.

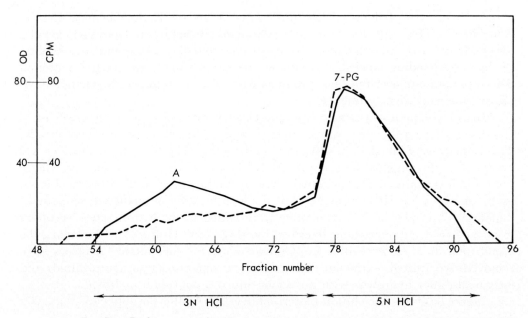

FIG. 7b. Rechromatography of maximum in the adenine region after application of 2-¹⁴C-di-*n*-propylnitrosamine (see Fig. 7a), 70 mg RNA + 7 mg inactive 7-propylguanine added. A, adenine; 7-PG, 7-propylguanine; ...., CPM/min; ———, optical density. Dowex 50 WX8.

μCi/388 mg/kg 1-¹⁴C-di-*n*-propylnitrosamine. It can be seen from this figure that the radioactive peak between adenine and guanine corresponds with the optical densitiy of the added 7-methylguanine, whereas the formation of 7-propylguanine is not clearly visible, because of the adenine labeling. The formation of 7-methylguanine was proven by the exact correspondence of radioactivity and optical densitiy, when the fractions between adenine and guanine were rechromatographed (Fig. 6b). As can be seen from Fig. 6c, which illustrates the rechromatography of fractions in the adenine region, after the addition of 7-propylguanine on the Dowex-50 WX 8, enabling a good separation of adenine and 7-propylguanine, there is a radioactive peak corresponding to the optical density of 7-propylguanine. The relatively low activity of this peak is due to an experimental error. Since the formation of 7-propylguanine could not be detected clearly in the first separation, most of the fractions containing the radioactive 7-propylguanine were discarded.

In agreement with the proposed mechanism of nitrosamine metabolism, it can be seen from Fig. 7a that no 7-methylguanine is formed after the application of 400 mg/2,060 μCi/kg 2-¹⁴C-di-*n*-propylnitrosamine. However, a distinct radioactive maximum in the adenine region can be observed, which correlates with the optical density of 7-propylguanine after rechromatography of those fractions and the addition of the latter compound (Fig. 7b).

In Fig. 8a, the elution pattern of liver RNA after the application of 371 mg/ 3,125 μCi/kg 1-¹⁴C-*n*-butylnitrosamine and the addition of inactive 7-methylguanine to the hydrolysate is illustrated. As can be seen from this figure, the main reaction product is 7-methylguanine. Again a small radioactive peak can be observed after the adenine region, which could be correlated with the optical density of 7-butyl-guanine after rechromatography of those fractions on the Dowex-50 WX 8, as is shown in Fig. 8b.

Table 1 shows the specific activity of the RNA and also what proportion of this activity is due to its biological incorporation into the pyrimidine bases, the specific activity of liver proteins and the total lipid extracts separated into neutral lipids and fatty acids after the application of 1- or 2-^{14}C-di-n-propylnitrosamine, respectively.

TABLE 1. Comparison of ^{14}C-Incorporation 16 hr after Application of 1- or 2-^{14}C-Di-n-propylnitrosamine (dpm/mg)

Substances and dosages	Time (hr)	Spec. act. RNA	Biol. incorporation into pyrimidines calculated from spec. act.	Protein	Total lipid extracts	Neutral lipids	Free fatty acids
388 mg/2,000 μCi/kg Di-n-propyl-nitrosamine 1-^{14}C	16	152	94	529	74	394	76
400 mg/2,060 μCi/kg Di-n-propyl-nitrosamine 2-^{14}C	16	805	731	2,900	1,095	11,200	80
Ratio of labeling 2-^{14}C PNA/1-^{14}C PNA		5.3	7.8	5.5	14.8	28.0	1

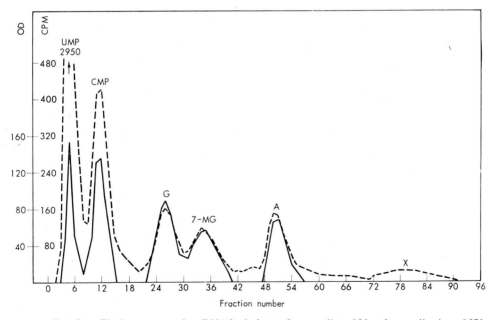

FIG. 8a. Elution pattern of an RNA hydrolysate from rat liver 16 hr after application of 371 mg/3,125 μCi/kg 1-^{14}C-di-n-butylnitrosamine, 50 mg RNA + 5 mg inactive 7-methylguanine added. UMP, uridinemonophosphate; CMP, cytidinemonophosphate; G, guanine; 7-MG, 7-methylguanine; A, adenine; X, 7-butylguanine?; ----------, CPM/min; ———, optical density. Dowex 50 WX2.

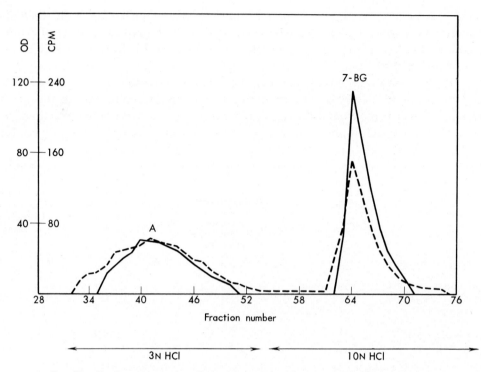

FIG. 8b. Rechromatography of adenine and the following fractions after application of 1-^{14}C-di-*n*-butylnitrosamine (see Fig. 8a), 80 mg RNA+8 mg 7-butylguanine added. A, adenine; 7-BG, 7-butylguanine; ----------, CPM/min; ——, optical density. Dowex 50 WX8.

It can be seen from this table also that the application of di-*n*-propylnitrosamine, labeled in the 2-position, leads to a considerably increased incorporation of the activity in the pyrimidine bases, the proteins and the neutral lipids, when compared with the labeling obtained after the application of the 1-^{14}C-labeled compound. Even though these results support the proposed mechanism of nitrosamine degradation, according to which a labeled, activated acetic acid might be formed after the application of 2-^{14}C-di-*n*-propylnitrosamine, the fact that no difference in the labeling of free fatty acids is observed excludes a direct correlation between nitrosamine and fatty acid metabolism.

Since these experiments showed that, besides the formation of 7-methylguanine after the application of di-*n*-butyl- and di-*n*-propylnitrosamine, small amounts of 7-propyl- or 7-butylguanine were formed, which are eluted after adenine (see Fig. 9), it seemed likely that in the experiments investigating cyclic nitrosamines (*4, 6*) in which only 7-methylguanine was found, small amounts of other alkylated guanine derivatives might have been overlooked. Also since the formation of an alkylating intermediate from cyclic nitroso compounds must involve the cleavage of the ring system, it seemed likely that an analysis of the reaction products with nucleic acids would reveal whether methylation and alkylation are due to a successive or alternative pathway.

The formation of 7-methylguanine after application of tritium-labeled nitroso-

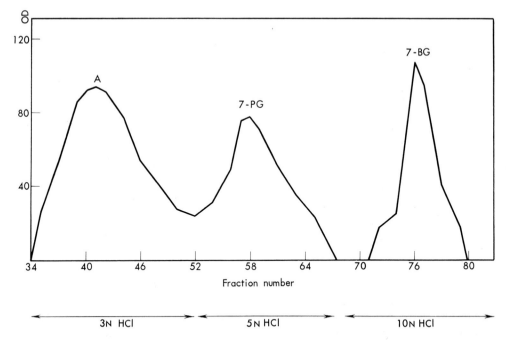

FIG. 9. Elution pattern of a mixture of 5 mg adenine, 5 mg 7-propylguanine and 5 mg 7-butylguanine, on Dowex-50 WX8 column (200–400 mesh), using a 3–10 N HCl gradient. A, adenine; 7-PG, 7-propylguanine; 7-BG, 7-butylguanine. Dowex 50 WX8.

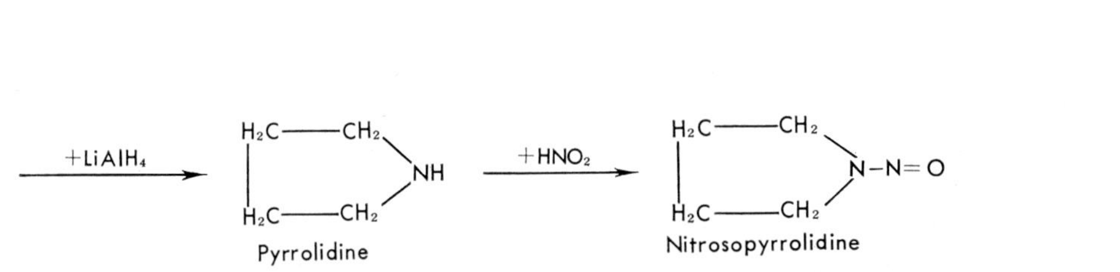

FIG. 10. Synthesis of 2,5- or 3,4-^{14}C-1-N-nitrosopyrrolidine.

pyrrolidine was described by Lee and Lijinsky (4). Hence, the alkylating activity of nitrosopyrrolidine was reinvestigated in male Sprague-Dawley rats with the appropriate ^{14}C-labeled nitroso compounds. 2,5- or 3,4-^{14}C-N-Nitrosopyrrolidine was synthesized from 1,4- or 2,3-^{14}C-succinic acid by the following route (Fig. 10). The overall yield of nitrosopyrrolidines was 35–40%, when this reaction was carried out

TABLE 2.   Specific Activity of RNA from Rat Liver after an Application of 2, 5- or 3, 4-
^{14}C-N-Nitrosopyrrolidine

Substances and dosages	Time (hr)	Spec. Act. (dpm/mg RNA)
40 mg/kg Pentothal 650 mg/1,954 μCi/kg Nitrosopyrrolidine 2,5-^{14}C	16	790
40 mg/kg Pentothal 650 mg/1,535 μCi/kg Nitrosopyrrolidine 3,4-^{14}C	16	1097
102 mg/770 μCi/kg Nitrosopyrrolidine 2, 5-^{14}C	12	240
104 mg/1,048 μCi/kg Nitrosopyrrolidine 3,4-^{14}C	16	1270

on a mM scale.   Table 2 illustrates the specific activity of RNA from rat liver after application of both compounds.   In the first two experiments, the same dosages as given by Lee and Lijinsky (4) were used.   A pentothal pretreatment of the animals was required to prevent neurotoxic effects.

Figure 11a shows the elution pattern of an RNA hydrolysate after application of 650 mg/1,594 μCi/kg 2,5-^{14}C-nitrosopyrrolidine and the addition of inactive 7-methylguanine.   As can be seen from this figure, a radioactive maximum is found between guanine and adenine which, however, did not correspond to the optical density of added 7-methylguanine.   Since Lee and Lijinsky (4) said that besides 7-methylguanine small amounts of a radioactive compound were formed which, according to its Rf-value, could be identical with 7-ethylguanine, the fractions containing the radioactivity were rechromatographed after the addition of both 7-methyl- and 7-ethylguanine (Fig. 11b).   As can be seen from Fig. 11b, the main reaction product from 2,5-^{14}C-nitrosopyrrolidine was not identical with either of these two compounds.

Figure 12a shows the elution pattern of a hydrolysate of RNA from rat liver after the application of 650 mg/1,535 μCi/kg 3,4-^{14}C-nitrosopyrrolidine.   Again a radioactive peak between adenine and guanine can be observed that is not identical with 7-methyl- or 7-ethylguanine, as can be seen from Fig. 12b, which illustrates the rechromatography of this peak after the addition of both these compounds.   However, it is obvious from these experiments that the same reaction product is formed after the application of the differently labeled compounds.   This indicates that this reaction product must contain at least two carbon atoms from the heterocyclic ring system.   (In these early studies the radioactivity of fractions following the adenine was not determined.)   Since the gas-chromatographic analysis of those ^{14}C-labeled nitrosopyrrolidines, which has been carried out by Dr. Lijinsky, revealed that the substances applied contained less than 0.1% impurities, it seemed unlikely that this radioactive peak observed in the RNA hydrolysates was formed from this minute amount of impurities.

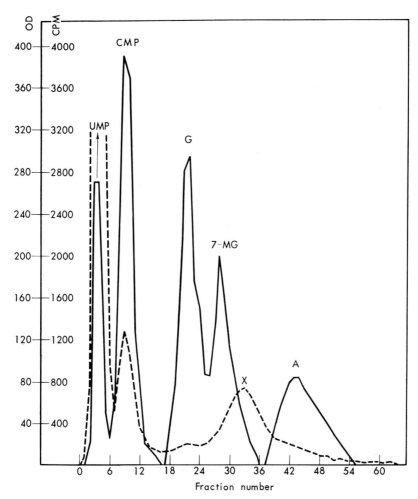

FIG. 11a. Elution pattern of an RNA hydrolysate from rat liver 16 hr after application of 650 mg/1,594 μCi/kg 2,5-¹⁴C-1-N-nitrosopyrrolidine, 55 mg RNA + 5.5 mg inactive 7-methylguanine added. A, adenine; 7-MG, 7-methylguanine; G, guanine; CMP, cytidine monophosphate; UMP, uridine monophosphate; ----------, CPM/min; ———, optical density. Dowex 50 WX.

As was already shown, the elongation of the aliphatic chain of the 7-alkylguanine derivative resulted in an increase in basicity of this compound. (7-Methyl- and 7-butylguanine are eluted before, whereas 7-propyl- and 7-butylguanine are eluted after the adenine containing fractions.) It, therefore, seemed possible that the unknown radioactive compound formed after the application of nitrosopyrrolidine could be identical with a 7-(Ω-carboxyalkyl)guanine, because the introduction of a carboxyl group into the aliphatic chains should increase the acidity of such a 7-alkylguanine derivative.

As can be seen in Fig. 13, two possible pathways of nitrosopyrrolidine degradation leading to such compounds can be formulated. After β-oxidation of the ring system, 7-methyl- and 7-(2-carboxyethyl)guanine should be expected as reaction pro-

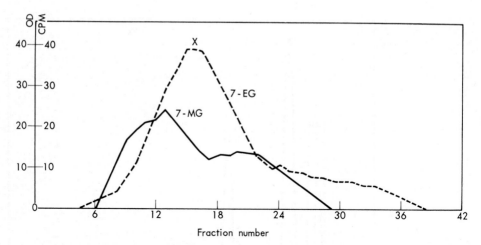

FIG. 11b. Rechromatography of fractions between adenine and guanine (see Fig. 11a), after an application of 2,5-^{14}C-1-N-nitrosopyrrolidine, with inactive 7-methyl- and 7-ethylguanine added. 7-MG, 7-methylguanine; 7-EG, 7-ethylguanine; ⸱⸱⸱⸱⸱⸱⸱⸱, CPM/min; ⸺, optical density. Dowex 50 WX.

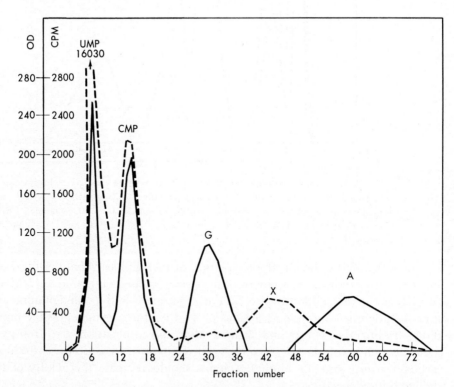

FIG. 12a. Elution pattern of an RNA hydrolysate after application of 650 mg/1,535 μCi/kg 3,4-^{14}C-1-N-nitrosopyrrolidine, with 45 mg RNA added. CMP, cytidinemonophosphate; UMP, uridinemonophosphate; A, adenine; G, guanine; ⸱⸱⸱⸱⸱⸱⸱⸱, CPM/min; ⸺, optical density. Dewex 50 WX.

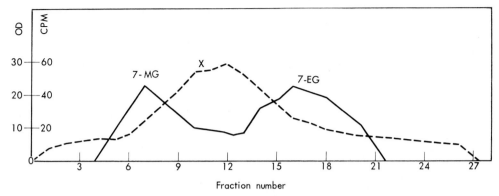

FIG. 12b. Rechromatography of fractions between adenine and guanine (see Fig. 12a) after an application of 3,4-^{14}C-1-N-nitrosopyrrolidine and the addition of 7-ethyl- and 7-methylguanine. 7-MG, 7-methylguanine; 7-EG, 7-ethylguanine; ---------, CPM/min; ———, optical density. Dowex 50 WX.

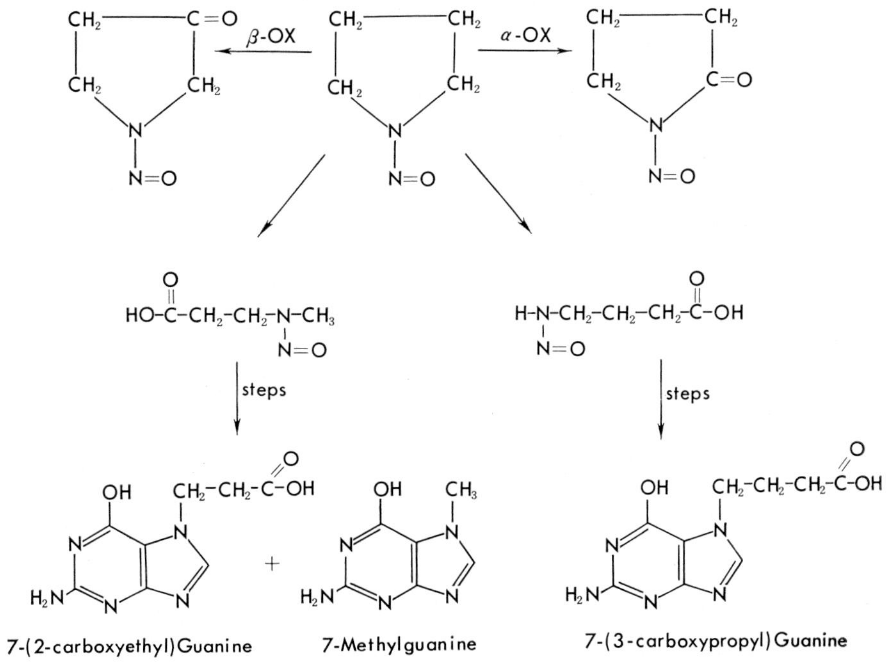

FIG. 13. Possible reaction products to be formed after α- or β-oxidation of nitrosopyrrolidine.

ducts with the genetic material, and α-oxidation should lead to the formation of 7-(3-carboxypropyl)guanine. Since the formation of 7-methylguanine had not been observed after the application of nitrosopyrrolidine and 7-(2-carboxyethyl)guanine (5) could not be separated from guanine on the Dowex columns used in these experiments, we tried to identify the unknown product as 7-(3-carboxypropyl)guanine. This compound was synthesized by reacting the ethyl ester of 4-iodobutyric acid with guanosine in dimethylformamide, followed by hydrolysis of the reaction product

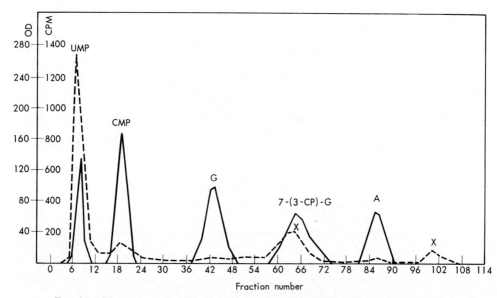

FIG. 14. Elution pattern of an RNA hydrolysate after an application of 102 mg/770 μCi/kg 2,5-^{14}C-1-N-nitrosopyrrolidine 12 hr after an application, with 100 mg RNA + 15 mg inactive 7-(3-carboxypropyl)guanine added. CMP, cytidinemonophosphate; UMP, uridine monophosphate; A, adenine; G, guanine; 7-(3-CP)-G, 7-(3-carboxypropyl)guanine; ----------, CPM/min; ————, optical density. Dowex 50 WX.

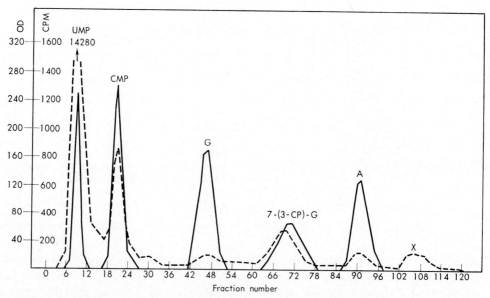

FIG. 15. Elution pattern of an RNA hydrolysate after the application of 104 mg/1,048 μCi/kg 3,4-^{14}C-1-N-nitrosopyrrolidine, with 40 mg RNA + 5 mg inactive 7-(3-carboxypropyl)guanine added. CMP, cytidinemonophosphate; UMP, uridinemonophosphate; A, adenine; G, guanine; 7-(3-CP)-G, 7-(3-carboxypropyl)guanine; ----------, CPM/min; ————, optical density. Dowex 50 WX.

with 3N HCl and separation of the compound from guanine on a Dowex column.

It can be seen from Figs. 14 and 15, which show the elution pattern of RNA hydrolysates from rat liver after the application of 102 mg/770 μCi/kg 2,5-^{14}C-1-N-nitrosopyrrolidine and 104 mg/1,048 μCi/kg 3,4-^{14}C-1-N-nitrosopyrrolidine and the addition of 7-(3-carboxypropyl)guanine, that the radioactive maximum found between adenine and guanine does not correspond with the optical densitiy of this added compound.   Hence, the identity of the unknown reaction product with 7-(3-carboxypropyl) guanine must be excluded.   It can be seen from both figures that another radioactive maximum can be observed in those fractions eluted after the adenine.   No attempts have yet been made to identify this product.

DISCUSSION

The experiments presented here were designed to explain the unexpected formation of 7-methylguanine after the application of various cyclic N-nitrosamines, according to the theory that higher alkylated or cyclic nitrosamines are degraded *in vivo* to methyl-alkyl- or dimethylnitrosamines, which are known to have strong methylating properties (*9*).   In agreement with this assumption it could be demonstrated that the application of both 1-^{14}C-di-*n*-propyl- and 1-^{14}C-di-*n*-butylnitrosamine led to the formation of 7-methylguanine, whereas this reaction product was not observed, when 2-^{14}C-di-*n*-propylnitrosamine was applied.   However, the results obtained, when the alkylating activity of -2,5-^{14}C and 3,4-^{14}C-N-nitrosopyrrolidine were investigated, do not support this theory.   It is clear that the main reaction products formed after the application of both nitrosopyrrolidines, which could not be identified until now, are not identical with 7-methylguanine, even though the formation of small amounts of these compounds cannot be excluded.

Since the formation of 7-methylguanine was not observed after the application of diethylnitrosamine, but was found to be the main reaction product after the application of both di-*n*-propylnitrosamine and di-*n*-butylnitrosamine, one is led to believe that 7-methylguanine might be the main reaction product, if the formation of this compound depends on the number of carbon atoms in the heterocyclic ring systems.   The identification of those unknown products, obtained after the application of N-nitrosopyrrolidines, and the investigation of the alkylating action of other ^{14}C-labeled cyclic nitrosamines might finally give more insight into these rather complex reactions of nitrosamine metabolism.

APPENDIX

With the exception of the following synthesis, experimental details of the data reported here have been recently described (Krüger, F. W. Metabolismus von Nitrosaminen *in vivo*. I. Über die β-Oxidation aliphatischer Di-*n*-alkylnitrosamine: Die Bildung von 7-Methylguanin neben 7-Propyl- bzw. 7-Butylguanin nach Applikation von Di-*n*-propyl- oder Di-*n*-butylnitrosamin. Z. Krebsforsch., *76*: 145–154, 1971).

Synthesis of 2,5-^{14}C- and 3,4-^{14}C-1-N-Nitrosopyrrolidine

1,4- or 2,3-^{14}C-Succinic acid was supplied by the Radio Chemical Centre, Amersham, and diluted with an inactive material to 236 mg (1 mM), and then dissolved in 4.5 ml of concentrated ammonium hydroxide. This solution was poured in small portions into a 5 ml retort and the water was carefully distilled off. After all of the solvent had been removed, the retort was heated with a free spirit flame and the succine imide formed, distilled. After this, the reaction vessel was split off mechanically and the remainder of succine imide in the retort's arm was removed with hot ethanol. The alcohol was evaporated under reduced pressure. The succine imide was dried *in vacuo* and then dissolved in 15 ml of anhydrous tetrahydrofurane. This solution was then added drop by drop to a boiling suspension of 600 mg LiAlH$_4$ in 50 ml anhydrous ether. The reaction mixture then was refluxed for 3 hr. After which, the excess of LiAlH$_4$ was destroyed by the careful addition of 15 ml of 30% aqueous NaOH and then extracted 10 times with 100 ml of ether. The combined ether extracts were acidified with anhydrous HCl and then evaporated to dryness. To the residual 6 ml of water, 2 ml of anhydrous acetic acid and 5 ml of a solution of 30% potassium nitrite in water were added. The reaction mixture was then kept for 1 hr at 25°C and cooled down with an ice/NaCl mixture. After this, 10 ml of 65% KOH in water were added and the reaction mixture was distilled to dryness. The yield of nitrosopyrrolidine in the distillate was determined by ultraviolet spectroscopy. Repeated synthesis of nitrosopyrrolidine at this scale gave yields between 35 and 44%. The aqueous solution showed the characteristic ultraviolet absorption spectra of 230 and 337 nm (pH 7).

Analysis of Labeled Nitrosopyrrolidine by GLC-Chromatography *

Two μl of each solution was injected into a 6 ft by 1/8 in stainless steel column, containing 80 to 100 mesh chromosorb W coated with 8.4% diethyleneglycol succinate. The inlet temperature was 190°C, the column temperature 110°C, the outlet temperature 170°C, and the flame ionization detector was at 340°C. The carrier gas flow rate (helium) was about 50 ml per min. With the attenuator setting such that the main peak due to nitrosopyrrolidine was off scale, no other significant peaks could be observed either before or after the appearance of the main peak, even at a setting five times as sensitive. Two minute peaks with very small retention times were found, but these represented less than 0.1% of the nitrosopyrrolidine peak.

Synthesis of 7-(3-Carboxypropyl)guanine

Two g of ethyl ester of 4-iodobutyric acid and 2 g of guanosine were heated in 10 ml dimethylformamide for 30 min at 130°C. After this the solvent was removed

---

* GLC-chromatogrophy was carried out by Dr. W. Lijinsky, the Eppley Institute for Research in Cancer, Omaha, Nebr., U.S.A.

in vacuo and the residue was refluxed for 2 hr with 50 ml of 3 N HCl. Then, after cooling, it was extracted three times with 100 ml of ether. The aqueous layer was treated with active charcoal, filtered and evaporated to dryness. The residue was dissolved in 10 ml of 1 N HCl. This solution was absorbed on a Dowex-50 WX 2 column (20 × 2 cm) and then eluted with 1 N HCl. Fractions, appearing after the guanine and having a characteristic absorption spectrum of 250 and 271 nm resp., were collected and evaporated to dryness. The residue was dissolved in 5 ml H_2O and adjusted to pH 3 with a few drops of 12% Na_4OH. The precipitate was filtered and recrystallized from 25 ml water. MP 274° (decomp.) yielded 135 mg.

calc. C=45.5%   found   C=45.7%
      H=4.64%   H=4.83%
      N=29.5%   N=29.44%

Rf 0.19 (*n*-propanol-water=75: 25 descending)

Ultraviolet absorption was:

pH 1	250; 271 nm	(infl.)
pH 7	283; 346	,,
pH 11	283; 346	,,

This work has been supported by the Verein zur Förderung der Krebsforschung in Deutschland e.V.

I would like to thank Dr. W. Lijinsky for carrying out the GCL-chromatography of labeled N-nitrosopyrrolidines and Dr. M. G. Burdon for his help in the preparation of this manuscript.

REFERENCES

1. Druckrey, H., Preussmann, R., Ivankovic, S., und Schmähl, D. Organotrope carcinogene Wirkungen bei 65 verschiedenen N-Nitroso-Verbindungen an BD-Ratten. Z. Krebsforsch., *69*: 103, 1967.
2. Heath, D. F., and Mattocks, A. R. Preparation of Labelled Dialkylnitrosamines and Improved Preparation of N-Methyl-*n*-butylamine. J. Chem. Soc., *1961*: 4226.
3. Kidson, C., Kirby, K. S., and Ralph, R. K. Isolation Characteristics of Rapidly Labelled RNA from Normal Rat Liver. J. Mol. Biol., *7*: 312, 1963.
4. Lee, K. Y., and Lijinsky, W. Alkylation of Rat Liver RNA by Cyclic N-Nitrosamines *in vivo*. J. Natl. Cancer Inst., *37*: 401, 1966.
5. Lijinsky, W., Loo, J., and Ross, A. E. Mechanism of Alkylation of Nucleic Acids by Nitrosodimethylamine. Nature, *218*: 1174, 1968.
6. Lijinsky, W., and Ross, A. E. Alkylation of Rat Liver Nucleic Acids not Related to Carcinogenesis N-Nitrosamines. J. Natl. Cancer Inst., *42*: 1095, 1969.
7. Magee, P. N., and Farber, E. Toxic Liver Injury and Carcinogenesis. Methylation of Rat Liver Nucleic Acids by Dimethylnitrosamine *in vivo*. Biochem. J., *83*: 114, 1962.
8. Magee, P. N., and Hultin, T. Toxic Liver Injury and Carcinogenesis. Methylation of Proteins of Rat Liver Slices by Dimethylnitrosamine *in vitro*. Biochem. J., *83*: 106, 1962.
9. Magee, P. N., and Lee, K. Y. Cellular Injury and Carcinogenesis. Alkylation of

Ribonucleic Acid of Rat Liver by Diethylnitrosamine and N-butyl-methyl-nitros-amine *in vivo*.   Biochem. J., *91*: 35, 1964.

10. Swann, P. F., and Magee, P. N.   Nitrosamine-induced Carcinogenesis.   The Alkylation of Nucleic Acids of the Rat by N-Methyl-N-nitrosourea, Dimethylnitros-amine, Dimethylsulphate and Methylmethansulphonate.   Biochem. J., *110*: 39, 1968.

11. Swann, P. F., and Magee, P. N.   Comparison between the Ethylation of Nucleic Acids by Diethylnitrosamine, Ethyl-methansulphonate, and N-Ethyl-N-nitrosourea and the Carcinogenic Activity of Each Compound.   10 Internat. Cancer Congress, Houston, Abstracts, p. 1, 1970.

12. Roberts, J. J., and Warwick, G. P.   The Reaction of β-Propiolactone with Guano-sine, Deoxyguanylic Acid and RNA.   Biochem. Pharmacol., *12*: 1441, 1963.

13. Rose, F. L.   *In*; Walpole, A. L. and Spinks, A. (eds.),   The Evaluation of Drug Toxicity, p. 116, Churchill, London, 1958.

Discussion of Paper by Dr. Krüger

DR. HEIDELBERGER: You mentioned 7-(2-carboxyethyl)guanine. This compound was shown several years ago by Roberts and Warwick to be the product of β-propiolactone alkylation of RNA.

DR. KRÜGER: I know that and have cited it in the paper.

DR. MAGEE: We have also observed 7-methylguanine in liver nucleic acids of rats treated with ^{14}C-dibutylnitrosamine. Very recently we have studied the liver nucleic acids of rats treated with ^{14}C-nitrosomorpholine and found no evidence of 7-methylguanine in the liver RNA.

DR. KRÜGER: Yes, I know that and have cited it in my paper in Z. Krebsforsch., *76*: 145, 1971, as a personal communication.

DR. MIRVISH: We injected tritium-labeled diethylnitrosamine into rats and found in their urine not only the expected 7-ethylguanine, but also a great deal of 7-methylguanine (Mirvish, S. and Sidransky, G., Biochem. Pharmacol., 1971, in press). We concluded that small amounts of labeled dimethylnitrosamine or methyl-alkyl-nitrosamine may have been present as impurities in the labeled diethylnitrosamine. Since dimethylnitrosamine produces far more 7-alkylation of guanine than does diethylnitrosamine, a small amount of methyl-containing nitrosamine would produce disproportionately large amounts of 7-methylguanine. However, it seems clear that radioactive impurities were not involved in your results, in view of your methods of radioactive synthesis.

DR. KRÜGER: We have not investigated the urine after the application of DENA. But the only compound found in RNA by Magee was 7-ethylguanine.

DR. WEISBURGER: What are the quantitative aspects of RNA labeling? How much of the activity in special peaks accounts for the total activity in RNA? Those experiments in the literature which prove only total RNA activity could be quite misleading.

DR. KRÜGER: We have not exactly calculated the amount of 7-methylguanine formed after application of the ^{14}C-nitrosamines. But it can be seen in Table 1 and from the elution patterns that the main part of the ^{14}C-activity is biologically incorporated into the pyrimidine bases.

DR. SUGIMURA: Was the experiment using ^{14}C-labeled butylnitrosamine at the 1 or 2 carbon? This experiment should give information to prove your hypothesis.

DR. KRÜGER: We have only examined the alkylating action of 1-^{14}C-di-n-butyl-nitrosamine because 2-^{14}C-butyric acid is not available on the market.   But we have found a way to synthesize

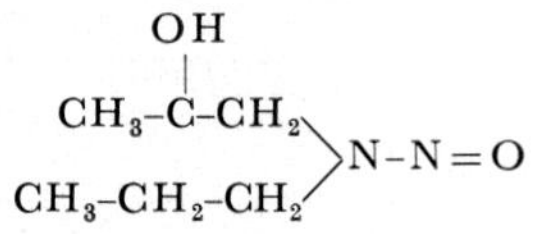

$$CH_3\text{-}\underset{\underset{\displaystyle OH}{|}}{C}\text{-}CH_2 \diagdown$$
$$CH_3\text{-}CH_2\text{-}CH_2 \diagup N\text{-}N=O$$

labeled in α- or β-position.   This might give clear results, if 7-methylguanine is formed after the application of the 1-^{14}C-labeled compound and if this is a real intermediate in di-n-propylnitrosamine metabolism.

DR. ISHIDATE: Have you any evidence that dialkylamine is convertible to the corresponding alkyl-acylnitrosamine in vivo?

DR. KRÜGER: No, we have not established this yet.   But Dr. Okada pointed out that

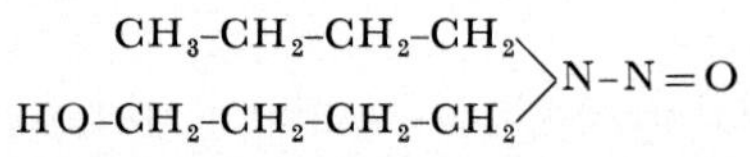

$$CH_3\text{-}CH_2\text{-}CH_2\text{-}CH_2 \diagdown$$
$$HO\text{-}CH_2\text{-}CH_2\text{-}CH_2\text{-}CH_2 \diagup N\text{-}N=O$$

is converted to the corresponding carboxylic acid.   If this is true, it is possible that my findings that 1-^{14}C-di-n-propylguanine leads to the formation of 7-MG, whereas the 2-^{14}C compound does not, could also be explained by the following reaction:

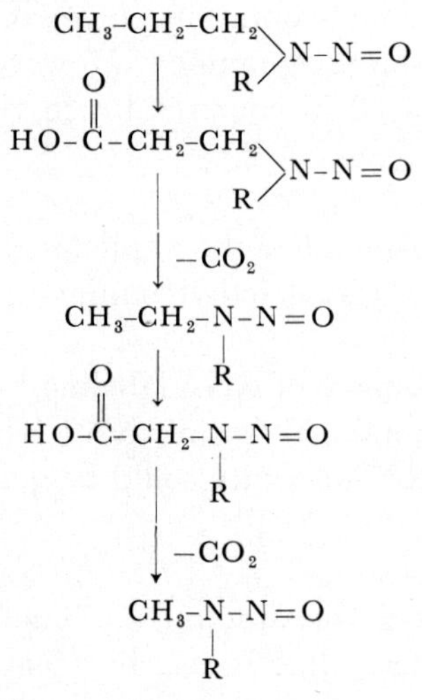

$$CH_3\text{-}CH_2\text{-}CH_2 \diagdown$$
$$\underset{R}{\diagup} N\text{-}N=O$$

$$\downarrow$$

$$HO\text{-}\underset{\underset{\displaystyle O}{\|}}{C}\text{-}CH_2\text{-}CH_2 \diagdown$$
$$\underset{R}{\diagup} N\text{-}N=O$$

$$\downarrow -CO_2$$

$$CH_3\text{-}CH_2\text{-}N\text{-}N=O$$
$$\underset{R}{|}$$

$$\downarrow$$

$$HO\text{-}\underset{\underset{\displaystyle O}{\|}}{C}\text{-}CH_2\text{-}N\text{-}N=O$$
$$\underset{R}{|}$$

$$\downarrow -CO_2$$

$$CH_3\text{-}N\text{-}N=O$$
$$\underset{R}{|}$$

even though 7-MG should also be observed after the application of diethylnitrosamine.   But this was not found by Magee and Lee.

DR. DRÜCKREY: If the carboxylated chain is degraded by β-oxidation (either in the nitrosamine or in the alkylated guanine), then different results are to be expected with even or odd numbered alkyl chains.   Have you observed such differences?

DR. KRÜGER: Yes, these differences can be expected.

The Action of Alkylating Mutagens and Carcinogens on Nucleic Acids: N-Methyl-N-nitroso Compounds as Methylating Agents

P. D. Lawley

Chester Beatty Research Institute, Institute of Cancer Research, Pollards Wood Research Station, Nightingales Lane, Chalfont St. Giles, Bucks, England

The alkylating agents include some of the chemically simplest carcinogens and are, therefore, of particular interest with respect to the elucidation of the molecular mechanisms of carcinogenesis. Methylating agents are of further interest, because biomethylation is a fundamental natural process. Nucleic acids are methylated *in vivo* by both the chemical and enzymic pathways. In RNA the sites of biomethylation and chemical methylation overlap to some extent (Srinivasan and Borek, 1966), but this does not appear to be true for DNA.

The nucleic acid targets of the methylating carcinogens may be of significance for several reasons a priori. Cellular DNA may be important because somatic mutations can be induced; many carcinogens other than alkylating agents are known to react with DNA *in vivo* in target organs (Lawley, 1966). Furthermore, for those carcinogens which require metabolism in order to exert their biological effects, the reactive metabolites may be alkylating agents (as with N,N-dialkyl-nitrosamines, Magee and Barnes, 1967), aralkylating agents (as with aromatic hydrocarbons, Dipple, Lawley and Brookes, 1968), or arylating agents (as with certain aromatic amines, Miller and Miller, 1966). Thus, for a wide range of carcinogens, comparisons with the simple alkylating agents will be useful in studying the mode of action.

In all cases studied, the carcinogens or their active metabolites also reacted with RNA *in vivo*. It is conceivable, therefore, that RNA could be a significant cellular target. Some alkylating agents are mutagens for RNA viruses (Singer and Fraenkel-Conrat, 1969). Most naturally occurring tumor viruses contain RNA, and these are known to induce provirus in the DNA of target cells (Mizutani and Temin, 1970). But it is not known whether the reaction of cellular RNA (most likely of the mRNA type) with carcinogens could cause such a process to occur.

Apart from intrinsic interest as a potential cellular target, the reactions of RNA with carcinogens are instructive for comparisons with DNA. The differences in the reactions with the various types of cellular nucleic acids could possibly aid in defining which ones are the significant cellular targets by comparing carcinogens of different potencies in this respect.

The present work was stimulated by the findings that, whereas alkylating agents in general are weak carcinogens (Brookes and Lawley, 1964), some alkylating agents, such as N-methyl-N-nitrosourea, could be potent carcinogens (*cf.*, Magee and Barnes, 1967). These latter agents were expected, on the basis of their chemical structures, to be activated chemically, rather than metabolically, in their reactions with cellular material. However, their mode of activation was expected to be different from that of many alkylating agents.

The broad subdivision of such agents into those of the SN2 and SN1 types is due to Ingold (1953, 1970). The simple concept is that the SN2 reagents form transition complexes with nucleophiles, hence, the bimolecular connotation. The SN1 agents, on the other hand, were thought to react by a dissociative rather than by an associative mechanism, and the rate-determining step was considered to be their ionization. More recent theories have abandoned the clear-cut distinction outlined above, and have attributed the differences between the various reagents to the relative rates of ion-pair formation and of the reaction of the ion-pair with the nucleophile (Sneen and Larsen, 1969). However, the distinction between SN1 and SN2 types is still pertinent to the present discussion.

In the present case, the typical SN2 reagents considered are dimethyl sulphate and methyl methanesulphonate. The reagents which are thought to react in part through the SN1 mechanism are N-methyl-N-nitrosourea (MNUA) and N-methyl-N'-nitro-N-nitrosoguanidine (MNNG).

Figure 1 compares the chemical activation of MNUA with the metabolic activation of N,N-dimethylnitrosamine. In both cases, the reactive intermediate monomethylnitrosamine, or methyldiazohydroxide, is generated. This may be supposed to react *per se*, or to ionize to give $CH_3N_2^+$, which may also react or further dissociate yielding the CH_3^+ ion.

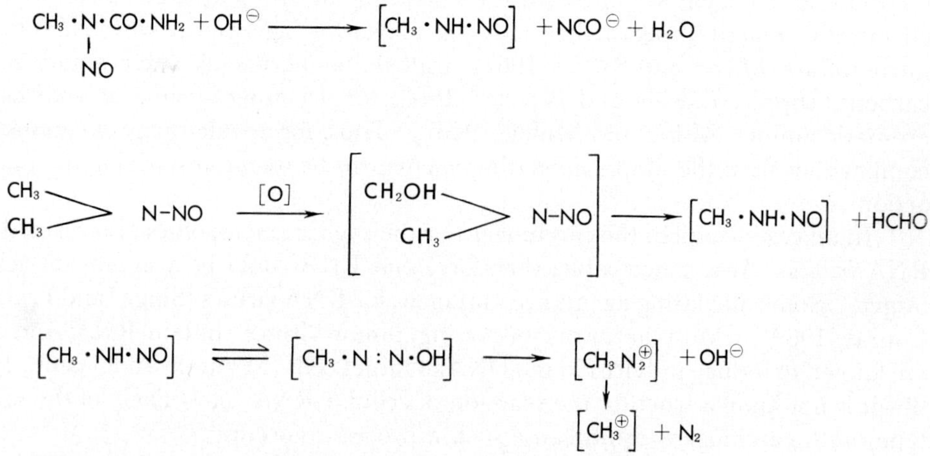

$$CH_3 \cdot N \cdot CO \cdot NH_2 + OH^\ominus \longrightarrow \left[CH_3 \cdot NH \cdot NO \right] + NCO^\ominus + H_2O$$
$$\overset{|}{NO}$$

$$\frac{CH_3}{CH_3}\!\!> N-NO \xrightarrow{[O]} \left[\frac{CH_2OH}{CH_3}\!\!> N-NO \right] \longrightarrow \left[CH_3 \cdot NH \cdot NO \right] + HCHO$$

$$\left[CH_3 \cdot NH \cdot NO \right] \rightleftharpoons \left[CH_3 \cdot N : N \cdot OH \right] \longrightarrow \left[CH_3 N_2^\oplus \right] + OH^\ominus$$
$$\downarrow$$
$$\left[CH_3^\oplus \right] + N_2$$

Fig. 1. Mode of activation of N-methyl-N-nitrosourea (MNUA) by alkali-catalyzed hydrolysis and of N,N-dimethylnitrosamine (DMN) by metabolic oxidation.

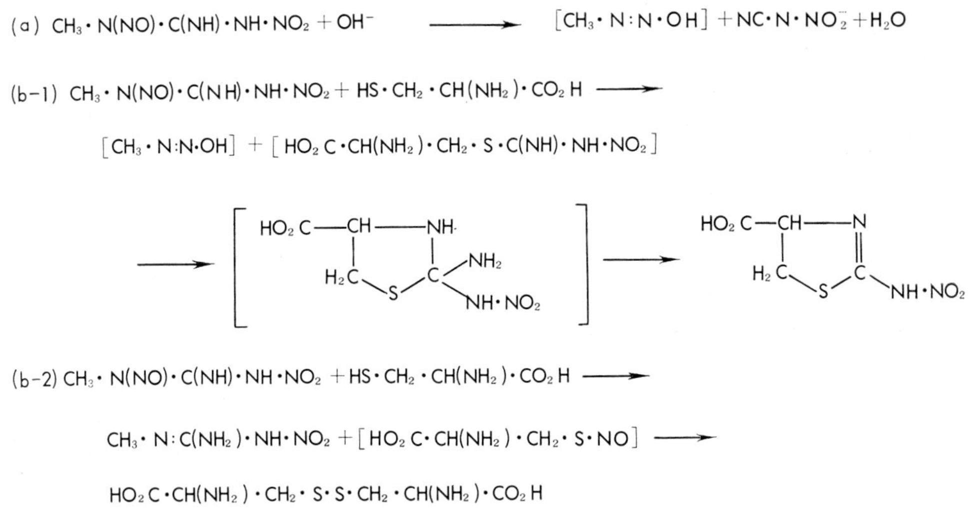

(a) $CH_3 \cdot N(NO) \cdot C(NH) \cdot NH \cdot NO_2 + OH^- \longrightarrow [CH_3 \cdot N:N \cdot OH] + NC \cdot N \cdot NO_2^- + H_2O$

(b-1) $CH_3 \cdot N(NO) \cdot C(NH) \cdot NH \cdot NO_2 + HS \cdot CH_2 \cdot CH(NH_2) \cdot CO_2 H \longrightarrow$

$[CH_3 \cdot N:N \cdot OH] + [HO_2 C \cdot CH(NH_2) \cdot CH_2 \cdot S \cdot C(NH) \cdot NH \cdot NO_2]$

(b-2) $CH_3 \cdot N(NO) \cdot C(NH) \cdot NH \cdot NO_2 + HS \cdot CH_2 \cdot CH(NH_2) \cdot CO_2 H \longrightarrow$

$CH_3 \cdot N:C(NH_2) \cdot NH \cdot NO_2 + [HO_2 C \cdot CH(NH_2) \cdot CH_2 \cdot S \cdot NO] \longrightarrow$

$HO_2 C \cdot CH(NH_2) \cdot CH_2 \cdot S \cdot S \cdot CH_2 \cdot CH(NH_2) \cdot CO_2 H$

FIG. 2.   Mode of activation of N-methyl-N′-nitro-N-nitrosoguanidine (MNNG) by (a), alkali-catalyzed hydrolysis; (b-1), reaction with thiol at electron-deficient C-atom; (b-2), reaction with thiol at nitroso group.   Note that (a) and (b-1) lead to the methylating species, mono-methylnitrosamine or methyldiazohydroxide; (b-2), yields a radical.

The activation of MNNG in aqueous media is similar to that of MNUA (Fig. 2), but activation through reaction with thiols also occurs (Lawley and Thatcher, 1970; McCalla, Reuvers and Kitai, 1968; Schulz and McCalla, 1969).   When the methods for studying the action of thiols, as used with MNNG *in vitro*, were applied to MNUA, no significant increase in the rate of hydrolysis of MNUA at pH 7 was found with cysteine (P. D. Lawley and J. V. Frei, unpublished data).   This finding suggests that MNUA, which reacts more rapidly than MNNG at a neutral pH in the absence of thiol (Garrett, Goto and Stubbins, 1965), would not be activated to a significant extent by thiols *in vivo*, and that such a process is not required for the carcinogenic action of nitroso compounds in general.

Some authors had previously suggested that diazomethane was the active agent in methylations by N-methyl-N-nitroso compounds, but the findings of Lijinsky, Loo and Ross (1968) showed that with CD_3-labeled DMN *in vivo* the methyl group entered 7-methylguanine intact.   Lingens, Haerlin and Süssmuth (1971) have reported analogous findings for MNNG and DNA in *Escherichia coli*.   It seems likely, therefore, that methylations by N-methyl-N-nitroso compounds in general are mediated by the methyldiazonium ion.   It would, in fact, be expected that diazomethane in aqueous media would itself react as its cation (Lawley, 1968).

It appears, therefore, that the differences between the N-methyl-N-nitroso compounds and the typical SN2 methylating agents should be attributed to their mechanisms of reaction.   It is also expected that the nitroso compounds would resemble the Ingold SN1 reagents.   In dealing with reactions of such agents at relatively low degrees of alkylation of nucleic acids, the obvious criterion to apply in seeking to test this hypothesis would be based on the concepts that, whereas the SN2 agents react with nucleophilic centers to extents positively correlated with their nucleophilicity, SN1 agents, according to the simplest theory, attack all nucleophiles to an equal extent, depending only on their concentration. Of course, this last assumption is rarely confirmed. Some degree of selectivity is almost invariably found, but the SN1 type of reagent would be expected to attack a wider spectrum of groups in a composite of various nucleophilic sites, such as that presented by nucleic acids.

In the following section, evidence showing that the supposed SN1 reagents do attack a different and wider spectrum of groups in nucleic acids and, in particular, that they react with O-atom sites as well as with ring-N-atoms, is presented. In the last section, the possible significance of these findings for the mode of biological action of these agents is discussed.

Methylation of Nucleic Acids by MNUA or MNNG: Comparisons with DMS and MMS

Clearly the first requisite for the study of methylations of nucleic acids by carcinogens is the availability of sensitive and reliable analytical techniques. These have been adequate previously for the detection of major products, but the recent

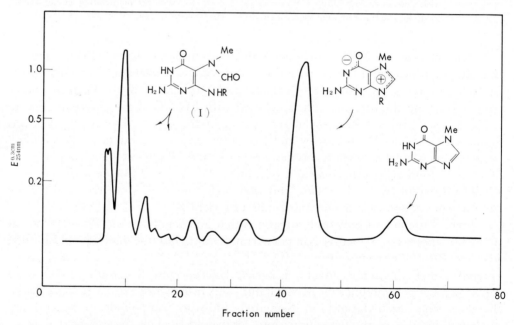

Fig. 3. Hydrolysis of 7-methyl-GMP to yield derivatives of 2-amino-4-hydroxy-5-methylformamido-6-ribosylaminopyrimidine (I) by alkali-catalyzed hydrolysis or 7-methylguanine by acid catalyzed hydrolysis. 7-Methyl-GMP was obtained by methylation of GMP and isolated by chromatography on Dowex-1 (formate form) eluted with water. The hydrolysate was prepared under the conditions used for degradation of RNA to nucleosides, *i.e.*, treatment with ribonuclease (100 μg/ml), spleen phosphodiesterase (0.1 units/ml at pH 6), and wheat germ acid phosphatase (0.5 units/ml), for 16 hr at 37°C. It was then chromatographed on Dowex-50 (NH₄⁺ form) (60 × 1.5 cm), eluted with 0.3m-ammonium formate, pH 8.9, 6.4 ml fractions. The products were identified by their characteristic UV absorption spectra.

interest in minor products has stimulated a review of methods and proposals for improved techniques (*cf.*, Brookes and Lawley, 1971). Recently, Lawley and Shah (1972) have compared analyses of methylated RNA's at the nucleoside and base levels.

The following methods have proved valuable for the degradation of RNA: (a) digestion with ribonuclease, phosphodiesterase (either spleen phosphodiesterase at pH 6 or venom at pH 8), and phosphomonoesterase; (b) KOH, then phospho-monoesterase; (c) HCl, giving purine bases and pyrimidine nucleotides; and (d) HClO$_4$, giving purine and pyrimidine bases. With DNA, apart from the enzymatic method, hydrolysis in 0.1 M-HCl to liberate purine bases has proved useful (Lawley and Thatcher, 1970).

It has been found that no one method yields all minor products in a suitable form. The reasons are that the alkylated nucleoside residues in nucleic acids are in several instances unstable either to alkali (as 1-, 3-, 7-alkyladenosine; 3-alkylcytidine or -uridine; 7-alkylguanosine) or to acid (O^6-alkylguanosines are dealkylated).

7-Alkylguanosines are unstable at any pH (Lawley and Brookes, 1963), yielding derivatives of 2,6-diamino-5-alkylformamido-4-hydroxypyrimidine by imidazole ring fission catalyzed by alkali, or the free base 7-alkylguanine by acid-catalyzed hydrolysis (Fig. 3). It should be noted that 7-methylguanosine cannot be recovered quantitatively from enzymatic digests of methylated RNA, since some of this product inevitably appears as pyrimidine derivatives of the type specified. Unfortunately, their precise nature is not known. Under the conditions used for the chromato-graphy of nucleosides, dephosphorylated 7-methylguanylic acid was found to yield several components. The UV spectra of the products were virtually identical, and corresponded to those of compounds of type (I) of Fig. 3, with presumably various radicals R derived from β-ribofuranosyl during the imidazole ring-opening process. These products may well be in equilibrium with each other in aqueous media, since if they are isolated on chromatograms and rerun, single peaks do not result.

It is, therefore, essential to isolate several methylated purines and pyrimidines by acid hydrolysis. But with RNA this method destroys O^6-alkylpurines, although they can be liberated from DNA by a mild acid treatment.

The question then arises whether all the products can be separated adequately. Again no one method proved satisfactory. The much used chromatography on Dowex-50 (H$^+$ form) eluted with HCl does not separate 3-methyladenine from 7-methylguanine, but 1- and 7-methyladenines are separable. If adenine itself has to be separated (as in nucleic acid methylated *in vivo*, which has incorporated some label from the methyl-labeled alkylating agent), this method would not be adequate.

For nucleoside separations, the use of Dowex-50 (NH$_4^+$ form) was investigated. We found that the elution of 7-methylguanosine at pH 6.6 was not satisfactory, but that the bases could be usefully separated at this pH. For nucleoside separations, pH 8.9 was satisfactory (*cf.*, Junowicz and Spencer, 1969).

It is possible here to give a limited selection of data to illustrate the type of results obtained. Generally [^{14}C]methyl-labeled alkylating agents have been used, but ^{3}H-labeling appears to be satisfactory, although the efficiency of counting is, of course, lower. In order to identify a new component recently found in methylated

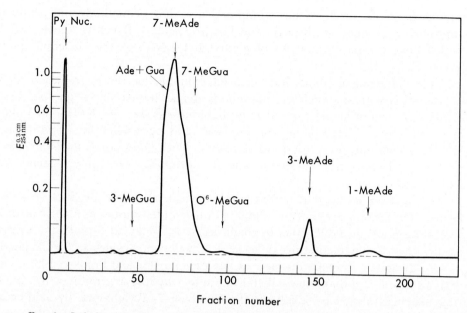

FIG. 4. Isolation of minor products of methylation of salmon sperm DNA (50 mg) with N-methyl-N-nitrosourea (2.4 g in 10 ml aqueous solution maintained at pH 7, 37°C, in a pH-stat). The methylated DNA was hydrolyzed in 0.1 M-HCl at 70°C and the purines liberated were chromatographed on Dowex-50 (NH₄⁺ form), 60 × 1.5 cm eluted with 0.3 M-ammonium formate, pH 6.65, 6.4 ml fractions. The products were identified by their characteristic UV spectra, and by running the authentic purines separately on the column to determine their positions of elution. " Py Nuc " denotes pyrimidine nucleotide material.

TABLE 1. Molar Proportions of Methylation Products in RNA

Reagent material treated type of RNA	MNUA RNA μ2-RNA	DMS RNA μ2-RNA	MNUA reticulocytes rRNA	DMS reticulocytes rRNA	MNUA phage μ2 μ2-RNA	MMS phage R17 R17-RNA
Extent of methylation (mmol/mol RNA P)	13	0.1	2	25	4	0.3
1-Methyladenine	2	13	2	9	2	12
3-Methyladenine	1	1	n.d.	1	n.d.	1
7-Methyladenine	2.5	1.5	2.5	1	3	2
3-Methylcytosine	2	12	2	9	1.5	7
3-Methylguanine	1	0.4	n.d.	0.5	n.d.	n.d.
7-Methylguanine	77	60	80	74	67	72
O⁶-Methylguanine	3.5	<0.2	3.5	<0.2	3.8	<0.2

[C¹⁴] Methyl-labeled reagents were used, and the proportion of total radioactivity eluted in column chromatograms together with UV-absorbing peaks of appropriate marker bases or nucleosides was estimated. The values quoted are generally averages of several determinations; n. d. denotes not determined. Methods for hydrolysis and chromatography are described and assessed in the text.

nucleic acids, *viz.*, 3-methylguanine (Lawley, Orr, and Shah, 1972), UV spectroscopy of unlabeled material was used, as shown in Fig. 4. It should be noted that the extent of methylation required to demonstrate the peaks of the minor methylation

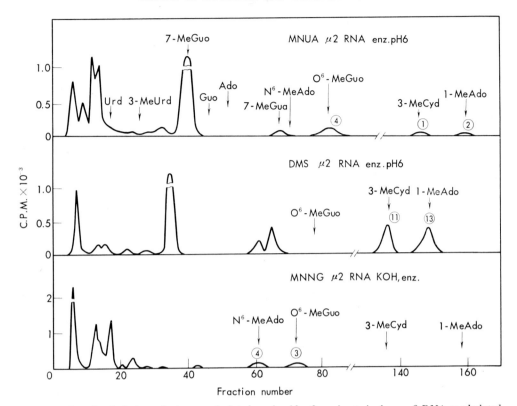

Fig. 5. Isolation of minor methylated nucleosides from bacteriophage $\mu2$-RNA methylated with N-[^{14}C]methyl-N-nitrosourea (MNUA) (13 mmol methyl/mol RNA-P), di-[^{14}C]methyl sulphate (DMS) (1.2 mmol/mol RNA-P) or N-[^{14}C]methyl-N′-nitro-N-nitrosoguanidine (17 mmol/mol RNA-P). The MNUA- and DMS-RNA (about 2 mg, more than 20,000 c.p.m.) were hydrolyzed enzymatically as described in Fig. 3. The MNNG-RNA was hydrolyzed to nucleotides with 0.3 M-KOH at 37°C, then with bacterial alkaline phosphatase (3 units/ml) at pH 9. Chromatography was as described for Fig. 3. The positions of the [^{14}C]methyl-labeled nucleosides were determined by the positions of the UV-absorbing peaks of added marker nucleosides, shown by the arrows. After the position shown as a break in the fraction number axis, elution was continued with 1 M-ammonium formate, pH 8.9. The ringed numbers show the proportion of radioactivity in each product.

products was excessive in comparison with those likely to be encountered *in vivo*.

Several types of RNA have been investigated by *in vitro* methylation at relatively low degrees, using isotopically labeled agents. Similar proportions of products are generally found for a given agent, irrespective of whether isolated RNA or whole cells were methylated. For example, in Table 1, methylations of RNA in rabbit reticulocytes and $\mu2$ bacteriophage are compared with those of isolated RNA.

The examples of chromatograms shown illustrate various aspects as follows. In Fig. 5 the separation of the nucleosides derived from methylated $\mu2$ bacteriophage RNA by enzymatic digestion at pH 6 is shown. The main features demonstrated are that both MNUA and MNNG yield O⁶-methylguanosine, whereas DMS does not. Moreover, the proportions of 1-methyladenosine and of 1-methylcytidine in

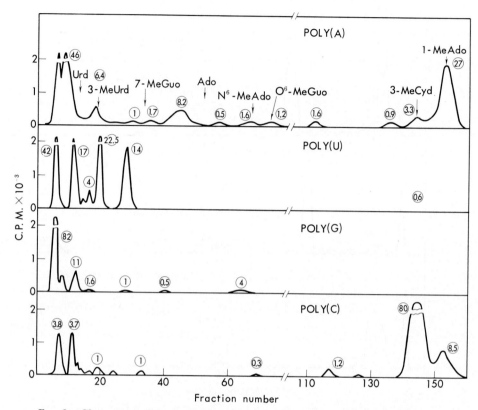

Fig. 6. Chromatography of nucleosides from degradation of homopolyribonucleotides, methylated by N-[^{14}C]methyl-N-nitrosourea, by the enzymatic procedure described in Fig. 3. It should be noted that poly (G) was not degraded by this procedure. Poly (A) yields some 1-methyladenosine; poly (U), some 3-methyluridine; poly (C), mainly 3-methylcytidine. The extent of methylation was about 10 mol methyl/mol polynucleotide-P.

MNUA- or MNNG-RNA are much lower than those in DMS-RNA. It will also be noted that, as expected, KOH hydrolysis of RNA destroys these latter products; 1-methyladenosine is converted into N^6-methyladenosine, but O^6-methylguanosine is not affected.

In Fig. 6 typical results from enzymatic digestion of MNUA-treated homo-polyribonucleotides at pH 6 and chromatography at pH 8.9 are shown. It can be seen that, as expected, poly (G) cannot be degraded. The remaining polynucleo-tides show that in poly (A) 1-methyladenosine is the principal product, the other derivatives not being detected by this method. In poly (U), some 3-methyluridine is found. But, as will be discussed later, the N-3 atom of uridine is relatively unreac-tive toward alkylating agents, in general, and its alkylation may be due to the partial acidic ionization of poly (U) at the reaction pH of 8. Poly (C) yields mainly 3-methylcytidine, which like 1-methyladenosine, is well separated from other products in this chromatographic system because of its relatively high pK$_a$ value.

This chromatographic method, Dowex-50 (NH$_4^+$ form) at pH 8.9, is thus useful for isolating certain minor products, derived from alkylation at N-1 of adenine, N-3

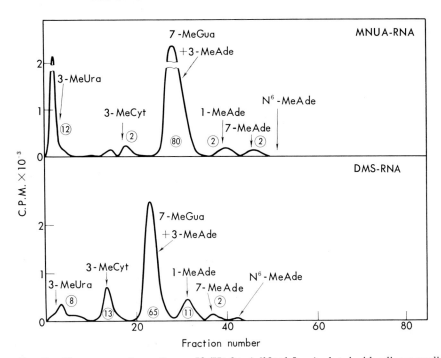

FIG. 7. Chromatography on Dowex-50 (H⁺ form) (10 × 1.5 cm), eluted with a linear gradient of 0.75–2.5 M-HCl (600 ml), of purine and pyrimidine bases obtained from perchloric acid-hydrolysates (72% [w/v] HClO₄, 1 hr, 100°C) of [¹⁴C]methylated bacteriophage μ2-RNA (cf., Fig. 5 for chromatography of nucleosides from these methylated RNA's). It will be noted that the principal product, 7-methylguanine, is not separated from 3-methyladenine by this system, but the use of other systems (cf., Fig. 8) shows that 3-methyladenine is about 1% of the total methylation products. It should also be noted that the first peak is not 3-methyluracil, which other systems show to be less than 1% of the total products.

of cytosine and O-6 of guanine residues. Appropriate methods for hydrolysis are available, but it should be noted that one sample of spleen phosphodiesterase did cause some de-O-methylation of O⁶-methylguanosine. This indicates a possibility of deaminase activity in this type of commercial product. Venom phosphodiesterase may, therefore, be preferable for degradation of methylated RNA to show the presence of O⁶-methylguanosine.

Apart from O⁶-methylguanine, which is demethylated in acid, the methylated bases of interest here are stable enough to enable the appropriate acid hydrolysis of RNA to be used. It was found, however, that 1 N-HCl at 100°C for 1 hr did partially convert 1-methyladenine into a product eluted from the Dowex-50 (H⁺ form) together with 7-methyladenine. Hydrolysis with perchloric acid is, therefore, preferable in order to obtain bases from RNA. With DNA, 0.1 M-HCl at 70°C can be used to liberate purines (cf., Fig. 4).

As an alternative chromatographic method to the previously used Dowex-50 (H⁺ form) eluted with HCl (illustrated in Fig. 7), Dowex-50 (NH₄⁺ form) is useful for separating bases (cf., Fig. 4, at pH 6.65; Fig. 8, at pH 8.9). Here again the differences in positions of eluted bases reflect their different pK$_a$ values; the more basic

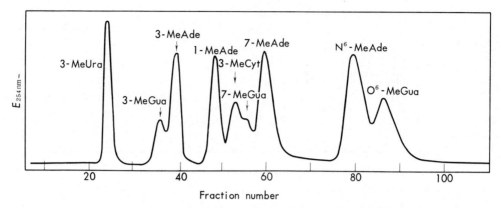

Fig. 8. Use of Dowex-50 (NH_4^+ form), eluted with 0.3 M-ammonium formate, pH 8.9, to separate purine and pyrimidine bases (these are marker bases only).

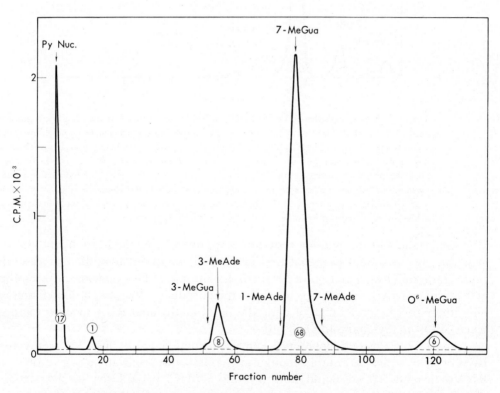

Fig. 9. Chromatography of purines from salmon sperm DNA, methylated at pH 7 with N-[14C]methyl-N-nitrosourea (2 mmol/mol DNA-P) and hydrolyzed with 0.1 M-HCl, 70°C.

1- and 3-methyladenines are eluted at pH 6.65 well after 7-methyladenine. Figure 9 shows that the presence of O^6-methylguanine in an acid-hydrolysate of MNUA-DNA can be well demonstrated by use of Dowex-50 (NH_4^+ form) at pH 8.9. The presence of 3-methylguanine (in methylated poly (G), Fig. 10) is also shown by this method, and its use for methylated poly (A) and poly (U) is illustrated in Fig. 11.

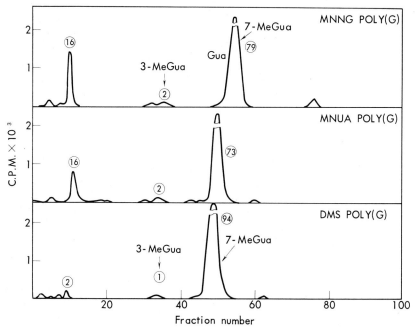

FIG. 10.   Chromatography of [¹⁴C]methylated purines from poly (G), methylated at pH 8 with ¹⁴C-labeled MNUA, MNNG or DMS, hydrolyzed with HClO₄ (note that O⁶-methylguanine is destroyed under these conditions of hydrolysis; 3-methylguanine is stable).   Chromatography, the same as for Fig. 8.

The principal conclusions drawn from the applications of the various techniques were as follows.   The nitroso compounds NMUA and MNNG closely resembled each other and methylations by either reagent were not significantly different.   But the sulphonates DMS and MMS, which also closely resembled each other, fell into a separate category.   The nitroso compounds were distinguished by their ability to methylate the O-6 atom of guanine, more so in DNA (7% of total products) than in RNA (3.5%).   But they showed less tendency to methylate N-1 of adenine, N-3 of cytosine and N-3 of uridine.   In DNA (native) they methylated N-3 of adenine to about half the extent given by DMS or MMS.   In poly (A), N-7 of adenine was almost as reactive as N-1 toward MNUA or MNNG, but much less so toward DMS or MMS.   This conclusion applies also for methylations of RNA.

Some questions remain for further study, concerning mainly the reactions at pyrimidine sites and in the sugar-phosphate chain.   The ability of MNUA and its analogues to methylate O-atoms in the guanine of nucleic acids suggests the possibility that O-atoms of pyrimidines or of ribose or phosphate residues can be methylated.

Mustard gas was shown to alkylate the terminal phosphate groups of poly (U) by Abell, Rosini and Ramseur (1965), but intrachain phosphodiester groups were not alkylated.   The facile hydrolysis at a neutral pH of a triester derived from uridylic acid (Brown and Todd, 1955) suggests that if phosphotriesters were formed in RNA they would hydrolyze at a neutral pH, and that presumably either

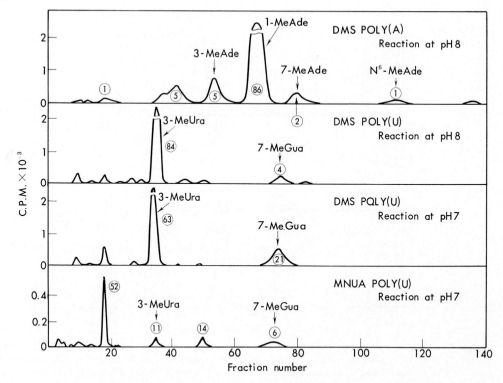

FIG. 11. Influence of reagent or of pH on methylation of homopolyribonucleotides. The [14C]methylated polymers were hydrolyzed with $HClO_4$ and chromatographed in the same way as Fig. 8. 7-Methylguanine evidently derives from guanylic acid residues present as impurities in poly (U).

the alkyl group would be lost, or the macromolecular chain would be cleaved.

Studies of bacteriophage RNA alkylated by mustard gas, DMS or MNUA showed that only the last named of the three reagents caused degradation of RNA (Shooter, 1971; Lawley, Shooter, House and Shah, 1971). It was notable, however, that about ten alkylations per RNA molecule of the phage sufficed to inactivate plaque formation, and that less than one-fifth of the lethality of MNUA toward the phage was due to chain breakage. It is unclear whether this breakage is due to phosphotriester formation. Rosenkranz, Rosenkranz and Schmidt (1969) found that MNUA, N-methyl-N-nitrosourethane and N,N-dimethylnitrosamine can produce single-strand breaks in DNA, and suggested that these were not caused by methylation.

Suggestions have been made from time to time that methylations of DNA could cause direct chain fission through phosphotriester formation (e.g., Rhaese and Freese, 1969), but other studies have not supported this view (e.g., Uhlenhopp and Krasna, 1971). Chemical studies have shown that phosphotriesters of thymidylic acid can be made using diazoalkanes (Scheit, 1967; Holy and Scheit, 1967), and as predicted by Brown and Todd (1955), these were found to be relatively stable during both acid and alkaline hydrolysis, e.g., ammonia (at unstated pH) caused slow hydrolysis, and the product was stable in 80% acetic acid at room temperature (Scheit, 1967).   Clearly, there are still discrepancies regarding the possible contribution of phosphotriester breakdown to the degradation of methylated DNA at neutral pH, which appears to result mainly, if not entirely, from depurination.

At the present time, therefore, no definitive evidence can be stated for phosphotriester formation in methylated RNA or DNA.   But some of the data suggest that the proportion of methylation products, not accounted for as known methylated bases and eluted early from columns, is in fact greater with MNUA than with DMS. As examples, Figs. 7, 10 and 11 may be quoted.   The data of Fig. 11 are particularly instructive with reference to methylated poly (U).   The sample of poly (U) used here evidently contained a small proportion of guanine, since some 7-methylguanine was obtained on methylation.   The amount of 7-methylguanine would not be expected to vary much with pH, but the yield of 3-methyluracil might well increase at pH 8, since unionized uridine is relatively unreactive, compared with the anionic form.

The main features of the data showed that, as expected, the proportion of 3-methyluracil to 7-methylguanine was higher for a reaction with DMS at pH 8 than for a reaction at pH 7.   But an additional finding was that the proportions of the products from MNUA were quite different from those with DMS.   MNUA evidently shows less tendency to react at the N-3 position of uridine than does DMS. Also, it shows more tendency to give products eluted early from the column and possibly derived from reaction with the sugar-phosphate groups.

Alternatively, MNUA may show a greater tendency to react with the O-atoms of pyrimidines to give products demethylated in acid, but such products have yet to be detected.

TABLE 2.   Summary of Principal Differences between the Reactions with Nucleic Acids of N-Methyl-N-nitroso Compounds (MNUA or MNNG) and of Methyl Sulphonates (DMS or MMS)

Product	Remarks
1-Methyladenine	Minor product in RNA with both types of reagent, but DMS gives more than MNUA.
	In DNA (native) very little is given by either; relatively more in denatured DNA.
3-Methyladenine	In RNA a very minor product with both types.
	In DNA the principal minor product, but MNUA gives less than DMS.
7-Methyladenine	A minor product with both agents; somewhat more with MNUA.
3-Methylcytosine	In RNA about the same amount as 1-methyladenine; again DMS gives more than MNUA. In DNA (native) very little is detected.
3-Methylguanine	In both nucleic acids a very minor product; MNUA gives rather more than DMS; much less than 3-methyladenine in DNA; about the same in RNA.
7-Methylguanine	Major product with both types of reagent in both nucleic acids.
O^6-Methylguanine	Not detected as a product from DMS; with MNUA the third most abundant product; twice as much in DNA as in RNA.
3-Methylthymine, or 3-Methyluracil	Not detected in DNA with either agent; can be found in RNA or poly(U) relatively more with DMS than with MNUA; probably from reaction of ionized form.
Phosphotriester	MNUA degrades RNA; possibly due to phosphotriester formation; DMS does not. Generally methylated DNA is not degraded by alkylation *per se*.

The principal differences between the two classes of methylating agents typified by MNUA and DMS are summarized in Table 2.

Methylations of Nucleic Acids in vivo

The relatively small amount of data available on *in vivo* methylations of nucleic acids suggests that, as expected, the differences between the classes of reagents are found *in vivo* as *in vitro*. Most of the data on minor methylation products from nitroso compounds has been obtained for N,N-di[^{14}C]methylnitrosamine injected into rats; liver nucleic acids were then isolated and analyzed.

The data of Lawley, Brookes, Magee, Craddock, and Swann (1968) showed that the proportions of 3-methyladenine in DNA isolated 5 hr after the administration of the nitrosamine were about the same as for MNUA-DNA or MNNG-DNA obtained by *in vitro* reaction, or in the case of MNNG-DNA, by treatment of mammalian cells in culture. This proportion (about 8%) was significantly lower than for DMS-methylated DNA (about 20%). The principal feature of the results for *in vivo* methylated RNA was that the proportions of 1-methyladenine and of 3-methylcytosine obtained were lower in DMN-RNA than in DMS-RNA.

It will be noted, therefore, that some of the distinguishing features of MNUA *in vitro* are also found for DMN *in vivo*. It remained to be established whether the more notable distinction, that MNUA (or MNNG) could yield O^6-methylguanine, was also a feature of the action of DMN. This has, in fact, been found to be true in collaborative work by the present author and Dr. P. J. O'Connor of the Paterson Laboratories, Christie Hospital and Holt Radium Institute, Manchester, England. Ribosomal RNA isolated from the liver of rats 5 hr after an injection of [^{14}C]DMN was shown to contain 3–4% of O^6-methylguanosine in the methylation products. The differences previously noted, that the proportions of 1-methyladenine and 3-methylcytosine were relatively low (around 1%), have also been confirmed.

It now appears that the previous suggestion (Lawley, Brookes, Magee, Craddock, and Swann, 1968), that these lower proportions reflect the involvement of the N-1 of adenine and N-3 of cytosine residues in hydrogen bonding in RNA, is a misinterpretation. The differences now appear to be more plausibly attributed to variations between the mode of reaction of the active methylating species derived from metabolized DMN, MNUA or MNNG and that of DMS or MMS.

With regard to methylations of RNA *in vivo* by MMS, Whittle (1969) reported that 1-methyladenine and 3-methylcytosine could be identified in rat liver RNA, following a single i.p. injection. The more recent data of O'Connor and Lawley (unpublished) show that the proportions of these minor bases is about 9% for each, *i.e.*, about the same as for RNA treated *in vitro*, but O^6-methylguanosine was not detected.

With regard to the methylations of DNA *in vivo* by MNUA, Frei (1971) has shown that O^6-methylguanine is a product (in bone marrow, spleen, thymus, kidney, liver and lung of mice). He also noted that what he termed " excess " 3-methyladenine (in proportions exceeding about 15%) was found in some organs, notably, bone marrow, spleen and thymus.

Thus, from the limited amount of data available at the time of writing, the broad conclusion that the principal differences between nitroso compounds and MMS are found to be the same *in vivo* as *in vitro* may be reiterated.

Possible Biological Implications of in vivo Methylations

The significance of the differences between the two classes of methylating agents with regard to nucleic acid methylations can, at present, only be speculated upon. Probably the most significant feature is the one pointed out by Loveless (1969): MNUA most likely owes its ability to induce mutations by the " transition " mis-pairing mechanism (Watson and Crick, 1953) to its capacity for alkylating the O-6 atom of guanine in guanine nucleosides.   The forms of methylated guanine nucleo-side residues which have been proposed as possible causes of miscoding are shown in Fig. 12.

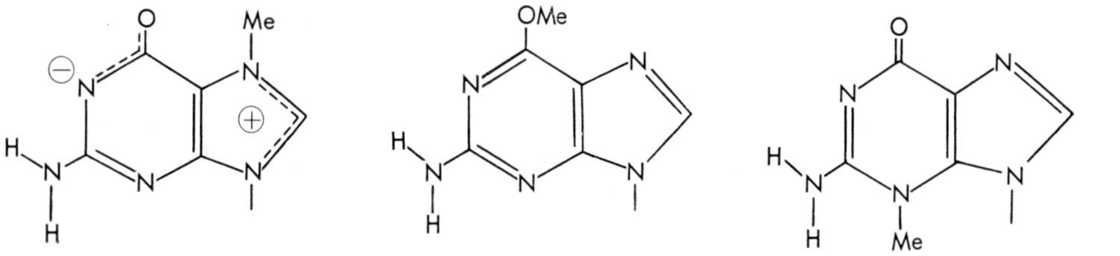

Ionized 7-Methylguanine   Neutral O^6-Methylguanine   Amino-form 3-Methylguanine

Fig. 12.   Possible " miscoding " forms of methylguanine residues in nucleic acids.   References: 7-methylguanine, Lawley and Brookes, 1961; O^6-methylguanine, Loveless, 1969; 3-methyl-guanine, Lawley, Orr, and Shah, 1972.   The term "miscoding" refers to the possibility that these tautomeric forms could establish hydrogen bonds with the "anomalous bases," thymine or uracil, rather than with their "normal" partner, cytosine, in the base-pairing scheme of Watson and Crick (1953).

Several reasons have been advanced why the first proposal, miscoding by ion-ized 7-alkylguanine residues, is not satisfactory.   It does not explain why only a limited number of alkylating agents are mutagenic for extracellularly treated T-even phages (Loveless and Hampton, 1969), where the main mechanism would be ex-pected to be the " transition " type.   No evidence for miscoding by 7-substituted guanine residues has been found (*e.g.*, with RNA templates, Wilhelm and Ludlum, 1966; Ludlum, 1970; with DNA templates, Hendler, Fürer and Srinivasan, 1970), although, of course, the " true " DNA polymerase has yet to be tested in this respect. [It should be noted here that Ludlum and Wilhelm [1968] did find evidence for miscoding by methylated poly (C), but the molecular mechanism was not obvious.]

The second type of mispairing base, here represented by O^6-methylguanine, " fixes " the anomalous tautomeric configuration previously proposed for the ionized form of 7-alkylguanosine.   Not only could this account for mutagenesis in phage systems by MNUA (Loveless and Hampton, 1969), but it is also attractive to ex-trapolate the applicability of this mechanism to include all SN1 reagents, such as ethyl and isopropyl methanesulphonates.   These agents, as tested in barley and *E. coli*, proved more efficient mutagens than MMS (Veleminsky, Osterman-Golkar, and Ehrenberg, 1970), and are known to react at the O-6 position of guanine residues in DNA (Lawley and Orr, unpublished data).

Further evidence for the biological significance of O-6, as opposed to N-7, methylation of guanine comes from the finding that O^6-methylguanine is " excised " from *E. coli* DNA but 7-methylguanine either is not, or is only to a very limited extent (Lawley and Orr, 1970).   Possibly the repair enzyme " recognizes " the potentially miscoding group.

The third potential cause of anomalous Watson-Crick hydrogen-bonding is that of the amino form of 3-methylguanine.   This product is given by both MNUA and MMS, but in a smaller proportion than O^6-methylguanine by MNUA (about one-tenth as much); and it could be thought to provide a mechanism for the occasional mispairing by either class of methylating agent.   Since this base in the imino form would probably pair normally, and the predominant tautomeric form is not known, the possibility of its causing " transitions " could well be less than its total extent in DNA, and maybe even zero.   It is not at present known whether this base is " excised " by repair enzymes.

It should, of course, be stressed that transition mispairing is unlikely to be the sole mechanism by which methylating agents cause mutations.   As with UV-induced mutations, repair errors may be a significant factor in bacterial and eukaryotic systems (*cf.*, Witkin, 1969).

In this connection, it is of interest that recent work on the action of methylating agents on mammalian cells has suggested that the MNUA- and DMS-types of reagent differ in a further respect—that they can induce different types of repair, possibly because of their distinctive modes of reaction with DNA (Plant and Roberts, 1971).

To revert to the initial stimuli of this work, it is pertinent to enquire whether any plausible relationship between the carcinogenic potency of methylating agents and their modes of reaction with nucleic acids can be discerned.   Clearly, this will depend, among other factors, on a further definition of the relationship between degrees of methylation in target tissues and the induction of tumors.   The indications are that for some target organs, such as the kidney of the rat, a positive correlation exists between the ability of alkylating carcinogens to induce tumors and their ability to alkylate O-6 atoms of guanine in nucleic acids (Swann and Magee, 1968, 1969).

These findings suggest, in turn, a positive correlation between the ability of carcinogens to induce transition mutations and carcinogenic potency; and further, a positive correlation of the latter with the ability to induce anomalous base-pairing in the Watson-Crick sense, which could apply to DNA-RNA or RNA-RNA interactions as well as the DNA-DNA interactions of classical mutagenesis.

Whether the apparently weaker carcinogenic potency of the DMS-type of methylating agent can be ascribed to some less probable mispairing mechanism, such as that of 3-alkylguanines, is, of course, much more speculative.   If a mutagenic mechanism of tumor initiation is considered, there are, as mentioned, other mechanisms worthy of consideration, for example, those involving repair errors. These may stem from other effects of the methylation of DNA, such as depurination.

The concepts outlined here, regarding differences in the mutagenic mechanisms of the methylating agents, might be in accord with the work of Malling and de Serres (1969), relating the carcinogenicity and mutagenicity of these agents. They were led to the conclusion that compounds which induce a high proportion of mutants in which the specific gene product has an altered function are stronger carcinogens than compounds which induce a high proportion of mutants with nonfunctional gene products. If the first class of mutations are more likely to result from the operation of the " transition " mechanism, whereas the second class are more likely to result from depurinations or repair errors, causing deletions, this distinction could, therefore, be interpreted in terms of the known reactions of the methylating agents with DNA.

The possible implication of " derepression " of a tumor RNA virus in the action of MNUA in adult inbred Swiss mice has been discussed by Frei (1971). Here again the ability of this carcinogen to form O^6-methylguanine in DNA *in vivo* was noted. But a somewhat unexpected finding was that in tissues thought to be involved in the induction of thymic lymphoma (likely to be of viral etiology) the significant feature was the formation of relatively high proportions (more than 15%) of 3-methyladenine.

There are thus many interesting pointers to the possible correlations between nucleic acid methylations and tumor induction. Their significance remains to be elucidated by further investigations.

SUMMARY

N-Methyl-N-nitroso compounds, typified here by N-methyl-N-nitrosourea (MNUA) or N-methyl-N'-nitro-N-nitrosoguanidine (MNNG), differ significantly from simpler methylating agents, such as dimethyl sulphate (DMS) or methyl methanesulphonate (MMS). These differences can be attributed to the mechanisms of reaction of the two groups of compounds. The nitroso compounds react through intermediates derived from monomethylnitrosamine and can be classified as SN1 reagents in part; DMS and MMS appear to typify SN2 reagents. These differences are reflected in the spectrum of minor products of methylation of nucleic acids produced by the two types of agents. The nitroso compounds, unlike MMS or DMS, can methylate the O-6 atom of guanine residues, but they show less tendency to react at the N-1 atom of adenine or at the N-3 of cytosine. Both types of agent react to a small extent at the N-3 of guanine and the N-7 of adenine, the nitroso compounds rather more than MMS or DMS.

Some possible implications of these reactions for the biological action of methylating agents are discussed herein. The ability of nitroso compounds to methylate the O-6 of guanine could account for their mutagenic potency, since this would be expected to cause mispairing in the Watson-Crick scheme and thus induce " transition " mutations. The 3-methylguanine residue in the amino form could also permit mispairing, but if this occurred it would be less probable than for O^6-methylguanine.

This work was supported by grants to the Chester Beatty Research Institute, Institute of Cancer Research, Royal Cancer Hospital, from the Medical Research Counctil and the Cancer Research Campaign. I wish to thank Dr. P. J. O'Connor of the Paterson Laboratories, Christie Hospital and Holt Radium Institute, Manchester, and Dr. K. V. Shooter, Mr. D. J. Orr, and Mr. S. A. Shah of this Institute, for permission to quote from work unpublished at the time of writing.

REFERENCES

1. Abell, C. W., Rosini, L. A., and Ramseur, M. R. Alkylation of Polyribonucleotides: The Biological, Physical and Chemical Properties of Alkylated Polyuridylic Acid. Proc. Natl. Acad. Sci., *54*: 608–615, 1965.

2. Brookes, P., and Lawley, P. D. (Carcinogenesis by) Alkylating Agents. Brit. Med. Bull., *20*: 91–95, 1964.

3. Brookes, P., and Lawley, P. D. *In*; Hollaender, A. (ed.), Chemical Mutagens: Principles and Methods for Their Detection, I. pp. 121–144, Plenum Press, London and New York, 1971.

4. Brown, D. M., and Todd, A. R. *In*; Cohn, W. E., and Davidson, J. N. (eds.), The Nucleic Acids, Part I, pp. 409–445, Academic Press, New York, 1955.

5. Dipple, A., Lawley, P. D., and Brookes, P. Theory of Tumour Initiation by Chemical Carcinogens: Dependence of Activity on Structure of Ultimate Carcinogen. Eur. J. Cancer, *4*: 493–506, 1968.

6. Frei, J. V. Tissue-dependent Differences in DNA Methylation Products of Mice Treated with Methyl-labelled Methylnitrosourea. Int. J. Cancer, *7*: 436–442, 1971.

7. Garrett, E. R., Goto, S., and Stubbins, J. F. Kinetics of Solvolyses of Various N-Alkyl-N-nitrosoureas in Neutral and Alkaline Solutions. J. Pharm. Sci., *54*: 119–123, 1965.

8. Hendler, S., Fürer, E., and Srinivasan, P. R. Synthesis and Chemical Properties of Monomers and Polymers Containing 7-Methylguanine and Investigation of Their Substrate or Template Properties for Bacterial DNA or RNA Polymerases. Biochemistry, *9*: 4141–4152, 1970.

9. Holy, A., und Scheit, K. A. Methylierung von Dinucleosidphosphaten mit Diazomethan. Biochim. Biophys. Acta, *138*: 230–240, 1967.

10. Ingold, C. K. Structure and Mechanism in Organic Chemistry, Chapter VII, Second Edition, pp. 421–555, G. Bell and Sons, Edinburgh, 1970.

11. Junowicz, E., and Spencer, J. H. Rapid Separation of Nucleosides and Nucleotides by Cation-exchange Chromatography. J. Chromatogr., *44*: 342–348, 1969.

12. Lawley, P. D. Effects of Some Chemical Mutagens and Carcinogens on Nucleic Acids. Prog. Nucleic Acid Res. Mol. Biol., *5*: 89–131, 1966.

13. Lawley, P. D. Reaction of N-Methyl-N-nitrosourethane and N-Methyl-N'-nitro-N-nitrosoguanidine with DNA to Yield 7-Methylguanine and 3-Methyladenine at Neutral pH. Nature, *218*: 580–581, 1968.

14. Lawley, P. D., and Brookes, P. Further Studies on the Alkylation of Nucleic Acids and their Constituent Nucleotides. Biochem. J., *89*: 127–138, 1963.

15. Lawley, P. D., Brookes, P., Magee, P. N., Craddock, V. M., and Swann, P. F. Methylated Bases in Liver Nucleic Acids from Rats Treated with Dimethylnitrosamine. Biochim. Biophys. Acta, *157*: 646–648, 1968.

16. Lawley, P. D., and Orr, D. J. Specific Excision of Methylation Products from DNA

of *Escherichia coli* Treated with N-Methyl-N'-nitro-N-nitrosoguanidine.   Chem. Biol. Interactions, *2*: 154–157, 1970.

17. Lawley, P. D., Orr, D. J., and Shah, S. A.   Reaction of Alkylating Mutagens and Carcinogens with Nucleic Acids: N-3 of Guanine as a Site of Alkylation by N-Methyl-N-nitrosourea and Dimethyl Sulphate.   Chem. Biol. Interactions, *4*: 431–434, 1971.

18. Lawley, P. D., and Shah, S. A.   Methylation of RNA by Dimethyl Sulphate, Methyl Methanesulphonate, N-Methyl-N-nitrosourea, and N-Methyl-N'-nitro-N-nitrosoguanidine-Comparison of Chemical Analyses at the Nucleoside and Base Levels.   Biochem. J., *128*: 117–132, 1972.

19. Lawley, P. D., Shooter, K. V., House, W. L., and Shah, S. A.   Methylation of μ2 Bacteriophage RNA by the Carcinogen N-Methyl-N-nitrosourea: Evidence for O-Methylation.   Biochem. J., *122*: 22, 1971.

20. Lawley, P. D., and Thatcher, C. J.   Methylation of DNA in Cultured Mammalian Cells by N-Methyl-N'-nitro-N-nitrosoguanidine: the Influence of Cellular Thiol Concentrations on the Extent of Methylation and the N-Oxygen Atom of Guanine as a Site of Methylation.   Biochem. J., *116*: 693–697, 1970.

21. Lijinsky, W., Loo, J., and Ross, A. E.   Mechanism of Alkylation of Nucleic Acids by Nitrosodimethylamine.   Nature, *218*: 1174–1175, 1968.

22. Lingens, F., Haerlin, F., and Süssmuth, R.   Mechanism of Mutagenesis by MNNG: Methylation of Nucleic Acids by CD_3-Labeled MNNG in Presence of Cysteine and in Cells of *Escherichia coli*.   FEBS Lett., *13*: 241–242, 1971.

23. Loveless, A.   Possible Relevance of O-6 Alkylation of Deoxyguanosine to Mutagenicity and Carcinogenicity of Nitrosamines and Nitrosamides.   Nature, *223*: 206–207, 1969.

24. Loveless, A., and Hampton, C. L.   Inactivation and Mutation of Coliphage T2 by N-Methyl- and N-Ethyl-N-nitrosourea.   Mutation Res., *7*: 1–12, 1969.

25. Ludlum, D. B.   Properties of 7-Methylguanine-containing Templates for RNA Polymerase.   J. Biol. Chem., *245*: 477–482, 1970.

26. Ludlum, D. B., and Wilhelm, R. C.   RNA Polymerase Reactions with Methylated Polycytidylic Acid Templates.   J. Biol. Chem., *243*: 2750–2753, 1968.

27. Magee, P. N., and Barnes, J. M.   Carcinogenic Nitroso Compounds.   Advan. Cancer Res., *10*: 163–246, 1967.

28. Malling, H. V., and de Serres, F. J.   Mutagenicity of Alkylating agents.   Ann. N.Y. Acad. Sci., *163*: 788–800, 1969.

29. McCalla, D. R., Reuvers, A., and Kitai, R.   Inactivation of Biologically Active N-Methyl-N-nitroso Compounds in Aqueous Solution: Effect of Various Conditions of pH and Illumination.   Can. J. Biochem., *46*: 807–811, 1968.

30. Miller, E. C., and Miller, J. A.   Mechanisms of Chemical Carcinogens: Nature of Proximate Carcinogens and Interactions with Macromolecules.   Pharmacol. Rev., *18*: 805–838, 1966.

31. Mizutani, S., and Temin, H. M.   RNA-dependent DNA Polymerase in Virions of Rous Sarcoma Virus.   Cold Spring Harbor Symposia, *35*: 847–849, 1970.

32. Osterman-Golkar, S., Ehrenberg, L., and Wachtmeister, C. A.   Reaction Kinetics and Biological Action in Barley of Monofunctional Methanesulphonic Esters.   Radiat. Botany, *10*: 303–327, 1970.

33. Plant, J. E., and Roberts, J. J.   Novel Mechanism for Inhibition of DNA Synthesis Following Methylation: Effect of N-Methyl-N-nitrosourea on HeLa Cells.   Chem. Biol. Interactions, *3*: 337–342, 1971.

34. Rhaese, H. J., and Freese, E.   Chemical Analysis of DNA Alterations.   IV. Reactions of Oligonucleotides with Monofunctional Alkylating Agents Leading to Backbone Breakage.   Biochim. Biophys. Acta, *190*: 418–433, 1969.

35. Rosenkranz, H. S., Rosenkranz, S., and Schmidt, R. M.   Effects of Nitrosomethylurea and Nitrosomethylurethan on the Physical Chemical Properties of DNA.   Biochim. Biophys. Acta, *195*: 262–265, 1969.

36. Scheit, K. H.   Benzylester von Desoxydinucleosidphosphaten und 5′-0-(ß,ß,ß) Trichloräthylphosphorylthymidylyl-(3′-5′)-thymidylyl-(3′-5′) thymidin.   Tetrahedron Lett., *33*: 3243–3247, 1967.

37. Schulz, U., and McCalla, D. R.   Reactions of Cysteine with N-Methyl-N-nitroso-*p*-toluenesulphonamide and N-Methyl-N′-nitro-N-nitrosoguanidine.   Can. J. Chem., *47*: 2021–2027, 1969.

38. Shooter, K. V.   Some Aspects of the Interaction of Carcinogenic and Mutagenic Agents with Purines in Nucleic Acids.   Jerusalem Symposia on Quantum Chemistry and Biochemistry, *4*: 509–518, 1972.

39. Singer, B., and Fraenkel-Conrat, H.   Role of Conformation in Chemical Mutagenesis.   Prog. Nucleic Acid Res. Mol. Biol., *9*: 1–29, 1969.

40. Sneen, R. A., and Larsen, J. W.   Substitution at a Saturated Carbon Atom.   X. Unification of Mechanisms SN1 and SN2.   J. Amer. Chem. Soc., *91*: 362–366, 1969.

41. Srinivasan, P. R., and Borek, E.   Enzymatic Alteration of Macromolecular Structure.   Prog. Nucleic Acid Res. Mol. Biol., *5*: 157–189, 1966.

42. Swann, P. F., and Magee, P. N.   Nitrosamine-induced Carcinogenesis.   The Alkylation of Nucleic Acids of the Rat by N-Methyl-N-nitrosourea, Dimethylnitrosamine, Dimethyl Sulphate and Methyl Methanesulphonate.   Biochem. J., *110*: 39–47, 1968.

43. Swann, P. F., and Magee, P. N.   Induction of Rat Kidney Tumours by Ethyl Methanesulphonate and Nervous Tissue Tumours by Methyl Methanesulphonate and Ethyl Methanesulphonate.   Nature, *223*: 947–948, 1969.

44. Uhlenhopp, E. L., and Krasna, A. I.   Alterations in the Structure of DNA on Chemical Methylation.   Biochemistry, *10*: 3290–3295, 1971.

45. Veleminsky, J., Osterman-Golkar, S., and Ehrenberg, L.   Reaction Rates and Biological Action of N-Methyl- and N-Ethyl-N-nitrosourea.   Mutation Res., *10*: 169–174, 1970.

46. Watson, J. D., and Crick, F. H. C.   Genetical Implications of the Structure of DNA.   Nature, *171*: 964–967, 1953.

47. Whittle, E. D.   Methylation of Rat-liver RNA *in vivo* by Methyl Methanesulphonate.   Biochim. Biophys. Acta, *195*: 381–388, 1969.

48. Wilhelm, R. C., and Ludlum, D. B.   Coding Properties of 7-Methylguanine.   Science, *153*: 1403–1405, 1966.

49. Witkin, E. M.   Ultraviolet-induced Mutation and DNA Repair.   Ann. Rev. Microbiol., *23*: 487–514, 1969.

Discussion of Paper by Dr. Lawley

DR. KRÜGER: According to the first slide you showed, both DMN and MNU reacted through an SN1 mechanism.   If this is so, the methyl cation formed *in vivo* by both compounds will react with all cell components which have nucleophilic activity.   Have you any explanation why DMN causes liver tumors and MNU does not, since the amount of methylated cell components must be the same?

DR. LAWLEY: There does not seem to be an adequate explanation at present.   But possibly the detailed distribution of methylation products in the cell may differ with different agents, *cf.*, Graffi's report on preferential methylation of mitochondrial versus nuclear DNA.   (See also the remarks by Dr. Magee on DMN carcino-genesis.)

DR. MAGEE: Referring to Dr. Krüger's question.   I would like to discuss the pro-blem of the failure to induce liver tumors by a single dose of dimethylnitrosamine, as I described it in my paper.   Although methyl methanesulphonate is not muta-genic in Loveless's system, it is a potent mutagen in other situations.   How can this be explained?

DR. LAWLEY: In Loveless's system, it is almost certain that the mutations are mainly induced by the " transition " mechanism (*cf.*, the review by Krieg in Prog. Nucleic Acid Res., 2:).
    In whole cells, mutations may result from " repair error " (*cf.*, Witkin, Howard-Flanders).   Repair could be stimulated by depurination, or could involve the exci-sion of bases other than O^6-alkylguanine, or be stimulated by chain breakage.   To a small extent, " transition " mutation could result from the mispairing of 3-methyl-guanine, if this does exist in the amino form in DNA.   Other mutations could re-sult from deletions, following depurinations or chain breakages.

DR. HEIDELBERGER: In our published work (Corbett *et al.*, Mol. Pharmacol., 1971) on mutagenicity, we found deletion and frameshift mutations in T4 bacteriophage, as well as transition mutants.   Incidentally, although N-acetoxy-AAF reacts in the test tube almost entirely with guanine, its mutagenicity to T4 results from an attack on adenine, not guanine.

DR. LAWLEY: Yes, others have also reported deletions and frameshifts, but only to relatively small extents (*cf.*, Krieg). But the major part of the phage mutations would be expected to be " transitions." It has not yet been proven that these result from mispairing of O^6-methylguanine, but GC pairs are generally found to be the mutated sites with EMS.

DR. WEISBURGER: That the situation is obviously more complex is proven by the fact that larger carcinogens of the aromatic amine type like AAF or 4NQO metabolites, which were discussed yesterday, interact with the 8-position of guanylic acid and, in a minor way, with adenylic acid. Is there any evidence of arylation at O-6 of guanylic acid with such agents as AAF or 4NQO metabolites?

DR. LAWLEY: I know of no evidence for arylation at O-6 of guanine. But Szybalski *et al.* reported that AAF derivatives could induce phage mutations by the " transition " mechanism, presumably following arylation of purines at C-8.

DR. KUROKI: If you put methylated guanosine or adenosine into the medium in any cell system, can it be incorporated into DNA or RNA? This type of experiment seems to make clear the possible role of these compounds in mutagenesis and carcinogenesis.

DR. LAWLEY: We (Lawley and Thatcher, unpublished) looked for the incorporation of ^{3}H-labeled O^6-methylguanine into nucleic acids of *E. coli* or of hamster embryo cells in culture, but did not detect it.

Dr. Chu (University Chemical Laboratory, Cambridge, U.K.) found a weakly positive mutagenic effect of this base at relatively high doses in the ϕ 80 reversion system. In contrast to 7-methylguanine, it seems possible that O^6-methylguanine could, like adenine, be converted to nucleotides *in vivo*. But Montgomery, who first designed O^6-methylguanine as a potential antimetabolite, found it to have only a very weakly toxic action in mice. Dr. Shooter of our Institute was unable to convert this base into a nucleoside diphosphate, using an enzymic system that can do this with adenine. We are now trying to make O^6-methyl-GDP chemically with a view to making poly (O^6-methyl-G).

Possible Mechanisms of Carcinogenesis and Mutagenesis by Nitrosamines

P. N. Magee

Courtauld Institute of Biochemistry, Middlesex Hospital Medical School, London, England

Interest in the biological actions of N-nitroso compounds, particularly carcinogenesis and mutagenesis, has increased rapidly in the past few years. Since the reviews by Magee and Barnes (25) and by Druckrey and his colleagues (7) in 1967, a large amount of new work has been published, some of which has been reviewed (23, 24, 28). Much of the more recent work has been concerned with the possible hazards to human health which might arise from the presence of nitrosamines in the environment or from their formation from secondary or tertiary amines and nitrites in the body (11, 17, 24, 38). The significance of the presence of nitroso carcinogens in the human environment is difficult to assess, particularly where the amounts concerned are very small. Better understanding of the mechanisms of the biological actions of these compounds may be of value in evaluating their possible hazards for man. For this reason, as well as for its intrinsic scientific interest, work aimed at improving this understanding has continued. In this communication, recent studies in this field by the author and his colleagues will be described and discussed.

The Role of Alkylation of Cellular Components in the Biological Actions of N-Nitroso Compounds

Although several nitrosamides and nitrosamines have been shown to alkylate nucleic acids and proteins of animal and bacterial cells *in vivo* (4, 19, 26, 27, 45, 50) the significance of these alkylation reactions is not clear. It is not known whether alkylation is responsible entirely, in part, or not at all for the biological actions of the nitrosamines.

Doubts of the role of alkylation in carcinogenesis by the nitroso compounds have been based on two objections. Until recently the available evidence suggested that the carcinogenic potency of the known biological alkylating agents was insufficent to explain the very powerful actions of the nitrosamines and claims were made that some cyclic nitrosamines could not undergo the necessary metabolic activation to produce the required alkylating intermediate (*1*).

The first objection has been countered by the work of Swann and Magee (*46*), who showed that the alkylating agents, methyl and ethyl methanesulphonate, particularly the latter, were effective carcinogens. They induced tumors of rat brain and kidney, respectively, which were similar to those induced in these organs by nitroso compounds. In these experiments, the alkylating agents were administered in one or a small number of large doses near to the lethal level, and the animals were then left without further treatment. This procedure was based on one previously found effective with nitrosamines.

Renal tumors produced by ethyl methanesulphonate occurred in about 50% of the surviving animals, leaving no doubt about its carcinogenicity. With methyl methanesulphonate the incidence of nervous system tumors was only about 5%, raising doubts about its significance, although tumors of the brain and nerves in untreated rats are very rare indeed. Recently, however, Dr. P. Kleihues (personal communication) has administered methyl methanesulphonate by the transplacental route and, although the experiment is still in progress, has confirmed that this compound is carcinogenic for the rat nervous system.

The other objection to alkylation as a mechanism of nitrosamine carcinogenesis by cyclic nitrosamines has been supported by some, but not all, subsequent evidence. Lee and Lijinsky (*16*) reported alkylation of rat liver RNA by some cyclic N-nitrosamines *in vivo* which indicated that metabolic opening of heterocyclic rings must have occurred. However, subsequently Lijinsky and Ross (*18*) failed to detect nucleic acid alkylation with some carcinogenic cyclic nitrosamines, but did find it with non-carcinogenic compounds. All the above work was done with tritium labeled materials. Very recently Mr. Bernard Stewart, working in the author's laboratory, has studied the metabolism of N-nitrosomorpholine labeled in the 2 or 3 position of the ring and has found that, with each sample, more than 80% of the radioactivity injected into rats was excreted in the urine during a period of 30 hr following administration.

In both cases, however, rather more than 3% of the injected radioactivity appeared in the expired CO_2 during this period, indicated that metabolic opening of the heterocyclic ring must have occurred (*43*). Liver RNA from these rats was radioactive and was analyzed by ion-exchange chromatography after acid hydrolysis. Work in progress reveals little incorporation of radioactivity into the major purine bases and some radioactive peaks unrelated to the major nucleic acid components. These peaks may indicate the presence of alkylated bases, but further work is necessary to substantiate this.

Metabolism of Nitrosamines in vitro and Its Implications for Their Organotropic Carcinogenic Action

The metabolism of dialkylnitrosamines *in vitro* has been discussed by Magee and Barnes (*25*). It appears that microsomal enzyme systems similar to those responsible for the metabolism of many other foreign compounds, including carcinogens, are present in the liver and other organs. In the experience of the author, however, the metabolism of dimethylnitrosamine is considerably less active than that of aminopyrine by microsomal preparations incubated under the same conditions. Metabolism by tissue slice preparations, however, can be readily measured by incubation with the nitrosamine labeled with radioactive carbon and determination of the amount of radioactive CO_2 produced using conventional Warburg techniques.

Such experiments have been done by Dr. R. Montesano (*32*), who has compared the metabolism of dimethyl- and diethylnitrosamine by tissue slices from various organs of rat and hamster. The reason for this choice of carcinogens and species was that diethylnitrosamine is a very potent carcinogen in the respiratory tract of hamsters (*6, 33*), but the dimethyl compound does not appear to induce any respiratory tumors in this species (*49*). Both nitrosamines induced liver tumors when fed to both species. The results of these experiments are shown in Figs. 1 and 2.

With both the compounds in the rat the liver was the most active organ and the kidney showed lower activity but greater than with the other organs. The activity of the liver relative to the other organs was considerably less with dimethyl- than with diethylnitrosamine. In the hamster the metabolism of diethylnitrosamine by lung tissue was remarkably high, being slightly more active even than the liver. With dimethylnitrosamine, however, there was no such high metabolic activity by the respiratory tissue. Since $^{14}CO_2$ production is taken as a measure of the rate of

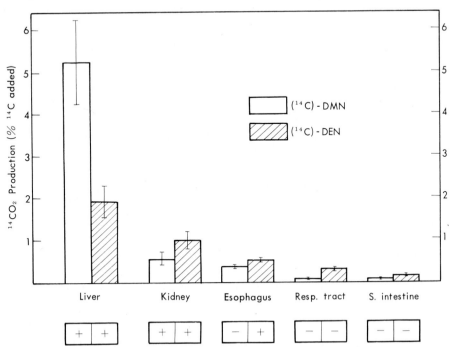

FIG. 1. Metabolism *in vitro* of (^{14}C) dimethyl- and (^{14}C) diethylnitrosamine. Production of $^{14}CO_2$ form [^{14}C]dimethylnitrosamine (DMN) and [^{14}C]diethylnitrosamine (DEN) incubated with rat tissue slices *in vitro*.

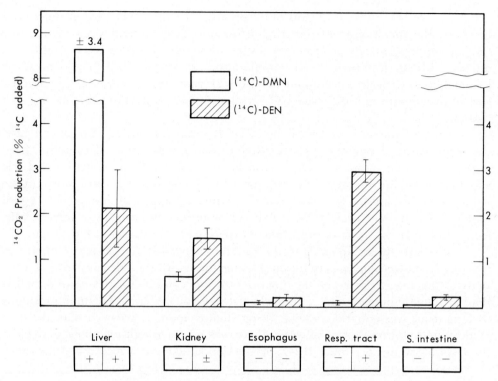

FIG. 2.   Production of $^{14}CO_2$ from [^{14}C] DMN and [^{14}C] DEN incubated with hamster tissue slices *in vitro*.

metabolism of the nitrosamine, it is clearly possible that some stage in the metabolic pathway, other than the initial one, could be rate-limiting.

Since the metabolism of the alkyl groups of the nitrosamines is thought to pass through the corresponding alcohols and aldehydes (*25*), experiments were made to determine the rates of metabolism of methanol and ethanol, and formate and acetate in tissue slices from hamster and rat.   Although some differences were found, none appeared adequate to explain the remarkably high level of activity of the hamster lung in the metabolism of diethylnitrosamine.   It is, therefore, con-cluded that the different rates of $^{14}CO_2$ production from the two nitrosamines by the tissues from rat and hamster do reflect differences in their rates of metabolism. These differences in metabolism may play an important role in determining the organ specificity of the different nitrosamines.   Further experimental work will show whether this concept can be extended to include other examples of the organo-tropic action of the nitrosamines.

The Possible Significance of Alkylation of N-7 of Guanine of Nucleic Acids for Carcinogenesis by Nitroso Compounds and Alkylating Agents

Since the first demonstration by Lawley and Wallick (*14*), it has been repeatedly confirmed that the predominant site of alkylation of both DNA and RNA by a number of alkylating agents is the N-7 position of guanine (*12*).   This predominance is usually very marked, with alkylation at this position accounting for 70 to 80% or more of the total.   It is also well established that alkylation occurs at other sites on guanine and on other bases.   Much of the chemical work on identification of the different alkylated bases has been done with relatively high concentrations of the alkylating agents acting on isolated nucleic acids *in vitro*.

When viruses are treated with alkylating agents, however, the proportions of the bases alkylated may differ from those when the same agent reacts with the isolated nucleic acid (*41*).   In the case of microorganisms, mammalian cells in culture and after treatment of the intact animal, the complicating factor to toxicity occurs, and the extent of alkylation of nucleic acids or any other cellular macromolecule is limited by the survival of the organism.   Methylation of DNA of rat liver *in vivo* by maximally tolerated doses of dimethylnitrosamine produced about 80% 7-methylguanine and considerably smaller amounts of 1-methyladenine (about 7%), 3-methyladenine (about 8%), and 3-methylcytosine (about 4%).   This pattern of alkylation corresponds fairly closely with that observed after the reaction of isolated nucleic acids *in vitro* with methyl methanesulphonate (*13*).

The predominance of alkylation of guanine on the 7-position obviously suggested that this reaction might have particular significance for carcinogenesis, mutagenesis and the other biological actions of these compounds and this possibility has been investigated by Swann and Magee who looked for correlations between the alkylation of rat nucleic acids *in vivo* by various nitroso and non-nitroso alkylating agents and the induction of tumors by the same compounds (*45, 47*).

With dimethylnitrosamine there was a reasonably good correlation between the organs showing most 7-methylguanine and those at which tumors appear, *i.e.*, liver, kidney and—to a lesser extent—lung.   The only real discrepancy was that the maximal level of alkylation in the liver.   In this organ tumors very rarely, if ever, appear in the adult rat after a single dose of dimethylnitrosamine, although continued feeding of this compound is powerfully carcinogenic.   This discrepancy remains to be explained, and it is interesting that the liver of the newborn rat is quite susceptible to tumor induction by a single dose of dimethylnitrosamine (*48*).

Thus the organotropy of dimethylnitrosamine appeared to be related to the organs in which most alkylation occurred and it also appeared probable that this, in turn, was related to the sites at which metabolism of the nitrosamine was greatest. Experimental evidence in support of this suggestion has been presented above. In similar experiments the amounts of 7-methylguanine were determined in different organs of rats treated with N-nitrosomethylurea and these were compared with the sites of tumor formation.   With this compound the levels of conversion of guanine to 7-methylguanine were about the same in all the organs studied (about 0.08–0.15 mol %, with RNA slightly higher than DNA).   Although tumors did not appear in all the organs of rats of the same strain receiving the same dose of N-nitrosomethylurea, they were found at several sites including stomach, small and large intestine, kidney, skin and jaw (*15*).   Since the carcinogen was administered in nearly lethal doses in these experiments, and it is known to induce tumors in other organs, including the brain, when given by multiple smaller doses (7), it was concluded that there was also a reasonably good correlation between the sites of tumor induction and methylation on the 7-position of guanine in the nucleic acids by N-nitrosomethylurea.

An interesting feature to emerge from these results was that the extent of conversion of guanine to 7-methylguanine in the kidneys of the rat was virtually the same with dimethylnitrosamine and with N-nitrosomethylurea, both of which induce morphologically indistinguishable tumors in this organ. These findings seemed to be quite consistent with a possible causative role for guanine alkylation in the induction of tumors. They suggested that other methylating agents might also induce renal and other tumors in the rat if they could be given in doses high enough to produce a similar level of nucleic acid alkylation without being too toxic to the animal. Since the pattern of nucleic acid methylation by methyl methanesulphonate *in vitro* was quite similar to that obtained with dimethylnitrosamine *in vivo* (*13*) the former agent was chosen for study. After administeration to rats in doses near to the limit of toxicity, methyl methanesulphonate gave rise to a level of nucleic acid methylation which, as measured by conversion of guanine to 7-methylguanine, was similar or slightly greater than that obtained with the nitrosamines, although the reaction with DNA was rather greater than that with RNA. Since these levels of alkylation occurred in rat kidney, tumor induction in this organ by single doses of methyl methanesulphonate should have occurred if it was causally related to

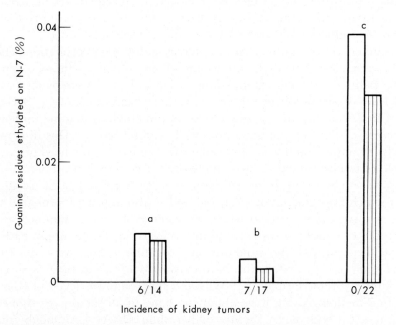

FIG. 3. Comparison between the amount of 7-ethylguanine produced in nucleic acids of rat kidney by single doses of (a) diethylnitrosamine (280 mg/kg), (b) N-nitrosoethylurea (150 mg/kg) and (c) ethyl methanesulphonate (275 mg/kg) with the carcinogenic activity in rat kidney of a similar dose of each compound. Although a single dose of ethyl methanesulphonate did not produce kidney tumors, three doses did.

alkylation on the 7-position of guanine.   However, as mentioned above, no kidney tumors were induced by methyl methanesulphonate, only a small number of nervous system tumors.   These findings, therefore, were inconsistent with a simple relationship between carcinogenesis and 7-methylation of guanine in total nucleic acids of the organs.

In contrast to the lack of renal carcinogenicity by methyl methanesulphonate, ethyl methanesulphonate readily induced kidney tumors after three separate large doses (46).   A comparison was therefore made by Dr. P. F. Swann of the extent of formation of 7-ethylguanine in rats treated with diethylnitrosamine, N-nitrosoethylurea and ethyl methanesulphonate respectively (47).   As shown in Fig. 3 the extent of 7-ethylation by a single dose of ethyl methanesulphonate, which induced no kidney tumors, was considerably greater than that by the two nitroso compounds which were powerfully carcinogenic in this organ.   Again, as with the methylating agents, there appeared to be no obvious correlation between alkylation on the 7-position of guanine and tumor induction.

In spite of this lack of correlation between the major product of nucleic acid alkylation and the induction of tumors, the above findings do not give any clear indication that alkylation plays no part in nitrosamine carcinogenesis unless it can be shown that alkyl alkanesulphonates also act by some other mechanism, since alkylation of cellular components is a common property of both types of compound.   The possibility that the nucleic acids are not the crucial cellular targets in carcinogenesis must also be kept in mind, although this would be more difficult to postulate for interaction with DNA in mutagenesis.   If, however, correlations are sought between carcinogenesis and reaction with nucleic acids at other sites on guanine and on other bases, there is an increasing number of possibilities.   The important work of Loveless (20) emphasizes the possible biological significance of O–6 alkylation of guanine and the studies of Ludlum and Wilhelm (22), which will be discussed below, draw attention to the 3-position of cytosine.   Work is in progress in our laboratory and several others, notably that of Dr. P. D. Lawley, as reported at this symposium, on the occurrence and extent of alkylation at different positions of the nucleic acids.   It remains to be seen whether any clear correlation with the biological actions of the various types of alkylating agent will emerge.   Although the currently available evidence does not support an important biological significance for alkylation at the 7-position of guanine, this reaction can be of considerable value in determining which organs are capable of metabolizing nitrosamines, since these compounds themselves do not react with cell components.

Effects of Nitrosamides and Alkylating Agents on Template Functions of Synthetic Polynucleotides

In view of the inherent difficulties in attempting to assess the relative importance of reactions at different sites in nucleic acids *in vivo* for their biological functions, it is desirable to explore alternative approaches.   One such alternative is to study the effects of the reaction of proximate carcinogens and mutagens on synthetic polynucleotide templates (*10, 21, 22, 42*).   These templates provide information for the synthesis of a new strand of RNA type polymer when they are incubated with RNA polymerase and suitable substrates. Changes produced by alkylation in the templates can be detected as differences in the composition of the product polymers. This system has been used by Ludlum to study the properties of 7-methylguanine-containing templates (21). Polyribonucleotides containing 7-methylguanylic acid were used to determine the base-pairing properties of 7-methylguanine in templates for RNA polymerase. Experiments with copolymers of uridylic acid and 7-methyl-guanylic acid (prepared by polymerization with polynucleotide phosphorylase) indicated that 7-methylguanine could still pair normally with cytosine to produce copolymers of adenylic and cytidylic acids. When copolymers of cytidylic and 7-methylguanylic acids were incubated with GTP and UTP, some abnormal base-pairing did occur between 7-methylguanine and uracil. However, this abnormal pairing was also observed at about the same level between guanine itself and uracil, and it was concluded that the base-pairing properties of 7-methylguanine and guanine were very similar in this system. These results are consistent with the lack of correlation between the levels of alkylation on the 7-position of guanine and carcino-

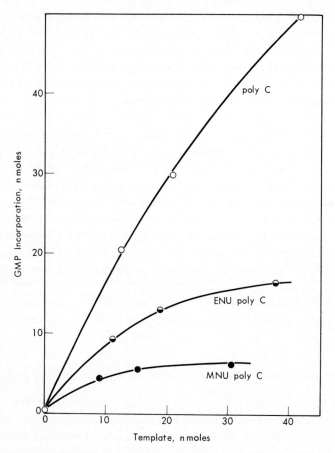

FIG. 4.   Effect of treatment of poly C template with N-nitrosomethyl- or N-nitrosoethylurea on GMP incorporation into polymer with RNA polymerase *in vitro*.

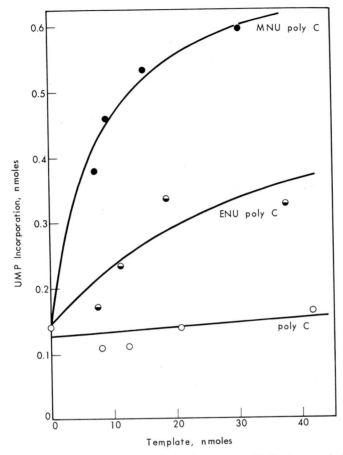

FIG. 5. Effect of treatment of poly C template with N-nitrosomethyl- or N-nitrosoethylurea on UMP incorporation into polymer with RNA polymerase *in vitro*.

genesis discussed above and support the conclusion that alkylation of nucleic acids at this site may have relatively unimportant biological significance. When, however, polycytidylic acids were partially methylated by incubation with methyl methanesulphonate and used as templates for RNA polymerase anomalous results were obtained. Under these conditions the presence of methylated cytidylic acid residues in the template led to the formation of a copolymer of uridylic and guanylic acids as shown by their reduced ability to act as a template for the formation of polyguanylic acid and the appearance of abnormal polymerization of uridylic acid (*22*). Analysis of the methylated polycytidylic acid showed that most of the methylation was in the form of 3-methylcytosine. By this criterion, therefore, alkylation of nucleic acids on the 3-position of cytosine might be expected to have greater biological significance than on the 7-position of guanine.

Similar experiments to test the effects of incubation of polycytidylic acids with nitrosamides and nitrosamines have been recently carried out by Dr. D. B. Ludlum and the author. The effects of incubation with N-nitrosomethyl- and N-nitrosoethylurea on polymerization of guanylic and uridylic acids are shown in Figs. 4 and

5.   The inhibitory effect on GMP incorporation and the anomalous stimulation of UMP incorporation are similar to those resulting from incubation of poly C templates with methyl methanesulphonate (22).   In contrast, the reaction of polycytidylic acid with methylurea or with dimethyl- or diethylnitrosamine or N-nitrosomorpholine at concentrations of about 0.1 M had no detectable effect on its template activity.   These results are consistent with the idea that some of the biological activities of the nitroso compounds are mediated by their capacity to alkylate nucleic acids and they support the conclusion that the dialkyl and cyclic nitrosamines require metabolic activation for biological activity (21a).

Mutagenesis by Nitroso Compounds

a)   Bacteria
     Since the observation of the potent mutagenic action of N-nitroso-N-methyl-N'-nitroguanidine (nitrosoguanidine) in bacteria by Mandell and Greenberg in 1960 (30), this compound and other nitrosamides have been recognized to be among the most powerful of known mutagens (25, 31, 36, 54).   The nitrosamides are mutagenically active in bacteria, yeasts, *Neurospora*, plants and *Drosophila* but the nitrosamines have generally been reported to be inactive in all the above organisms except *Drosophila*.   This difference in the behavior of the two classes of compound has been explained by the requirement for metabolic activation by the nitrosamines and the lack of this requirement by the nitrosamides (36).   As with carcinogenesis, however, the situation is not clear-cut.   Relatively high concentrations of dimethylnitrosamine have been reported to be mutagenic in *E. coli* (37) and several nitrosamines were found active in the plant *Arabidopsis* (51, 52).   It has also been suggested that the unchanged molecule of nitrosoguanidine may be mutagenic (3, 30) and that this accounts wholly or partly for its activity.   Other evidence suggests that the nitrosamides become mutagenic by release of alkylating decomposition products (31, 39, 40, 55).   It has also been suggested that their mutagenic activity at acid pH may be due to the formation of nitrous acid (55).   The situation with mutagenesis is thus comparable to that with carcinogenesis by the nitroso compounds in that much of the evidence favors alkylation as the biochemical mechanism, but other reactions involving the unchanged molecule or other decomposition products may also be involved.   In an attempt to clarify this situation and perhaps gain information relevant to the biological actions of the nitroso carcinogens in other systems, Dr. Stella Neale has recently studied effects of pH on nitrosamide-induced mutations in *E. coli* (35).
     Powerful mutagenic effects, as measured by the induction of revertants to tryptophan prototrophy in *E. coli* A58, were observed with N-nitrosomethyl- and N-nitrosoethylurea but higher concentrations of methylurea and of dimethyl- and diethylnitrosamine had no detectable effect nor had similar concentrations of N-nitrosomorpholine (not shown in Table 1).   These results are shown in Table 1, which also shows that nitrosoguanidine, as expected, was highly effective at a lower concentration than the nitrosoalkylureas and that the toxicity of the guanidine derivative was higher.

TABLE 1.   Induction of Revertants to Tryptophan Prototrophy in *E. coli* A58

	Time of exposure (hr)	Survivors initial cell no. (%)	Number of revertants per 10^8 survivors
Spontaneous reversion	4	100	0.5
10mM Methylurea	4	100	0.5
2.5mM N-Nitroso-N-methylurea	1	>95	125
2.5mM N-Nitroso-N-ethylurea	1	>95	298
10.0mM N, N′-Dimethyl-N-nitrosamine	4	>95	0.5
10.0mM N, N′-Diethyl-N-nitrosamine	4	>95	0.5
0.3mM N-Methyl-N′-nitro-N-nitrosoguanidine	1	62	266

Cells, 3×10^9ml, were exposed to the test compound at pH 7.0, 37°C.

TABLE 2.   Effect of Nitrosamide Pretreatment on Induction of Revertants to Leucine Prototrophy in *E. coli* C600

	pH Cell system	Number of reversion per 10^8 viable cells
A 5mM N-Methyl N-nitrosourea Nitrosamide pretreatment		
,,	7.9	3600
100% decay, pH 7.9 in dark	7.9	2
,,	6.0	4200
100% decay, pH 6.0 in dark	6.0	2
,,	5.0	116
50% decay, pH 5.0 in dark	5.0	50
100% decay, no buffer in light	6.0	2
B Spontaneous reversion	6.0	2

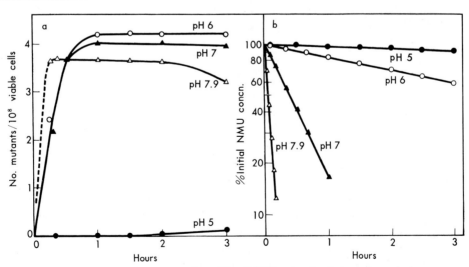

FIG 6.   The effect of pH on reversion of *E. coli* C600 to leucine-independence during exposure to an initial concentration of 5 mM N-nitrosomethylurea.   (a) Reversion expressed as number of revertants induced per 10^8 survivors after subtraction of number of spontaneous revertants. (b) Concentration of residual N-nitrosomethylurea as a percentage of the initial value.

The effects of pretreatment of *E. coli* with N-nitrosomethylurea at different pH values on the induction of revertants to leucine prototrophy in *E. coli* C600 are shown in Table 2.   There was little difference in the mutagenic activity in the range from pH 6.0 to pH 7.9 but at pH 5 it was drastically reduced.   The table also shows that mutagenesis was abolished by allowing the nitrosamide to decompose completely.   The above results are of interest because of the very different rates of decomposition of N-nitrosomethylurea which are shown in Fig. 6b.   The decay rate of the nitrosamide clearly decreased markedly with decreasing pH but, as shown in Table 2, the number of revertants was virtually constant between pH 7.9 and 6.0. The rate of induction of reversions in *E. coli* C600 by 5 mM nitrosomethylurea at 37° was followed, at various pH values, over a period of 3 hr as shown in Fig. 6a.   The maximum number of mutations was induced within 15 min at pH 7.9 and in 60 min at pH 6.0.   There appeared to be no direct correlation between the decay rate of the nitrosamide (Fig. 6b) and the induction of reversions.   The number of reversions induced was, however, directly proportional to the initial nitrosamide concentration for both N-nitrosomethyl- and N-nitrosoethylurea (Fig. 6a).   It should be noted that, for a given initial concentration, N-nitrosoethylurea was a more effective mutagen than the methyl derivative.

It can be concluded from these results, which are in agreement with the work of others, that the dialkyl and cyclic nitrosamines and also methylurea are not mutagenic under the conditions used.   The effects of different pH values on the mutagenic activity of the nitrosamides are difficult to interpret and do not clarify the nature of the active mutagenic molecule.   Work is in progress to determine the extent of DNA alkylation under the various conditions of the assays for mutagenesis.

b)   Mammals

An attempt, using the dominant lethal test in the mouse (*2, 9*), to assess the mutagenic potential of N-nitrosomethylurea for the mammal has been made by Mr. H. B. Waynforth and Mr. R. Parkin.   Methyl methanesulphonate, which is known to be active in this test (*8, 34*), was used as a positive control.   The results of the assay are shown in Fig. 7.   N-Nitrosomethylurea proved to be mutagenic in the mouse by the criterion of this method but it was less effective than an approximately molar equivalent dose of methyl methanesulphonate.   This result is in contrast with the considerably more powerful carcinogenic effect of N-nitrosomethylurea discussed above.   The possibility was considered that the nitrosamide may have failed to reach the germ cells in the testis in concentrations comparable to those attained by methyl methanesulphonate which is rapidly distributed throughout the organs of the body, including the testis (*5*).   The distribution of N-nitrosomethylurea after intraperitoneal injection into mice was studied using a polarographic method for its estimation in the tissues.   Because of the very short halflife of the compound in the body (*44*), however, this method was rather unsatisfactory and the alkylation of the nucleic acids in the testis was investigated, using [^{14}C]nitrosomethylurea, and compared with that produced by methyl methanesulphonate, using conversion of guanine to 7-methylguanine as the index of methylation.   As shown in Table 3, the amount of 7-methylguanine was

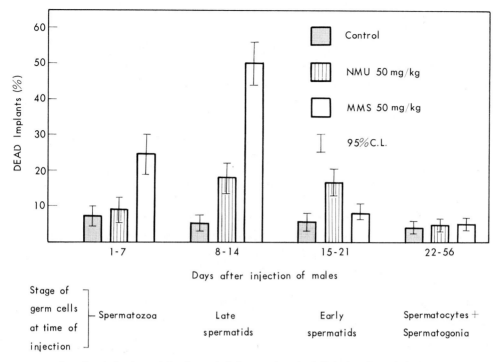

FIG. 7. Induction of dominant lethal mutations in Balb/c female × C57Bl male mice by N-nitrosomethylurea (NMU), 50 mg/kg, and by methyl methanesulphonate (MMS), 50 mg/kg.

somewhat greater with the nitrosamide than with methyl methanesulphonate, indicating that penetration of the latter to the genetic material was probably equally as good as with the former compound.

The cyclic nitrosamine, N-nitrosomorpholine, failed to induce dominant lethal mutations in mice under the conditions used. This result is of interest because the same compound, which is a potent carcinogen was found positive in the host-mediated assay for mutagenesis using *Salmonella typhimurium* in Swiss mice, although negative for the bacterium alone (*53*).

The observations with N-nitrosomethylurea suggest that about the same concentration of the biologically active molecule is needed in the germ and somatic cells for the induction of mutagenesis and carcinogenesis respectively.

TABLE 3. Percentage of Guanine Converted to 7-Methylguanine Following Administration of NMU or MMS at 50mg/kg

		NMU		MMS		Ratio NMU : MMS	
		DNA	RNA	DNA	RNA	DNA	RNA
Testis	Expt. 1	0.037	0.042	0.013	0.008	2.9	5.3
Testis	2	0.025	0.029	0.017	0.012	1.4	2.4
Colon	1	0.082	0.089	0.022	0.014	3.7	6.2

CONCLUSIONS

In spite of some conflicting evidence, it seems probable that carcinogenesis and mutagenesis by N-nitroso compounds are mainly mediated by decomposition product of these agents but it cannot be excluded that the unchanged molecules may also play a part. Experiments on metabolism of some nitrosamines by tissue slices *in vitro* suggest that the organotropic actions of these carcinogens may be determined by the capacity of the organs in which tumors are induced to metabolize them. The nature of the biologically active decomposition products of the nitrosamines has not been established but much of the available evidence suggests that the formation of an alkylating agent may be an important step. Because of the lack of correlation between the extent of alkylation on the 7-position of guanine in the nucleic acids of different organs and the sites at which tumors are induced, it seems unlikely that this is a crucial reaction in carcinogenesis. The biological relevance of alkylation at other sites on nucleic acid bases is not known and merits further detailed study. The use of alkylated polynucleotide templates for nucleic acid polymerases *in vitro* may be of value in elucidating the sites of nucleic acid alkylation that may be important for carcinogenesis or mutagenesis.

SUMMARY

Experiments on the metabolism of dimethyl- and diethylnitrosamines by tissue slices from rat and hamster tissues *in vitro* are described. In rat tissues, the most rapid metabolism of both nitrosamines occurred with liver slices, other organs showing varying lesser activities. With hamster tissues, the lung was slightly more active than the liver for diethylnitrosamine but the pattern with dimethylnitrosamine was similar to that in the rat. The possible relevance of these results to the organotropic carcinogenic activities of the nitrosamines is discussed.

The extent of conversion of guanine to 7-ethylguanine was measured in the kidney and other organs of rats given single large doses of diethylnitrosamine, N-nitrosoethylurea or ethyl methanesulphonate. The levels of ethylation on this position did not correlate with the carcinogenic activity. This result is in agreement with earlier work involving the corresponding methylating compounds.

Some effects of treatment of polycytidylic acids with nitrosamides on their template function for RNA polymerase *in vitro* are described. Inhibition of GMP incorporation and anomalous stimulation of UMP incorporation were observed and their possible biological implications are discussed. Effects of varying pH on the mutagenic action of nitrosamides on *E. coli* are reported.

The number of mutants produced was relatively constant, although the rate of decomposition of the nitrosamides varied considerably with pH. Nitrosamines tested for mutagenesis were all inactive. N-Nitrosomethylurea induced dominant lethal mutation in mice but was less active than methyl methanesulphonate which is in contrast with their relative carcinogenic potencies. These findings are discussed in relation to the part played by the metabolism or decomposition of these compounds in their biological activities and the possible significance of alkylation reactions with special reference to alkylation of nucleic acids.

REFERENCES

1. Argus, M. F., Arcos, J. C., and Hoch-Ligeti, C. Studies on the Carcinogenic Activity of Protein-denaturing Agents: Hepatocarcinogenicity of Dioxane. J. Natl. Cancer Inst., *35*: 949–958, 1965.

2. Bateman, A. J. Testing Chemicals for Mutagenicity in the Mammal. Nature, *210*: 205–206, 1966.

3. Cerda-Olmeda, E., and Hanawalt, P. C. Diazomethane as the Active Agent in Nitroguanidine Mutagenesis and Lethality. Molec. Gen. Genetics, *101*: 191–202, 1968.

4. Craddock, V. M. Reaction of the Carcinogen Dimethylnitrosamine with Proteins and with Thiol Compounds in the Intact Animal. Biochem. J., *94*: 323–330, 1965.

5. Cumming, R. B., and Walton, M. F. Fate and Metabolism of Some Mutagenic Alkylating Agents in the Mouse. I. Ethyl Methanesulfonate and Methyl Methanesulfonate at Sublethal Dose in Hybrid Males. Mutation Res., *10*: 365–377, 1970.

6. Dontenwill, W., und Mohr, U. Carcinome des Respirationstractus nach Behandlung von Goldhamstern mit Diäthylnitrosamin. Z. Krebsforsch., *64*: 305–312, 1961.

7. Druckrey, H., Preussmann, R., Ivankovic, S., und Schmähl, D. Organotrope carcinogene Wirkungen bei 65 verschiedenen N-Nitroso-Verbindungen an BD-Ratten. Z. Krebsforsch., *69*: 103–201, 1967.

8. Ehling, U. H., Cumming, R. B., and Malling, H. V. Induction of Dominant Lethal Mutations by Alkylating Agents in Male Mice. Mutation Res., *5*: 417–428, 1968.

9. Epstein, S. S., and Shafner, H. Chemical Mutagens in the Human Environment. Nature, *219*: 385–387, 1968.

10. Hendler, S., Furer, E., and Srinivasan, P. R. Synthesis and Chemical Properties of Monomers and Polymers Containing 7-Methylguanine and an Investigation of Their Substrate or Template Properties for Bacterial Deoxyribonucleic Acid or Ribonucleic Acid Polymerases. Biochemistry, *9*: 4141–4153, 1970.

11. Lancet, *1*: 1071–1072, (1968), Nitrites, Nitrosamines and Cancer.

12. Lawley, P. D. Effects of Some Chemical Mutagens on Nucleic Acids. Progr. Nucleic Acid Res. Mol. Biol., *5*: 89–131, 1966.

13. Lawley, P. D., Brookes, P., Magee, P. N., Craddock, V. M., and Swann, P. F. Methylated Bases in Liver Nucleic Acids from Rats Treated with Dimethylnitrosamine. Biochim. Biophys. Acta, *157*: 646–648, 1968.

14. Lawley, P. D., and Wallick, C. A. The Action of Alkylating Agents on Deoxyribonucleic Acid and Guanylic Acid. Chem. & Ind., 633, 1957.

15. Leaver, D. D., Swann, P. F., and Magee, P. N. Induction of Tumours in the Rat by a Single Oral Dose of N-Nitrosomethylurea. Brit. J. Cancer, *23*: 177–187, 1969.

16. Lee, K. Y., and Lijinsky, W. Alkylation of Rat Liver RNA by Cyclic N-Nitrosamines *in vivo*. J. Natl. Cancer Inst., *37*: 401–406, 1966.

17. Lijinsky, W., and Epstein, S. S. Nitrosamines as Environmental Carcinogens. Nature, *225*: 21–23, 1970.

18. Lijinsky, W., and Ross, A. E. Alkylation of Rat Liver Nucleic Acids not Related to Carcinogenesis by N-Nitrosamines. J. Natl. Cancer Inst., *42*: 1095–1100, 1969.

19. Lingens, F., Haerlin, R., and Sussmuth, R.   Mechanism of Mutagenesis by N-Methyl-N'-nitro-N-nitrosoguanidine (MNNG).   Methylation of Nucleic Acids by N-Trideuteriomethyl-N'-nitro-N-nitrosoguanidine (Dz-MNNG) in the Presence of Cysteine and in Cells of *Escherichia coli*.   FEBS Lett., *13*: 241–242, 1971.

20. Loveless, A.   Possible Relevance of O-6 Alkylation of Deoxyguanosine to the Mutagenicity and Carcinogenicity of Nitrosamines and Nitrosamides.   Nature, *223*: 206–207, 1969.

21. Ludlum, D. B.   The Properties of 7-Methylguanine-containing Templates for Ribonucleic Acid Polymerase.   J. Biol. Chem., *245*: 477–482, 1970.

21a. Ludlum, D. B., and Magee, P. N.   Reaction of Nitrosoureas with Polycytidylate Templates for Ribonucleic Acid Polymerases.   Biochem. J., *128*: 729–731, 1972.

22. Ludlum, D. B., and Wilhelm, R. C.   Ribonucleic Acid Polymerase Reactions with Methylated Polycytidylic Acid Templates.   J. Biol. Chem., *243*: 2750–2753, 1968.

23. Magee, P. N.   *In vivo* Reactions of Nitroso Compounds.   Ann. N.Y. Acad. Sci., *163*: 717–730, 1969.

24. Magee, P. N.   Toxicity of Nitrosamines: Their Possible Human Health Hazards.   Fd. Cosmet. Toxicol., *9*: 207–218, 1971.

25. Magee, P. N., and Barnes, J. M.   Carcinogenic Nitroso Compounds.   Advan. Cancer Res., *10*: 163–246, 1967.

26. Magee, P. N., and Farber, E.   Toxic Liver Injury and Carcinogenesis.   Methylation of Rat Liver Nucleic Acids by Dimethylnitrosamine *in vivo*.   Biochem. J., *83*: 114–124, 1962.

27. Magee, P. N., and Hultin, T.   Toxic Liver Injury and Carcinogenesis.   Methylation of Proteins of Rat Liver Slices by Dimethylnitrosamine *in vivo*.   Biochem. J., *83*: 106–114, 1962.

28. Magee, P. N., and Swann, P. F.   Nitroso Compounds.   Brit. Med. Bull., *25*: 240–244, 1969.

29. Magee, P. N., and Vandekar, M.   Toxic Liver Injury.   The Metabolism of Dimethylnitrosamine *in vitro*.   Biochem. J., *70*: 600–605, 1958.

30. Mandell, J., and Greenberg, J.   A New Chemical Mutagen for Bacteria, 1-Methyl-3-nitro-1-nitrosoguanidine.   Biochem. Biophys. Res. Commun., *3*: 575–577, 1960.

31. Marquardt, H., Zimmermann, F. K., und Schwaier, R.   Die Wirkung Krebsauslosender Nitrosamine und Nitrosamide auf das Adenin-6-45-Ruckmutationsystem von *Saccharomyces cerevisiae*.   Z. Vererbungsl., *95*: 82–96, 1964.

32. Montesano, R., and Magee, P. N.   Metabolism of Nitrosamines by Rat and Hamster Tissue Slices *in vitro*.   Proc. Amer. Assoc. Cancer Res., *12*: 14, 1971.

33. Montesano, R., and Saffiotti, U.   Carcinogenic Response of the Respiratory Tract of Syrian Golden Hamsters to Different Doses of Diethylnitrosamine.   Cancer Res., *28*: 2197–2210, 1968.

34. Mouschen, J.   Mutagenesis with Methyl Methanesulfonate in Mouse.   Mutation Res., *8*: 581–588, 1969.

35. Neale, S.   Effect of pH and Temperature on Nitrosamide-induced Mutation in *Escherichia coli*.   Mutation Res., *14*: 155–164, 1972.

36. Pasternak, L.   Untersuchungen über die mutagene Wirkung vershiedener Nitrosamin- und Nitrosamid Verbindungen.   Arzneim.-Forsch., *14*: 802–804, 1964.

37. Pogodina, O. N.   On the Mutagenic Action of Some Carcinogens Belonging to the Group of Nitrosamines.   Tsitologiya, *8*: 503–509, 1969.

38. Sander, J.   Kann Nitrit in der menschlichen Nahrung Ursache einer Krebsentstehung durch Nitrosaminbildung sein?   Arch. Hyg. Bakt., *151*: 22–28, 1967.

39. Schwaier, R. Vergleichende Mutationsversuche mit sieben Nitrosamiden im Rückmutationstest an Hefen. Z. Vererbungsl., *97*: 55–67, 1965.

40. Schwaier, R., Zimmermann, F. K., and von Laer, U. The Effect of Temperature on the Mutation Induction in Yeast by N-Alkyl-nitrosamides and Nitrous Acid. Z. Vererbungsl., *97*: 72–74, 1965.

41. Singer, B., and Fraenkel-Conrat, H. Chemical Modification of Viral Ribonucleic Acid. VIII. The Chemical and Biological Effects of Methylating Agents and Nitrosoguanidine in Tobacco Mosaic Virus. Biochemistry, *8*: 3266–3269, 1969.

42. Singer, B., and Fraenkel-Conrat, H. Messenger and Template Activities of Chemically Modified Polynucleotides. Biochemistry, *9*: 3694–3701, 1970.

43. Stewart, B. W., and Magee, P. N. Effect of a Single Dose of Dimethylnitrosamine on Biosynthesis of Nucleic Acid and Protein in Rat Liver and Kidney. Biochem. J., *125*: 943–952, 1971.

44. Swann, P. F. The Rate of Breakdown of Methyl Methanesulphonate, Dimethyl Sulphate and N-Methyl-N-nitrosourea in the Rat. Biochem. J., *110*: 49–52, 1968.

45. Swann, P. F., and Magee, P. N. Nitrosamine-induced Carcinogenesis: the Alkylation of Nucleic Acids of the Rat by N-Methyl-N-nitrosourea, Dimethylnitrosamine, Dimethyl Sulphate and Methyl Methanesulphonate. Biochem. J., *110*: 39–47, 1968.

46. Swann, P. F., and Magee, P. N. Induction of Rat Kidney Tumours by Ethyl Methanesulphonate and Nervous Tissue Tumours by Methyl Methanesulphonate and Ethyl Methanesulphonate. Nature, *223*: 947–948, 1969.

47. Swann, P. F., and Magee, P. N. The Alkylation of N-7 of Guanine of Nucleic Acids of the Rat by Diethylnitrosamine, N-Ethyl-N-nitrosourea and Ethyl Methanesulphonate. Biochem. J., *125*: 841–847, 1971.

48. Terracini, B., and Magee, P. N. Renal Tumours in Rats Following Injection of Dimethylnitrosamine at Birth. Nature, *202*: 502–503, 1964.

49. Tomatis, L., Magee, P. N., and Shubik, P. Induction of Liver Tumours in the Syrian Golden Hamster by Feeding Dimethylnitrosamine. J. Natl. Cancer Inst., *33*: 341–345, 1964.

50. Turberville, C., and Craddock, V. M. Methylation of Nuclear Proteins by Dimethylnitrosamine and by Methionine in the Rat *in vivo*. Biochem. J., *124*: 725–739, 1971.

51. Veleminsky, J., and Gichner, T. The Mutagenic Activity of Nitrosamines in *Arabidopsis thaliana*. Mutation Res., *5*: 429–431, 1968.

52. Veleminsky, J., and Gichner, T. Two Types of Dose-response Curves in *Arabidopsis thaliana*. Mutation Res., *12*: 65–70, 1971.

53. Zeiger, E., and Legator, M. S. Mutagenicity of N-Nitrosomorpholine in the Host-mediated Assay. Mutation Res., *12*: 469–471, 1971.

54. Zimmermann, F. K. Genetic Aspects of Carcinogenesis. Biochem. Pharmacol., *20*: 985–995, 1971.

55. Zimmermann, F. K., Schwaier, R., and von Laer, U. The Influence of pH on the Mutagenicity in Yeast of N-Methyl-nitrosamides and Nitrous Acid. Z. Vererbungsl., *97*: 68–71, 1965.

Discussion of Paper by Dr. Magee

DR. LAWLEY: I think that the significance of the radioactivity eluted early from columns in acid hydrolysates of nucleic acids labeled *in vivo* should be regarded with some caution.   In our experience, and in that of others, when the extent of reaction or of incorporation, of labeled material is low, a relatively large proportion of apparently nonspecific radioactivity elutes early from the columns.

With regard to the miscoding by methyl-poly C, there is some disagreement between Ludlum and Fraenkel-Conrat and Singer.   Both find miscoding in the RNA polymerase system, but this is a rather " unnatural " system, involving the use of Mn^{2+}.   Fraenkel-Conrat and Singer did not find miscoding in Nirenberg's system for amino acid incorporation, using methyl-poly C.

DR. MAGEE: We would agree that some of the material which elutes early from the columns is nonspecific radioactivity but not necessarily all of it.   The fact remains that the common feature of our results with nucleic acids alkylated *in vivo* is this early eluting material, and we feel that it may contain components of significance.   It is true that O–6 alkylated guanines would have been lost with our procedures.

I also accept your point that our results with methyl-poly C must be interpreted with great caution, but I still feel that this type of approach has value in attempting to determine the biological significance of alkylation on different positions of different bases.

DR. HEIDELBERGER: Have you chromatographed the urine of rats given nitrosomorpholine in order to have another measure of metabolism?

DR. MAGEE: Not yet.   This is very recent work and we will certainly chromatograph the urine as soon as possible.   Fortunately, we have samples containing large amounts of radioactivity.

DR. HEIDELBERGER: If we consider the initiation of 2-stage carcinogenesis of the skin, we find that there is great specificity of binding to DNA, RNA, and proteins.   β-Propiolactone has a 1,000-fold higher dose for initiation than DMBA.   It is also bound 1,000-fold more.   If binding to DNA is important for skin initiation, then DMBA is 1,000,000-fold more specific than the DNA binding of β-propiolactone, because BPL alkylate the N-7 of guanine, as Boutwell has shown.   I believe that Dipple and Brookes have shown that carcinogenic hydrocarbons may react with amino groups of nucleic acids.

DR. MAGEE: I entirely agree that there may be specific sites of interaction with DNA which may be crucial for the biological consequences of the interaction with different carcinogens and mutagens.

DR. WEISBURGER: The differences in biological activities in relation to biochemical behavior may be due to differences in the repair mechanism in the liver and kidney between young adults and newborn rats.

The liver is important for metabolism, and sometimes also in the production of transport forms.

DR. MAGEE: It certainly appears that the liver of the adult rat is more resistant to the carcinogenic action of single doses of nitrosamines than that of the newborn animal.

I agree that this may reflect some form of " repair " mechanism in the adult which has not developed in the newborn. This may be DNA repair, but it may be also that the adult liver has a greater capacity for repairing or recovering from damage to other systems.

You are, of course, right in saying that the liver may not only produce locally active carcinogenic metabolites, but also transport forms which may undergo further activation in other organs.

DR. LAWLEY: With regard to Dr. Heidelberger's remarks, Dipple et al. have shown that 7-bromomethylbenzen[a]anthracene reacts with nucleic acid amino groups (Biochemistry, in press).

With regard to the material eluted early from the column, in our experience, the radioactivity elutes before uracil or thymine, and it seems unlikely that it is located in pyrimidines.

DR. NAKAHARA: This is a rather unsophisticated question, but I would like to know what type of kidney tumors are produced. To be more specific, in the slide you showed, there was a huge tumor in the right kidney, while the left kidney was normal, or, at least, any tumors present were quite small. Is this the usual way in which your kidney tumors are produced?

DR. MAGEE: There are two distinct types of kidney tumors induced by these agents. One is an epithelial tumor, either adenoma or adenocarcinoma. There has been much disagreement about the other type which has been variously described as anaplastic, interstitial, nephroblastoma, stromal nephroma and angiosarcoma.

It is quite usual to observe a very large tumor in one kidney and no apparent tumor or only a very small one in the other kidney. I have no explanation for this.

DR. DAWE: I am interested in the possibility that metabolism of the nitrosamine compounds might occur in one cell type, such as, the connective tissue of an organ (i.e., kidney), while the carcinogenic effect might be manifested in another, such as, the epithelium of that same organ. Do you have evidence bearing on this question?

DR. MAGEE: This is a very interesting question, but unfortunately our present methods do not provide an answer, because our metabolic studies are all done with slices or homogenates of whole organs.

DR. MIRVISH: The rather small amount of binding found for nitrosomorpholine may be made more important by the relatively long time during which this nitroso compound remains in the body, since a reaction with nucleic acids could occur anytime during this whole period.   Do you agree?

DR. MAGEE: Yes I do agree.   As I indicated, the biological behavior of nitroso-morpholine appears to be very similar to that of diethylnitrosamine.   Therefore, it is possible that the smaller amount of binding with the morpholine derivatives may be at the more biologically important sites.

Studies on N-Nitrosation Reactions: Kinetics of Nitrosation, Correlation with Mouse Feeding Experiments, and Natural Occurrence of Nitrosatable Compounds (Ureides and Guanidines)

Sidney S. Mirvish

The Eppley Institute for Research in Cancer, University of Nebraska Medical Center, Omaha, Nebraska, U.S.A.

It was suggested by Druckrey (*8*) and Sander (*37*) that N-nitroso compounds might be formed under the acidic conditions of the stomach, and that this process could be a significant source of carcinogens for man, even though N-nitroso compounds might not be present as such in food.   The N-nitroso compounds include nitrosamines, nitrosamides (*e.g.*, nitrosoureas and nitrosourethans), nitrosoamidines (*e.g.*, N-methyl-N-nitroso-N'-nitroguanidine) and nitrosocyanamides.   The nitrosamides, nitrosoamidines and nitrosocyanamides contain the group $O=N-N-C=X$ ($X=N$ or O) and, unlike the nitrosamines, produce diazoalkanes or carbonium ions in alkaline solution.   Probably because of similar reactions in producing alkylating agents *in vivo*, these compounds often act as carcinogens at the site of application (*7*), unlike the nitrosamines, which probably require enzymic activation and typically act at distant sites.   Some nitrosamides and related compounds induce adenocarcinomas of the glandular stomach in experimental animals, similar to the usual type of gastric cancer in man.   Thus, these tumors were induced by methylnitrosourea and methylnitrosourethan in guinea pigs (*5*); N-methyl-N-nitroso-N'-nitroguanidine in rats, hamsters, and dogs (*51*); and N-methyl-N-nitroso-N'-acetylurea in rats (*6*).

Gastric cancer in man varies widely in incidence and is particularly common in Japan, Chile, Finland and Iceland (*60*).   In 1964–65, the age-adjusted death rate for both males and females was seven times higher in Japan than for whites in the United States, and the rate in the latter but not the former group is decreasing with time (*47*).

A particularly high incidence of gastric cancer occurs in areas of Great Britain and Japan with peaty, waterlogged or alluvial soils.   This variation suggests that extrinsic agents are involved in the etiology of the disease.   Sato *et al.* (*44, 45*) presented evidence that gastric cancer is associated with the high intake of salted fish and vegetables in Japan, and salted fish and meat products in Europe.   Others postulated an association with high intakes of rye, barley, oats and other starchy food, e.g., in Norway (30). In view of the results in animals, a significant factor in the etiology of human gastric cancer might possibly be the production of carcinogenic nitrosamides in the stomach by acid-catalyzed nitrosation, followed by a local carcinogenic action *in situ*.

In this paper, I shall review and attempt to correlate our work on the kinetics of N-nitrosation reactions, and on the induction of tumors in Swiss mice by feeding nitrite together with amines or ureas. I shall also discuss the natural occurrence of nitrosatable compounds, especially alkylureas and alkylguanidines.

Kinetics of Nitrosation Reactions

We confirmed earlier findings that nitrosation of dimethylamine follows the kinetics given by Eqs. 3 and 4 (26).

$$2\ HNO_2 \rightleftharpoons N_2O_3 + H_2O \tag{1}$$

$$R_2NH + N_2O_3 \longrightarrow R_2N \cdot NO + HNO_2 \tag{2}$$

$$rate = k_1 \times [R_2NH] \times [HNO_2]^2 \tag{3}$$

$$rate = k_2 \times [\text{total amine}] \times [\text{total nitrite}]^2 \tag{4}$$

The active nitrosating agent is nitrous anhydride (N_2O_3), formed reversibly from two molecules of HNO_2. The reaction rate is proportional to the amine and N_2O_3 concentration (Eq. 2) and hence to the square of HNO_2 concentration (Eq. 1). In Eq. 3, we use the concentrations of nonionized amine and free nitrous acid both of which vary with pH, and k_1 is independent of the pH. In Eq. 4 we use the total concentrations of dimethylamine and nitrite, and k_2 (the stoichiometric rate constant) depends on the pH.

k_2 and the reaction rate show maximum values at pH 3.4 for the following reason: For each 1-unit drop of pH in the pH range 3.4–9, the concentration of nonionized amine decreases about tenfold, and that of nonionized HNO_2 increases about tenfold. Because the reaction rate is proportional to the nonionized amine concentration, but to HNO_2 concentration *squared*, the rate increases tenfold for each 1-unit drop in pH. Below the pK_a of HNO_2 at pH 3.36, the nitrite is almost completely converted to HNO_2. The main effect of a further lowering of pH is the continuing drop in nonionized amine concentration, causing a decrease in the reaction rate. Incidentally, this discussion shows that there is no sharp pH limit for nitrosation. It can occur slowly at a pH of 5 or even 6 (as observed for dimethylamine (26)).

We recently studied the nitrosation of 6 secondary amines (Table 1, top 6 rows) using ultraviolet (UV) absorption of the nitrosamines to measure the reaction. The nitrosations followed Eqs. 3 and 4 at the optimum pH of about 3.0. k_2 at pH 3 (which indicates relative nitrosation rates under standard conditions) increased 185,000 times on proceeding from piperidine (pK_a; 11.2) to piperazine (pK_a; 5.57), *i.e.*, from the strongest to the weakest base. k_1 at pH 3 varied only fourfold, showing that the nonionized species of these 6 amines have rather similar reactivities (but

TABLE 1. Rate Constants for the Nitrosation of Some Secondary Amines and Amino Acids

Amine	pK_a	Optimum pH	k_2[a]	$k_1 \times 10^{-6}$ [a]
Piperidine	11.2	3.0	0.027	8.6
Dimethylamine	10.72	3.4	0.10	8.9
N-Methylbenzylamine	9.54	3.0	0.67	4.8
Morpholine	8.7	3.0	14.8	15.0
Mononitroso-piperazine	6.8	3.0	400.	5.0
Piperazine	5.57	3.0	5000.	3.7
L-Proline	—	2.25	2.9	—
L-Hydroxyproline	—	2.25	23.0	—
Sarcosine	—	2.5	13.6	—

[a] Values at the optimum pH, in $moles^{-2} l^2 min^{-1}$.

note the high k_1 for morpholine). k_1 rose several-fold as the pH was dropped from 5 to 1, indicating that at pH < 3 nitrosation was proceeding not only according to Eqs. 3 and 4, but also by other reactions. Our results confirm the finding of Sander et al. (42) that the less basic an amine is, the more readily it is nitrosated. The main difference between the nitrosation of different amines thus lies in the proportion of reactive nonionized amine at pH 3; and this, in turn, depends on the basicity of the amine.

Nitrosation of the amino- acids proline, hydroxyproline and sarcosine (N-methylglycine) proceeded at an optimum pH of 2.25–2.5 (Table 1, last 3 rows) and not 3 as for the amines. Reaction at the optimum pH followed Eq. 4, i.e., the rate was proportional to amino- acid concentration and nitrite concentration squared. However, k_1 increased much more rapidly as the pH dropped than for the secondary amines. The probable reason for these differences is the complicated ionization of amino- acids, since there are 4 molecular species, $-NH_2^+-COOH$, $-NH_2^+-COO^-$, $-NH-COOH$ and $-NH-COO^-$, of which only the last two (with nonionized -NH-) are nitrosatable. The k_2 values show that at the optimum pH hydroxyproline and sarcosine are nitrosated at rates similar to that for morpholine (i.e., at 130–230 times the rate for dimethylamine), and that proline is nitrosated at about one-fifth of the rate for morpholine. Since proline and hydroxyproline are components of proteins, the kinetic findings would be disturbing if the nitroso derivatives turn out to be carcinogenic.

The nitrosation of alkylureas and N-alkylurethans proceeds rapidly (27, 41). The reaction rate, which increases about tenfold for each 1-unit drop in pH from 3 to 1, does not show a pH maximum, and follows Eqs. 7 and 8 (27). The main nitrosating agent is probably the nitrous acidium ion, $(H_2NO_2)^+$. For methylurea nitrosation, the rate is proportional to the methylurea and nitrous acidium ion concentration (Eq. 6), which, in turn, is proportional to the hydrogen ion and nitrous acid concentration (Eq. 5). k_3 (like k_1) depends on the ionization of nitrite and, hence, on pH. k_4 does not depend on the ionization of methylurea, since this is almost completely nonionized above pH 2 ($pK_a = +0.9$ (35)).

$$H^+ + HNO_2 \rightleftharpoons (H_2NO_2)^+ \tag{5}$$

$$RNH \cdot CO \cdot R' + (H_2NO_2)^+ \longrightarrow RN(NO) \cdot CO \cdot R' + H_2O + H^+ \tag{6}$$

$$rate = k_3 \times [RNH \cdot CO \cdot R'] \times [HNO_2] \times [H^+] \tag{7}$$

$$rate = k_4 \times [RNH \cdot CO \cdot R'] \times [total\ nitrite] \times [H^+] \tag{8}$$

k_3 in moles^{-2} l^2 min^{-1} was 630 for methylurea, 180 for ethylurea, 22 for N-methylurethan (ethyl N-methylcarbamate), 6.1 for N-ethylurethan, 43 for citrulline, and 2.5 for hydantoin. The simple alkylnitrosoureas and N-alkyl-N-nitrosourethans are known to be powerful carcinogens, but the nitroso derivatives of citrulline and hydantoin (synthesized by us and identified as N-δ-nitroso-L-citrulline and 1-nitroso-hydantoin) have not yet been tested.

The nitrosation of methylguanidine was then examined (27). Prolonged nitrosation under strongly acidic conditions gave a 35% yield of methylnitrosourea. When methylguanidine (0.05 M) was reacted with nitrite (0.05 M) at pH 1 and 25°C for 1 hr, methylene chloride extracts showed absorption peaks due to a volatile new compound, methylnitrosocyanamide. After reacting for a longer period, the UV spectrum gradually changed to that of methylnitrosourea. Spectral analysis showed that the yield of methylnitrosocyanamide reached a maximum of 2% (from methylguanidine) at 3 hr and then fell, and that methylnitrosourea continued rising until a 7% yield was reached at 10 hr.

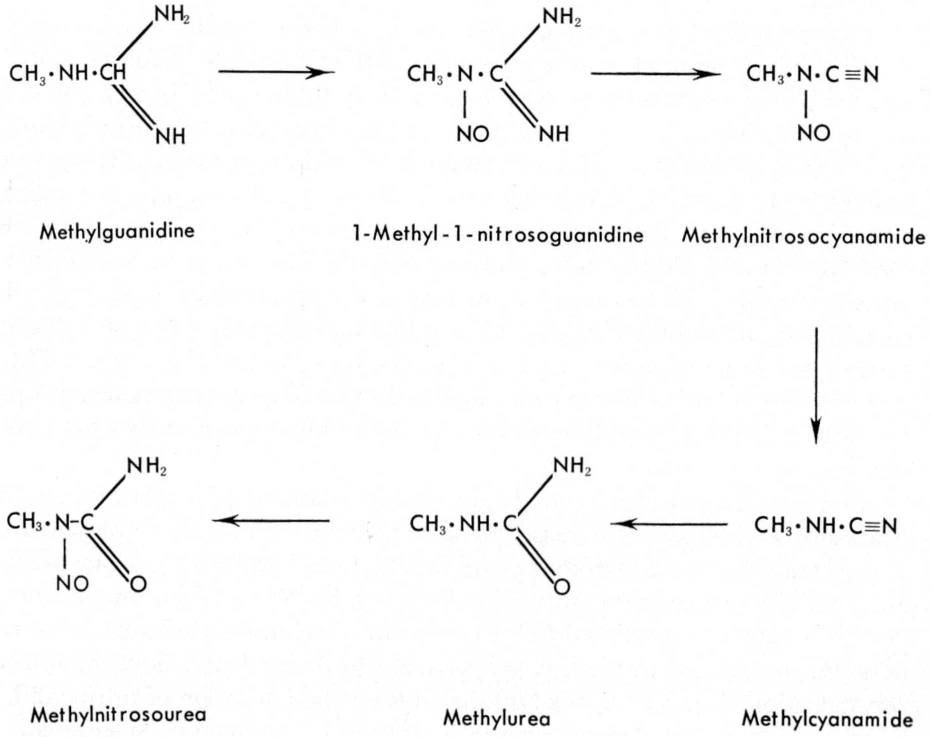

FIG. 1. Nitrosation of methylguanidine.

Methylnitrosocyanamide was also prepared by nitrosation of methylcyanamide, but could not be fully purified. However, ethylnitrosocyanamide was obtained analytically pure by nitrosation of ethylcyanamide. In cold dilute sulfuric acid, the nitrosocyanamides liberate nitrous acid and slowly produce the corresponding nitrosoureas. In alkali, ethylnitrosocyanamide is converted into diazoethane and cyanate (Mirvish, Nagel, and Sams, in preparation).

Nitrosation of methylguanidine also gave a third UV-absorbing product that is not extracted by methylene chloride, decomposes when solutions are evaporated to dryness, appears to be readily converted under mildly basic conditions to methylnitrosocyanamide, and may be the unknown 1-methyl-1-nitrosoguanidine (27). The isomeric 1-methyl-3-nitrosoguanidine has been synthesized by reduction of 1-methyl-3-nitroguanidine with Zn/HCl (4). The postulated route for methylguanidine nitrosation is given in Fig. 1. The formation of methylnitrosocyanamide is reminiscent of the production of nitrocyanamide from N-methyl-N-nitroso-N'-nitroguanidine (21).

The kinetics for methylguanidine nitrosation to give methylnitrosourea appear to obey Eq. 8, with $k_4=0.24$ moles^{-2}l^{2}min^{-1} at pH 2. This is only 0.045% of k_4 for the formation of methylnitrosourea from methylurea. When the guanidino-amino- acids arginine and N-a-acetylarginine were nitrosated under strongly acidic conditions, butanol extracts showed UV maxima similar to those of nitrosocitrulline, indicating that nitrosoureas were produced. The reaction rates were similar to that for methylguanidine nitrosation (27).

Occurrence of Nitrosatable Compounds in Nature

In order to decide whether *in vivo* production of N-nitroso compounds is relevant to cancer in man, it is important to know the distribution in nature and especially in food of nitrite, nitrate (if it is reduced to nitrite), and nitrosatable compounds. As far as we know, the last group comprises chiefly the secondary amines, ureas, carbamates, and guanidines. Since certain nitrosoureas induce gastric cancer in animals, the natural occurrence of ureas could be of particular relevance for human gastric cancer.

Little is known about the distribution in nature of secondary amines other than dimethylamine, which occurs in fish, but is very slowly nitrosated (Table 1). Some secondary amines are used as drugs (*e.g.*, piperazine) or food additives (*e.g.*, morpholine) (12, 23). The production of dialkylnitrosamines by the nitrosation of tertiary amines was recently discussed by Lijinsky *et al.* (22).

With respect to amino- acids with secondary amino groups, proline occurs combined in most proteins, and hydroxyproline in collagen. Free sarcosine was first observed in starfish by Kossel in 1915. Relatively large amounts were found in the muscles of cartilaginous (46) and ganoid (55) fish, and in the hepato-pancreas of the South African rock lobster (33). Cartilaginous fish also contain much betaine (N-trimethylglycine) (46), for which sarcosine is presumably a precursor.

N-Alkylcarbamates are not known to occur in nature, but are widely used as tranquilizers, insecticides and weed-killers (25). Despite the occurrence of large

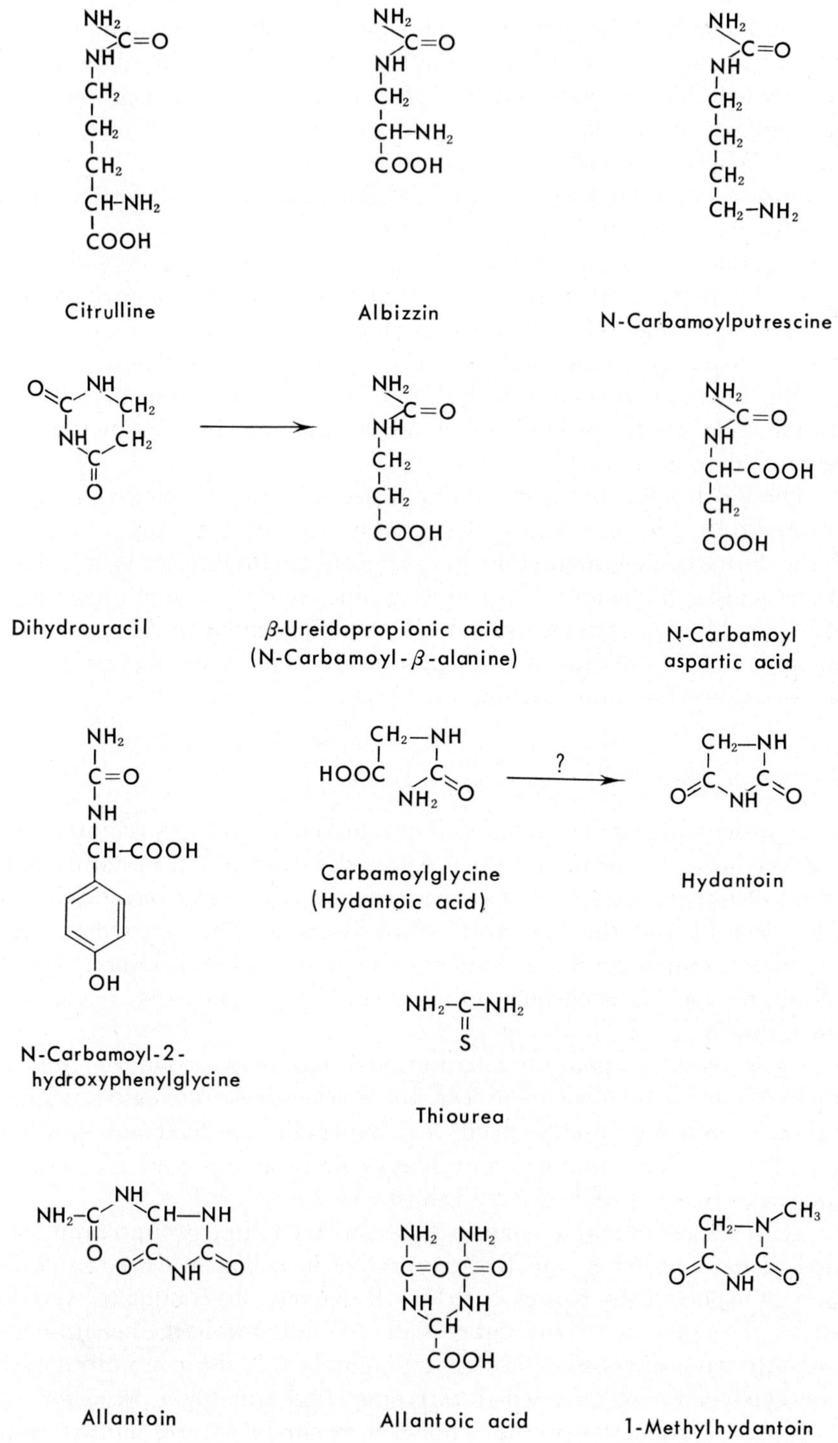

FIG. 2. Naturally occurring ureides.

amounts of urea in urine and also fungi (*53*), simple alkylureas have not yet been found in nature.

In 1877, methylurea was reported to be a urinary metabolite of methylamine in rabbits, but not dogs (*59*). We found no methylurea in the urine of adult rats injected with 100 mg of methylamine·HCl. The method of analysis involved chromatography of the urine on Dowex-50 columns (adsorption from 0.1 N NaCl, elution with 0.25 M formate buffer, pH 3.75), which separated urea plus methylurea as one fraction, and then nitrosation (urea is destroyed). The resulting methylnitrosourea was extracted with ether and estimated by the nitrobenzylpyridine method (*36*). The detection limit corresponded to a 1% conversion of the methylamine.

Urea compounds (ureides) also containing other functional groups occur fairly widely in both plants (*9, 53*) and animals (Fig. 2 and underlined compounds). They are related metabolically to amino- acids, purines or pyrimidines, and appear to be produced by (1) hydrolytic de-imidation of guanidines catalyzed by bacterial de-imidases, or (2) carbamoylation of primary amines catalyzed by transcarbamoylases, with carbamoyl phosphate providing the carbamoyl (NH_2·CO-) group. We shall not list compounds in which urea forms part of a resonating ring system, *e.g.*, uracil, xanthine and uric acid, since these three compounds do not seem to be nitrosated (as indicated by the absence of new UV peaks under nitrosating conditions).

L-Citrulline is a component of the Krebs urea metabolic cycle, and occurs in plants, *e.g.*, watermelons (50 mg/kg wet wt.) (*56*) and green peppers (350 mg/kg wet wt.) (*32*). The amount increases after infection of watermelon with a fungus (*13*). During the brewing of soy sauce (which takes several weeks), the highly salted soybean extract accumulates free arginine (up to 4 g/l) and citrulline (up to 1.3 g/l) (*34*). Fresh and flue-cured tobacco leaves with the condition of " frenching " contain up to 1 g citrulline/kg wet wt. (*54*). *Albizzin* (L-2-amino-3-ureidopropionic acid) is a lower homolog of citrulline, occurring in plants of the Mimosa family (*11*).

The gut microorganism *Streptococcus faecalis* converts agmatine (decarboxylated arginine) by de-imidation to *N-carbamoylputrescine* and then to putrescine (*29*). Pea seedling homogenate and ornithine carbamoyl-transferase prepared from the homogenate acts on putrescine to give N-carbamoylputrescine (*18*). Barley seedlings form N-carbamoylputrescine when fed with agmatine (*49*), and potassium-deficient barley and clover accumulate putrescine and agmatine (*50*). *N-Carbamoyl-2-p-hydroxyphenylglycine* occurs in broad bean leaves (1.0 g/kg dry wt.) (*9*). *Hydantoin* was isolated from sugar beet sprouts by von Lippman in 1898. It possibly arose as an artefact from *hydantoic acid* (N-carbamoylglycine) (*9*). *1-Methylhydantoin* (which should not be nitrosatable) is formed by bacterial de-imidation of creatine (*52*), and is present in deteriorated whale meat (*31*). *Thiourea* (which should not yield a nitroso derivative) occurs in various species of Laburnum plants (*19, 58*).

N-Carbamoylaspartic acid is an intermediate in pyrimidine biosynthesis. Uracil is catabolized in the liver to give *dihydrouracil* and then *β-ureidopropionic acid* (N-carbamoyl-*β*-alanine). Both metabolites are present in rat urine (*3*). *Dihydrouracil* also occurs as a minor base in transfer RNA and as the free base in the brain (*24*). Similarly, thymine is metabolized to *dihydrothymine* and *β-ureido-isobutyric acid* (*10, 57*), but these have apparently not been detected in urine.

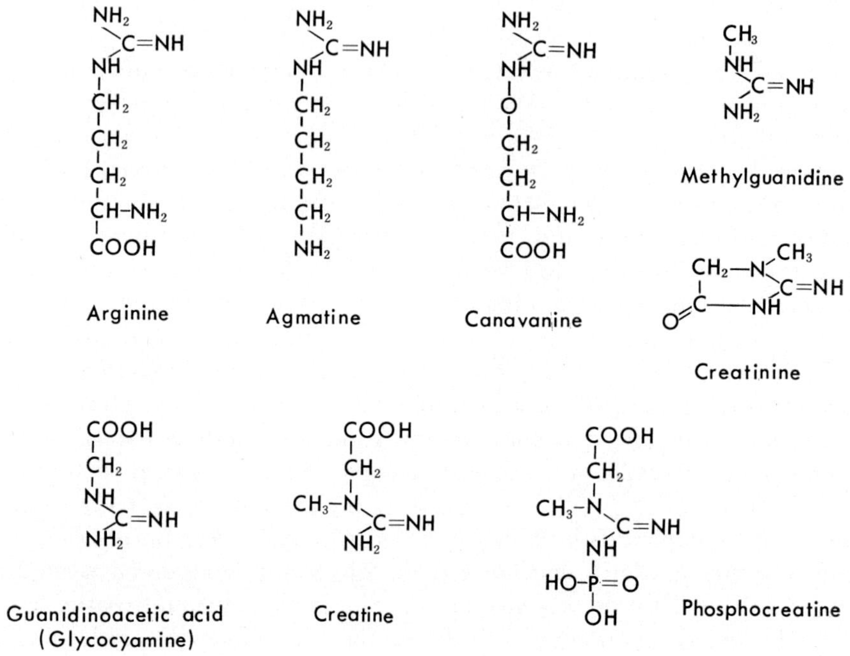

Fig. 3. Naturally occurring guanidines.

Uric acid is degraded by uricase and allantoinase to give first *allantoin*, and then *allantoic acid*; both of which occur widely in plants (*2, 53*). Allantoin occurs in normal human blood plasma and urine (10–30 mg/24 hr). However, preliminary experiments indicate that nitrosation of allantoin does not yield an N-nitroso derivative. Alkylureas and cyclic ureas are also widely used as drugs (*41*).

Turning to the guanidines (Fig. 3), *methylguanidine* was reported in the early 1900's to occur in fresh and decaying meat, fish, and urine. These reports are suspect, since it was shown that methylguanidine is produced from creatine and creatinine by the silver salts used in the isolation. However, after this factor was eliminated, methylguanidine was still detected in fresh beef, fish rays, cod, sardines, and sharks (60–1,900 mg/kg fresh wt.) (*16, 17, 20, 43*). Other naturally occurring guanidines are *arginine, creatine, creatinine, phosphocreatine, guanidinoacetic acid* (*i.e.,* glycocyamine, an intermediate in creatine synthesis and a normal constituent of urine), *agmatine* (produced by bacterial decarboxylation of arginine), and the oxyguanidine *canavanine* (occurs in jack beans and soybeans).

The slow nitrosation of methylguanidine, arginine and N-α-acetylarginine suggests that only small amounts of the carcinogenic nitrosoureas may be produced by direct intragastric nitrosation of alkylguanidines. Perhaps, more significantly, bacterial de-imidation of alkylguanidines could occur during food storage under non-sterile conditions. This could be followed by intragastric nitrosation of the resulting alkylureas.

Induction of Lung Adenomas in Mice by Feeding Nitrite and Amines or Ureas

Sander and co-workers (*38–40, 42*) and Ivankovic and Preussmann (*14*) induced tumors in rats by feeding them sodium nitrite together with various secondary amines and alkylureas. In later studies, Greenblatt, Mirvish and So (*12*) treated Swiss mice with sodium nitrite in the drinking water and four secondary amines in the food. Mice treated with nitrite plus morpholine, piperazine or N-methylaniline developed 1.4–1.8 lung adenomas/mouse. Negative results were observed in a group treated with nitrite plus dimethylamine, and in groups fed the amines or nitrite alone. Mice fed the corresponding nitrosamines showed 2–6 adenomas/mouse. Mirvish, Greenblatt and Kommineni fed sodium nitrite and methylurea or ethylurea to Swiss mice at molar doses similar to those used for the amines, and obtained 4.0–4.3 adenomas/mouse. Mice fed methylurea or ethylurea alone gave negative results (see; J. Natl. Cancer Inst., *48*: 1311–1315, 1972).

The lung adenoma test is particularly suitable for quantitative comparisons (*48*). We could roughly estimate the fraction of amine nitrosated in the amine plus nitrite groups by comparing the tumor yield with that in groups receiving the corresponding nitrosamines (Table 2). Piperazine is nitrosated to give mononitroso-

TABLE 2. Comparison of Estimated and Calculated Nitrosation in the Mouse Stomach

Compound	k_2[a]	Percent amine or urea nitrosated			Percent nitrite used[c]	Partition coefficient[d]
		Estimated from adenoma yield	Calculated from kinetics	Maximum[b]		
Dimethylamine	0.1	<0.04	0.001	5	0.005	0.01
Morpholine	14.8	0.27	0.26	5	1.3	0.01
Piperazine	5000	1.6	4.5	5	22.5	0.01
N-Methylaniline	—[e]	2.0	20.0	20	3.8	3.0
	k_4[a]					
Methylurea	630	—[f]	2.4	5	12.0	0.01
Ethylurea	180	—[f]	0.83	5	4.2	0.01

[a] In moles^{-2}l^{2}min^{-1}.

[b] Assuming 75% of the nitrite disappears.

[c] Calculated percent nitrite used to nitrosate the amine or urea, without correction for disappearance of the nitrite.

[d] Methylene chloride : water partition coefficient at pH 3.

[e] Nitrosation is too rapid to estimate k_2.

[f] Not estimated since the nitrosoureas were not administered as positive controls.

and then dinitroso-piperazine. The first nitrosation is more rapid than the second, since the k_2 for piperazine is higher than the k_2 for mononitrosopiperazine (Table 1). In the piperazine plus nitrite group, therefore, tumorigenesis was probably due to the mononitroso derivative; and the estimated conversion is based on the tumorigenic activity of this compound (unpublished results).

Correlation between Chemical and Biological Results

We then calculated the percent of nitrosation of the amines and ureas that might be expected to occur in the mouse stomach on the basis of the kinetic results, and compared these figures with the estimates based on tumor yield (28). In the calculations, we assumed that (1) the food can be regarded as a homogeneous aqueous solution weighing 1.0 g/ml; (2) the stomach contained equal volumes of food (containing amine or urea), ingested water (containing nitrite), and gastric juice; (3) the food and water were consumed at the same time; (4) the mixture was in the glandular portion of the stomach for 1 hr at pH 3 and 37°C; (5) the nitrite disappears in the stomach due to acid-catalyzed decomposition and reaction with food constituents, so that the average concentration for the 1 hr is 25% of the initial value (Mirvish and Kommineni, unpublished results on rats); and (6) k_2 at 37°C is twice k_2 at 25°C. These assumptions give lower nitrosation values than those used before (27). Based on assumptions (2) and (5), the final concentrations of amine/urea and nitrite are, respectively, 1/3 and 1/12 of the original values in the food or water, i.e., 24.17 mM amine or urea and 1.208 mM nitrite.

Since for most groups a fivefold molar excess of amine or urea to nitrite was used, and 75% of the nitrite is assumed to decompose, the 100% yield based on the remaining undecomposed nitrite corresponded to a 5% yield from the amine or urea. The latter is the " maximum " yield in Table 2, column 5. A lower dose of N-methylaniline was used since it induced methemoglobinemia. Thus here the final amine concentration was 6.04 mM and the maximum yield was 20% of the amine. The calculations were based on Eqs. 4 and 8, using integration where necessary. The results are expressed as percent amine or urea and percent nitrite.

These calculations and the estimations from tumor yield agree well for dimethylamine, where no nitrosation was predicted and no tumors were induced, and for morpholine, where the calculated and estimated values for the nitrosation were 0.26% and 0.27% of the amine. Piperazine is very readily nitrosated and the calculated nitrosation is 4.5% (close to the maximum of 5%), which perhaps does not differ excessively from the estimated value of 1.6%. N-Methylaniline is nitrosated so rapidly that the reaction rate in 0.002 M perchloric acid is determined only by the rate of formation of nitrous anhydride from nitrous acid (Eq. 1) (15). Thus, the calculated nitrosation of N-methylaniline is close to the 20% maximum, whereas the estimate from the tumor yield was 2%.

The low yield for N-methylaniline may be due to the extraction of nonionized amine by dietary fats, which would remove the amine from the aqueous solution where nitrosation occurs. The partition coefficient of N-methylaniline was found to be 3 : 1 for methylene chloride : pH 3 buffer and 43 : 1 for methylene chloride : pH 4 buffer. Under the same conditions, the other amines and the ureas were almost entirely partitioned into the water phase (Table 2, last column), Presumably, only the nonionized species of the amines is extracted by methylene chloride, and the high partition coefficient of N-methylaniline is due to the low pK_a of 4.85, which allows a relatively large fraction of the amine to be nonionized (and, hence, extractable) at pH 3–4.

It turns out that for equal rates of nitrosation at pH 3 and 1.208 mM nitrite (the assumed final conditions in the stomach), $k_4 = 1.2 \times k_2$. Thus, k_2 and k_4 can approximately be compared directly, and methylurea and ethylurea should be nitrosated at rates between those for morpholine and piperazine (Table 2, column 2). Calculations suggest that 2.4% of the methylurea and 0.83% of the ethylurea would be nitrosated (maximum=5%), but the actual conversion cannot be estimated since the nitrosoureas themselves were not fed.

In the studies by Sander *et al.* (*38–40, 42*) and Ivankovic and Preussmann (*14*), tumor were induced in rats by feeding them nitrite together with the amines, morpholine, N-methylbenzylamine (but not diethylamine), and the ureas, methylurea, ethylurea, N,N'-dimethylurea and 2-imidazolidone. These results are in qualitative agreement with the kinetic data (Table 2), except that the positive results for N-methylbenzylamine (*39*) were unexpected in view of its rather slow nitrosation. Additional factors not considered in our calculations are (1) catalytic effects on the nitrosations, *e.g.*, by sulfate (*27*), phosphate (*27*), and thiocyanate (*1*) ions (the last is a normal constituent of saliva); (2) decomposition of nitrosamines and especially nitrosamides; (3) possible removal of amine from aqueous solution by precipitation as insoluble salts; and (4) physiological effects of the amine, urea or nitrite on gastric secretion and emptying.

CONCLUSIONS

The kinetic results show which types of nitrogen compound are likely to be readily nitrosatable. These include weakly basic secondary amines (*e.g.*, morpholine, piperazine, N-methylaniline), some *free* amino-acids with secondary amino groups (hydroxyproline, sarcosine), alkylureas and N-alkylcarbamates. The presence in food of even small concentrations of these compounds would be disturbing if the N-nitroso derivatives are strongly carcinogenic and sufficient nitrite is present, because of the possibility of intragastric nitrosation and also of nitrosation during food storage especially under acidic conditions. Less readily nitrosatable compounds, *e.g.*, strongly basic secondary amines (piperidine, dimethylamine), free proline, and alkylguanidines (methylguanidine, arginine) are less likely to be nitrosated in significant amounts, unless relatively large concentrations occur in the food.

The natural occurrence of 16 urea derivatives (ureides), mostly in unknown amounts, suggests that their nitrosation could be significant, though nitrosation of these compounds do not all appear to give N-nitroso derivatives. Moreover, the carcinogenicity of these derivatives is in all cases unknown [nitrosocitrulline is remarkably nontoxic (*27*)]. The occurrence of 8 guanidine compounds could also be significant, since alkylguanidines can give rise to alkylnitrosoureas either by slow direct nitrosation or by bacterial conversion to alkylureas during food storage, followed by nitrosation of the alkylureas.

Correlations between the kinetic data and results of the mouse experiments generally support the view that N-nitroso compounds, which presumably induced the lung tumors, were produced by nitrosation in the mouse stomach. The various assumptions and complicating factors, *e.g.*, physiological variables in the stomach, decomposition of the nitrite, fat extraction of the amines, and catalysis by anions, will hopefully be of use in predicting the amount of N-nitroso compounds likely to be produced in the human stomach from different amines or ureas. Our results, especially the negative results obtained with dimethylamine plus nitrite, are consistent with the view that these nitrosations are acid-catalyzed chemical reactions occurring in the stomach, and not enzyme-catalyzed reactions occurring in tissues or gut bacteria.   The kinetic results may also be useful for predicting the formation of N-nitroso compounds in stored food.

It seems clear that quantitative analysis of foods for nitrite and nitrosatable compounds may be the most important factor in deciding whether or not intragastric nitrosation is significant for the etiology of human cancer of the stomach and other organs.   The geographic distribution of gastric cancer (see Introduction) may help to suggest foods which should be analyzed.

This discussion has emphasized the possible hazard involved in the natural occurrence of nitrosatable compounds in food.   However, similar principles should apply to the use of drugs or food additives containing nitrosatable groups, especially if large amounts are consumed on a continuous basis.   For example, it seems reasonable to suggest that when drugs such as piperazine, which can readily be nitrosated to yield carcinogenic N-nitroso derivatives, are administered, the patient should avoid food containing large amounts of nitrite, *e.g.*, certain green vegetables and nitrite-preserved meat and fish.   (The drug might also be given with ascorbic acid, which reacts with nitrite—Mirvish, Wallcave, Eagen, and Shubik, Science, *177*: 65–68, 1972).

SUMMARY

The kinetics of nitrosation were studied for 6 secondary amines (piperidine, dimethylamine, N-methylbenzylamine, morpholine, mononitrosopiperazine, piperazine), 3 amino- acids (proline, hydroxyproline, sarcosine), 4 ureides (methylurea, ethylurea, citrulline, hydantoin), 2 carbamates (N-methyl- and N-ethyl-urethan), and 3 guanidines (methylguanidine, arginine, N-α-acetylarginine).   A new class of N-nitroso compounds, *viz.*, nitrosocyanamides, was prepared by nitrosation of methylguanidine and methyl- and ethylcyanamide.   The natural occurrence of 16 ureides and 8 guanidines is reviewed.

Sodium nitrite was fed to Swiss mice in the drinking water, together with 4 secondary amines and 2 ureas given in the food.   Lung adenomas were induced in 5 of the 6 groups.   Percent nitrosation *in vivo*, as estimated from the yield of lung adenomas, was compared with percent nitrosation calculated from the rate constants, after making certain assumptions about conditions in the stomach.   The agreement was fairly satisfactory, except for the lower-than-expected results for N-methylaniline, perhaps due to the extraction of nonionized amine by fats.   The significance of these results is discussed with respect to intragastric nitrosation as a possible factor in the etiology of human cancer, especially gastric cancer.

I wish to thank Drs. P. Shubik, W. Lijinsky, M. Greenblatt and L. Wallcave for their very helpful discussions, Mr. J. Sams and Miss Cecilia Chu for their efficient technic alassistance, Mrs. Marline Gerrity for literature searches, and Miss Sharon Lasley for secretarial help.   The work was supported by Public Health Service Contract PH 43–68–67 from the National Cancer Institute, a contract from the International Agency for Research in Cancer, Lyon, France, and grant BC-19 from the American Cancer Society.

REFERENCES

1. Boyland, E., Nice, E., and Williams, S. K. The Catalysis of Nitrosation by Thiocyanate from Saliva. Food Cosmetics Toxicology, In press.

2. Brunel, A., et Capelle, G. Sur l'Importance Biologique des Uréides Glyoxyliques ches les êtres Vivants. 1.-L'Allantoïne et l'Acide Allantoïque chez les Végétaux. Bull. Soc. Chim. Biol., *29*: 427–445, 1947.

3. Crokaert, R. Carbamoyldérivés d'Acides Aminés d'Intérêt Biologique. Bull. Soc. Chim. Biol., *43*: 1317–1329, 1961.

4. Davis, T. L., and Rosenquist, E. N. Studies in the Urea Series. XV. Transformations of Nitrosoguanidine, Alkylnitrosoguanidines, N-R,N'-R'-Dialkylguanidines. J. Amer. Chem. Soc., *59*: 2112–2115, 1937.

5. Druckrey, H., Ivankovic, S., Bücheler, J., Preussmann, R., und Thomas, C. Erzeugung von Magen- und Pankreas-Krebs beim Meerschweinchen durch Methylnitroso-Harnstoff und -Urethan. Z. Krebsforsch., *71*: 167–182, 1968.

6. Druckrey, H., Ivankovic, S., und Preussmann, R. Selektive Erzeugung von Carcinomen des Drüsenmagens bei Ratten durch orale Gabe von N-Methyl-N-nitroso-N'-acetylharnstoff (AcMNH). Z. Krebsforsch., *75*: 23–33, 1970.

7. Druckrey, H., Preussmann, R., Ivankovic, S., und Schmähl, D. Organotrope carcinogene Wirkungen bei 65 verschiedenen N-Nitroso-Verbindungen an BD-Ratten. Z. Krebsforsch., *69*: 103–201, 1967.

8. Druckrey, H., Steinhoff, D., Beuthner, H., Schneider, H., und Klärner, P. Prüfing von Nitrit auf toxische Wirkung an Ratten. Arzneim.-forsch., *13*: 320–323, 1963.

9. Eagles, J., Laird, W. M., Matai, S., Self, R., Synge, R. L. M., and Drake, A. F. N-Carbamoyl-2-(*p*-hydroxyphenyl)glycine from Leaves of Broad Bean (*Vicia faba* L.). Biochem. J., *121*: 425–430, 1971.

10. Fink, R. M., Fink, K., und Henderson, R. B. β-Amino Acid Formation by Tissue Slices Incubated with Pyrimidines. J. Biol. Chem., *201*: 349–355, 1953.

11. Gmelin, R., Strauss, G., und Hasenmaier, G. Über neue Aminosäuren aus Mimosaceen. Z. Phys. Chem., *314*: 28–32, 1959.

12. Greenblatt, M., Mirvish, S. S., and So, B. T. Nitrosamine Studies: Induction of Lung Adenomas by Concurrent Administration of Sodium Nitrite and Secondary Amines in Swiss Mice. J. Natl. Cancer Inst., *46*: 1029–1034, 1971.

13. Hadwiger, L. A., and Hall, C. V. The Relation of Pigmentation and Free Amino Acid Content with Resistance to Colletotrichum Lagenarium in Watermelons. Plant Disease Reporter, *45*: 373–374, 1961.

14. Ivankovic, S., und Preussmann, R. Transplazentare Erzeugung maligner Tumoren nach oraler Gabe von Äthylharnstoff und Nitrit an Ratten. Naturwissenschaften, *57*: 460, 1970.

15. Kalatzis, E., and Ridd, J. H. Nitrosation, Diazotisation, and Deamination. XII. The Kinetics of N-Nitrosation of N-Methylaniline. J. Chem. Soc., 529–533, 1966B.

16. Kapeller-Adler, R., and Krael, J. Untersuchungen über die Stickstoffverteilung in den Muskeln verschiedener Tierklassen. I. Biochem. Z., *221*: 437–460, 1930.

17. Kapeller-Adler, R., und Krael, J. Untersuchungen über die Stickstoffverteilung in der Muskeln verschiedener Tierklassen. II. Über die Stickstoffverteilung im Rochen- und Haifischmuskel. Biochem. Z., *224*: 364–377, 1930.

18. Kleczkowski, K., and Wielgat, B. Carbamoylation of Putrescine in Plant Material. Bull. Acad. Pol. Sci., *16*: 521–526, 1968.

19. Klein, G., and Farkass, E.   Microchemical Detection of Alkaloids in Plants.   XIV. Cytisine.   Oesterr. Bot. Z., *79*: 107–124, 1930.

20. Komarow, S. A.   Über das Vorkommen des präformierten Methylguanidins im Muskelgewebe.   Biochem. Z., *211*: 326–351, 1929.

21. Lawley, P. D., and Thatcher, C. J.   Methylation of Deoxyribonucleic Acid in Cultured Mammalian Cells by N-Methyl-N′-nitro-N-nitrosoguanidine.   Biochem. J., *116*: 693–707, 1970.

22. Lijinsky, W.   Formation of Carcinogenic Nitrosamines by Reaction of Drugs with Nitrite.   *In*; Analysis and formation of nitrosamines, International Agency for Research in Cancer, Lyon, France, 1971.

23. Lijinsky, W., and Epstein, S. S.   Nitrosamines as Environmental Carcinogens. Nature, *225*: 21–23, 1970.

24. Minard, F. N., and Grant, D. S.   5,6-Dihydrouracil: Its Occurrence and Metabolism in Rat Brain.   Biochim. Biophys. Acta, *209*: 255–257, 1970.

25. Mirvish, S. S.   The Carcinogenic Action and Metabolism of Urethan and N-Hydroxyurethan.   Advan. Cancer Res., *11*: 1–42, 1968.

26. Mirvish, S. S.   Kinetics of Dimethylamine Nitrosation in Relation to Nitrosamine Carcinogenesis.   J. Natl. Cancer Inst., *44*: 633–639, 1970.

27. Mirvish, S. S.   Kinetics of Nitrosamide Formation from Alkylureas, N-Alkylurethans, and Alkylguanidines: Possible Implications for the Etiology of Human Gastric Cancer.   J. Natl. Cancer Inst., *46*: 1183–1193, 1971.

28. Mirvish, S. S.   Kinetics of N-Nitrosation Reactions in Relation to Tumorigenesis Experiments with Nitrite plus Amines or Ureas.   *In*; Analysis and formation of nitrosamines.   International Agency for Research in Cancer, Lyon, France, 1971.

29. Møller, V.   Simplified Tests for Some Amino Acid Decarboxylases and for the Arginine Dihydrolase System.   Acta Pathol. Microbiol. Scand., *36*: 158–172, 1955.

30. Muñoz, N., and Asvall, J.   Time Trends of Intestinal and Diffuse Types of Gastric Cancer in Norway.   Int. J. Cancer, *8*: 144–157, 1971.

31. Nakai, T., Uchijima, S., and Koyama, M.   Paper Chromatography of 3-Methylhydantoic Acid and 1-Methylhydantoin, Possible Intermediates of Microbial Degradation of Creatine and Creatinine.   J. Chromatogr., *53*: 406–408, 1970.

32. Navarro, F., Rodriguez, A., et Sancho, J.   Estudio Quimicofisico de las Especies " Capsicum."   II.   Cromatografia en Papel de los Amino-Acidos.   An. Real. Soc. Espan. Fis. Quim., *58B*: 571–574, 1962.

33. Novelle, L., and Schwartz, H. M.   Occurrence and Distribution of Sarcosine in the Rock Lobster.   Nature, *173*: 450, 1954.

34. Ogasawara, T., Ito, K., Abe, N., and Homma, H.   Basic Amino Acids of Soy Sauces and Seasoning Liquids.   II.   The Quantitative Changes of L-Arginine in the Process of Soy Sauce Brewing.   Nippon Nogei Kagaku Kaishi, *37*(4): 208–213, 1963.

35. Perrin, D. D.   Dissociation Constants of Organic Bases in Aqueous Solution, Butterworths, London, 1965.

36. Preussmann, R., Schneider, H., und Epple, F.   Untersuchungen zum Nachweis alkylierender Agentien.   II.   Der nachweis verschiedener Klassen alkylierende Agentien mit einer Modifikation der Farbreaktion mit 4-(4-Nitrobenzyl)-pyridin (NBP).   Arzneim.-Forsch., *19*: 1059–1073, 1969.

37. Sander, J.   Kann Nitrit in der menschlichen Nahrung Ursache einer Krebsentstehung durch Nitrosaminbildung sein?   Arch. Hyg. Bakt., *151*: 22–28, 1967.

38. Sander, J.   Induktion maligner Tumoren bei Ratten durch orale Gabe von N,N′-Dimethylharnstoff und Nitrit.   Arzneim.-Forsch., *20*: 418–419, 1970.

39. Sander, J. B., und Bürkle, G. Induktion maligner Tumoren bei Ratten durch gleichzeitige Verfütterung von Nitrit und sekundären Aminen. Z. Krebsforsch., *73*: 54–66, 1969.

40. Sander, J., und Bürkle, G. Induktion maligner Tumoren bei Ratten durch orale Gabe von 2-Imidazolidinon und Nitrit. Z. Krebsforsch., *75*: 301–304, 1971.

41. Sander, J., Bürkle, G., Flohe, L., und Aeikens, B. Untersuchungen *in vitro* über die Möglichkeit einer Bildung cancerogener Nitrosamide im Magen. Arzneim.-Forsch., *21*: 411–414, 1971.

42. Sander, J., Schweinsberg, F., und Menz, H. P. Unterschungen über die Entstehung cancerogener Nitrosamine im Magen. Hoppe-Seyler's Z. Physiol. Chem., *349*: 1691–1697, 1968.

43. Sasaki, A. Über die Extraktivstoffe des Sardinenfleisches (Maiwasi: *Sardinia melanostica*). Tohoku J. Exp. Med., *34*: 561–570, 1938.

44. Sato, T., Fukuyama, T., Suzuki, T., Takayanagi, J., Murakami, T., Shiotsuki, N., Tanaka, R., and Tsuji, R. Studies of the Causation of Gastric Cancer. II. The Relation between Gastric Cancer Mortality Rate and Salted Food Intake in Several Places in Japan. Bull. Inst. Public Health (Japan), *8*: 187–198, 1959.

45. Sato, T., Fukuyama, T., Suzuki, T., Takayanagi, J., and Sakai, Y. Studies on the Causation of Gastric Cancer. Intake of Highly Brined Foods in Several Places with High Mortality Rate in Europe. Bull. Inst. Public Health (Japan), *10*: 9–17, 1961.

46. Schaefer, H. Free Amino Acids and Related Compounds in the Muscles of Chimaera and Some Elasmobranchs and Invertebrates. Helgolaender Wiss. Meeresuntersuch., *8*: 280–286, 1962.

47. Segi, M., Kurihara, M., and Matsuyama, T. Cancer Mortality for Selected Sites in 24 Countries. Dept. of Public Health, Tohoku University School of Medicine, Sendai, Japan, 1969.

48. Shimkin, M. B., Wieder, R., McDonough, M., Fishbein, L., and Swern, D. Lung Tumor Response in Strain A Mice as a Quantitative Bioassay of Carcinogenic Activity of Some Carbamates and Aziridines. Cancer Res., *29*: 2184–2190, 1969.

49. Smith, T. A., and Garraway, J. L. N-Carbamoylputrescine—An Intermediate in the Formation of Putrescine by Barley. Phytochemistry, *3*: 23–26, 1964.

50. Smith, T. A., and Richards, F. J. The Biosynthesis of Putrescine in Higher Plants and Its Relation to Potassium Nutrition. Biochem. J., *84*: 292–294, 1962.

51. Sugimura, T., Fujimura, S., Kogure, K., Baba, T., Saito, T., Nagao, M., Hosoi, H., Shimosato, Y., and Yokoshima, T. Production of Adenocarcinomas in Glandular Stomach of Experimental Animals by N-Methyl-N'-nitro-N-nitrosoguanidine. Gann Monograph, *8*: 157–196, 1969.

52. Szulmajster, J. Bacterial Degradation of Creatinine. II. Creatinine Desimidase. Biochim. Biophys. Acta, *30*: 154–163, 1958.

53. Tracey, M. V. Urea and Ureides. *In*; Paech, K. and Tracey, M. V. (eds.), Moderne Methoden der Pflanzen Analyse, vol. 4, pp. 119–141, Springer Verlag, Berlin, 1955.

54. Tso, T. C., Engelhaupf, M. E., and Sorokin, T. P. Chemical Changes Associated with Tobacco Frenching. Tobacco Science, *8*: 154–157, 1964.

55. Vul'fson, P. L. Nitrogenous Extractives in Fish Muscles. Biokhimiya, *26*: 300–304, 1961.

56. Wada, M. Über Citrulline, eine neue Aminosäure im Pressaft der Wassermelone, Citrullus vulgaris Schrad. Biochem. Z., *224*: 420–429, 1930.

57. Wallach, D. P., and Grisolia, S.   The Purification and Properties of Hydropyrimidine Hydrase.   J. Biol. Chem., *226*: 277–288, 1957.
58. Wehmer, C., and Hadders, M.   *In*; Kleins J. (ed.), Handbuch der Pflanzenanalyse, vol. 4, p. 222, Springer Verlag, Berlin, 1933.
59. Williams, R. T.   Detoxication Mechanisms, Second ed., Chapman & Hall Ltd., London, 1959.
60. Wynder, E. L., Kmet, J., Dungal, N., and Segi, M.   An Epidemiological Investigatino of Gastric Cancer.   Cancer, *16*: 1461–1496, 1963.

Discussion of Paper by Dr. Mirvish

DR. SUGIMURA: Could you give me any information on the carcinogenicity of nitrosocitrulline? You said that there was a great deal of it in Japanese food.

DR. MIRVISH: I have no information.

Induction of Tumors by Nitrite and Secondary Amines or Amides

Johannes SANDER, Gernot BÜRKLE, and Fritz SCHWEINSBERG

Hygiene-Institut, University of Tübingen, West Germany [J. S., F. S.]; Medizinisches Strahlen Institute, University of Tübingen, West Germany [G. B.]

In vitro experiments in our laboratory (Sander, Schweinsberg, and Menz, 1968; Sander, Bürkle, Flohe, and Aeikens, 1971) have shown that of the many organic nitrogen-containing compounds which are nitrosable under laboratory conditions, only a few readily form nitrosamines or nitrosamides under biological conditions. With secondary amines it was found that, due to a salt formation, a high basicity protected the nitrogen atom from the attack of the nitrosating agent. The lower the basicity of the secondary amine the easier it was to achieve nitrosation in diluted acid solutions. With increasing acid concentration, a higher proportion of the nitrite is converted in N_2O_3, which is the nitrosating agent under the conditions of the experiment. At the same time, however, the salt formation of the amines is enhanced. This was the reason that an optimal pH value for the nitrosation of the secondary amines was found to be about pH 3. Higher acid concentrations lowered the nitrosamine yield, as well as lower hydrogen ion concentrations.

Tertiary amines and nitrite also react under acidic conditions to form nitrosamines. For the simple aliphatic tertiary amines at 100°C the best yields are obtained at pH 3.3, as was found for the nitrosation of secondary amines. The tertiary amines however react 200 times slower than the corresponding secondary amines (Schweinsberg and Sander, 1972). Alkylamides show a very low basicity. Therefore, we did not find a pH-optimum for the nitrosation, but the yield increased with the lowering of the pH of the reaction medium.

The nitrosation products of secondary and tertiary amines are very often stable and thus can accumulate in the environment and in food. The nitroso derivatives of alkylamides, however, are often quite unstable; and therefore, are most important when they occur *in vivo* rather than in the environment. *In vivo* experiments concerning the formation of nitrosamines, as well as nitrosamides, are of interest not only because the precursors of these compounds may often be ingested by humans, but also because in the stomach an optimum pH for the nitrosation reaction is often found.

Druckrey, Steinhoff, Beuthner, Schneider, and Klaerner (1963) were the first to attempt tumor induction by concurrent application of nitrite and a secondary amine to experimental animals. These authors used diethylamine, which is strongly basic. They found no tumors, although the experiments extended over the whole life-span of the animals, including the F_1 and F_2 generations.

We repeated and extended these experiments but with amines of different basicity, and also with alkylamides of different structures (Sander and Bürkle, 1969; Sander and Bürkle, 1971; Sander, 1970, 1971a, b). Before beginning the experiments, the pH of the stomach contents of our rats and mice was measured to make sure that it was suitable for the nitrosation reaction. In the forestomach, pH values were found to be between 5.0 and 7.0. However, in the glandular part near the pylorus, the pH was between 1.5 and 2.5, which is near the nitrosation optimum.

EXPERIMENTS

Experiments with Secondary Amines of Varying Basicity

Experiments with rats

Secondary amines of low basicity (N-methylaniline and indole)—Five groups of 16 to 32 female rats were used in the experiments with N-methylaniline. The first group was an untreated control. The second group received the standard diet to which 1% of sodium nitrite was added. Group 3 received the same feed but with 0.09% of N-methylaniline in place of the nitrite. Group 4 was given the standard diet containing 1% of sodium nitrite and 0.03% of methylaniline. In the fifth group the dosage of amine was reduced to 0.015%. These diets were continued for a period of 117 days.

The combined addition of nitrite and amine to the diet exhibited a marked inhibitory effect on the growth of the young rats. Within 783 days after the end of the treatment, all the animals in Groups 4 and 5 died from tumors, most of which were located in the esophagus or the nasal cavity. These tumors were not observed in Groups 1 to 3. Histologically, the tumors of the esophagus of rats proved to be papillomas and squamous cell carcinomas. The tumors in the nasal cavity had the histologic pattern of esthesioneuroepitheliomas.

In another experiment, indole was given in a 0.5% concentration for 120 days to 6 rats. Nitrite was administered in the drinking water in a concentration of 0.5%. No tumors were observed within 2 years, probably either because no N-nitroso derivatives were formed in the stomach or because these compounds are not carcinogenic.

Secondary amines of moderate basicity (morpholine and methylbenzylamine)—Morpholine (0.5%) plus nitrite (0.5%), added to the feed for 56 days, caused the death of every one of the 8 rats within 270 days. The animals died from tumors of the liver. Focal nodular hyperplasias, adenomas derived from hepatic cells and bile duct cystadenomas were found. Some tumors had a cell arrangement in trabeculae with invasive and destructive growth. In other multinodular lesions, there was a papillary or tubular aspect or a cholangiolar type of carcinoma. A few tumors of multicentric origin showed a highly undifferentiated aspect, and even vasoformative

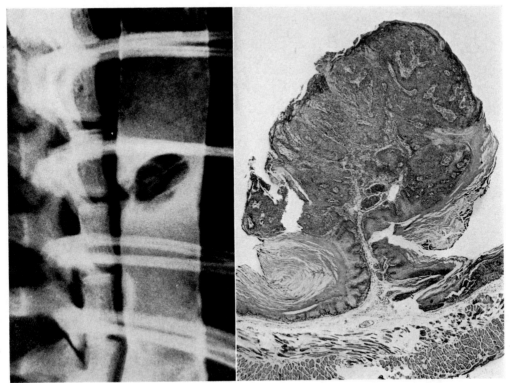

Fig. 1. Roentgen appearance of a squamous cell papilloma in the esophagus of a rat. Double contrast examination. (Tumor induction: Standard diet, containing 0.25% methylbenzylamine and 0.32% sodium nitrite, administered for 152 days. Examination was 221 days after the beginning of the experiment.) [left]

Fig. 2. Histologic section of the projecting nodular lesion, shown in Fig. 1. It is a benign tumor with a branched papillary structure without evidence of invasive growth. ×27. [right]

neoplasms with malignant endothelial lining cells with the well-known pattern of malignant haemangioendotheliomas were seen. Similar tumors have been described by other authors who applied nitrosomorpholine (Bannasch *et al.*, 1964).

In the experiments done with methylbenzylamine and nitrite, we examined not only whether tumor induction might be possible, but also what doses of this naturally occurring amine and nitrite are necessary to induce tumors when added to the diet for a limited period of time. In the first experiments groups of 8 rats, each received a diet containing 0.5% methylbenzylamine and 0.5% sodium nitrite for a period of 56 and 28 days, respectively. All animals in these groups died within 220 and 312 days, respectively, from esophageal tumors. The pathologic-anatomic examination showed several different lesions. In the esophagus of the rats, there was a formation of focal subepithelial inflammatory changes and formations to varing degrees of acanthosis, hyperkeratosis and anomalous tumor-like hyperplasias of squamous epithelium. These things were seen in association with single or, in most cases, multiple nodules. Most of them were well-differentiated papillary lesions (Figs. 1 and 2), but there were nodular tumors too, which had the macroscopic and

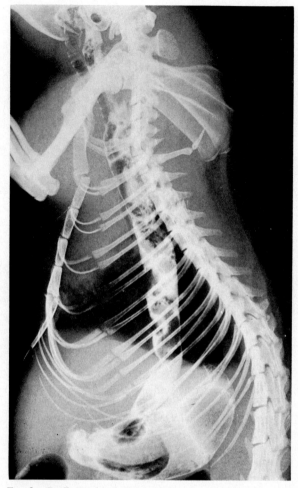

FIG. 3.   Radiographic double contrast examination of the esophagus in a rat, showing multiple filling defects.   Post mortem there were—corresponding to the roentgen finding—multiple epithelial tumors and hyperplasias.   (Tumor induction: The same as in Fig. 1.)

histologic appearance, the atypical epithelium and the invasive growth of squamous cell carcinomas (Fig. 4).

In another experiment, 8 groups of rats were treated for 152 days with a diet containing 0.25% methylbenzylamine.   The control group was given no nitrite; the 7 other groups received sodium nitrite in concentrations ranging from 0.01 to 0.32%.   In 4 of the groups receiving the diet with 0.08 to 0.32% nitrite, all of the animals died from esophageal cancer;   The length of time for death was relative to the nitrite dose;   e.g., in the 0.32% group, all 4 animals died within 100 days after the end of the application, while in the 0.08% group, all the rats died within 600 days.   In all groups in which the nitrite addition to the feed was 0.06% or less (8 rats/group), not one rat died within 28 months.   At this time the animals were killed.   No tumors of the esophagus were found.

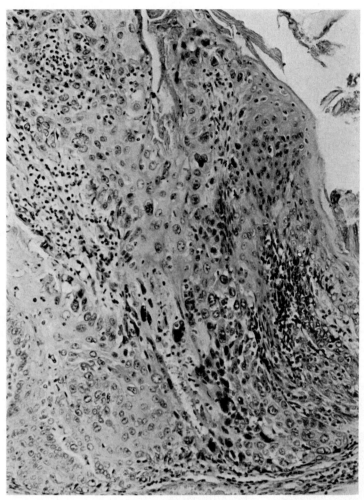

FIG. 4.   The margin of a squamous cell carcinoma in the esophagus of a rat.   At the right of the photomicrograph there is evidence of cell atypia with mitotic figures and individually keratinized cells.   At the left, the epithelium of the esophagus is well-differentiated.   × 140.

In the above-mentioned experiments, the amine and nitrite were mixed with the feed along with a sufficient amount of water to make a plastic mass.   Although the reaction was nearly neutral, a small portion of the amines could be nitrosated in the food outside the stomach.   Therefore, tumor induction in these groups was due to the combined effects of an intragastral and an extragastral nitrosamine formation.

In several of the experiments the animals were used also to work out radiological methods for an early and reliable diagnosis of tumor size and location.   These methods, which have to be applicable several times to the same animals without affecting their health, as well as be relatively simple and usable with a large test animal series, have been described elsewhere (Bürkle, 1971; Bürkle, Sander, Bürkle, and Vergau, 1971).   However, we want to include here some of the radiological pictures which directly apply to our nitrosamine research.

Secondary amines of high basicity (diethylamine, piperidine, N-methylcyclohexylamine)—
In these groups (8 rats each), 0.5% sodium nitrite and 0.5% of one of the amines were
mixed with the diet.   This mixture was fed to the rats for 76 days.   The nitroso
derivatives of all of these amines are known to be very effective carcinogens in the
rat and reveal also a strongly toxic effect.   Nitrosation, even only a small proportion, of the amines should, therefore, have been detectable not only by the induction
of tumors, but also by symptoms of toxicity.   The toxic effect on the growth of the
young rats did not exceed that found for the amount of nitrite alone.   No tumors
were induced within an observation time of 380 days in the groups receiving nitrite
and diethylamine or piperidine.   In the group treated with N-methylcyclohexylamine, a single carcinoma of the esophagus was found in one animal.   Because
tumors of the esophagus are extremely rare in untreated rats and because N-methyl-
N-nitrosocyclohexylamine is known to induce esophageal cancer, it is believed that
this tumor was due to the formation of a very low amount of this nitrosamine.

Experiments with secondary amines which are components of drugs—To one group of
5 rats a diet was fed which contained 1% folic acid for 197 days.   The drinking water
contained 1% sodium nitrite.   No tumors were observed within 2 years in this group,
as well as, in another group of 6 rats who received feed mixed with 0.3% morpholine
salicylate and drinking water with 0.5% sodium nitrite for a period of 120 days.

In a group of rats receiving a diet containing 0.5% piperazine and 0.5% sodium
nitrite, all the animals died within 3 weeks from the toxic effect of the reaction pro-

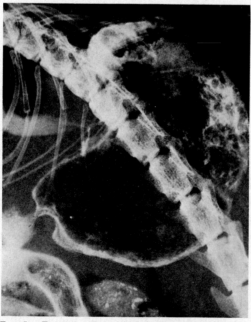

FIG. 5.   Example of a radiologic double contrast examination of the stomach of a mouse.
There are multiple tumors in the forestomach; the histologic examination revealed multicentric
papillomas.   (Tumor induction: Feed with 0.2% methylbenzylamine and 0.15% sodium
nitrite for 23 days.   Roentgen examination on the 278th day.)

duct.   No tumors were observed, of course, in this short time.   Greenblatt, Mirvish, and So (1971), however, have demonstrated that lung adenomas can be induced by feeding piperazine and nitrite concurrently to mice.

Experiments with mice

Secondary amines of moderate basicity (N-methylbenzylamine and morpholine)—Several groups of mice (10 to 60 mice/group) were fed a standard diet containing N-methyl-benzylamine and nitrite in different concentrations.   In every group which received a diet containing at least 0.1% N-methylbenzylamine and 0.15% sodium nitrite for at least 16 days, all the mice developed squamous cell carcinomas and papillomas of the forestomach (Figs. 5 and 6).   Approximately half the mice had, in addition, papillomas of the esophagus.   In the group with the lowest dose (16 days on a diet containing 0.1% N-methylbenzylamine and 0.1% sodium nitrite), only 3 mice died from carcinomas of the forestomach.   The mice in this group died from lung adenomas.   Some also had small papillomas in the forestomach.

Morpholine itself, as well as the combination of morpholine and nitrite, was more toxic to mice than to rats.   Therefore, the addition of 0.5% morpholine and 0.5% sodium nitrite to the feed had to be limited to a period of 12 days.   In the case

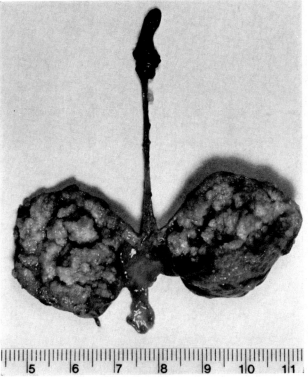

Fig. 6.   Huge tumor (squamous cell carcinoma) in the forestomach of a mouse.   The esophagus shows a benign papilloma.   (Tumor induction: The same as in Fig. 5.)

of 0.2% morpholine and 0.15% sodium nitrite, the diet could be given for 20 days. Within a year all of these mice developed multiple adenomas of the lung. But the livers were free of tumors.

Experiments with a Tertiary Amine

Because of the natural occurrence of so many tertiary amines and because there are so many drugs which are tertiary amines, we examined the effect of 0.5% triethyl-amine in the diet when applied concurrently with 0.5% sodium nitrite. We did not observe a toxic effect in a group of 6 rats, exceeding that of nitrite alone, although the dose of the amine was quite high and diethylnitrosamine, which was expected to form, is very toxic. Tumors have not yet (within a year) been induced. The results show, however, that a high proportion of the amine was not transformed into the nitrosamine. Meanwhile Lijinsky, Conrad and Van de Bogart (1971) have demonstrated *in vitro* that several drugs with similar structures as tertiary amines

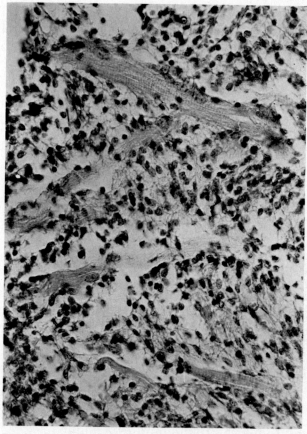

FIG. 7. Destruction of striated muscle fibers in the surroundings of a malignant neurinoma arising from the 10th intercostal nerve. (Tumor induction: 0.3% methylurea in the drinking water and 0.3% sodium nitrite in the diet. Post mortem examination 312 days after the beginning of the experiment.) ×140.

may react with nitrite to produce nitrosamines. This indicates that by using other tertiary amines a positive result might be obtained with the animal experiments. More *in vitro* and *in vivo* experiments in this direction will have to be done, especially with concentrations which correspond to the human condition.

Experiments with Alkylamides

Application of urea derivatives and nitrite

Methylurea, ethylurea, 1,3-dimethylurea or ethyleneurea have been fed to rats concurrently with nitrite. One compound was always dissolved in the drinking water, while the other was added to the diet in different concentrations, as shown in Table 1. The combined application of the ureas and nitrite in high doses proved to be highly toxic to the rats, an effect which was not found when the ureas were given without nitrite. Unless the doses of these ureas or of nitrite were low, tumors were produced in the animals. Similar to results obtained by application of the corresponding N-nitrosoureas, neoplasms of the nervous system (Fig. 7) and of the kidneys prevailed.

The tumors of the kidneys ranged from less than 1 to 30 mm in diameter. Their incidence was unbilateral and bilateral. The microscopic examination revealed tissue structures with great variability. The mean histological feature of the tumors was a scant loose connective tissue stroma which had undergone a myxomatous change in some areas. Scattered in the loose connective tissue, tubules of neoplastic

TABLE 1. Groups of Rats Treated with Alkylureas and Nitrite

Feed additive	Water additive	Animals with tumors
0.3% Methylurea	—	0/5
0.1% ,,	0.1% NaNO$_2$	0/5
0.1% ,,	0.3% ,,	0/5
0.3% ,,	0.1% ,,	3/5
0.3% ,,	0.3% ,,	5/5
0.3% NaNO$_2$	0.1% Methylurea	3/5
0.3% ,,	0.3% ,,	5/5
0.3% ,,	0.9% ,,	5/5
0.45% Ethylurea	—	0/5
0.45% ,,	0.5% NaNO$_2$	3/3
—	0.3% Dimethylurea	0/5
0.3% NaNO$_2$	—	0/5
0.3% ,,	0.1% Dimethylurea	5/5
0.3% ,,	0.3% ,,	5/5
0.1% ,,	—	—
0.1% ,,	0.05% NaNO$_2$	4/6
0.1% ,,	0.1% ,,	6/6
0.05% ,,	0.05% ,,	5/6
0.05% ,,	0.1% ,,	5/6

Duration of application, 56 days; observation period, 2 years.

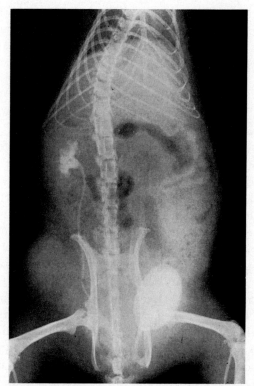

FIG. 8.   Urographic examination of a rat.   The left kidney does not show.   In the post mortem, destruction of the renal parenchyma by a nephroblastoma was found.   (Tumor induction: 0.1% ethyleneurea in the feed and 0.12% sodium nitrite in the drinking water for 150 days. Roentgen examination on the 289th day after the beginning of the experiment.)

epithelium or residual tubules, separated glomeruli (Fig. 9) and cystic spaces are present.   The tubules are often surrounded with a whorled pattern of bundles of fibroblasts (Fig. 10).   The renal neoplasms have a striking resemblance to human nephroblastoma.

It should be pointed out that in the several hundred rats used in the positive feeding experiments with secondary amines or alkylamides, cancer of the glandular stomach was never found.   Long-term experiments are now underway to determine the minimum doses of nitrite and alkylureas sufficient to induce tumors.   Within one year most animals in the groups receiving high doses of an alkylurea and nitrite died from tumors.   However, in a group of 6 rats receiving only 0.05% ethyleneurea and 0.05% sodium nitrite for 150 days, only 2 developed tumors, while not one of the 24 rats died within 1 year when the concentration of both compounds were reduced to 0.025%, although given permanently.

Other alkylamides and nitrite

Methylacetamide, glycylglycine, 6-methyluracil or methylguanidine in concentrations of 1% were added to the diet of groups with 4 rats each.   The animals received simultaneously drinking water containing 1% sodium nitrite.   This ap-

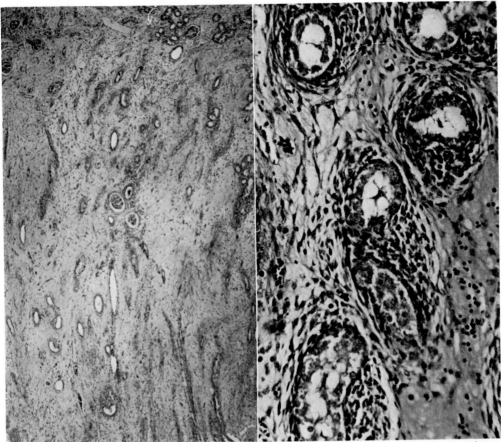

FIG. 9.   Histologic section of a nephroblastoma with loose connective tissue stroma undergoing myxomatous changes in some areas.   Throughout the tumor there are scattered tubules and glomerula.   (Tumor induction: The same as in Fig. 8.)   ×56.   [left]

FIG. 10.   Higher magnification of some tubules, separated by a scant connection tissue stroma. At the right of the photomicrograph a myxomatous area is present.   In the surroundings of tubules, there is a whorl formation of undifferentiated cells and fibroblasts.   Tumor induction: The same as in Fig. 8.)   ×140.   [right]

plication lasted from 57 days to 96 days.   No tumors were induced within one and a half years and no toxic reaction exceeding that of nitrite alone was observed. It should be pointed out, of course, that if in such experiments no tumors are produced, this does not necessarily mean that no carcinogenic nitroso compound was formed.   It can only be said that the doses were not sufficient to induce tumors within the time of the experiment.

Ethyleneurea and nitrate

Drinking water with 0.2% sodium nitrate and feed containing 0.2% ethyleneurea were given to a group of 6 rats to determine if nitrite might be formed *in vivo* resulting in a nitrosation of the amide.   No toxic reaction nor tumors have been observed in this group during the first year of the experiment.

Experiments with Thiocyanate as a Possible Catalyst

It has been known for many years that some ions (*i.e.*, SCN^-, I^-, Br^-, Cl^-) catalyze the nitrosation reaction.   Boyland, Nice and Williams (1971) pointed out that this reaction might cause an increase of nitrosamine formation *in vivo*.   We are now conducting feeding experiments to determine whether an addition of sodium thiocyanate (a widespread substance) will enhance the yield of nitroso derivatives *in vivo*.   Amines which had not induced tumors in previous experiments, as well as amines and amides which had given positive results, were used.   These experiments have been underway for only 6 months, so it is still too early to expect tumor formation.   However, an increased formation of nitrosamines or nitrosamides would have been detectable by toxic reactions.

The concentrations of sodium thiocyanate were 0.1 or 0.3% in the diet.   The development of the body weight has been compared in this experiment in groups of 6 rats each (Table 2).   No influence of the thiocyanate was detected in most groups.   Only with 0.05% N-methylaniline and 0.1% nitrite was an increased toxic effect noted in the presence of 0.3% thiocyanate.

The reason for this result is probably not that the thiocyanate is not effective as a catalyzing agent in the rat stomach.   Since the gastric juice of rats already contained a certain amount of SCN^-, a further addition of it is probably effective only in certain ranges of concentrations of the amines and nitrite.   Parallel experiments with human

TABLE 2. Development of the Body Weight—Groups of 6 Rats Each under Application of Secondary Amines, Nitrite and Thiocyanate

Feed	Body weight		
	15 days	30 days	76 days
0.5% DEA/HCl	159	185	230
0.5% DEA/HCl 0.5% NaNO$_2$	167	200	220
0.5% DEA/HCl 0.5% NaNO$_2$ 0.3% NaSCN	165	187	220
0.1% MBA 0.1% NaNO$_2$	167	188	226
0.1% MBA 0.1% NaNO$_2$ 0.3% NaSCN	160	186	234
0.05% MA	149	172	234
0.05% MA 0.1% NaNO$_2$	121	146	148
0.05% MA 0.1% NaNO$_2$ 0.3% NaSCN	112	120	117
0.05% MA 0.3% NaNO$_2$	108	108	106
0.05% MA 0.3% NaNO$_2$ 0.3% NaSCN	109	108	105
0.05% MA 0.3% NaSCN	134	170	213

DEA, Diethylamine;   MBA, N-Methlbenzylamine;   MA, N-Methylaniline.

gastric juice indicate, however, that in man an additional source of thiocyanate might well contribute to an increased formation of nitroso compounds. The thiocyanate concentration of the stomach juice was very often found to be too low to give a maximal catalysis of the nitrosation reaction. This was true for smokers as well as for nonsmokers.

CONCLUSION

The experiments showed that nitrosation of certain nitrogen containing organic compounds can take place *in vivo* and that the resulting nitrosamines or nitrosamides can be produced in sufficient amounts to induce cancer. The minimal doses of nitrite which proved to be necessary to induce tumors, when given concurrently with suitable amino compounds, were not much higher than those allowed to be used as a food additive. Furthermore, these minimal concentrations were much lower than the nitrite concentrations described by many authors for some foodstuffs in which a bacterial nitrite formation takes place. The amount of nitrite which is incorporated by man, including also the bacterial nitrite formation in the oral and nasal cavity and under pathological conditions in the stomach, the small intestine or the urine and the inhalation of nitrous gases as well as ingestion of NO_2^-, should allow a formation of nitroso compounds sufficient to induce cancer. However, we do not as yet know enough about the occurrence of nitrosable compounds. Nor do we know enough about the possible carcinogenic action of nitroso derivatives of many amines and amides which are known to be ingested as natural components of food and as drugs or as pollutants.

SUMMARY

In vivo examinations showed that from the many amines and amides which may be found in the human environment, in food, and in drugs, only a few are easily nitrosated under conditions prevailing in the human organism, especially in the stomach.

Experiments in rats and mice were done to demonstrate that tumors can be induced by feeding these amines simultaneously along with nitrite. According to the results of the *in vitro* experiments, the animals developed cancer when N-methylaniline, N-methylbenzylamine, morpholine, methylurea, ethylurea, ethyleneurea or 1,3-dimethylurea were applied. But no carcinogenesis was observed with several other amino compounds and nitrite.

REFERENCES

1. Bannasch, P., und Mueller, H. A. Lichtmikroskopische Untersuchungen über die Wirkung von N-Nitrosomorpholin auf die Leber von Ratte und Maus. Arzneim.-Forsch., *14*: 805–814, 1964.
2. Boyland, E., Nice, E., and Williams, K. The Catalysis of Nitrosation by Thiocyanate from Saliva. Food Cosmet. Toxicol., *9*: 639–643, 1971.

3. Bürkle, G.   Informationsgewinn durch Röntgendiagnostik am kleinen Laboratoriumsnagetier bei Tumorinduktions- und Therapieversuchen. Ref. Deutscher Krebskongress Hannover, 9.30–10.2, 1971. In press.

4. Bürkle, G., Sander, J., Bürkle, V., und Vergau, W.   Radiologische Untersuchungsmethoden zur Frühdiagnose und Verlaufsbeurteilung experimentell induzierter Tumoren bei Ratte und Maus. Fortschr. Röntgenstr., *114*: 698–709, 1971.

5. Druckrey, H., Steinhoff, D., Beuthner, H., Schneider, H., und Klärner, P.   Prüfung von Nitrit auf chronisch toxische Wirkung an Ratten. Arzneim.-Forsch., *13*: 320–325, 1963.

6. Greenblatt, M., Mirvish, S., and So, B. T.   Nitrosamine Studies: Induction of Lung Adenomas by Concurrent Administration of Sodium Nitrite and Secondary Amines in Swiss Mice. J. Natl. Cancer Inst., *46*: 1029–1034, 1971.

7. Sander, J.   Induktion maligner Tumoren bei Ratten durch orale Gabe von Nitrit und N, N'-Dimethylharnstoff. Arzneim.-Forsch., *20*: 418, 1970.

8. Sander, J.   Weitere Versuche zur Tumor-Induktion durch orale Applikation niederer Dosen von N-Methylbenzylamin und Nitrit. Z. Krebsforsch., *76*, 93–96, 1971a.

9. Sander, J.   Untersuchungen über die Entstehung kanzerogener Nitrosoverbindungen im Magen von Versuchstieren und ihre Bedeutung für den Menschen. Arzneim.-Forsch., In press.

10. Sander, J., und Bürkle, G.   Induktion maligner Tumoren bei Ratten durch gleichzeitige Verfütterung von Nitrit und sekundären Aminen. Z. Krebsforsch., *73*: 54–66, 1969.

11. Sander, J., und Bürkle, G.   Induktion maligner Tumoren bei Ratten durch orale Gabe von 2-Imidazolidinon und Nitrit. Z. Krebsforsch., *75*: 301–304, 1971.

12. Sander, J., Bürkle, G., Flohe, L., und Aeikens, B.   *In vitro* Untersuchungen über die Möglichkeit einer Bildung kanzerogener Nitrosamide im Magen. Arzneim.-Forsch., *21*: 411–414, 1971.

13. Sander, J., Schweinsberg, F., und Menz, H.-P.   Untersuchungen über die Entstehung kanzerogener Nitrosamine im Magen. Hoppe-Seyler's Z. Physiol. Chem., *349*: 1691–1697, 1968.

14. Schweinsberg, F., und Sander, J. Hoppe-Seyler's Z. Physiol. Chem.,.   In press.

Discussion of Paper by Drs. Sander et al.

Dr. Sugimura: In your experiment using citrulline and sodium nitrite, you obtained 2 tumors out of 8 animals.   Where were these tumor located?

Dr. Sander: One was a mammary tumor, the other was located in the leg.   Although these tumors have not yet been examined microscopically, they appeared to be malignant tumors.

Dr. Magee: What are the implications of your results for cancer in man?

Dr. Sander: In my opinion, the results of my animal experiments demonstrate that there is a very real possibility that tumor induction by ingestion of nitrite and nitrosable amino compounds might occur in man.   I think that these positive animal experiments should be considered as a warning, in spite of the fact that we do not yet know enough about the occurrence of nitrosable amino compounds in the content of the human stomach and in spite of the fact that we do need more information on the carcinogenic activity of the reaction products of amino compounds that are known to be ingested.

Dr. Weisburger: Did you see colon cancer in animals given nitrite and methylurea?   Is there any evidence of the formation of nitrosamines or nitrosamides in organs other than the stomach by bacterial action, especially at a neutral pH?

Dr. Sander: There were two cases of tumors in the small intestine, but no colon tumors appeared in any of the experiments.   Up until now there has been no evidence that bacteria in the colon might nitrosate amines or amides by forming nitrite from ingested nitrate.   In an experiment which is going on now, no tumors have developed in rats within the first year after application of 0.2% ethyleneurea and 0.2% sodium nitrate.

Dr. Nakahara: Without any intention of detracting from the merits of your experiments, I want to call attention to the well-known fact that lung adenoma and mammary tumors occur spontaneously fairly commonly in mice.   In the evaluation of long-term carcinogenesis experiments, this point should be kept in mind.

Dr. Sander: In these experiments the adenomas of the lung arose much earlier than in the control groups. It has been observed that such an early production of these tumors, which do occur normally later in the life of the animal, is caused by many carcinogens. In the experiments described here, the early induction of the adenomas was used as an indicator demonstrating the formation of the carcinogenic nitroso compound *in vivo*.

DR. MIRVISH: In answer to the question raised by Dr. Nakahara, we used the induction of lung adenomas in mice merely as an *indicator* of the formation of N-nitroso compounds. Our animal experiments agree with the idea that nitrosation occurs only as an acid-catalyzed reaction in the stomach. I do not see the need to assume that nitrosation is catalyzed by bacteria, unless convincing evidence is presented. Hill in London (personal communication) has observed nitrosation in the urinary bladder, after infection with *E. coli*, probably due to the acidic pH. So, this can be considered as an alternative site of chemical *in vivo* nitrosation.

Secondary Amines, Nitrites and Nitrosamines in Japanese Foods

Morizo Ishidate*, Akio Tanimura, Yoshio Ito, Ayako Sakai,
Hiroko Sakuta, Taro Kawamura, Keiichi Sakai,
Fumio Miyazawa, and Hiroshi Wada

National Institute of Hygienic Sciences, Tokyo, Japan

In considering the geographical distribution of cases of cancer, it seems probable that the normal daily food intake of people in a certain area may be a major etiological factor in certain types of human cancer, especially those of the digestive tract and liver.

The normal diet of Japanese people differs greatly from those of people in other countries, particularly, western countries. In Japan fish and fish products are the main source of protein. Furthermore, in Japan methods of cooking differ from those in other countries. For instance, roast fish is frequently eaten.

Thus, it is interesting and important to study the nitrosamine contents of different Japanese foods, because this class of compounds is known to be carcinogenic. It is also important to measure the amount of secondary amines and nitrites present, since these are precursors of nitrosamines both *in vivo* (9) and *in vitro*.

The procedures used for estimating these compounds were developed in the National Institute of Hygienic Sciences, Tokyo. The data shown in the following tables were compiled from results obtained in different laboratories.

Figure 1 shows details of the method used for preparation of different samples and their fractionations (3).

Figure 2 shows the two methods originally used for estimating these compounds. The first method is the nitrosation method, developed by Uno (12) and modified by Tanimura *et al.* (2). The second method is Dyer's method and our modification of it (4). Comparative studies on the two procedures showed that our modification of Uno's method was better for simultaneous estimation of nitrosamines. So, we used it in this work. Nitrosamines could be detected with a sensitivity of approximately 0.001 μmole/g, which is equivalent to 0.05 ppm.

Table 1 shows the level of secondary amines in some marine fish commonly

* Present address: Tokyo Biochemical Research Institute, Toshima-ku, Tokyo, Japan

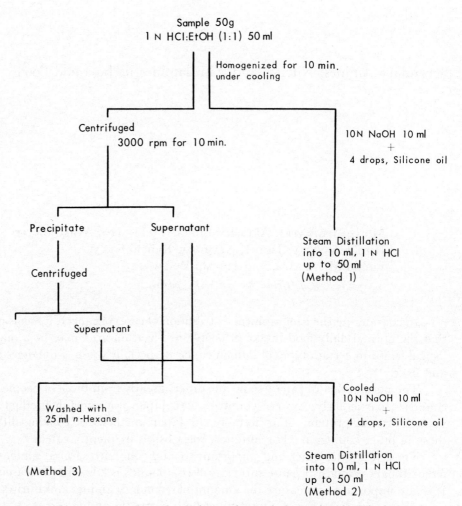

Fig. 1. Extraction procedure of secondary amines and nitrosamines from foods.

1. Modified Uno's Method

$$\underset{R_2}{\overset{R_1}{>}}NH \overset{NO_2'}{\longrightarrow} \underset{R_2}{\overset{R_1}{>}}N\text{-}NO \underset{BuOH}{\overset{HCl}{\longrightarrow}} HNO_2$$

$$\xrightarrow[C_{10}H_7\text{-}NH\text{-}CH_2CH_2\text{-}NH_3]{H_2N\text{-}C_6H_4SO_2NH_2} \text{Red Color at 552 m}\mu \text{ in BuOH}$$

2. Modified Dyer's Method

$$\underset{R_2}{\overset{R_1}{>}}NH + CS_2 + 1/2Cu^{+2} + NH_3$$

$$\longrightarrow SC\underset{NR_1R_2}{\overset{S-Cu/2}{<}} +NH_4^+ \text{ at 435 m}\mu \text{ in CHCl}_3$$

Fig. 2. Determination procedure of secondary amines in foods.

eaten in Japan, before and after roasting for 20 min.   These data show that the level of secondary amines, such as dimethylamine, usually increases during roasting.   In the mackerel pike (Sanma) and sardine, which are the most common fish eaten in Japan, the dimethylamine content increases more than tenfold during roasting.

Table 2 shows the amine content of some other fish and fish roe (6).   The amine contents of the roe are extremely high, even in the raw state.

Figure 3 shows the amine content of raw, boiled and roasted meat products. The amine content in beef, pork and chicken is relatively low, while that in mutton is high (7).

Boiling meat caused an increase in its amine content.   Pressed ham and sausage

TABLE 1.   Secondary Amines in Raw and Roasted Fishes[a] (μmole per sample(g), average of 3 samples)

Sample		Raw	Roasted[b]
Herring	(Nishin)	0.29	0.68
Mackerel pike	(Sanma)	0.07	1.23
Tuna	(Maguro)	0.12	0.15
Mackerel	(Saba)	0.05	0.54
Swordfish	(Mekajiki)	0.13	0.23
Yellowtail	(Inada)	0.06	0.35
Perch	(Suzuki)	0.01	0.12
Scorpionfish	(Menuke)	0.05	0.36
Lockington	(Hokke)	0.07	0.25
Rock trout	(Ainame)	0.12	0.32
Gurnard	(Kanagashira)	0.04	0.14
Cod	(Tara)	0.18	0.48
Plaice	(Karei)	0.02	0.50
Sardine	(Iwashi)	0.13	1.08

[a]   ( ), Calculated as dimethylamine, ppm.
      Detection limit, 0.01 μmole/g (0.5 ppm).
[b]   Roasted in toaster *ca*. 20 min and calculated the reduction of weight.

TABLE 2.   Secondary Amines in Raw and Roaated Fishes

Sample		Raw	Roasted
Shrimp	(Ebi)	0.10	—
Crab	(Kani)	0.01	0.04
Cuttlefish	(Yari-ika)	0.01	0.15
Abalone	(Awabi)	0.01	0.04
Ascidian	(Hoya)	0.07	—
Oyster	(Kaki)	0.00	0.01
Corbicula	(Shijimi)	0.01	0.01
Pollack roe	(Sukesodara-Tarako)	2.59	4.57
Cod roe	(Tarako)	3.40	3.20
Sea urchin	(Uni)	0.09	0.23
Seminal vesicle of cod	(Kiku)	0.34	—
Mackerel roe	(Saba-tamago)	0.52	—

Nitrosamines were not detected in these samples by this procedure.

both had a high amine content, possibly because they usually contain whale and/or tuna fish.   On the other hand, ham and bacon contained relatively small amounts.

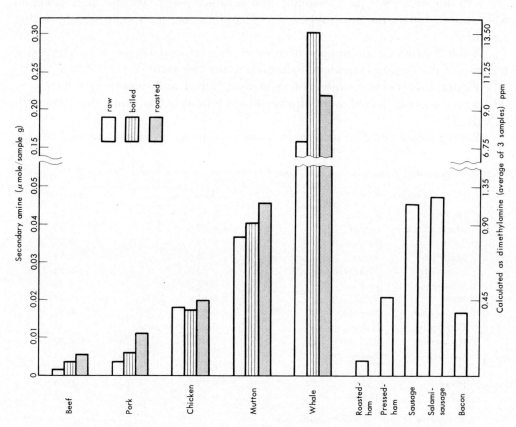

FIG. 3.   Secondary amines in raw, roasted and boiled meats and meat products.

TABLE 3.   Secondary Amines in Dried, Smoked or Canned Fishes (μmole/g)

Sample	Dried	Smoked	Canned
Sardine	0.33		
Small Sardine	0.82		
Cod	5.27		
Cuttlefish	5.27	3.45	
Flaked Bonito	3.88		
Boiled Salmon			1.06
Oiled Sardine			3.99
Oiled Tuna			0.29
Boiled Mackerel			1.25
Cuttlefish with Soy			8.19
Salted Shrimp			0.31
Crab			0.50

Calculated as dimethylamine, average 3 samples.
Detection limit: 0.01 μmole/g=0.5 ppm.

Table 3 shows the amount of secondary amines in dried, smoked or canned fish (7). It can be seen that the processing of fish, either by drying, smoke-drying or canning, results in a large increase in the amine content, *e.g.*, the drying and canning of sardines caused a five- to sevenfold increase in the amine content. This was

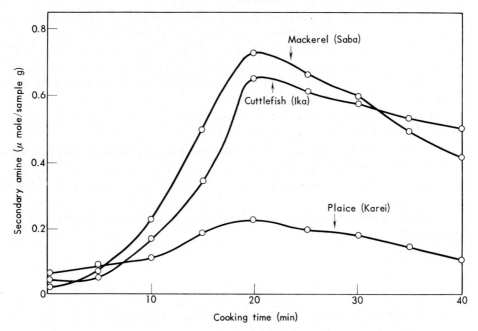

FIG. 4. Relationship between formation of secondary amines and cooking time.

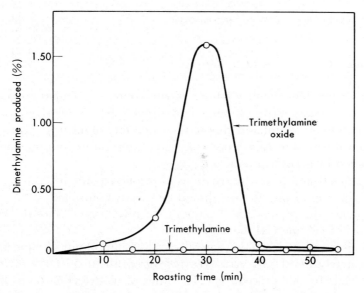

FIG. 5. Dimethylamine produced from trimethylamine and trimethylamine oxide by roasting.

especially noticeable in cuttlefish where the values increased as much as 500–700 times the value in raw cuttlefish.

Figure 4 shows the relationship between secondary amine formation and the cooking time of mackerel, cuttlefish and plaice (5). The amine content increased steadily for 20 min and then decreased gradually.

Similar results were obtained with roasting. It was also found that the secondary amine content of fish increased to a higher level than that of meat with roasting. Fish are known to contain trimethylamine (TMA), trimethylamine oxide (TMAO), choline and betaine, along with dimethylamine (DMA). Therefore, experiments were made to see whether the DMA could be produced from these four amines by roasting.

TMAO was found to be the only one of the four amines that was converted to DMA, and its conversion rate was only 1.58% (5).

In 1960, Miyahara reported that dried cuttlefish, sardines and mackerel contained 2,000, 1,900 ppm of TMAO (8).

Figure 5 shows the relationship between the conversion rate of TMAO and the roasting time.

Table 4 shows the nitrite contents in various kinds of food measured in our laboratory (1).

TABLE 4.   Nitrite Content in Foods (ppm)

1.	Vegetables:	Most of samples	1.0
		Exception: Lettuce, boiled corn and beans	(5.0)
2.	Pickled vegetables:	Salted cucumber	9.0
		Juice	96.0
		Leaf mustard	3.9
3.	Cereals:	Wheat flour	3.8
		Flour	10.0
		Macaroni, noodle flour, soy-bean flour	10.0–15.0
4.	Meat products:	Wiener sausage (white)	12–18
		(red)	64–80
		Fish sausage	18–24
		Press ham	14–29
5.	Dried fishes:	Small sardine	8–30

Preserving vegetables increased their nitrite content. Similar increases were also observed in cereals, meat products and dried fish. A relatively low nitrite content in certain foods is probably due to the instability of nitrites. However, it is well known that nitrite is readily produced in situ from nitrate and that the latter is widely distributed in natural products.

From these facts and from the reactions of secondary amines, it is felt that the addition of nitrite and nitrate to food should be strictly controlled.

Table 5 shows the presence and amounts of nitrosamine (mostly DMNA) in about 150 kinds of commercial foods (10).

The method for microdetermination of trace amounts of nitrosamine in food has not been adequately developed yet. We recovered about 50–60% of the added DMNA from foods by our procedure. The limit of its detection on a TLC plate with ninhydrin was 0.2 μg.

TABLE 5. Nitrosamine in Commercial Foods

Foods	Number of samples	Number of samples contanining nitrosamine	Kind of nitrosamine
Fish sausage	10	0	
Pork sausage	10	0	
Salami sausage	3	0	
Wiener sausage	20	0	
Frankfurter sausage	3	0	
Bologna sausage	3	0	
Pressed ham	*20*	*6*	DM[b]
Boneless ham	3	0	
Roasted ham	3	0	
Bacon	3	0	
Corned beef	3	0	
Hamburger	*3*	*1*	DM
Dried Mackerel pike	*3*	*1*	
Salted salmon roe	*20*	*7*	DM (trace)
Salted cod roe	20	0	DE (trace)
Nitrite added cod roe[a]	*3*	*3*	DM, DE
Smoked cod	3	0	
Smoked salmon	3	0	
Smoked herring	3	0	
Dried small sardine	10	0	
Mushroom	3	0	

a) Treated with 1% sodium nitrite solution for 24 hr.

b) DM, dimethylnitrosamine; DE, diethylnitrosamine.

DMNA was detected in 6 out of 20 samples of pressed ham containing pork, whale and/or tuna fish. DMNA and DENA were detected in 7 out of 20 samples of salted salmon roe, in which nitrite was used as a color fixative, though there was only a trace amount of nitrosamine.

The amount of DMNA in the pressed ham was estimated as approximately 15–25 ppb. No nitrosamine was detected in salted cod roe, purchased in markets. But when treated with nitrite, the roe showed over 1 ppm, *i.e.*, 40 times more DMNA, including DENA.

In 1967, Terracini *et al.* (*11*) reported that a diet containing 2 ppm DMNA produced hepatomas in 1 out of 26 rats; and a diet 5 ppm produced 8 hepatomas out of 74 rats. Let us assume tentatively that the dose of 2 ppm is the minimal carcinogenic dose in rats and one-tenth of this dose is the maximal noncarcinogenic dose possible. The actual amount of DMNA in a 20 g diet of this maximal noncarcinogenic dose may be estimated as 40 μg per rat. This is equivalent to 16 μg per kg wt., assuming the weight of the rat to be 1/4 kg. Then if a safety factor of 100 is taken into account, the estimated safe daily dose for a man is about 8 μg per 50 kg body wt.

The highest content of DMNA in the food, obtained so far, was estimated as 0.025 μg/g in pressed ham. Therefore, the threshold value will be reached upon taking 320 g of this food (see Table 6).

This is an amount which is far from hazardous, but the possibility should not be

TABLE 6.   Discussion on the Carcinogenicity of DMNA

1)	Minimum carcinogenic dose/day (Terracini, Magee, and Barnes, Brit. J. Cancer, *31*: 559, 1967)		2 ppm/rat
	2 ppm : 1/26, Rat hepatoma		0.04 mg/rat
	5 ppm : 8/74		(as 20g-food)
	10 ppm : 2/5		
	20 ppm : 15/23		*0.16* mg/kg
2)	Maximum non-carcinogenic dose		($\times 1/10$)
			16 μg/kg
3)	Safe daily dose		($\times 1/100$)
			8 μg/*50*kg
4)	Maximum content of DMNA in foods		*0.025* μg/g
5)	3)/4) : 8 μg/0.025		*320* (g)

overlooked that further nitrosamine may be produced *in vivo* from secondary amines and nitrite, under certain conditions.

The relationship between the high incidence of cancer of the digestive tract and liver in Japan and the daily food intake requires further investigation.

REFERENCES

1. Harada, M., Nakamura, Y., and Tanimura, A.   Studies on Nitrosamines in Foods. IX.   Nitrite Contents in Japanese Foods.   J. Food Hyg. Soc. Japan, In press.
2. Ito, Y., Sakuta, H., Takada, H., and Tanimura, A.   Studies on Nitrosamines in Foods.   VI.   Comparison of Two Extraction and Determination Methods of Secondary Amines.   J. Food Hyg. Soc. Japan, *12*: 399–403, 1971.
3. Ito, Y., Sakuta, H., Takada, H., and Tanimura, A.   Studies on Nitrosamines in Foods.   VII.   Increment of Secondary Amines in Foods by Cooking or Processing. J. Food Hyg. Soc. Japan, *12*: 404–407, 1971.
4. Ito, Y., Sakuta, H., Yokota, S., Ayukawa, I., and Tanimura, A.   Studies on Nitrosamines in Foods.   III.   Extraction and Identification of Secondary Amines in Foods.   J. Food Hyg. Soc. Japan, *12*: 185–191, 1971.
5. Ito, Y., and Tanimura, A.   Studies on Nitrosamines in Foods.   II.   Colorimetric Determination of Secondary Amines and Nitrosamines.   J. Food Hyg. Soc. Japan, *12*: 177–184, 1971.
6. Kawamura, T., Sakai, K., Miyazawa, F., Wada, H., Ito, Y., and Tanimura, A. Studies on Nitrosamines in Foods.   IV.   Distribution of Secondary Amines in Foods. J. Food Hyg. Soc. Japan, *12*: 192–197, 1971.
7. Kawamura, T., Sakai, K., Miyazawa, F., Wada, H., Ito, Y., and Tanimura, A. Studies on Nitrosamines in Foods.   V.   Distribution of Secondary Amines in Foods. J. Food Hyg. Soc. Japan, *12*: 394–398, 1971.
8. Miyahara, S.   Isolation and Determination of Methylamines by Chromatography. J. Chem. Soc. Japan, *81*: 1158–1163, 1960.
9. Sakai, A., and Tanimura, A.   Studies on Nitrosamines in Foods.   *In vitro* and *in vivo* Formation of Dimethylnitrosamine.   J. Food Hyg. Soc. Japan, *12*: 170–176, 1971.

10. Sakai, A, and Tanimura, A.   Studies on Nitrosamines in Foods.   VIII.   Nitros-
    amines Detected in Foods.   J. Food Hyg. Soc. Japan, *12*: 485–488, 1971.
11. Terracini, B., Magee, P. N., and Barnes, J. M.   Hepatic Pathology in Rats on
    Low Dietary Levels of Dimethylnitrosamine.   Brit. J. Cancer, *21*: 559–570, 1967.
12. Uno, T., and Yamamoto, M.   Colorimetric Determination of Secondary Amines.
    Japan Analyst, *15*: 958–961, 1966.

Discussion of Paper by Drs. Ishidate et al.

DR. SAITO: Could you tell me how many ppm of secondary amine were detected in the experimental animal diet? In a typical experimental animal diet, about 15% fish meal is added. Therefore, my question is partly related to Dr. Sander's presentation.

DR. ISHIDATE: We have not yet tested the animal diet, but we intend to do it in the near future.

DR. MIRVISH: Did you ever detect any secondary amines other than dimethylamine and diethylamine in the food?

DR. ISHIDATE: We have never detected any other secondary amines besides dimethyl- and diethylamine, although our procedure is capable of finding even a trace (0.05 ppm) of an amine, such as pipyridine or methylphenylamine.

DR. PREUSSMANN: Which method do you use for nitrite determination?
Is the addition of nitrite and nitrate to food allowed in Japan; and if so, how much is allowed and in what commodities is it allowed?

DR. ISHIDATE: For nitrite determination, we used the modified Griess reaction.
Since last year the addition of nitrite to food has been strictly controlled. I am not certain how much is allowed, but perhaps about 200 ppm in fish roe and a residual amount in fish meal.

DR. HIGGINSON: This time-consuming and difficult analytical work on diets in man is most valuable, because it provides the only basis on which a sound correlation of epidemiological studies can be developed, in attempting to access the significance of secondary amines and nitrites in man.

DR. MAGEE: With regard to your last slide, I think that it is rather unwise to place too much reliance on the results obtained by Terracini, Barnes and myself. Our figure for the minimum carcinogenic level of dimethylnitrosamine was 2 ppm, but this was based on only 26 rats. If more animals had been used, it is possible that tumors might have been observed at lower levels. Unfortunately, we do not have much information on dose-response relationships at low levels of chemical carcinogens.

DR. ISHIDATE: Thank you for your comments, Dr. Higginson and Dr. Magee.

Problems and Recent Results in the Analytical Determination of N-Nitroso Compounds

R. PREUSSMANN and G. EISENBRAND

The German Cancer Research Center, Institute of Experimental Toxicology and Chemotherapy, Heidelberg, West Germany

The potent biological effects of a large number of organic N-nitroso compounds (nitrosamines and nitrosamides) include carcinogenicity, mutagenicity, teratogenicity and embryotoxicity among other acute and subchronic toxic effects. The occurrence of such compounds in the human environment has therefore caused rising concern in recent years. In view of the pronounced carcinogenic effects of such compounds, even low or very low quantities of environmental N-nitroso compounds must be considered a potential human health risk. The determination of the degree of human exposure, therefore, is of paramount importance in the field of nitrosamine research.

For the evaluation of the significance of an exposure to nitrosamines as a carcinogenic hazard, adequate analytical methods for the detection and determination of N-nitroso compounds are necessary. Such methods must be extremely sensitive, must give unequivocal and reproducible results and must cover a wide range of N-nitroso compounds, often with very different physico-chemical and stability properties. The usual criteria for analytical methods must be fulfilled, namely, specificity, sensitivity, accuracy and reproducibility.

Many of the methods used for nitrosamine analysis until recently did not fulfill such necessary requirements. Although the results obtained with such methods are not meaningless, it is clear that they must be repeated and confirmed (if possible) with improved methodology.

Much progress has been made in the last few years in the improvement of nitrosamine analysis. A summary will be given in this paper. The contributions of our own group will be given with more detail.

N-Nitroso Compounds as a Human Health Hazard

In the absence of direct and conclusive evidence about the activity of a chemical carcinogen in man, the question always arises whether animal experiments are relevant and whether such experimental evidence can be extrapolated to man. At the present moment we have no direct evidence of the carcinogenicity of an N-nitroso compound in man.   No long-term studies on exposed humans have been reported until now.

On the other hand, however, a very large number of experimental studies on chemical, biochemical, biological and toxicological properties with special emphasis on carcinogenic effects are available.   Summaries of this work have been published (Druckrey *et al.*, 1967; Magee and Barnes, 1967; Magee, 1971).   Almost 100 different compounds of this group have been tested up until now.   The great majority of them have shown more or less potent carcinogenic activity in animal experiments.

For example, dimethylnitrosamine has been investigated for carcinogenic activity in 6 animal species: mouse, hamster, rat, guinea pig, rabbit and rainbow trout.   In all these different species, the compound is a potent carcinogen.

The next higher homologue, diethylnitrosamine, has been even more extensively studied.   It has been shown to be a carcinogen in 12 animal species, including sub-human primates.   The 12 species are mouse, hamster, rat, guinea pig, rabbit, dog, pig, rainbow trout, the aquarium fish, Branchydanio rerio, grass parakeet and monkey.   So far no animal species tested has been found to be resistant to the carcinogenicity of this compound.

Methylnitrosourea, as an example of a nitrosamide, has been tested in mouse, hamster, rat, guinea pig, rabbit and dog.   It is a powerful carcinogen in all these animals.

Many of the other N-nitroso carcinogens have not been studied as extensively, but for almost all of them reliable and reproducible animal data are available.

There are further data which are relevant to the problem of extrapolation of animal data to man.   Since nitrosamines most likely require enzymatic activation to form the proximate and/or ultimate carcinogen (an alkylating agent ?), comparative metabolism in animal and man can give further evidence to facilitate the discussed extrapolation of animal data to man.   Montesano and Magee (1970) in a comparative *in vitro* study with dimethylnitrosamine showed that this compound is metabolized in a qualitatively similar manner in both human and rat liver.   Quantitatively, it was shown that the rate of metabolism in human liver slices was comparable to that in rat liver and that similar levels of nucleic acid methylation occur in both species.

Last, but not least, there is one direct observation in man, though not in regard to carcinogenicity.   Dimethylnitrosamine has induced acute toxic liver damage in exposed persons working with this compound in the chemical industry (Barnes and Magee, 1954).   Centrilobular necrosis is similarily produced in most animal species treated with high doses of nitrosamines in acute toxicity experiments.

All relevant data have been collected by a " Working Group on the Evaluation of Carcinogenic Risk of Chemicals to Man " under the auspices of the International Agency for Research on Cancer, Lyon, and will be published, complete with an extensive bibliography, in the near future.

Summarizing the presented evidence, it is clear that N-nitroso compounds act as carcinogens in many animal species, including subhuman primates.   Until now no animal species has been found to be resistant to the carcinogenic effect, as far as the most important representatives of this group of compounds are concerned.   The metabolism as well as the acute toxic effects are similar or identical in man and experimental animals.   Taking all facts into consideration, one can conclude that man will probably react in a manner similar to the experimental animals and that, therefore, *N-nitroso compounds are almost certainly carcinogenic in man.*   The opinion of Lijinsky and Epstein (1970) that nitrosamines and nitrosamides " seem to be a major class of carcinogens that are likely to be causally related to human cancer " is shared by many now.   The widespread concern about carcinogenic nitrosamines in the human environment is, therefore, justified.

A more difficult problem is what are the levels of nitrosamines which should be considered as dangerous to man.   This problem is closely related to the necessary sensitivity and detection limits of analytical methods and, therefore, is very important in the context of this paper.   In general, there is agreement that for carcinogens only a " zero tolerance " can be accepted in principle.   However, it is well-known that this concept is not always feasible in general practice.   Moreover, from the analytical point of view, " zero " is always a matter of analytical methodology, which is not a constant.   Therefore, a rough estimation of " no-effect " doses from animal experiments is necessary.

There is one dose-response study available for dimethylnitrosamine in the rat (Terracini *et al.*, 1967).   Dietary concentrations ranged between 2 and 50 ppm. At 2 and 5 ppm, incidences of liver tumors among survivors at 60 weeks were, respectively, 1/26 and 8/74.   Higher concentrations produced incidences where more than 70% of the rats had liver tumors.   Therefore, for continuous feeding studies, a concentration of 1 ppm in the diet could be considered a " threshold dose."   Single doses of 20 mg/kg body wt. are carcinogenic in the rat (Magee and Barnes, 1959).

A dose-response study, involving oral administration of diethylnitrosamine in the rat, was performed by Druckrey *et al.* (1963).   Daily doses ranged between 14.2 and 0.075 mg/kg in 9 dosage groups.   Total doses administered until death were between 65 and 64 mg/kg.   All doses higher than 0.15 mg/kg/day gave a tumor yield of 100%.   Doses of 0.15 mg/kg/day gave a tumor incidence of 27/30 liver carcinomas.   At 0.075 mg/kg/day, 20 rats lived longer than 600 days; 11/20 had benign or malignant tumors of the liver, the esophagus and/or hepatomas.   All 4 of the animals living longer than 940 days at this dose level had tumors.   Therefore, 0.075 mg/kg/day diethylnitrosamine, which corresponds approximately to 0.5–0.75 ppm in the diet, is clearly carcinogenic and above the " threshold concentration." The marginal effect dose could be estimated to be at 0.5 ppm.

It is a generally accepted international practice in establishing tolerated doses that a safety margin of 100 should be observed when extrapolating animal data to man.   *Therefore, a level of 5–10 ppb ($\mu g/kg$) should be considered as a " tolerable " dose of low-molecular weight nitrosamines.*   This is also logically *the concentration that must be detected and determined in a chemical analysis of such N-nitroso compounds in environmental media.*   This detection limit is generally accepted now.

It must be stressed, however, that such " calculations " are rather unsatisfactory and can by no means lead to " safe " levels of nitrosamines.   For one, it is well known that single-dose experiments with N-nitroso compounds have led to malignant tumors in animals.   Unfortunately, no dose-response studies for such experiments are available.   On the other hand, many experiments, especially those by Schmähl and his colleagues (1970) and Montesano and Saffiotti (1968), have shown that sub-threshold doses of diethylnitrosamine still give rise to tumors when administered to-gether with other carcinogens.   This synergistic, additive effect of different groups of chemicals with the same organotropic carcinogenic effect (syncarcinogenesis) clearly is similar to the human situation, where a population almost certainly is never ex-posed to only one single carcinogen, but to minute quantities of many different carcinogenic compounds.

Analytical Methods for N-Nitroso Compounds

Older methods

There are several analytical methods which give good results with pure com-pounds or in simple mixtures (*e.g.*, urine), but give equivocal or no results when ap-plied to complicated mixtures (*e.g.*, tobacco smoke condensate, most extracts from foodstuffs).   The following principles for the detection and determination of organic N-nitroso compounds have been used.

Photochemical splitting of the N-nitroso bond—Upon exposure to ultraviolet or visible light, nitrosamines in *neutral* aqueous or alcoholic solutions are split to form nitrite and secondary amines (Preussmann, 1964).   This method has been utilized for *staining methods on thin-layer chromatograms* (Preussmann *et al.*, 1964).   A good separation of nitrosamines can be obtained using silica gel plates and solvent mix-tures containing hexane/ether/dichloromethane.   The *Rf*-values of many nitros-amines are known.   Two spray reagents are used for the detection of N-nitroso compounds after irradiation of the plates with UV light:

1)   diphenylamine-palladium chloride, yielding blue to violet spots, and
2)   sulphanilic acid-1-naphthylamine, resulting in red to violet and/or green spots.

The detection of the secondary amine, formed after UV-splitting, is also possible on a plate with ninhydrin, resulting in blue spots (Kröller, 1967).

Specificity ranges of the reagents overlap in such a manner that positive results with at least two or all three reagents can be considered as selective for N-nitroso compounds.   However, it is known that false positive results can be obtained with certain compounds without N-nitroso structure (Preussmann *et al.*, 1964).   The lower detection limit, which is also affected by impurities, is 0.5 μg nitroso compound per spot.   In the analysis of complicated mixtures, adequate and extensive purification is a prerequisite before tentative characterisation by *Rf*-values is possible.

Under strictly controlled conditions, *quantitative colorimetric* determination of N-nitroso compounds in aqueous or methanolic solutions is possible (Daiber and Preussmann, 1964).   Nitrite formed after short-wave UV irradiation is quantitatively determined by the Griess reaction forming an azo dye.   The lower detection limit is 1 μg nitroso compound/ml.   The reaction is highly dependent on experimental conditions and, therefore, cannot be used in complicated mixtures (see Möhler and Mayrhofer, 1968).   The use of long-wave UV light, as suggested by Sander (1967), eliminates some of the difficulties.   But nitrite yields are only in the range of 30%, thus resulting in decreased sensitivity.   Adequate control experiments are always necessary for the reaction conditions used.

Polarography—N-Nitroso compounds can be determined quantitatively by polarographic reduction.   Nitrosamines (Heath and Jarvis, 1953; Lydersen and Nagy, 1967) as well as nitrosamides (Garrett and Cusimano, 1966; Schaper, 1970) can be estimated.   The method is sensitive (lower detection limit: appr. 0.25 μg/ml) and reliable.   It is excellent for the analysis of pure compounds or simple mixtures. The method however is not specific, and the results are difficult to evaluate in more complicated mixtures.   Pyrazines, for example, have been shown to have very similar polarographic (and gas chromatographic) behavior in comparison with nitrosamines (Kadar and Devik, 1970; Heyns and Koch, 1971).   To increase the reliability of results, differential polarography has been used, measuring with and without photolysis at an acid and neutral pH (Walters *et al.*, 1970).

Reduction and derivative formation of nitrosamines—Identification of nitrosamines by derivative formation has been carried out by reducing them to the corresponding asymmetric hydrazine with lithium alanate (Neurath *et al.*, 1964) or with Zn–HCl (Ender and Ceh, 1971).   The formation of characteristic hydrazones with 5-nitro-2-hydroxybenzaldehyde has been used (Neurath *et al.*, 1964).   Ender and co-workers estimate the formed hydrazine by colorimetry after it reacts with *p*-dimethyl-amino-benzaldehyde (Ender and Ceh, 1971).   The main disadvantage of the reduction method lies in the low and poorly reproducible yields of the hydrazine (Eisenbrand, 1970).

The main disadvantage of the methods discussed in this section is that they are not specific when applied to more or less complex mixtures and that results obtained with them are therefore questionable.   At this stage, the need for adequate and reproducible separation and isolation methods as well as highly specific methods for positive end determination of N-nitroso compounds was evident.

Recent analytical developments

With growing experience in the field of trace analysis of N-nitroso compounds, it became apparent that the problem must be considered from various aspects.   On the one hand, a subdivision of N-nitroso compounds into three different groups was necessary:

    a)   (steam)-volatile nitrosamines, comprising the low molecular weight dialkylnitrosamines and heterocyclic nitrosamines

    b)   nonvolatile nitrosamines, mainly alkyl nitrosamines, containing hydrophilic functional groups and

    c)   nitrosamides.

On the other hand, it also became quickly apparent that within the group of volatile nitrosamines, the analytical procedure had to be divided into at least two parts:

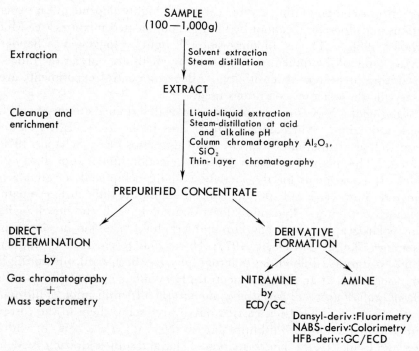

Fig. 1.   Flow sheet diagram for analysis of volatile nitrosamines.

a)   extraction, purification (cleanup) and enrichment and
b)   end determination by different methods.

Remarkable progress has been made in the last two to three years in the trace analysis of volatile nitrosamines at the 5–10 ppb level.   Adequate and reliable methods, though highly sophisticated, expensive and time-consuming, are available now.

Volatile nitrosamines—This group includes the most important nitrosamine carcinogens like dimethyl- and diethylnitrosamine, and cyclic representatives, such as nitrosopyrrolidine and nitrosopiperidine.   In Fig. 1 a flow sheet diagram is given with some details of the procedure as suggested by us.

Extraction, cleanup and enrichment: For *separation* from the product, mainly steam distillation from alkali or acid, or continuous solvent extraction, usually with dichloromethane, have been used by most authors working in the field (Ender and Ceh, 1967; Sen *et al.*, 1970; Eisenbrand *et al.*, 1970 a; Foreman *et al.*, 1969; Heyns and Koch, 1971; Kröller, 1967).   An interesting alternative has been suggested recently by Nunn and du Plessis (1971).   The sample is freeze-dried under strictly standardized conditions, and the distillate containing volatile nitrosamines is collected.   Reasonable to good recoveries have been obtained.   Another valuable method seems to be the digestion of the sample by refluxing with alcoholic KOH and subsequent steam distillation (Howard *et al.*, 1970).

Extraction methods with water (Ender and Ceh, 1967) and fractional distillation from aqueous methanol, containing 5% NaCl, and collecting a nitrosamine containing fraction appearing between the methanol and water fractions (Walters *et al.*, 1970) have a more limited applicability. Until now no recovery studies of nitrosamines present in an original sample are available. Therefore, the effectiveness of extraction methods cannot be estimated at the present moment. Further work is necessary in this regard. Recovery data, however, are available for nitrosamines added to samples.

For purification and cleanup, many different methods have been used. Our own group investigated several possible techniques with the aim of developing generally applicable methods in which a wide range of different nitrosamines were to be covered. In all such experiments particular attention must be paid to high recoveries, especially of the highly volatile lower nitrosamines (*e.g.*, dimethyl-, methylvinyl-nitrosamine). We investigated the following separation techniques.

Liquid-liquid partition between acetonitrile/n-heptane (Eisenbrand *et al.*, 1969). This solvent pair proved to be a valuable system for the enrichment of nitrosamines in the acetonitrile phase and for separating them from interfering lipophilic contaminants. Partition coefficients ($K_D = C_{acetonitrile}/C_{n-heptane}$) for several nitrosamines have been determined and are shown in Table 1. After three repeated distribution, 95% of all

TABLE 1. Distribution Coefficients K_D ($C_{acetonitrile}/C_{heptane}$) of Different N-Nitroso Compounds and Partition between Acetonitrile and *n*-Heptane

Nitrosamine	K_D	Nitrosamine	K_D
Dimethyl-	17.3	Methyl-2–hydroxyl-	32.0
Diethyl-	8.4	N-NO-morpholine	23.9
Di-*n*-pentyl-	2.6	N-NO-piperidine	8.8
Dicyclohexyl-	2.1	N-NO-pyrrolidine	17.3
Di-*n*-octyl-	0.5	N-NO-trimethylurea	19.6
Methylpentyl-	8.3		

nitrosamines are found in the acetonitrile phase with the exception of the highly lipophilic di-*n*-octylnitrosamine, which requires five extractions for quantitative transfer to the acetonitrile phase. This purification is to be recommended when material with high lipid contents is to be analyzed.

Steam distillation at alkaline, acid or neutral pH at reduced and atmospheric pressure (Eisenbrand *et al.*, 1970a). Since steam distillation is used in practically all steps of extraction and cleanup, a systematic study of recoveries under various experimental conditions was undertaken, using 16 different nitrosamines. The results, as shown in Table 2, demonstrate that this method, in fact, provides a very useful cleanup step. Dialkylnitrosamines up to a total of 12 carbon atoms (dihexylnitrosamine) for distillation *in vacuo* (12 mm) and up to a total of 16 carbon atoms (dioctylnitrosamine) for distillation at atmospheric pressure are recovered in the distillate with almost quantitative yields. The distillation from an 0.2 N acid medium does not result in any hydrolysis of nitrosamines and provides an effective separation from basic contaminants. Steam distillation at an acid pH should always be preceded by distillation from an alkaline medium to remove nitrosating agents possibly present in the sample. Such a contamination might lead to nitrosamine artifacts at distillation

TABLE 2.   Recoveries (%) of Heterocyclic, Dialkaryl-, and Alkaryl-N-nitrosamines by Distillation from Neutral, Alkaline and Acid Media

| Nitrosamine | Medium: | Water | | 0.2 N NaOH | | 0.2 N Tartaric acid | |
	Pressure:	Reduced	Atmosph.	Reduced	Atmosph.	Reduced	Atmosph.
I Di-methyl-nitrosamine		94	101	94	98	98	101
II Di-ethyl-		101	98	101	99	100	97
III Di-n-propyl-		98	96	99	98	100	97
IV Di-iso-propyl-		100	100	99	100	99	98
V Di-n-butyl-		100	96	100	98	100	100
VI Di-n-pentyl-		100	99	100	100	100	100
VII Di-n-hexyl-		98	99	100	100	96	99
VIII Di-n-octyl-		45	93	43	95	30	93
IX Methyl-vinyl-		94	90	89	89	88	78
X Methyl-n-butyl-		100	96	99	96	100	99
XI Methyl-n-pentyl-		99	96	101	96	100	97
XII Methyl-n-heptyl-		98	97	99	98	99	97
XIII Methyl-benzyl-		96	94	98	96	94	92
XIV N-Nitrosopyrrolidine		89	71	100	85	67	71
XV N-Nitrosopiperidine		98	97	100	99	97	98
XVI Methyl-2-hydroxyethyl-nitrosamine		29	29	27	14	16	—

from an acid pH.   As can be seen from Table 2, nitrosopyrrolidine reacts atypically. Distillation at reduced pressure is less destructive than distillation at atmospheric pressure.   This may be true also for other nitrosamines not investigated in this study.

Quantitative thin-layer chromatography as a cleanup method (Eisenbrand *et al.*, 1970b). As a further purification step, quantitative thin-layer chromatography (TLC) was investigated.   Preliminary experiments showed that losses of 50–100% for highly volatile nitrosamines occurred when working with conventional TLC conditions. Investigations of the reasons for such losses showed that the solvent used for spotting on the plate must have a low boiling point and be absolutely free of water; conditions for TLC also had an important influence.   Reproducible recoveries of better than 90%, even for highly volatile nitrosamines, can be obtained if the following conditions are maintained: 1) Dichloromethane is a suitable solvent for extraction of nitrosamines from aqueous solutions.   It is also suitable for spotting on the plate if well dried.   2) Evaporation of high solvent volumina should be done in a Kuderna-Danish evaporator to avoid losses by volatility.   3) TLC separation should be effected in the dark and at a temperature of 4°C. SiO_2-gel layers should have a thickness of not less than 0.6 mm.   4) Separated nitrosamines from a scratched-off solvent can be quantitatively removed by steamdistillation.

Column chromatography: Alumina columns adsorb nitrosamines quantitatively from unpolar solvents such as hexane.   Elution can be effected by using water and aqueous methanol (Eisenbrand, 1970).   Very good separations of nitrosamines have been obtained with Sephadex LH-20, eluting with methanol-water (50: 50). An elution chromatogram is shown in Fig. 2.   This method, however, is easily disturbed by certain impurities in a sample (Eisenbrand *et al.*, 1970c).

Other purification methods, used by various groups, include acid ion exchange (Foreman *et al.*, 1969), Acid-Celite 545 (Howard *et al.*, 1970), and polyamide ion

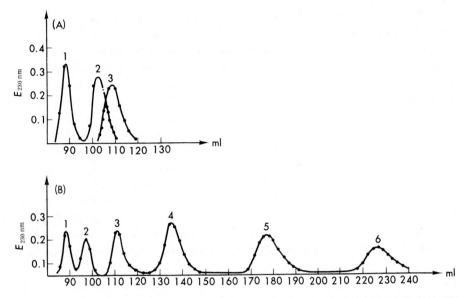

FIG. 2. Gel chromatography on Sephadex LH-20. Column, Sephadex LH-20, 100×100 mm; eluent, methanol-water (1: 1), 4.3 ml/h; sample volume, 0.5 ml. (A) $1 \doteq 19.4$ μg methylethylnitrosamine, $2 \doteq 26.4$ μg methylbutylnitrosamine, $3 \doteq 25.3$ μg methylpentylnitrosamine. (B) $1 \doteq 10.5$ μg dimethylnitrosamine, $2 \doteq 14$ μg diethylnitrosamine, $3 \doteq 21.5$ μg di-n-propylnitrosamine, $4 \doteq 50$ μg di-n-butylnitrosamine, $5 \doteq 74$ μg di-n-pentylnitrosamine, $6 \doteq 52$ μg di-n-hexylnitrosamine.

exchange (Sen *et al.*, 1970) chromatography, mainly to remove basic impurities. Nitrosamines are easily adsorbed from aqeuous distillates on charcoal. This would be an excellent cleanup method, if desorption gave better recoveries. Desorption has been tried with boiling methanol (Walters *et al.*, 1970) and by steam-distillation (Ender and Ceh, 1967).

Gas liquid chromatography (GLC): Gas liquid chromatography is now almost invariably used as a final method of separation and purification before end determination of nitrosamines. A great number of different columns have been used (for a survey, see Wasserman, 1971). The use of capillary columns has been recommended by Heyns and Röper (1971). Flame ionization, as well as thermal conductivity detectors, has been used for unspecific detection. A recent development has led to the use of more selective detector systems: Howard *et al.* (1970) use alkali flame ionization with a potassium chloride salt tip and Fiddler *et al.* (1971) use it with a rubidium sulfate salt tip as nitrogen-selective indicator systems. In the absence of amines, the Coulson detector can be used as an almost specific nitrosamine detector system. The nitrosamine is pyrolyzed to NH_3 and measured by conductimetry. The sensitivity is in the nanogram region (Rhoades and Johnson, 1970; Issenberg and Tannenbaum, 1971; Crosby *et al.*, 1971).

GLC with specific nitrosamine detection systems is certainly very promising as a method for end determination of nitrosamines. At the present moment, more experience with such systems is necessary.

End determination: The need for an unequivocal end determination of traces of carcinogenic nitrosamines in food and other samples must be stressed again and again.   It is dangerous to depend only on retention times, *Rf*-values or polarographic waves for establishing the identity of traces of such compounds isolated from complex mixtures.   These techniques are nonspecific and confirmation by *mass spectrometry* for the determination of the nitrosamines *per se* or derivative formation and adequate determination of such derivatives is absolutely necessary.

Mass spectrometry: The mass spectra of nitrosamines have been recorded (Schroll *et al.*, 1967).   Either the NO^+ ion mass (29,997) or the molecular ions can be used for identification.   The molecular ions in many cases are more abundant than the NO^+ ions and probably also more specific.   Sensitivity of detection depends upon the type of apparatus used and the working conditions, but usually lies in the range of 0.01–0.5 μg (Telling *et al.*, 1971; Heyns and Röper, 1971).   By direct coupling of GLC and mass spectrometry, a good separation technique is combined with an optimum in specificity.   Therefore, the combination GLC-MS at the present moment offers the best method for direct determination of nitrosamines.   Results obtained can be considered as reliable.   The technique is sophisticated, expensive and not available in all laboratories.   This is certainly a serious restriction, but there can be no doubt that GLC–MS is the best means of identification of an N-nitroso compound at the present moment.

Derivative formation: *Nitramines*.   The oxidation of nitrosamines to the corresponding dialkylnitramines can be performed in model experiments with good and reproducible yields, using trifluoroperacetic acid:

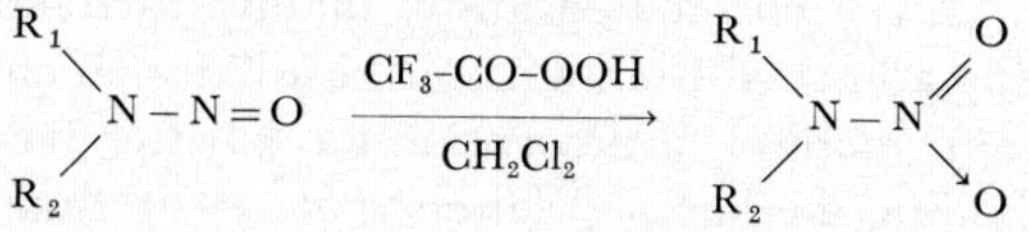

The main advantage of this method is that nitramines are extremely sensitive to electron capture detection and can be separated easily in gas liquid chromatography (Sen, 1970; Althorpe *et al.*, 1970).   Increases in sensitivity by a factor between 100 and 1,000 can be obtained, compared with flame ionization detection of nitrosamines. About 15–20 picograms of dimethylnitrosamine can thus be detected.

Application of the method to food samples, which is possible, has shown, however, that extensive purification is necessary before the method can be applied to food extracts.   The technique should be useful in laboratories where no mass spectrometer is available or where extremely low levels of nitrosamines must be detected.

Amine derivatives.   Our own group found recently (Eisenbrand and Preussmann, 1970) that nitrosamines can be converted to the corresponding secondary amines under very mild conditions using hydrobromic acid in glacial acetic acid:

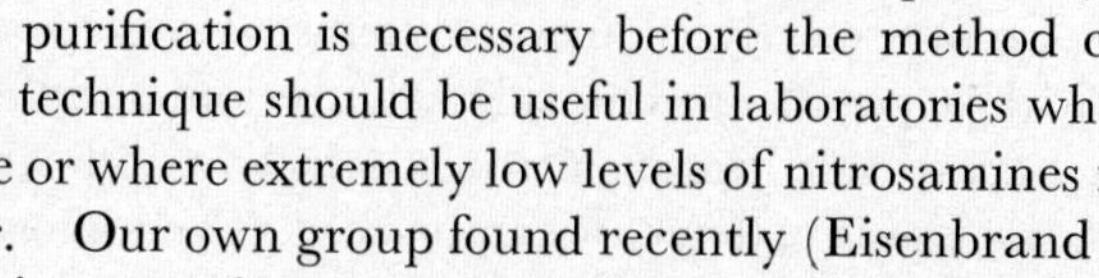

TABLE 3. Denitrosation of Nitrosamines with HBr in Acetic Acid with Yields and Sensitivity of Colorimetric Determination of Liberated NO^+

Nitrosamine	% Yield	Sensitivity $\mu g/ml$
Dimethyl-	99.2	0.85
Diethyl-	97.7	1.16
Di-n-propyl-	99.5	1.48
Di-n-pentyl-	99.3	2.13
Di-iso-propyl-	100.5	1.48
Methyl-ethyl-	100.3	1.00
Methyl-n-butyl-	99.4	1.32
Methyl-n-pentyl-	97.6	1.48
Methyl-2-hydroxyethyl-	102.3	1.19
Methyl-phenyl-	98.1	1.55
Dibenzyl-	100.3	2.58
N-NO-pyrrolidine	99.8	1.44
N-NO-piperidine	98.3	1.30
N-NO-morpholine	98.3	1.32
Methyl-vinyl-	92.8	1.05

The reaction conditions have been optimized, and it can be shown that 15 min at room temperature or 3 min at 50°C warrant a quantitative splitting of the nitrosamine. The HBr concentration was 1.5% in the end volume of the sample. The released nitrosylbromide can be determined quantitatively by colorimetry of a formed azo dye. Some results are given in Table 3, showing the yields in percent of the theory and the sensitivity of the colorimetric response in $\mu g/ml$. Linear calibration curves have been obtained with all nitrosamines investigated, showing that this new colorimetric determination of nitrosamines can be used for quantitative work.

Recent unpublished results have shown that the colorimetric detection of the

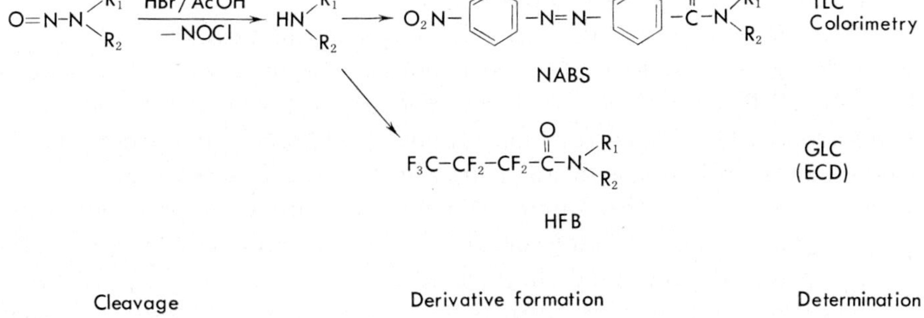

FIG. 3. Determination of nitrosamines by derivative formation.

released nitrosylbromide gives rise to some difficulties when impurities are present in the sample. Olefines, especially, seem to react very quickly with nitrosylbromide added to the double bond.

The essential advantage of the new method rests in the possibility of identification and quantitative determination of the liberated amine after quantitative denitrosation with HBr by formation of suitable derivatives. At the present moment, we are investigating the following possibilities (Fig. 3).

1) Reaction with 1-dimethylamino-naphthaline-5-sulfochloride (Dansyl-chloride) to the corresponding sulfonamides with intensive fluorescence.
2) Reaction with 4'-nitroazobenzenecarboxylic acid chloride (NABS-chloride) to form colored amides with a high molar extinction coefficient.
3) Reaction with heptafluorobutyric acid chloride (HFB-chloride) to form carbonic acid amides with high sensitivity in the electron capture detection in GLC.

In general, satisfactory to good yields in the reaction of the acid chlorides with the liberated amines can be obtained.

An ion exchange method for the selective isolation of the liberated amines, which simplifies and improves the entire cleanup procedure, has recently been developed. The type of ion exchange material used in this step is crucial. Poor recoveries resulted when polystyrene/divinylbenzene copolymers were used. SE cellulose, on the other hand, proved to be very suitable because of its hydrophilic character, and quantitative recoveries of amines were obtained.

Crucial to all methods using amine derivatives for the analysis of nitrosamines is the removal of interfering secondary amines. For example, traces of secondary amines, which must be removed very carefully before use, were found in analytical grade methanol.

The *Dansyl method*, at the present moment, is being investigated as a rapid screening method for nitrosamines at low levels in food. After cleanup and HBr cleavage, the formed Dansyl derivative is separated by TLC. A mixture from 5 nitrosamines (dimethyl- to dipentylnitrosamine) was easily separated and detected because of their strong green fluorescence upon irradiation with filtered long-wave UV light (350 nm). The lower limit of detection is less than 1 nmole. This method seems to be well suited for screening purposes because of its simplicity. It must be emphasized, however, that unequivocal results can only be obtained if contamination from secondary amines is scrupulously excluded.

The *HFB method* has also been elaborated in the meantime (Eisenbrand, 1971). Excellent gas chromatographic separation can be obtained. The lower detection limit for HFB derivatives was determined to about 100–200 picograms, using the tritium foil ECD. This corresponds to about 10–12 nmole for nitrosamines. Linearity studies within 1–100 ng indicate a straight line relationship of the detector response with the quantity of HFB amide. Furthermore, the GLC-MS coupling technique was successfully applied to the specific and highly sensitive detection of HFB derivatives. Dimethyl- and diethylnitrosamines, added at the 10 ppb level to 200 g samples of wheat flour, were easily detected and recovered by the mass spectrometer focused to detect the perfluoropropylium ion mass at m/e 169.

Total recoveries of nitrosamines added to wheat flour were 65–85%, after adequate cleanup.

Thus, it can be stated that adequate, sensitive and reliable methods for the analysis of volatile nitrosamines are available now.   These methods are still rather complicated, time-consuming, expensive and require highly sophisticated instrumental equipment.   If the proper conditions are met, nitrosamine analysis offers no serious problems any longer.

Nonvolatile nitrosamines and nitrosamides

For these groups of carcinogens, the situation is clearly not as satisfactory as for volatile nitrosamines.   Research is just beginning on these groups of carcinogens.

No work has as yet been done on the isolation of nonvolatile nitrosamines and on the purification of extracts.   Difficulties are forseen in this field in view of the relative instability of, e.g., nitrososarcosine and nitrosoproline, which decarboxylate under certain conditions.

Detection can probably be effected by the same methods used for volatile nitrosamines.   In fact, one study by Johnson and Walters (1971) has shown that several nonvolatile nitrosamines are hydrolyzed in high yields by HBr in acetic acid in the same way as described for volatile nitrosamines and nitrosamides (Eisenbrand and Preussmann, 1970).   Released nitrite was estimated, but of course, the formed parent amine can also be analyzed with adequate methods.

Much further work has to be done in the analytical field as well as with the biological activities of nonvolatile nitrosamines.   Many of the products that might occur in food samples treated with nitrite have not yet been investigated in animal experiments.

Still more difficulties are to be expected with nitrosamides in view of the well-known instability of some representatives, especially at an alkaline pH.   No systematic research on the chemical analysis for this important group of chemical carcinogens is available at present.

The acid-catalyzed hydrolysis, however, has been used for the determination of certain nitrosamides, e.g., the cancer chemotherapeutic agent 1,3-bis-(2-chloroethyl)-1-nitrosourea (BCNU) (Loo and Dion, 1965) and streptozotocin, a naturally occurring antibiotic and a methylnitrosourea derivative (Forist, 1964).   The method is based on the ready liberation of nitrous acid from the nitrosoureas with diluted mineral acids at slightly elevated temperatures (50°C).   The released nitrous acid is determined colorimetrically, according to well-known methods (formation of azo dyes).

Schaper (1970) in our laboratory in Freiburg undertook a study to investigate the general applicability of this analytical procedure.   Working with 11 different nitrosamides, she showed that the method worked well with all of the nitrosamides she investigated.   The optimal reaction conditions have been found, the nitrite release by percent of the theory and the sensitivity have been determined (Table 4). For all nitrosamides, linear standardization curves have been obtained, showing that the method can be used for quantitative work.   It was shown too that under strictly standardized reaction conditions the colorimetric determination is also possible in

TABLE 4.   Nitrite Release in Percent of Theory and Sensitivity of Colorimetric Determination of Different Nitrosamine

Compound	Number of experiment	% Nitrite release	Sensitivity (μg/ml end volume)
Nitrite	8	100±1	0.262
N-Metyl-N-nitroso-N'-acetylurea	9	99±1	0.384
N-Metyl-N-nitrosourea	8	99±2	0.272
N-Ethyl-N-nitroso-N'-acetylurea	13	98±1	0.425
N-Ethyl-N-nitrosourea	10	102±1	0.300
N-Pentyl-N-nitrosourea	5	98±1	0.425
N-Methyl-N-nitrosobiuret	5	87±2	0.441
N, N'-Dimethyl-N-nitrosourea	5	82±3	0.373
N-Methyl-N-nitro-N-nitrosourea	5	78±4	0.494
N-Methyl-N-nitroso-p-toluenesulfonamide	5	73±4	0.770
N, N', N'-Trimethyl-N-nitrosourea	5	66±1	0.520
N-Methyl-N-nitrosourethane	11	50±4	0.692

the presence of biological material such as urine, blood, serum and organ homogenates.   The method almost certainly cannot be used for more complex analytical samples.   It might be used, however, after adequate cleanup to release the parent amide which could be determined by specific methods, since the amide itself is very probably a stable compound.   Finally, it should be mentioned that hydrolysis with diluted aqueous acids is rather selective for nitrosamides.   Typical nitrosamines are completely stable under the reaction conditions used and do not interfere with the analysis.

Occurrence of N-Nitroso Compounds in the Human Environment

Today there can be no doubt that N-nitroso compounds do occur in the human environment.   The evidence available has been summarized (Eisenbrand and Marquardt, 1969).   Therefore, we just want to mention that N-nitroso compounds can be naturally occurring compounds (streptozotocin and alanosine, antibiotics from microorganisms, p-nitrosomethylaminobenzaldehyde in mushrooms).   No systematic survey on naturally occurring N-nitroso compounds is available.   In certain regions of the Transkei in South Africa, which are high incidence cancer areas, dimethylnitrosamine was found in the fruit of a solanaceous bush, which is used in food (du Plessis et al., 1969).

The presence of trace amounts of volatile nitrosamines in certain samples of wheat, unburnt tobacco, dairy products and smoked and nonsmoked meat and fish products has been reported.   As mentioned already, these results were obtained with analytical methods, giving equivocal results.

With the improved methods available now for volatile nitrosamines, some of these reports have been checked.   After the cleanup, nitrosamine end determination was confirmed by mass spectrometry and/or derivative formation.   Some hitherto unpublished results were reported at a recent joint meeting of the International Agency for Research on Cancer, Lyon, and the German Cancer Research Center on "Analysis and Formation of Nitrosamines " in Heidelberg.   The studies reported show the presence of very small quantities of volatile, low molecular weight nitrosamines in a number of commodities, *e.g.*, several types of cooked and uncooked meats, certain cheeses, nitrite-treated marine fish, maize and beans.   The levels of contamination were generally less than 10 μg/kg, and the nitrosamines found were dimethyl- and diethylnitrosamine with some evidence of N-nitroso-pyrrolidine and -piperidine.   Evidence was presented at the meeting indicating higher concentrations of dimethylnitrosamine in one source of soybean oil.

CONCLUSION

These are only the very first results of the application of improved methods for the analysis of nitrosamines in environmental samples.   Systematic investigations of these problems have just begun.   The assessment of carcinogenic risk for man from environmental N-nitroso compounds, however, cannot be done by analysis of these compounds alone.   As has been described by Sander and Mirvish during this meeting, N-nitroso compounds can also be formed from inactive precursors, secondary and tertiary amines and amides and nitrosating agents, such as nitrite, nitrate and nitrous gases.   These precursors also must be detected and determined in the attempt to evaluate the health risk of these compounds.   This task is tremendous, but feasible.   It is hoped that many research institutes all around the world will cooperate to solve this important problem.

REFERENCES

1.   Althorpe, J., Goddart, D. A., Lissons, D. J., and Telling, G. M.   The Gas Chromatographic Determination of Nitrosamines at the Picogram Level by Conversion to Their Corresponding Nitramines.   J. Chromatogr., *53*: 371–373, 1970.
2.   Barnes, J. M., and Magee, P. N.   Some Toxic Properties of Dimethylnitrosamine.   Brit. J. Indust. Med., *11*: 167–174, 1954.
3.   Crosby, N. T., Foreman, J. K., Palframan, J. F., and Sawyer, R.   The Determination of Volatile Nitrosamines in Food Products at the 1–50 Parts per 10⁹ Level.   Paper given at a Meeting, "Analysis and Formation of Nitrosamines," Heidelberg, 1971.
4.   Daiber, D., und Preussmann, R.   Quantitative colorimetrische Bestimmung organischer N-Nitroso-Verbindungen durch photochemische Spaltung der Nitrosaminbindung.   Z. Anal. Chem., *206*: 344–352, 1964.
5.   Druckrey, H., Preussmann, R., Ivankovic, S., und Schmähl, D.   Organotrope carcinogene Wirkung bei 65 verschiedenen N-Nitroso-Verbindungen an BD-Ratten.   Z. Krebsforsch., *69*: 103–200, 1967.
6.   Druckrey, H., Schildbach, A., Schmähl, D., Preussmann, R., und Ivankovic, S.   Quantitative Analyse der carcinogenen Wirkung von Diäthylnitrosamin.   Arzneim.-Forsch., *13*: 841–851, 1963.
7.   Du Plessis, L. S., Nunn, J. R., and Roach, W. A.   Carcinogen in a Transkeian Bantu Food Additive.   Nature, *222*: 1198–1199, 1969.
8.   Eisenbrand, G.   Zur Spurenanalytik cancerogener Nitrosamine.   Doctoral Thesis, University Freiburg/Br., 1970.
9.   Eisenbrand, G.   Determination of Volatile Nitrosamines at Low Levels in Food by Acid-catalyzed Denitrosation and Derivative Formation of the Resulting Amines.

Paper given at a Meeting on "Analysis and Formation of Nitrosamines," Heidelberg, 1971.

10. Eisenbrand, G., v. Hodenberg, A., and Preussmann, R. Trace Analysis of N-Nitroso Compounds. II. Steam Distillation at Neutral, Alkaline and Acid pH under Reduced and Atmospheric Pressure. Z. Anal. Chem., 251: 22–24, 1970a.

11. Eisenbrand, G., und Marquardt, P. Über die Problematik des Vorkommens von N-Nitroso-Verbindungen in der Nahrung. Med. und Ernährung, 10: 73–75, 1969.

12. Eisenbrand, G., Marquardt, P., and Preussmann, R. Trace Analysis of N-Nitroso Compounds. I. Liquid-liquid Distribution in Acetonitrile/n-Heptane as Cleanup Method. Z. Anal. Chem., 247: 54–55, 1969.

13. Eisenbrand, G., und Preussmann, R. Eine neue Methodik zur kolorimetrischen Bestimmung von Nitrosaminen nach Spaltung der N-Nitrosogruppe mit Bromwasserstoff in Eisessig. Arzneim.-Forsch., 20: 1513–1517, 1970.

14. Eisenbrand, G., Spaczynski, K., und Preussmann, R. Spurenanalyse von N-Nitroso-Verbindungen. III. Quantitative Dünnschicht-Chromatographie von Nitrosaminen. J. Chromatogr., 51: 503–509, 1970b.

15. Eisenbrand, G., Spaczynski, K., and Preussmann, R. Separation of Carcinogenic Nitrosamines on Sephadex LH-20. J. Chromatogr., 47: 304–306, 1970c.

16. Ender, F., and Ceh, L. Occurrence and Determination of Nitrosamines in Foodstuffs for Human and Animal Nitrition. In; Alkylierend wirkende Verbindungen, Second Conference, pp. 83–91, Freiburg, 1967.

17. Ender, F., and Ceh, L. Conditions and Chemical Reaction Mechanisms by which Nitrosamines May Be Formed in Biological Products with Reference to Their Possible Occurrence in Food Products. Z. Lebensm.-Unters. Forsch., 145: 133–142, 1971.

18. Fiddler, W., Doerr, R. C., Ertel, J. R., and Wasserman, A. E. Determination of N-Nitrosodimethylamine in Ham by Gas-liquid Chromatography with an Alkali Flame Ionization Detector. J. Ass. Offic. Anal. Chem., 54: 1160–1163, 1971.

19. Foreman, J. K., Walker, E. A., and Palframan, J. F. In; Report of the Government Chemist, H. M. Stationery Office, Great Britain, 1969.

20. Forist, A. Spectrophotometric Determination of Streptozotocin. Anal. Chem., 1338, 1964.

21. Garrett, E. R., and Cusimano, A. G. Polarography of Various N-Alkyl-N-nitroso-ureas. J. Pharm. Sci., 55: 702–710, 1966.

22. Heath, D. F., and Jarvis, J. A. E. Polarographic Determination of Dimethyl-nitrosamine in Animal Tissues. Analyst, 80: 613–619, 1955.

23. Heyns, K., und Koch, H. Zur Frage der Entstehung von Nitrosaminen bei der Reaktion von Monosacchariden mit Aminosäuren (Maillard-Reaktion). Z. Lebensm.-Unters. Forsch., 145: 76–84, 1971.

24. Heyns, K., und Röper, H. Ein spezifisches analytisches Trenn- und Nachweis-verfahren für Nitrosamine durch Kombination von Capillargaschromatographie und Massenspektrometrie. Z. Lebensm.-Unters. Forsch., 145: 69–75, 1971.

25. Howard, J. W., Fazio, T., and Watts, J. O. Determination of N-Nitrosodimethyl-amine (DMNA) in Smoked Fish. Application to Smoked Nitrite-treated Chub. J. Ass. Offic. Anal. Chem., 53: 269, 1970.

26. Issenberg, P., and Tannenbaum, S. R. Approaches to Determination of Volatile and Nonvolatile N-Nitroso Compounds in Foods and Beverages. Paper given at a Meeting on "Analysis and Formation of Nitrosamines," Heidelberg, 1971.

27. Johnson, E. M., and Walters, C. L.   The Specificity of the Release of Nitrite from N-Nitrosamines by Hydrobromic Acid.   Anal. Lett., *4*: 383–386, 1971.

28. Kadar, R., and Devik, O. G.   Pyrazines as Interfering Substances in the Determination of Nitrosamines in Roasted Foods.   Acta Chem. Scand., *24*: 2943–2948, 1970.

29. Kröller, E.   Untersuchungen zum Nachweis von Nitrosaminen in Tabakrauch und Lebensmitteln.   Deut. Lebensm. Rundschau, *10*: 303–305, 1967.

30. Lijinsky, W., and Epstein, S. S.   Nitrosamines as Environmental Carcinogens.   Nature, *225*: 21–23, 1970.

31. Loo, T. L., and Dion, R. L.   Colorimetric Method for the Determination of 1,3-Bis(2-chloroethyl)-1-nitrosourea.   J. Pharm. Sci., *54*: 809–810, 1965.

32. Lydersen, D. L., und Nagy, K.   Polarographische Bestimmung von Dimethylnitrosamin in Fischprodukten.   Z. Anal. Chem., *230*: 277–282, 1967.

33. Magee, P. N.   Toxicity of Nitrosamines: Their Possible Human Health Hazards.   Food Cosmet. Toxicol., *9*: 207–218, 1971.

34. Magee, P. N., and Barnes, J. M.   Carcinogenic Nitroso Compounds.   Advan. Cancer Res., *10*: 163–246, 1967.

35. Möhler, K., und Mayrhofer, O. L.   Nachweis und Bestimmung von Nitrosaminen in Lebensmitteln.   Z. Lebensm.-Unters. Forsch., *135*: 313–318, 1968.

36. Montesano, R., and Magee, P. N.   Metabolism of Dimethylnitrosamine by Human Liver Slices *in vitro*.   Nature, *228*: 173, 1970.

37. Montesano, R., and Saffiotii, U.   Carcinogenic Response of the Respiratory Tract of Syrian Golden Hamsters to Different Doses of Diethylnitrosamine.   Cancer Res., *28*: 2197–2210, 1968.

38. Neurath, G., Pirrmann, B., und Dünger, M.   Identifizierung von N-Nitroso-Verbindungen und asymmetrischen Hydrazinen als 5-Nitro-2-hydroxy-benzol-Derivate und Anwendung im Mikromaßstab.   Chon. Ber., *97*, 1631–38, 1969.

39. Nunn, J. R., and du Plessis, L. S.   N-Nitrosamine Analysis.   I.   Estimation of Low Molecular Weight Alkyl-N-nitrosamines.   Paper given at a Meeting on "Analysis and Formation of Nitrosamines," Heidelberg, 1971.

40. Preussmann, R.   Zum oxydativen Abbau von Nitrosaminen mit Enzyme-freien Modell-Systemen.   Arzneim.-Forsch., *14*: 769–774, 1964.

41. Preussmann, R., Neurath, G., Wulf-Lorentzen, G., Daiber, D., und Hengy, H.   Anfärbemethoden und Dünnschicht-Chromatographie von organischen N-Nitroso-Verbindungen.   Z. Anal. Chem., *202*: 187–192, 1964.

42. Rhoades, J. W., and Johnson, D. E.   Gas Chromatography and Selective Detection of N-Nitrosamines.   J. Chromatogr., *8*: 616–617, 1970.

43. Sander, J.   Eine Methode zum Nachweis von Nitrosaminen.   Z. Phys. Chem., *348*: 852–854, 1967.

44. Schaper, F.   Zur Analytik von N-Alkyl-N-nitrosamiden.   Dipl.-Arbeit, Univ. Freiburg, 1970.

45. Schmähl, D.   Experimentelle Untersuchungen zur Syncarcinogenese.   Z. Krebsforsch., *74*: 457–466, 1970.

46. Schroll, G., Cooks, G., Klemmensen, P., and Lawesson, S. O.   The Mass Spectra of Nitroso Compounds.   Ark. Kemi, *28*: 413–422, 1967.

47. Sen, N. P.   Gas-liquid Chromatographic Determination of Dimethylnitrosamine as Dimethylnitramine at Picogram Levels.   J. Chromatogr., *51*: 301–304, 1970.

48. Sen, N. P., Smith, D. S., Schwinghammer, L., and Howsam, B.   Formation of Nitrosamines in Nitrite-treated Fish.   J. Inst. Canad. Techn. Aliment., *3*: 66–69, 1970.

49. Telling, G. M., Bryce, T. A., and Althorpe, J. Use of Vacuum Distillation and Gas Chromatography-Mass Spectrometry for Determination of Low Levels of Volatile Nitrosamines in Meat Products. J. Agr. Food Chem., *19*: 937–941, 1971.

50. Terracini, B., Magee, P. N., and Barnes, J. M. Hepatic Pathology in Rats on Low Dietary Levels of Dimethylnitrosamine. Brit. J. Cancer, *21*: 559–565, 1967.

51. Walters, C. L., Johnson, E. M., and Ray, N. Separation and Detection of Volatile and Nonvolatile N-Nitrosamines. Analyst, *95*: 485–489, 1970.

52. Wasserman, A. E. A Survey of Analytical Procedures for N-Nitrosamines. Paper given at a Meeting on "Analysis and Formation of Nitrosamines," Heidelberg, 1971.

Discussion of Paper by Drs. Preussmann and Eisenbrand

Dr. Dawe: Dr. Preussmann, would you anticipate any problem in identifying and quantitating the presence of nitrosamine compounds in the bottom sediments of harbors or estuaries, where bottom-feeding fish or filter-feeding shellfish might be expected to ingest such sediments? Would you expect the nitrosamines to adsorb to sediments much as they do to charcoal, and would this create a problem in deadsorption for purposes of analysis?

Dr. Preussmann: In principle I see no difficulties, if volatile nitrosamines are to be detected.   If the sediments have a high surface activity, however, difficulties might be expected, as far as quantitative determination is concerned.

Dr. Sugimura: Could you give me a rough idea about the dose level of dimethyl- or diethylnitrosamine in soybean oil, which you mentioned in the last part of your presentation?

Dr. Preussmann: The compound found was dimethylnitrosamine.   If I am not mistaken, the concentrations of DMNA in our sample of soybean oil was in the range of 0.1–1 ppm.   A short summary of that work has recently been published in J. Amer. Oil Chem. Soc.

Carcinogenicity of Benzene Hexachloride (BHC)

Hiroshi Nagasaki, Shosuke Tomii, Tomoichi Mega, Masao Marugami, and Nobuyuki Ito

Department of Hygiene, Nara Medical University, Nara, Japan [H.N., S.T., T.M.]; Cancer Center, Nara Medical University, Nara, Japan [M.M.]; First Department of Pathology, Nara Medical University, Nara, Japan [N.I.]

Recently, many observers have reported acute or chronic toxicity of organo-chloride pesticides, such as DDT, dieldrin, and benzene hexachloride (*11, 13*). One of the properties of benzene hexachloride which makes it an effective agricultural insecticide is the relatively persistent action of its residues. The distribution of benzene hexachloride in tissues, including fatty tissue of mammals, humans included, has been analyzed by several investigators (*10, 14, 15, 17, 20, 24*). Previously, Davis and Fitzhigh (*9*) and Tarjan and Kemeny (*23*) studied the tumorigenicity of DDT, aldrin, and dieldrin in mammals. However, the carcinogenicity of benzene hexachloride in mammals has not been examined. This paper reports studies on the chronic toxicity and carcinogenicity of benzene hexachloride and pathologic findings on examination of various organs of mice treated with benzene hexachloride. The residual level of benzene hexachloride in the liver of these animals was also measured.

MATERIALS AND METHODS

Seventy-four male dd-mice (Nippon Animal Farm, Osaka) weighing about 22.3 g were used. The animals were divided into four groups: Group 1, twenty mice fed on a basal diet NMF (Oriental Co. Ltd., Tokyo) supplemented with 660.0 ppm of benzene hexachloride composed of several isomers (Table 1); Group 2, twenty mice fed on a basal diet containing 66.0 ppm of benzene hexachloride; Group 3, twenty mice fed on a basal diet supplemented with 6.6 ppm of benzene hexachloride; Group 4, fourteen mice fed on a basal diet alone. All the animals were housed individually in aluminum cages in an air-conditioned room at 24°C, and received the experimental diets and tap water *ad libitum*. Each mouse was weighed once a week and its food intake was measured twice a week. The animals were fed nothing for 18 hr before they were killed with ether 24 weeks after the

TABLE 1.   Active Constituents of Benzene Hexachloride
(Sankyo Co., Tokyo) Added to Basal Diet (Oriental NMF)
for Group 1

α-isomer	439 ppm
β-isomer	75
γ-isomer	100
δ-isomer	42
Others	4
Total	660

start of the experiment, and their final weight was measured.   At autopsy the liver,
brain, heart, kidneys, spleen, and testis of each mouse were removed and weighed,
and pieces were taken for microscopic examination.   These pieces were fixed in 10%
formaldehyde solution and eosin, van Gieson, Mallory, and periodic acid-Schiff
stains.   The levels of each isomer in the liver of the experimental mice were analyzed by gas-liquid chromatography following the method prescribed in Official
Methods of Analysis of the Association of Official Agricultural Chemists (AOAC
method, 1965).

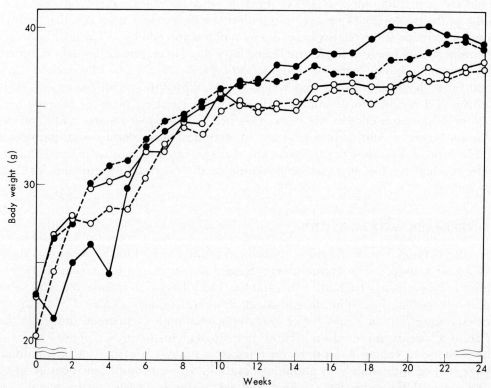

FIG. 1.   Growth curves of dd-mice treated with benzene hexachloride.   ●———●, 660.0
ppm BHC diet; ●--------●, 66.0 ppm BHC diet; ○———○, 6.6 ppm BHC diet; ○--------○,
control diet.

RESULTS

Growth Curves

The growth curves of the animals in each group are shown in Fig. 1.   Growth of mice receiving 66.0 ppm and 6.6 ppm of benzene hexachloride (Groups 2 and 3) was very similar to that of the control animals (Group 4).   Mice receiving 660.0 ppm of benzene hexachloride (Group 1) lost weight for the first 4 weeks and then gained weight steadily, and after 12 weeks the weight of animals in Group 1 was the highest among all the groups.

Food Consumption

The changes in weekly food consumption of the mice in each group are shown graphically in Fig. 2.   After 8 weeks, clear differences were seen between the groups. All experimental groups showed decreased food consumption, especially Group 1. The control group showed marked variation in food consumption but the level remained high during the whole experimental period.

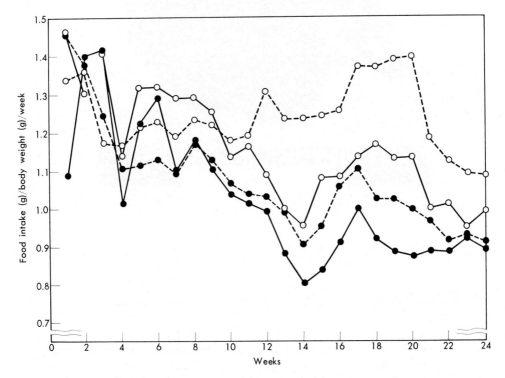

FIG. 2.   Changes in food intake of dd-mice treated with benzene hexachloride.   ●————●, 660.0 ppm BHC diet;   ●--------●, 66.0 ppm BHC diet;   ○————○, 6.6 ppm BHC diet;   ○--------○, control diet.

Liver Changes

In Group 1 (receiving 660 ppm of benzene hexachloride), tumors developed in the livers of all 20 mice.   In all these animals the liver increased in weight due to tumor growth, and had a rough surface with many large yellowish nodules of up to 1.0 cm in diameter (Fig. 3).   No tumors were seen in the livers of mice of Groups 2 (Fig. 4), 3, and 4.   However, the weights of their livers were more than in the control group, those of Group 1 being about 3.7 times those of control mice.   The liver weights and their percentages of the total body weights are showed in Table 2.

Microscopically, the nodules in the livers of all 20 mice in Group 1 were found to be hyperplastic nodules and hepatomas.   Hyperplastic nodules were sharply de-

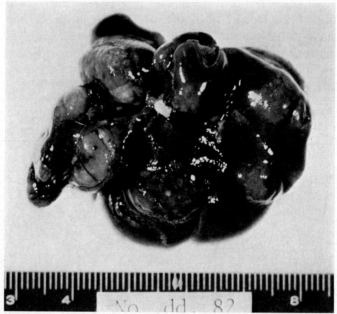

FIG. 3.   Multiple tumors in the liver of a mouse in Group 1 after 24 weeks.   All lobes have tumors.

TABLE 2.   Pathological Findings in the Livers of dd-Mice Treated with Benzene Hexachloride for 24 Weeks[a]

Group	Benzene hexachloride in diet[b] (ppm)	Number of mice	Body weight		Liver weight		Hepatoma incidence	
			Initial	Final	(g)	%/Body weight	Number	(%)
1	660.0	20	22.9±1.0	38.9±3.0	5.0±1.8	15.2±4.9	20/20	(100.0)
2	66.0	20	22.8±0.7	38.7±0.3	2.0±0.3	5.1±1.3	0/20	(0.0)
3	6.6	20	22.7±1.8	37.8±4.4	1.9±0.7	5.0±1.6	0/20	(0.0)
4	0.0	14	20.1±1.9	36.4±2.5	1.6±0.3	4.4±0.9	0/14	(0.0)

[a]   All figures indicate mean±S.D.

[b]   Benzene hexachloride was added to basal diet as described in the text.

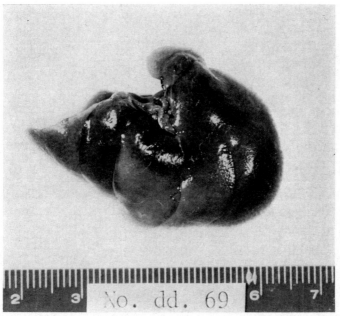

FIG. 4. Smooth surface of the liver of a mouse in Group 2 after 24 weeks.

marcated from the surrounding liver tissue, and these nodules contained a few sinusoids and blood vessels.   The cytoplasm was hypertrophic and nuclear irregularities of the cells were seen but mitotic figures were rare (Fig. 5).   In some adenomatous areas of tumors, dilated sinusoids were seen separated by narrow cords of cells. Large trabecular structures with distended sinusoids were frequently seen.   Cells in these areas had pyknotic and irregular nuclei (Fig. 6).   Some carcinomatous areas of hepatomas consisted of uniform neoplastic hepatic cord cells, and mitotic figures were frequent (Fig. 7).   Cells in nontumorous areas of the liver also had irregular nuclei.   However, proliferation of connective tissue or bile ducts and oval cell infiltration were not marked.   In Group 2, hypertrophic foci of liver parenchymal cells in centro-lobular areas were frequent (Fig. 8).   Some hypertrophic cells showed nuclear irregularities and mitotic figures.   However, no hyperplastic nodules or hepatomas were seen.   In Groups 3 and 4, no remarkable changes of the liver were observed.   The histopathological findings on the livers of the mice are summarized in Table 3.

TABLE 3. Histopathological Findings in the Livers of Mice Treated with Benzene Hexachloride for 24 Weeks

Group	Oval cell infiltration	Bile duct proliferation	Fibrosis	Cellular hyperplasia	Nodular hyperplasia	Hepatoma
1	+	±	−	⧺	⧺	⧺
2	−	−	−	⧺	−	−
3	−	−	−	±	−	−
4	−	−	−	−	−	−

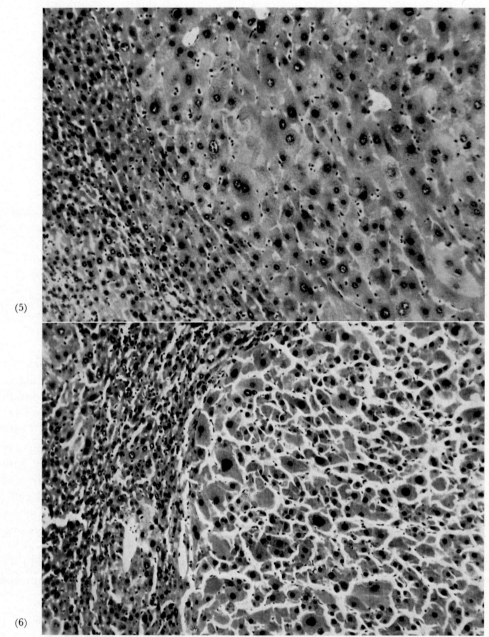

(5)

(6)

FIG. 5.   Liver of a mouse in Group 1 showing large hypertrophic cells with nuclear irregularities and few mitotic figures.   H-E.   ×100.

FIG. 6.   Small nodule sharply demarcated from the surrounding liver parenchymal tissues in the liver of a mouse in Group 1.   Cellular and nuclear irregularities and mitotic figures are seen in the area of hepatoma.   H-E.   ×100.

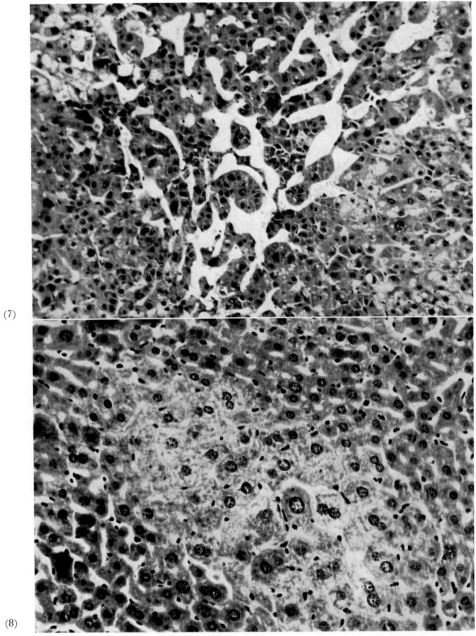

(7)

(8)

Fig. 7.   Trabecular arrangement of cells in an area of hepatoma in a mouse of Group 1.   H-E.
×100.
Fig. 8.   Slightly enlarged cells with nuclear irregularities in the liver of a mouse of Group
2.   H-E.   ×100.

Other Organs

Macroscopically, the brain, heart, lung, kidney, spleen, testis, stomach, intestine, and pancreas appeared essentially normal in all groups.   The weights of the brain, heart, two kidneys, spleen and testis are summarized in Table 4.   Microscopically, no remarkable changes were seen in any of these organs.

TABLE 4.   Changes of Organ Weight in Mice Treated with Benzene Hexachloride for 24 Weeks   [Mean S. D.]

Group	Number of mice	Organ weight (g)					
		Brain	Heart	l-Kidney	r-Kidney	Spleen	Testis
1	20	0.42±0.05	0.16±0.02	0.26±0.05	0.28±0.06	0.13±0.06	0.11±0.01
2	20	0.41±0.05	0.16±0.02	0.29±0.05	0.32±0.05	0.19±0.09	0.12±0.01
3	20	0.44±0.06	0.16±0.01	0.31±0.09	0.34±0.08	0.26±0.14	0.10±0.05
4	14	0·41±0.04	0.15±0.06	0.27±0.03	0.30±0.05	0.24±0.16	0.09±0.01

Total Intake of Benzene Hexachloride and Its Accumulation in Liver

The average total intake of benzene hexachloride per mouse in each group and the amounts of benzene hexachloride isomers accumulated in the liver are summarized in Table 5.   The average benzene hexachloride intake was 555.21 mg in Group 1, 59.06 mg in Group 2, and 6.20 mg in group 3.   In Group 1, the amounts of the α- and β-isomers accumulated reached very high levels.   In Group 2, the amounts of the α- and β-isomers accumulated were about 10% of those in Group 1 while in Group 3, they were about 20% of those in Group 2.   In all groups, the γ- and δ-isomers were present in only trace amounts.

TABLE 5.   Total Intake of Benzene Hexachloride by Mice in 24 Weeks and Its Accumulation in Liver (Method : AOAC)

Group	Total intake (mg/mouse)	Accumulation of isomer (ppm)			
		α	β	γ	δ
1	555.21	11.44	12.37	±	±
2	59.06	1.13	1.36	+	±
3	6.20	0.22	0.23	+	±
4	—	+	+	+	±

+, 0.03~0.01 ;   ±, 0.01>.

DISCUSSION

In the present work hepatomas were induced in high incidence in dd-mice on administration of benzene hexachloride for 24 weeks.   Induction of hepatomas in mice by the chemical carcinogens o-aminoazotoluene, 4-dimethylaminoazobenzene, N-nitrosodimethylamine and N-nitrosopiperidine have been reported by many observers (*1, 2, 5, 6, 18, 19, 21, 22*). Histologically the hepatomas induced in mice by benzene hexachloride appeared similar to those induced by other chemicals.

Previously, spontaneous liver tumors in mice were reported by several observers (*3, 4, 7*), but a very low incidence of these hepatomas was observed in dd-strain mice. This suggests that none of the present hepatomas developed spontaneously. Davis *et al.* (*9*) reported that hepatomas in mice developed on administration of aldrin or dieldrin for two years. Tarjan and Kemeny (*23*) found that the incidences of leukemias, pulmonary carcinomas, hepatomas and reticulo-sarcomas were higher in animals receiving DDT than in control animals. In the present work, benzene hexachloride induced hepatomas but not malignant tumors in other organs.

In the present study, technical benzene hexachloride was used which is composed of the α, β, γ, δ, and other isomers. After administration of benzene hexachloride for 24 weeks the amounts of the isomers accumulated in the livers of animals in the four groups were very different. The amounts of the α- and β-isomers were much higher than those of the γ- or δ-isomers. Davidow and Frawley (*8*) observed that benzene hexachloride administered to rats accumulated most in adipose tissue, brain, kidneys, liver, and muscle. They also observed a striking difference in the accumulations of the different isomers of benzene hexachloride in the rat. The α- and β-isomers of benzene hexachloride may be important in hepato-carcinogenesis in mice. The synergistic actions of mixtures of certain hepatic carcinogens have been observed by several investigators (*12, 16*), and a mixture of the α- and β-isomers of benzene hexachloride may also have a synergistic action in hepatic carcinogenesis in mice. The metabolic change of benzene hexachloride in mammals *in vivo* has been studied (*17*), but its mechanism of carcinogenesis is unknown, and further studies are needed to determine which isomer(s) is carcinogenic. Egan *et al.* (*10*) reported that the organo-pesticides, DDT, benzene hexachloride, and dieldrin, accumulated in human fat and human milk. Thus, statistical analyses should be made on the relation between the geographical distribution of cases of hepatoma and the residual levels of benzene hexachloride in man.

REFERENCES

1. Akamatsu, Y., and Ikegami, R. Induction of Hepatoma and Systemic Amyloidosis in Mice by 4-(Dimethylamino)Azobenzene Feeding. Gann, *59*: 201, 1968.
2. Akamatsu, Y., Takemura, T., Ikegami, R., Takahashi, A., and Miyajima, H. Growth Behavior of Hepatomas in *o*-Aminoazotoluene Treated Mice in Comparison with Spontaneous Hepatomas. Gann, *58*: 323, 1967.
3. Akamatsu, Y., Wada, F., and Ikegami, R. Transplantation of Spontaneous Hepatomas in C_3H Mice; Biological and Biochemical Studies. Gann, *60*: 145, 1969.
4. Andervont, H. B., and Dunn, T. B. Transplantation of Spontaneous and Induced Hepatomas in Inbred Mice. J. Natl. Cancer Inst., *13*: 455, 1952.
5. Andervont, H. B., and Edwards, J. E. Carcinogenic Action of Two Azo Compounds in Mice. J. Natl. Cancer Inst., *3*: 349, 1943.
6. Andervont, H. B., Grady, H. G., and Edwards, J. E. Induction of Hepatic Lesions, Hepatomas, Pulmonary Tumors, and Hemangioendotheliomas in Mice with *o*-Aminoazotoluene. J. Natl. Cancer Inst., *3*: 131, 1942.

7. Burns, E. L., and Schenken, J. R.   Spontaneous Primary Hepatomas in Mice of Strain C_3H a Study of Incidence, Sex Distribution and Morbid Anatomy.   Amer. J. Cancer, *39*: 25, 1940.

8. Davidow, B., and Frawley, J. P.   Tissue Distribution, Accumulation and Elimination of Isomers of Benzene Hexachloride.   Proc. Soc. Exptl. Biol. Med., *76*: 780, 1951.

9. Davis, K., and Fitzhigh, O. G.   Tumorigenic Potential of Aldrin and Dieldrin for Mice.   Toxicol. Applied Pharm., *4*: 187, 1962.

10. Egan, H., Goulding, R., Roburn, H., and Tatton, J. O'G.   Organochlorine Pesticide Residues in Human Fat and Human Milk.   Brit. Med. J., *10*: 66, 1965.

11. Fitzhigh, O. G., Nelson, A. A., and Frawley, J. P.   The Chronic Toxicities of Technical Benzene Hexachloride and Its Alpha, Beta, and Gamma Isomers.   J. Pharm. Exptl. Therap., *100*: 59, 1950.

12. Ito, N., Hiasa, Y., Konishi, Y., and Marugami, M.   The Development of Carcinoma in Liver of Rats Treated with *m*-Toluylene Diamine and the Synergistic and Antagonistic Effects with Other Chemicals.   Cancer Res., *29*: 1137, 1969.

13. Kostoff, D.   Induction of Cytogenetic Changes and Atypical Growth by Hexachlorocyclohexane.   Science, *109*: 467, 1949.

14. Laug, E. P., Nelson, A. A., Fitzhigh, O. G., and Kunzen, F. M.   Liver Cell Alteration and DDT Storage in the Fat of the Rat Induced by Dietary Levels of 1 to 50 ppm DDT.   J. Pharm. Exptl. Therap., *98*: 268, 1950.

15. Lillie, R. D., Smith, M. I., and Stahlman, E. F.   Pathologic Action of DDT and Certain of Its Analogs and Derivatives.   Arch. Pathol., *43*: 127, 1947.

16. MacDonald, J. C., Miller, E. C., Miller, J. A., and Rusch, H. P.   Synergistic Action of Mixtures of Certain Hepatic Carcinogens.   Cancer Res., *12*: 50, 1952.

17. Newland, L. W., Chesters, G., and Lee, G. B.   Degradation of γ-BHC in Simulated Lake Impoundments as Affected by Aeration.   J. Water Pollut. Cont. Fed., *41*: 174, 1969.

18. Nishizuka, Y., Ito, K., and Nakakuki, K.   Liver Tumor Induction by a Single Injection of *o*-Aminoazotoluene to Newborn Mice.   Gann, *56*: 135, 1965.

19. Sasaki, T., und Yoshida, T.   Experimentelle Erzeugung des Lebercarcinoms durch Fütterung mit *o*-Amidoazotoluol.   Virchows Arch. Pathol. Anat. Physiol., *295*: 175, 1935.

20. Selby, L. A., Newell, K. W., Hauser, G. A., and Junker, G.   Comparison of Chlorinated Hydro Carbon Pesticides in Maternal Blood and Placental Tissues.   Environmental Res., *2*: 247, 1969.

21. Shelton, E.   Hepatomas in Mice.   I.   Factors Affecting the Rapid Induction of a High Incidence of Hepatomas by *o*-Aminoazotoluene.   J. Natl. Cancer Inst., *16*: 107, 1955.

22. Takayama, S., and Oota, K.   Malignant Tumors Induced in Mice Fed with N-Nitrosodimethylamine.   Gann, *54*: 465, 1963.

23. Tarjan, R., and Kemeny, T.   Multigeneration Studies on DDT in Mice.   Food Cosmet. Toxicol., *7*: 215, 1969.

24. Vos, J. G., van der Maas, A., Musch, A., and Ram, E.   Toxicity of Hexachlorobenzene in Japanese Quail with Special Reference to Porphyria, Liver Damage, Reproduction, and Tissue Residues.   Toxicol. Applied Pharm., *18*: 944, 1971.

Discussion of Paper by Drs. Nagasaki et al.

Dr. Sanders: I note from your figure that the control mice in Group 4, which had received no BHC in their diet, contained traces of the α- and β-isomers in their livers after 24 weeks.   How would you explain this?

Dr. Nagasaki: Commercial stock diets are composed of agricultural products in Japan.   Trace amounts of BHC used as agricultural insecticide were accumulated in the stock diets of our experiment.

Dr. Tomatis: At what time were the evaluations of BHC levels in the liver carried out?   Could you evaluate the latency period for the appearance of hepatomas?   It appeared from your pictures that hepatomas presented different histological patterns!   Did you have metastases?

Dr. Nagasaki: The residual level of BHC was measured in the liver of the mice at 24 weeks.   There were no metastases in any of the animals of the experimental groups at 24 weeks.

Dr. Ishidate: You used the technical BHC mixture.   I wonder if the mixture contains an unknown substance of higher molecular weight.   I ask you if you have any information on carcinogenicity of each of the isomers of BHC in pure state?

Dr. Nagasaki: We are conducting further experiments using pure isomers of BHC.

Detection of Weak Carcinogenic Stimuli

Fred G. Bock

Roswell Park Memorial Institute, New York State Department of Health, Buffalo, New York, U.S.A.

Identification of carcinogens as potential causes of cancer in man can be thought of as consisting of two historical stages, and, it is hoped, one future stage. Potent carcinogens were first studied in man. A more sophisticated analysis of their effect in animals has now provided means for detecting potent carcinogenic stimuli before their action in man is apparent. Soon we should enter a third stage where even weak carcinogenic stimuli can be avoided.

For the purposes of this discussion, I choose to define potent carcinogenic stimuli as those that can produce tumors in at least 20% of the exposed population during the normal lifespan. I define moderate carcinogenic stimuli as those that produce tumors in 5–20% of the exposed population, and weak carcinogenic stimuli as those that produce tumors in fewer than 5% of the exposed population. I limit the term *carcinogen* to any agent that is, under appropriate conditions, a carcinogenic stimulus. Failure to make such distinctions has caused very many problems in communications, resulting in limitation of experimental progress. For example, benzo[a]pyrene (BP) is a strong carcinogen, but a 1 part per million solution of BP in a toxic non-volatile solvent is so weak a carcinogenic stimulus that it would probably defy detection. Nevertheless, a great deal of effort was expended to prove that cigarette smoke condensate (CSC) both did and did not contain this single compound. Today, we concede that BP is only one of the hydrocarbons in smoke, all of which combined cannot account for the activity of the whole CSC. Even now, however, we continue to see reports of " strong carcinogens " that have been detected in CSC at levels so low that their detection alone is a notable analytical achievement. In our analytical search for the ultimate carcinogen in tobacco tar, we tend to ignore classes of " weak carcinogens " that CSC may contain in quantity. We would probably save a great deal of effort by looking for the significant carcinogenic stimuli in this extremely complex mixture, rather than for " strong carcinogens " that may be present at levels so low as to be meaningless.

Our ability to detect carcinogens in man depends upon the intensity of the carcinogenic stimulus, the size of the population under study, the degree to which the population is controlled, and the incidence of the same tumors in presumably unexposed members of the same population. For potent or moderate carcinogenic stimuli, these limitations do not preclude success. Even small populations, such as occupation groups or closely knit cultural units, may suffice for potent stimuli. Moderate carcinogenic stimuli, such as cigarette smoke or tobacco extracts, have been detected in man, because very large populations were exposed to the agents. Weak carcinogenic stimuli, however, probably will not be detected in man during the foreseeable future, because the background tumor incidence will be high in comparison with the increased incidence caused by the carcinogen. This will be particularly true in cases where combinations of carcinogenic stimuli exhibit co-carcinogenic properties.

In the laboratory, identification of carcinogens is less difficult than it is in man. Often, concentrations higher than those met in the environment can be used. Thus a potent carcinogenic stimulus can be tested in the laboratory to study a weak stimulus in the environment. When this can be done, the effort required for the bioassays will not be excessive. On the other hand, if the environmental carcinogenic stimuli are weak and the carcinogens cannot be concentrated, the requirements for adequate routine bioassays may exceed the resources available for the task.

What are the factors that prevent us from concentrating the carcinogens in a weak environmental stimulus so that adequate laboratory studies might be undertaken? First of all, an unknown agent might be present in such low concentration that any test material would of necessity be a weak stimulus. For example, extracts of unburned cigarette tobacco (TE) at a concentration containing 0.6–0.8 g of solids per ml act as moderate tumor-promoting stimuli (4). That is, they will produce tumors in approximately 30% of mice that have been previously painted with 125 µg of DMBA. Without the DMBA pretreatment, the extracts are nearly inactive. Are the extracts true tumor promoters, or is their activity due to the presence of complete carcinogens? If the latter is the case, the carcinogenic stimulus of the extracts must be very weak; it was detected only in combination with a near-threshold level of DMBA. We could determine whether TE is indeed a weak carcinogenic stimulus by testing it in about 1,000 mice. To compare the potency of two extracts would require thousands of mice per assay. If we could concentrate the carcinogen, fewer mice would be required. The original extracts are thick syrups, however, and cannot be concentrated further. We are thus restricted in our studies of tobacco extracts, because the unknown active agents are present in very low concentration. Similar factors may limit the identification of weak carcinogenic stimuli in foodstuffs.

A second factor that can prevent raising the concentration of environmental carcinogens is toxicity. Some-time ago, Wynder and Wright suggested that the basic fraction of CSC has weak carcinogenic activity (32). We observed tumors in mice painted with DMBA followed by the ether-soluble bases of CSC. The numbers of tumors were small and of questionable statistical significance. Obviously we should test the bases at higher concentration to confirm or disprove the presence of carcinogens.   This is not possible, however, because the fraction contains so much nicotine that even moderate doses are lethal.   Nicotine has not yet been separated from the possible carcinogens.

The third factor that can limit adequate concentration of carcinogens for laboratory study is the economic cost.   It is not considered quite proper to suggest that cost limits progress in the prevention of death or disease in developed countries; nevertheless, costs can reach levels that prevent timely laboratory study.

This problem is again illustrated by studies with CSC.   We needed to design a bioassay for fractions of CSC that could ultimately identify the active agents in this material.   It was first necessary to determine how much effort and test material would be required.   For the purposes of the analysis, we made certain assumptions. We first assumed that we must detect any fraction of CSC that contains 10% or more of the activity of the crude material.   In the interest of economy, we could sacrifice any fraction exhibiting less than 10% of the total activity, in spite of the fact that such a fraction might be proportionately more active in human lungs than in mouse skin.   We further assumed that two mice bearing skin tumors are required in any experimental group to identify the respective test solution as potentially active. (Fortunately, we have not seen any skin tumors in control mice over the 18-month span of observation that we employ in our experiments.)   Our third assumption was that we should test each active fraction at two concentrations differing by a factor of two.   This would provide a very rough semiquantitative comparison of the relative importance of any active fractions that might be uncovered.   We would also test the starting CSC and " reconstituted CSC " to measure losses due to the chemical

TABLE 1.   Costs of Conventional Bioassays of Fractions of Cigarette Smoke Condensate

0.5 g of CSC per week per mouse (78 weeks)=50% tumors

~ 40 g of CSC per mouse=50% tumors

∴ The "A" from 40 g of CSC per mouse=5% tumors (p=0.05)

To produce two tumors 80% of the time with p=0.05 will require about 100 mice, and hence "A" from 4 kg of CSC.

A second dose level twice as high will require another 100 mice and 8 kg of CSC.

Additional fractions will require 200 mice each, but no more CSC.

To test crude CSC itself will require 200 mice and 6 kg of CSC (100 mice with 4 kg, and 100 with 2 kg).

Likewise, the " reconstituted CSC " will require 200 mice and 6 kg of CSC.

Positive controls are not required.

Total needs for 10 fractions (18-month experiment)

	Mice	CSC (kg)
Negative controls	100	0
CSC	200	6
10 Fractions	2,000	12
Reconstituted	200	6
Totals	2,500	24 kg (1,200,000 cigs.)

Total staff: 15½ man-years (5 technically trained).

The first follow-up study with 10 fractions would require 43 kg of CSC (2,100,000 cigs.) and 19 man-years (8 technically trained).

A second follow-up study would require 51 kg of CSC.

manipulations.   Lastly, we assumed that any primary fraction submitted to follow-up separations might contain only 80% of its active ingredients, the remainder being misplaced through incomplete separation.   Except for this reservation, we assumed 100% recovery.

In our experience, a dose of 40 g of CSC administered over a period of 18 months was required in order to produce tumors in approximately 50% of the animals.   We also knew from experience that with moderate to low doses of CSC, tumor incidence appears to be proportional to the dose employed.   Thus, if fraction A accounted for 1/10 of the activity of the CSC, it would provide about 1/10 as many tumors as CSC does.   If these facts and assumptions are valid, we would need 24 kg of CSC and 2,500 mice for the first study (Table 1).   The first follow-up experiment would require more CSC for tests of the starting and reconstituted materials plus 20% for incomplete recovery.   If losses were anticipated, appropriately larger quantities of material would be required.   Because of these requirements, progress in the identification of the active agents of CSC has been glacially slow.   It has been 18 years since CSC was shown to produce tumors in mice.   The active agents have not yet been identified.

Very weak carcinogenic stimuli *could* be studied with success if adequate support were provided to permit conducting tests with very large populations of animals. In the real world, however, where decisions depend on the relative pressures of alternative demands for resources, support for adequate large-scale screening to detect very weak carcinogenic stimuli does not seem likely.   This is particularly true if we seek to detect stimuli that are so weak that they can only modify an existing tumor incidence caused by a more potent stimulus, or to detect incomplete carcinogenic stimuli capable of carrying out only some of the steps leading to a malignant tumor.

If we cannot afford to support very large populations of experimental animals, how can we detect and identify weak carcinogenic stimuli that may be of considerable importance to man?   And how can we be most likely to detect incomplete carcinogens that might play a role in human cancer?

A major reduction in skin-painting costs has resulted from the use of mice pretreated with DMBA.   This experimental design offers two important advantages. First of all, it is possible to detect much weaker carcinogenic stimuli if the dose of DMBA is one that by itself will produce tumors only rarely (22).

The second major advantage is that, in addition to complete carcinogens, the bioassays will detect tumor-promoting agents that may be present in tobacco tar. A growing body of evidence suggests that in man, cigarette smoke acts as a co-carcinogen in combination with other agents, such as asbestos (24), ionizing radiation (1), and urban air pollutants (23).   There is some evidence that cigarette smoking acts as a tumor-promoting stimulus.   Doll suggested that the rapid decrease in lung tumor incidence in individuals who stop smoking is comparable to the dependence of promoting activity on the frequent application of croton oil (16).   East-cott (18) and Dean (14, 15) presented data indicating that the carcinogenic effects of cigarette smoke in man may depend on childhood environment, just as the effects of croton oil depend on the prior history of the experimental mice.   Of course, these data alone do not prove that cigarette smoke is a tumor-promoting agent in man. It appears prudent, however, to look at promoting activity in our laboratory studies of this material.

Using mice treated with 125 μg of DMBA permits a substantial saving in the quantities of CSC required for the assays. For crude CSC, the tumor yield is about four times as great in DMBA-treated mice as it is in untreated mice. Some of the savings, however, are apparent rather than real. Positive fractions will include not only complete carcinogens, but also tumor-promoting agents that by themselves do not produce many tumors—even at relatively high concentrations. Sooner or later, it is necessary to distinguish between these possibilities in order to evaluate the importance of the observations. Even so, these evaluations need be conducted only at the end of the series of stepwise fractionation procedures. As a consequence, the ultimate savings should be between 50 and 75% of the CSC otherwise required for assays using untreated mice. That is, we can obtain two to four times as much data for a given expenditure of effort. More important, potential tumor-promoting fractions will be disclosed by these tests, whereas they would be apparently negative in a conventional carcinogenesis assay.

Hoffmann and Wynder have utilized tumor-initiating tests of assays for subfractions of their B1 fraction (19). Their procedure requires still less material, but will detect only complete carcinogens or tumor-initiating agents. It will fail to detect tumor promoters. Takayama has tested tobacco tar by injection of newborn mice (27). Although this method is probably less specific than skin painting for contact carcinogens, it requires very little material. It may prove of substantial value in identifying carcinogens that may induce nonpulmonary cancer, or carcinogens that modify the principal contact carcinogens of CSC.

I would like now to discuss results of assays of fractions of CSC and extracts of unburned cigarette tobacco. The results indicate that combinations of agents are of very great importance, and that the complexities of multicomponent carcinogenesis are far more extensive than those of simple initiation and promotion. They suggest that all of the possible co-carcinogenic effects tabulated by Berenblum may have to be considered in any analysis of the effects of weak environmental carcinogenic stimuli.

Fractions of Cigarette Smoke Condensate

In a series of four fractionation schemes, Swain *et al.* prepared various fractions and subfractions of CSC for bioassay (11, 25, 26). The assays of the major fractions indicated that the ether-soluble weak acids were active, that the ether-soluble bases were of questionable activity, and that all three of the neutral subfractions were active (9). Work in other laboratories led us to expect that the weak acid fraction and the one neutral fraction that contained the polynuclear aromatic hydrocarbons (PAH) would be active (17, 29, 30). We did not expect that the other neutral subfractions would be active. To test our expectations, the total neutral fraction was separated into 10 subfractions by silicic acid chromatography. Four active subfractions were obtained (10). One of these was the most polar neutral subfraction (MPN). It was eluted from silicic acid with methanol; and when distributed between the two layers of a solvent system consisting of methanol, water, and petroleum ether, it remained in the aqueous methanol layer. The other three positive neutral subfractions were relatively nonpolar. One was eluted from silicic acid with petroleum ether and when partitioned between cyclohexane (CH) and dimethyl sulfoxide (DMSO), was found in the DMSO solution. Two active subfractions were eluted with 25% benzene in petroleum ether; after separation between CH and DMSO, both layers were active. These two fractions combined correspond roughly to the fraction B1 of Wynder and Hoffmann (30). Nearly all of the benzo[a]pyrene of CSC was found in the DMSO phase of the benzene-petroleum ether eluate (26).

When the biological activity of the reconstituted neutral fraction following silicic acid chromatography was compared with that of the starting neutral fraction from which it was obtained, it appeared that about three-fourths of the activity was probably lost during the separation procedure. Throughout the course of the experiment, fewer tumors were produced by the reconstituted neutrals equivalent to 60% crude CSC than were produced by the starting neutral material equivalent to only 15% CSC. Subsequent studies, which are still under way, suggest that a modified countercurrent distribution procedure can be employed to concentrate the active neutral subfraction without losses of activity (12). It might thus be possible to subject a less bulky material to chromatographic separation, so that the losses could be better controlled.

The neutral subfractions have not been available in sufficient quantity to test in mice that were not pretreated with DMBA. This must be done at some time to determine whether they are complete carcinogens or only tumor promoters. In the meantime, we have assayed the neutral subfractions for tumor-initiating activity (13). The most polar neutrals did not contribute to the production of tumors when mice were treated first with this fraction and then with repetitive applications of 12-O-tetradecanoyl phorbol-3-acetate (PMA). We conclude that the MNP acts as a tumor-promoting stimulus only. In contrast, the fraction containing BP was a potent tumor initiator when tested at concentrations representing the same quantity of crude CSC. These tests show that the fraction containing BP is both an initiator and a promoter and are in agreement with many other reports that similar fractions act both as initiators and as complete carcinogenic stimuli (6, 17, 29, 30).

The other two neutral fractions eluted from silicic acid at approximately the same point as BP fail to exhibit tumor-initiating activity when tested at the same relative concentrations. At these concentrations, however, their tumor-promoting activity was low. It is very possible that the dosage was insufficient to disclose the initiating activity of a weak carcinogenic stimulus.

The ether-soluble weak acid fraction could be tested at higher concentrations for complete carcinogenic activity. The weak acids equivalent to 82% CSC produced two tumors in 50 mice after 43 and 47 weeks of treatment (11). This number is small, but we have seen no skin tumors in thousands of control animals treated only with solvent for this period of time. Accordingly, we consider that the weak acid fraction is a weak complete carcinogenic stimulus and a potent tumor-promoting stimulus.

In summary, CSC contains two major fractions that act primarily as tumor-promoting stimuli, and three neutral fractions, one of which is a complete carcinogenic stimulus and the other two of which have not been adequately tested, but are, at least, tumor-promoting stimuli.

We have further examined the weak acid fraction by assaying both the steam distillate, which contains the simple phenols, and the residues remaining after steam distillation.   It has often been assumed that the promoting activity of the weak acids is due to their content of simple phenols.   We found, to our surprise, that the non-volatile residues possessed the bulk of the tumor-promoting activity (11).   Neither the steam distillate nor a synthetic mixture of simple phenols at concentrations greater than those of the weak acid fraction were effective tumor-promoting stimuli in the assay system.   The residues remaining after steam distillation contain several long-chain fatty acids.   Holsti has shown that 20% oleic acid was an effective tumor-promoting stimulus in his system (20).   Substantially less of the fatty acids were present in our weak acid solutions, and insufficient dose-response data are available to establish whether the fatty acids might account for the activity of this fraction in our system. Experiments are currently under way in our laboratory to explore this possibility.

The most polar neutral fraction is being fractionated further by Swain et al.   It may be possible to identify the class of compounds that account for this activity in the near future.

The weakly polar active fraction has been studied extensively by Hoffmann and Wynder as their fraction B1.   A combination of solvent separations designed to concentrate BP, followed by extensive chromatographic separation, provided 80 subfractions, many of which exhibited significant tumor-initiating activity (19). The active subfractions contained a large variety of compounds that might be suspected to possess such activity.   It seems possible that in the weakly polar neutrals, a " most important single agent " may not exist, but rather that the fraction contains a large number of complete carcinogens that act both as very weak carcinogenic stimuli and as moderate tumor-initiating stimuli.

What happens when we assay various combinations of these active fractions? To answer this question, we felt it necessary to pool the BP fraction together with the other fractions that appeared close to it in the silicic acid eluates.   This eliminated the possibility that two fractions containing the same active agents would be considered qualitatively different.   We thus were left with three completely different active materials: the weak acid fraction, which is primarily a tumor-promoting stimulus; the most polar neutral fraction, apparently a tumor-promoting stimulus only; and a weakly polar neutral fraction, which is a complete carcinogenic stimulus. These three fractions were tested alone and in various combinations in DMBA-treated mice.

When we added the weak acids to the weakly polar neutrals, the combination was much more potent than either fraction alone (Table 2).   In contrast, when the most polar neutrals were added to either of the weak acids or the weakly polar neutrals, the combination was no more active than the weak acids alone or the weakly polar neutrals alone.   The combination of all three agents was no more active than the combination of the weak acids with the weakly polar neutrals alone.

TABLE 2.   Summation of Fractions of CSC

Sample[a]	Number of mice with tumors at CSC equivalent dose (%)[b]		
	15	30	60
Crude CSC	36	19	
Total neutrals		18	29
WA		4	17
WPN		19	31
MPN		3	7
WA+WPN		32	44
WA+MPN		10	18
MPN+WPN		15	34
WA+WPN+MPN		30	42

[a]   CSC, cigarette smoke condensate;   WA, weak acids;   WPN, weakly polar neutrals;   MPN, most polar neutrals.

[b]   43 weeks, 50 mice per group.

Nakahara (21) and Berenblum (3) have discussed many possible interrelationships among carcinogenic stimuli.   The present data illustrate again the fact that complex interrelationships, even of agents within a single carcinogenic stimulus, may be critical in determining its activity.   We must ask ourselves whether it is important to identify and eliminate the MPN from cigarette smoke, or whether we should concentrate our attention on the weak acids and the weakly polar neutral fraction.   Certainly, if we wish to make cigarette smoke less hazardous for mice, we should do so.   Nevertheless, since we dare not rely completely on mouse skin assays, we must also study the most polar neutrals until we understand more completely their possible role in human disease.

What sort of results might we expect when the tars from two different types of cigarettes are compared?   Let us assume that CSC contains a combination of very weak carcinogenic stimuli and moderate tumor-promoting stimuli.   Under these conditions, if the amount of complete carcinogens is decreased, there ought to be a commensurate reduction in tumor incidence throughout the experiment.   If only the amount of tumor promoters is decreased, we might see a reduction in the tumor incidence early in the experiment, when the effect of promoters ought to be predominant.   This might then be followed by a normal rate of appearance of new tumors in the late stages of the experiment, when the level of complete carcinogens should play a more substantial role.   We have seen this type of result in two series of experiments (Fig. 1).   We know that the level of benzo[a]pyrene is the same in the two condensates;   but we cannot confirm our hypothesis by analysis of the tumor-promoting agents in the CSC, inasmuch as they remain unknown.

Accordingly, we have attempted to set up a model CSC solution containing both a complete carcinogen with initiating activity equal to that of CSC, and a tumor promoter with promoting activity equal to that of CSC.   Preliminary assays indicated that 30% CSC was equivalent to about 20 μg/ml BP as a tumor initiator.   Likewise, 30% CSC appeared to be equivalent to 1.3 μg/ml PMA as a tumor-promoting agent.

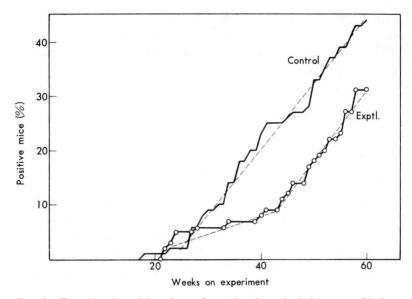

FIG. 1. Tumorigenic activity of experimental and standard cigarettes. Similar curves were obtained in two different experiments with a total of three experimental groups. Each group consisted of 100 mice painted 10 times a week with the heptane-soluble portion of the smoke condensate.

Under the circumstances, we prepared a solution of these two compounds at those levels, together with a series of solutions with reduced concentrations of the two co-carcinogens. Berenblum reported many years ago that concurrent administration of croton oil enhanced the tumorigenic activity of BP solutions (2), but his doses were many times higher than those we found to be comparable to CSC. We hoped to learn what might happen in conventional mouse skin assays if we should compare two types of CSC differing in concentration of either complete carcinogens or tumor-promoting agents. Unfortunately, the combination of BP and PMA was much more

TABLE 3. Tumorigenic Activity of Mixtures of BP and PMA

Test solution		N	20 Weeks		35 Weeks	
			Positive (%)	Tumor yield	Positive (%)	Tumor yield
30% CSC			0	0	6	0.6
BP	PMA					
(μg/ml)						
20	1.33	282	81	5.6		
20	0.67	281	19	0.6		
20	0.33	264	8	0.2	67	—
20	0.17	264	0.5	0.005	32	—
10	1.33	281	43	1.3		
10	0.67	280	14	0.2		
10	0.33	264	1	0.01	23	0.46
10	0.17	264	0	0	7	0.10

active than CSC, and our dosages were too high to be useful for this purpose.   Indeed, it appears that CSC is best mimicked by a solution containing 10 μg of BP and
0.17 μg of PMA per ml, *i.e.*, about one-half as much BP and one-fourth as much
PMA as is equivalent to CSC when tested separately (Table 3).   Clearly, the activity of CSC is not a simple summation of an initiating stimulus and a promoting
stimulus.

The behavior of the combined carcinogens of crude CSC in mouse skin is far different from what we could predict by adding the effects of its individual components
—even with the two-stage hypothesis of carcinogenesis.   On extrapolating from
mouse skin to human lung, differences in the biochemical responses of the species and
organs and differences in the penetration of various agents to and into target cells
make laboratory analysis of CSC tenuous indeed.   Does this mean that we have no
rational way to develop less hazardous cigarettes other than by simple filtration?
Not at all.   It does imply, however, that animal studies can only provide candidates
for further evaluation.   Cigarettes providing smoke less hazardous to mouse skin
should be developed in increasing numbers during this decade (*31*).   We would do
well to establish a human monitoring system that can evaluate these cigarettes as
soon as possible.

Extracts of Unburned Tobacco

It has been apparent for some time that the chewing of tobacco is associated
with oral cancer in man (*28*).   To develop a laboratory model for studying this
process, we extracted cigarette tobacco with aqueous barium hydroxide.   When
freed of the barium ion and neutralized, these extracts exhibited tumor-promoting
activity (*7*).   Although the total activity per cigarette was high, the solutions that
could be achieved were only moderate tumor-promoting stimuli.   They contained
0.6–0.8 g of solids per ml.   With half this concentration, the activity dropped below the level that could be detected consistently.   Higher concentrations of crude
extract are impossible.   It has thus been impossible to determine whether the extracts contained complete carcinogens or only tumor promoters.   To study the
process adequately, it was necessary to fractionate the extracts so that the active
agents could be applied in a more concentrated form.

The separations proved to be quite complex.   We first separated the extract
into one fraction with molecular weight greater than 1,200 and a second with molecular weight smaller than 1,200.   Neither fraction was active alone; but when the
two were recombined proportionately, the starting activity was recovered in full.
When the crude extract was separated according to solubility in 80% methanol,
both the methanol-soluble and methanol-insoluble fractions were inactive (*4*).
Again, when the two inactive fractions were recombined, the starting activity was
recovered.

The methanol-insoluble fraction was subjected to gel filtration, providing a
large-molecule fraction (m.w. > 1,200) and a small-molecule fraction (m.w. < 1200).
A combination of the large-molecule methanol-insoluble fraction with the methanol-
soluble fraction was active.   The large-molecule component comprised approxi-

TABLE 4.   Activity of Fractions of Tobacco Extracts

Test solution	Number of mice	Mice with tumors[a]	
		Number	%
DMBA+H$_2$O	40	0	0
DMBA+C. R.	40	23	58
L+3 bases	28	3	11
L+1 base	40	3	8
L+3 (acids+water-soluble neutrals)	40	0	0
L+1 (acids+water-soluble neutrals)	40	1	3
L+3 (butanol-soluble neutrals)	40	0	0
L+1 (butanol-soluble neutrals)	40	0	0
L+3 (butanol-soluble acids)	39	0	0
L+1 (butanol-soluble acids)	40	0	0
L+3 (water-soluble acids)	39	1	3
L+1 (water-soluble acids)	40	0	0

[a] 23 weeks.

mately 6% of the total weight of the extract; the methanol-soluble fraction comprised about 53% of the weight and all of the nicotine from the crude extract. Preliminary follow-up study of the methanol-soluble active component indicates that the active material is soluble in a mixture of benzene and methanol, and appears to be a basic compound (Table 4).   It thus appears with nicotine in its most refined state.   Nicotine itself, however, does not appear to be identical with the active agent.

As a result of a number of experiments, we have arrived at further tentative conclusions regarding the nature of the two active constituents.   The component of high molecular weight appears to be present in excess in commercial cigarette tobacco.   At least one of the components appears to be irreversibly precipitated by either strong acid or strong base, or else it is irreversibly bound to strong ion-exchange resins (8).   At least one of the agents, probably the fraction of high molecular weight, is introduced into the tobacco leaf during the process of curing (5).

These conclusions are consistent with the hypothesis that the agent of high molecular weight comprises tobacco pigments, polymeric materials that are often acidic. Whether this hypothesis is correct can be decided only when the respective fractions have been identified more fully.   We must also wait until the nicotine has been successfully removed from the methanol-soluble material before we can determine whether that fraction is a complete carcinogenic stimulus or a tumor-promoting stimulus, or whether it requires the fraction of high molecular weight even to function as a tumor-promoting stimulus.

We can, however, conclude that, like CSC, crude extracts of unburned tobacco owe their activity to combinations of weak stimuli that collectively behave differently than by simple addition of their separate activities.   In both cases, identification of individual components of the carcinogenic stimulus can be only a first step in understanding and preventing the tumorigenic effect.   A knowledge of how the components act in combination is essential.

Combinations of potential carcinogenic stimuli should also be considered as a cause for other environmental cancers.   Of all species, man is exposed to the greatest combinations of environmental stimuli. Assuming that tumor promotion by tobacco extracts does not depend on nicotine, do edible plant products contain the same agents or similar agents? Could one active agent be present in one food-stuff, and the other in a second? Under these circumstances, conventional laboratory assays of individual foods, either for carcinogenic activity or for tumor-promoting activity, would fail. Only bioassay of total diets would suffice. It is becoming apparent that we cannot adequately study these stimuli in isolated laboratory systems.

REFERENCES

1. Bair, W. J. Inhalation of Radionuclides and Carcinogenesis. *In*; Hanna, M. G., Jr., Nettesheim, P., and Gilbert, J. R. (ed.), Inhalation Carcinogenesis, pp. 77–101, USAEC Div. of Tech. Inform., Oak Ridge, Tenn., 1970.

2. Berenblum, I. The Cocarcinogenic Action of Croton Resin. Cancer Res., *1*: 44–48, 1941.

3. Berenblum, I. A Re-evaluation of the Concept of Cocarcinogenesis. Progr. Exptl. Tumor Res., *11*: 21–30, 1969.

4. Bock, F. G. The Nature of Tumor-Promoting Agents in Tobacco Products. Cancer Res., *28*: 2363–2368, 1968.

5. Bock, F. G. Tumor-Promoting Activity of Tobacco Extracts. J. Indian Med. Profes., *17*: 7561–7564, 1970.

6. Bock, F. G., and Moore, G. E. The Significance of Mouse Skin Tests of Cigarette Smoke Condensate. *In*; James, G. and Rosenthal, T. (ed.), Tobacco and Health, pp. 72–86, Springfield, Illinois, 1962.

7. Bock, F. G., Moore, G. E., and Crouch, S. K. Tumor-Promoting Activity of Extracts of Unburned Tobacco. Science, *145*: 831–833, 1964.

8. Bock, F. G., Shamberger, R. J., and Myers, H. K. Tumour-Promoting Agents in Unburned Cigarette Tobacco. Nature, *208*: 584–585, 1965.

9. Bock, F. G., Swain, A. P., and Stedman, R. L. Bioassay of Major Fractions of Cigarette Smoke Condensate by an Accelerated Technic. Cancer Res., *29*: 584–587, 1969.

10. Bock, F. G., Swain A. P., and Stedman, R. L. Composition Studies on Tobacco. XLI. Carcinogenesis Assay of Subfractions of the Neutral Fraction of Cigarette Smoke Condensate. J. Natl. Cancer Inst., *44*: 1305–1310, 1970.

11. Bock, F. G., Swain, A. P., and Stedman, R. L. Composition Studies on Tobacco. XLIV. Tumor-Promoting Activity of Subfractions of the Weak Acid Fraction of Cigarette Smoke Condensate. J. Natl. Cancer Inst., *47*: 429–436, 1971.

12. Bock, F. G., Swain, A. P., and Stedman, R. L. Unpublished.

13. Bock, F. G., Swain, A. P., and Stedman, R. L. Unpublished.

14. Dean, G. Lung Cancer Among White South Africans. Brit. Med. J., *2*: 852–859, 1959.

15. Dean, G. Lung Cancer in Australia. Med. J. Australia, *1*: 1003–1006, 1962.

16. Doll, R. Interpretations of Epidemiologic Data. Cancer Res., *23*: 1613–1623, 1963.

17. Dontenwill, W., Elmenhorst, H., Harke, H. P. Reckzeh, G., und Weber, K. H. Experimentelle Untersuchungen über die tumorerzeugende Wirkung von Zigarettenrauch-Kondensaten an der Mäusehaut. Z. Krebsforsch., *73*: 305–314, 1970.

18. Eastcott, D. F. The Epidemiology of Lung Cancer in New Zealand. Lancet, *1*: 37–39, 1956.
19. Hoffmann, D., and Wynder, E. L. A Study of Tobacco Carcinogenesis. XI. Tumor Initiators, Tumor Accelerators, and Tumor Promoting Activity of Condensate Fractions. Cancer, *27*: 848–864, 1971.
20. Holsti, P. Tumor Promoting Effects of Some Long Chain Fatty Acids in Experimental Skin Carcinogenesis in the Mouse. Acta Path. Microbiol. Scand., *46*: 51–58, 1959.
21. Nakahara, W. Critique of Carcinogenic Mechanism. Progr. Exptl. Tumor Res., *2*: 158–202, 1961.
22. Poel, W. E. Study of Methods for Abbreviating Carcinogenicity Bioassays. I. Enhancement of Neoplastic Response by Pretreating with a Potent Carcinogen. J. Natl. Cancer Inst., *25*: 1265–1277, 1960.
23. Royal College of Physicians. Air Pollution and Health, Pitman Medical and Scientific Publishing Co. Ltd., 1970.
24. Selikoff, I. J., Hammond, E. C., and Churg, J. Asbestos Exposure, Smoking, and Neoplasia. J. Amer. Med. Assoc., *204*: 106–112, 1968.
25. Swain, A. P., Cooper, J. E., and Stedman, R. L. Large Scale Fractionation of Cigarette Smoke Condensate for Chemical and Biologic Investigations. Cancer Res., *29*: 579–583, 1969.
26. Swain, A. P., Cooper, J. E., Stedman, R. L., and Bock F. G. Composition Studies on Tobacco. XL. Large Scale Fractionation of the Neutrals of Cigarette Smoke Condensate Using Adsorption Chromatography and Solvent Partitioning. Beiträge zur Tabakforsch., *5*: 109–114, 1969.
27. Takayama S. Carcinogenic Effect of Cigarette Tar Using Newborn ICR Mice. Gann, *61*: 297–298, 1970.
28. U. S. Public Health Service. The Health Consequences of Smoking. A Report of the Surgeon General, Washington, D.C., 1971.
29. Whitehead, J. K., and Rothwell, K. The Mouse Skin Carcinogenicity of Cigarette Smoke Condensate. Fractionated by Solvent Partition Methods. Brit. J. Cancer, *23*: 840–857, 1969.
30. Wynder, E. L., and Hoffmann, D. Tobacco and Tobacco Smoke; Studies in Experimental Carcinogenesis, Academic Press, Inc., New York, 1967.
31. Wynder, E. L., and Hoffmann, D. Less Harmful Ways of Smoking. J. Natl. Cancer Inst., In press.
32. Wynder, E. L., and Wright, G. A Study of Tobacco Carcinogenesis. I. The Primary Fractions. Cancer, *10*: 255–271, 1957.

Discussion of Paper by Dr. Bock

DR. HOSHINO: I'd like to ask you something about terminology.   Although you have proved the carcinogenicity of 30% CSC solution, you called it a low dose level promoter.   Therefore, it appears to me very confusing that the same substance was called by two different terms in the very same area of carcinogenesis.   These two terms, carcinogen and promoter, had been applied originally to two substances completely different in quality.   What do you think?

DR. BOCK: I like to distinguish between carcinogen and carcinogenic stimuli and tumor-promoting stimuli.   A carcinogen can act both as a carcinogenic stimulus or a tumor-promoting stimulus depending on the circumstances.   I apologize for lapses in terminology during my presentation.

DR. DRUCKREY: What was the proportion of carcinomas among the observed tumors?

DR. BOCK: Among the tobacco extract experiments, nearly every tumor was benign.   Among the mice treated with CSC fractions, there was a substantial number of carcinomas, generally in 10–25% of all positive animals.   Also there was a difference in the durations of the experiments.   The tobacco extract experiments lasted about six months, the CSC studies, more than a year.

DR. NAKAHARA: Carcinogenic phenomena include two fundamentally different biological processes.   One is that of cell cancerization, the process of normal cells being altered into cancer cells.   The other is the cell proliferation process.   With strong carcinogens you have both processes.   Weak carcinogens may not show tumor formation by themselves.   Initiators and promotors are merely phenomenological terms and do not refer to chemical entities.

When people speak of " initiation " and " promotion " I take them to mean the process of cell cancerization and cell proliferation, respectively.   If I am correct in this interpretation, I would expect that there are " initiating " and " promoting " substances—two different substances.   Could Dr. Bock, or anyone else, point out a promoter without carcinogenicity, or an initiator which only cancerizes normal cells without producing tumors?

Any organic chemist would expect the existence of two different substances, when he hears of " initiator " and " promoter."

Perhaps agreement can be reached if we use the terms simply in the convenient phenomenological sense, without any chemical basis whatever.   Otherwise, we have to face the contradiction of calling one and the same substance a powerful carcinogen (with " initiating " and " promoting " action) and a mere promoter when highly diluted.

DR. BOCK: I agree.   I think the problem of terminology is a serious one but I don't like to have so rigid a definition that it limits our consideration of the processes involved.   Therefore, I prefer the use of the term stimulus to refer to a process in an exposed population.

DR. WEISBERGER: I agree with the views presented by Professor Nakahara and Dr. Hoshino as well as Dr. Bock relative to detection of weak carcinogenic stimuli. However, distinction between promoters and initiators, while of theoretical interest, is of limited practical value in the light of human data.   Perhaps cell culture as discussed by Professor Katsuta will be useful to distinguish initators and promoters.

The human data do not worry about semantic problems.   It is important to detect weak stimuli to protect man.

DR. LAWLEY: Some German workers have reported alkylating activity in cigarette smoke condensates.   I wondered if you would care to comment on the possible significance of reactive compounds of this sort, which might be lost in your fractionation procedures.

DR. BOCK: Cigarette smoke is so complex that it would not surprise me if any type of carcinogen were found in it—assuming an analyst was prepared to spend a year or so on the search.   The critical question is how much is present and what its effect in the mixture represented by smoke might be.   Certainly, for mouse skin, the less stable carcinogens of smoke are not an important carcinogenic stimulus.   It is almost a theological question.   Do you believe that we should eliminate the mouse skin carcinogens or do you believe we should eliminate all strong carcinogens even if we cannot demonstrate they have any effect at the concentrations involved?

In vitro Studies on the Role of Epoxides in Carcinogenic Hydrocarbon Activation

Charles HEIDELBERGER

McArdle Laboratory for Cancer Research, Medical School, University of Wisconsin, Madison, Wisconsin, U.S.A.

It is a great honor to have been invited to participate in this symposium of the Princess Takamatsu Fund for Cancer Research, and to have the opportunity to renew my friendship with many colleagues from Japan and other countries. It is particularly appropriate that a symposium on chemical carcinogenesis should be held in Japan, the country where this subject had its birth and where so many distinguished contributions have been made. Among the leaders in these contributions is Professor Nakahara, the honorary chairman of this symposium.

For about 25 years I have been interested in the cellular and molecular mechanisms by which polycyclic aromatic hydrocarbons initiate the complicated and deadly process of carcinogenesis (*11, 12*). My colleagues and I have done much work on the interactions of labeled carcinogenic hydrocarbons with the DNA, RNA, and proteins of mouse skin. However, I became impressed with the limitations of working in whole animals and the necessity of freeing myself from this constraint. Accordingly, I set out to develop a system for studying chemical carcinogenesis *in vitro*. The lead I chose to follow came from the work of Lasnitski, and I spent an enjoyable and fruitful sabbatical in her laboratory in England. She grows mouse ventral prostate pieces in organ culture and upon the addition of carcinogenic hydrocarbons obtains histological changes suggestive of malignancy (*16*). However, such morphologically altered cultures did not induce tumors upon inoculation into isologous mice, as Dr. Röller and I found to our disappointment (*21*). But when these treated pieces were dispersed and put into cell culture, Dr. Iype and I obtained cell lines that did produce tumors in C3H mice (*13*).

When Dr. T. T. Chen joined my laboratory, he succeeded in culturing fibroblastic cells derived from C3H mouse prostates. These cells were not malignant and showed a very low incidence of spontaneous malignant transformation (*3*). When methylcholanthrene was added to such cells their growth characteristics changed, and at the same time they acquired the property of giving highly malignant

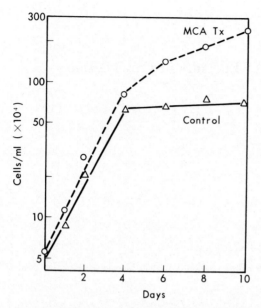

FIG. 1.   Saturation densities of control and MCA-transformed mouse prostate cells (4).

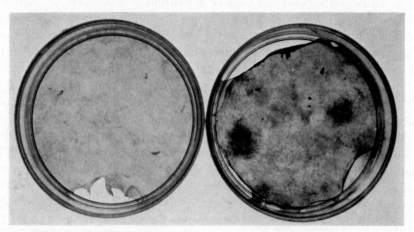

FIG. 2.   Fixed and stained dishes of mouse prostate cells after they have reached confluence. Control cells are on the left.   MCA-treated cells are on the right (5).

fibrosarcomas on injection into C3H mice (4).   The control nonmalignant cells grow until they reach a monolayer and then stop, as shown in Fig. 1, whereas the transformed malignant cells continue to grow after reaching a monolayer and have a higher saturation density.   Figure 2 shows the appearance of dishes of fixed and stained control cells on the left, and foci of piled-up transformed cells on the right. A high-power view of a fixed and stained control culture is shown in Fig. 3; note that there is only one layer of cells.   Figure 4 shows the edge of a piled-up colony of cells so thick that it is out of focus.   It then became necessary to find out whether the individual transformed foci could give rise to tumors on inoculation into mice.   The

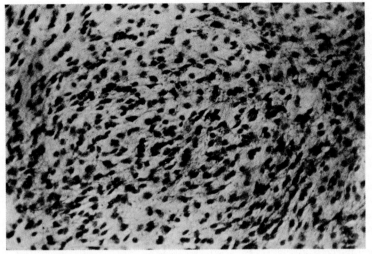

FIG. 3.   High-power view of fixed and stained confluent control cells (5).

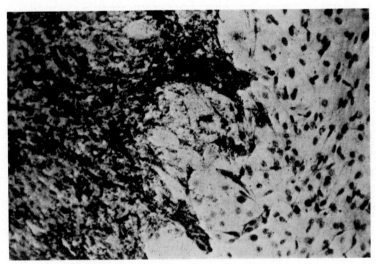

FIG. 4.   High-power view of the edge of a transformed colony (5).

TABLE 1.   The Production of Tumors in C3H Mice by Individual Piled-up Colonies in a Single Dish (5)

Area isolated	Number of cells inoculated/ mouse	Number of mice	Duration of observation (days)	Times of tumor appearance (days)	Number of tumors
Monolayer	1,000	4	150	—	0
Colony 1	500	3	60	30–60	3
Colony 2	500	3	60	30	1
Colony 3	500	3	60	30	1
Colony 4	500	3	60	30	1
Colony 5	500	3	60	30–60	2
Colony 6	500	3	60	30–60	2
Monolayer	1.000	3	150	—	0

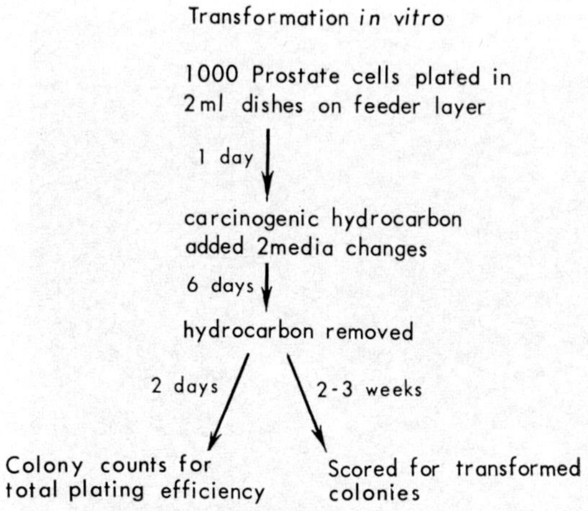

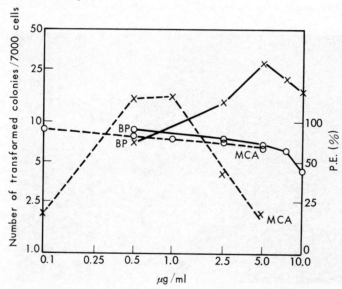

Transformation *in vitro*

1000 Prostate cells plated in
2 ml dishes on feeder layer

1 day

carcinogenic hydrocarbon
added 2 media changes

6 days

hydrocarbon removed

2 days   2-3 weeks

Colony counts for   Scored for transformed
total plating efficiency   colonies

FIG. 5.   Experimental set-up for quantitative studies of cytotoxicity and malignant transformation in mouse prostate cells.

FIG. 6.   Number of transformed colonies (×) and toxicity (○) produced by MCA and BP in mouse prostate cells (5).

experiment in Table 1 shows that 6 piled-up colonies from a single dish gave tumors in mice, whereas cells from the monolayer areas between the transformed colonies did not (5).   Therefore, we are fully justified in equating morphological transformation with malignant transformation.

The system was now ready to be made quantitative.   As shown in Fig. 5, 1,000 cells are plated in a dish and treated for one or six days with a carcinogenic hydrocarbon.   Two days after removal of the carcinogen, some of the dishes are fixed and stained to determine the plating efficiency, which is a measure of toxicity.   The other dishes are cultured until they become confluent and pile up; the number of piled-up transformed colonies is then counted.   The results of dose-response curves with methylcholanthrene (MCA) and benzpyrene (BP) are shown in Fig. 6.   Each compound produced an optimal frequency of transformation at a dose above which the transformation frequency decreased.   This, as can be seen from the lines with circles, was not due to toxicity, and the shapes of the curves show clearly that toxicity and malignant transformation are different processes.   A number of other carcinogenic and noncarcinogenic hydrocarbons were tested in the same way.   We found that there was an excellent correlation between the carcinogenic activity of a hydrocarbon and the frequency of transformed colonies it produced in this system (5).   Thus, in this sense, the model system appears to be related to the real world of *in vivo* chemical carcinogenesis.

Dr. Mondal then joined my laboratory from India and developed an elegant technique to obtain single individual prostate cells in separate dishes.   These single cells grew into clones, as shown in Table 2, with 72% efficiency.   When these cells grew to confluency and were allowed to pile up, there was a 5% incidence of spontaneous transformation in the solvent control clones.   However, at concentrations of MCA that produced no toxicity (as indicated by the cloning efficiency), 100% of the carcinogen-treated clones gave rise to transformed colonies in the dishes and to tumors in the mice (18).   This is an extraordinarily high efficiency of transformation and eliminates, at least in this system, a cellular mechanism of carcinogenesis that postulated a selection of pre-existing malignant cells.   Consequently, the chemical directly transforms nonmalignant into malignant cells.   Whether the chemical activates a latent oncogenic virus or its informational precursors or does the job of

TABLE 2.   Toxicity and Transformation Produced by MCA in Individual Single Cells (18)

Treatment	Cloning efficiency		Transformation	
0.5% Dimethyl sulfoxide, 6 days	18/25	72%	1/18	5.5%
MCA, 0.25 μg/ml, 6 days	6/10	60	2/6	33
MCA, 0.50 μg/ml, 6 days	9/14	64	8/9	88
MCA, 1.0 μg/ml, 6 days	26/36	72	26/26	100
MCA, 1.0 μg/ml, 1 day	13/21	62	13/13	100
MCA, 2.5 μg/ml, 6 days	11/16	68	11/11	100
MCA, 5.0 μg/ml, 6 days	12/22	55	8/12	67
MCA, 10.0 μg/ml, 6 days	12/28	43	8/12	67
MCA, 10.0 μg/ml, 1 day	11/25	44	8/11	72

Individual single cell
   ↓ MCA 1 mg/ml, 1 day
   ↓ 36 days
No piled-up colonies
Plate 400 cells in 10 dishes
   | 8 days
36 Clones isolated

33 Clones grown successfully

FIG. 7.   Recloning experiment (18).

carcinogenesis by itself is currently under study. We then inquired whether all the progeny of the single cell in the dish were transformed. The experiment shown in Fig. 7 was designed to answer this question. An individual single cell in a dish was treated for one day with MCA. After 36 days, when no piled-up colonies were evident, 400 cells were picked at random and plated in 10 dishes. Eight days later 36 colonies derived from single cells were isolated, of which 33 grew successfully. After some time, which was variable, all 33 clones gave rise to piled-up colonies. Thus, this recloning experiment proves that all of the progeny of the MCA-treated individual single cells became transformed, although at somewhat different rates.

It is well known that chemically induced tumors have characteristic antigens on the surface of the cells, and that these are individual and not cross-reacting. Dr. Mondal and I wished to determine whether the same situation obtains in our *in vitro* system. As shown in Table 3, 14 of 17 clones isolated from individual transformed

TABLE 3. Summary of the Immunological Studies of Individual
Chemically Transformed Clones of Mouse Prostate Cells *(19)*

17 Clones tested for immunogenicity.
    14 Antigenic, 1 non-antigenic, 2 uncertain.
 7 Pairs of antigenic clones from the same dish tested
    reciprocally for cross-reactivity.
        0 cross-reactive.
 3 Antigenic clones derived from 3 different dishes
    tested reciprocally for cross-reactivity.
        0 cross-reactive.

colonies were antigenic in transplantation tests; when 7 pairs of such clones from the same dish were tested reciprocally, no pairs were cross-reactive *(19)*. Therefore, the *in vitro* system behaves exactly analogously in this respect to the chemically induced tumors in mice, and gives us additional confidence in the validity of this model system. Dr. Mondal was also able to select, from highly malignant clones, variants of much lesser malignancy. These variants, Dr. M. J. Embleton found, have also lost their surface tumor-specific antigens.

I now wish to consider certain important metabolic aspects of hydrocarbon carcinogenesis. In recent years the concept has arisen, largely from the work of the Millers at the University of Wisconsin *(17)*, that compounds, in order to be active as carcinogens, must be chemically reactive as electrophiles. Although a few active carcinogens, such as the nitrosoureas, are chemically reactive, the majority of them are not and must be converted by metabolism in the target tissue or cells into a chemically reactive and ultimately carcinogenic form. The Millers have elucidated the chemistry of this process for several series of aromatic amine hepatocarcinogens *(17)*, but the nature of the chemical activation of carcinogenic hydrocarbons was unknown.

The initial stages in the metabolism of a typical aromatic hydrocarbon, benzanthracene, are shown in Fig. 8. It has been known for a long time that compounds such as this are converted into phenols, *trans*-dihydrodiols, and glutathione conjugates. In 1950 Boyland postulated that an epoxide might be the intermediate

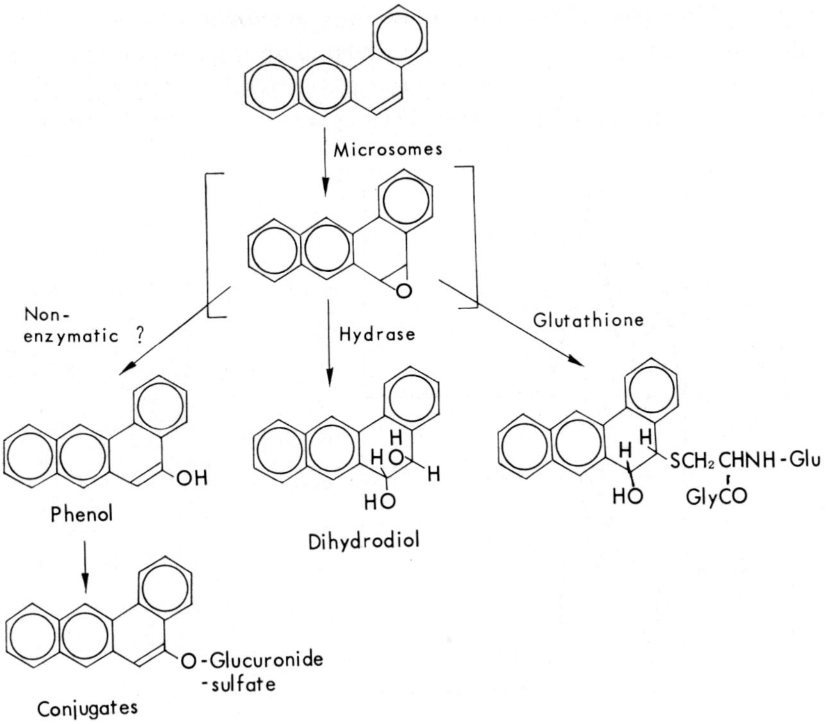

FIG. 8.   Sheme of the metabolism of benzanthracene.

in such metabolism (2).   However, when epoxides of carcinogenic hydrocarbons were tested for their ability to induce tumors in mice, they were found to be much less active than the parent hydrocarbons and hence were considered not to be the carcinogenically active metabolites.   More recently, however, Grover and Sims found that K-region epoxides of several hydrocarbons could bind with DNA and proteins in the test tube (9) and in cells in culture (8).   However, because of their great chemical reactivity, epoxides had not been isolated or shown to be produced from polycyclic hydrocarbons by metabolism.

Selkirk, Huberman, and I thought that such an isolation might be possible if we used the microsomal drug-metabolizing system that is known to hydroxylate such compounds.   The experiment we performed is shown in Fig. 9.   Radioactive dibenzanthracene (DBA) was incubated with rat liver microsomes in the presence of a large amount of nonradioactive DBA-epoxide for 5 min and rapidly extracted; the extract was quickly subjected to thin-layer chromatography.   As shown in part a, there was a nonradioactive spot of epoxide, and the radioactivity was found to be present as unchanged DBA and as phenols and dihydrodiols at the origin.   However, when the microsomes were heated at 55°C for 5 min in order to inhibit epoxide hydrase activity, incubation similar to that described above gave rise to a radioactive peak on the chromatogram that coincided with the nonlabeled epoxide (curve b).   When another aliquot of the extract from that incubation was treated with acid, the epoxide peak was converted into a phenol, a reaction that proves that the radioactivity in the epoxide region actually was an epoxide (curve c) (*22*). Thus, we have demonstrated that an epoxide is formed as an intermediate in the microsomal oxidation of an active carcinogenic hydrocarbon, DBA. It remained to determine whether an epoxide is the ultimately carcinogenic form of the hydrocarbon.

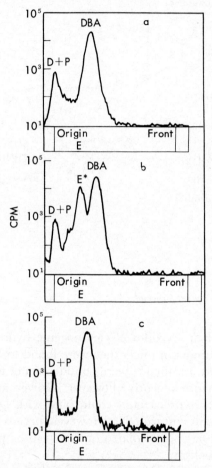

FIG. 9. Demonstration of an epoxide as an intermediate in the microsomal metabolism of DBA. See text for details (*22*).

Hamster embryo cells
  Primary or secondary
  500 or 5000 cells plated on feeder layer
  | 1 day
Treat with test compound
  | 7 day
  Fix and stain
  Score for plating efficiency and
  transformation of individual colonies

FIG. 10. Experimental set-up for quantitative transformation of hamster embryo cells in culture.

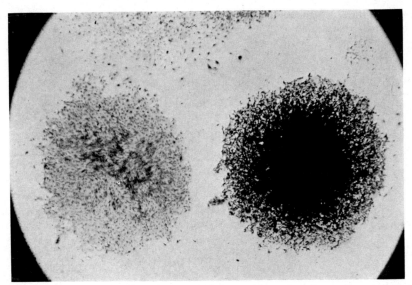

FIG. 11.   Morphology of fixed and stained colonies of hamster embryo cells.   A normal colony
is on the left, and a transformed colony is on the right.

I must now digress for a moment and describe the other system that has been
used for the quantitative study of chemical carcinogenesis *in vitro*.   This system was
first developed by Berwald and Sachs in 1965 (*1*) and its use extended by Huberman
and Sachs (*15*).   Dr. Huberman took leave from the Weizmann Institute in Israel
and spent two very productive years in my laboratory.   His system involves the use
of embryonic hamster cells, and the experimental set-up is shown in Fig. 10.   A small
number of hamster embryonic cells are plated on a feeder layer of irradiated rat cells.
One day later, the cells are treated with the test compound for seven days, and the
dishes are fixed and stained and scored for plating efficiency as a measure of toxicity,
and individual colonies are scored for transformation.   As shown in Fig. 11, a normal
colony on the left remains quite flat, whereas a transformed colony on the right piles
up to a thick mass and exhibits a characteristic criss-cross pattern of cells on the
edges of the colony.   Such morphologically transformed colonies have been picked
and shown to be malignant by the production of tumors on inoculation into hamsters
(*7*).

The hamster system has some advantages over the mouse prostate cell system in
that the cells are diploid and transformation can be scored in a shorter period of
time.   The mouse prostate cell system has the advantages that the nonmalignant
cells form permanent lines so that clones of malignant and nonmalignant cells can be
compared.

Dr. Huberman and I then compared in the hamster cell system, in collaboration
with Grover and Sims, several hydrocarbons and their K-region epoxides, *cis*-dihy-
drodiols, and phenols.   Representative data with the benzanthracene series are
shown in Table 4.   BA, which is a very weakly carcinogenic compound, produced
an insignificant incidence of toxicity and transformation.   Its epoxide, however,
did produce toxicity, but also a high level of transformation.   As shown in Table 5,

TABLE 4. Toxicity and Transformation Produced in Hamster Embryo Cells by BA and Its Epoxide *(10)*

Compound	Dose (μg/ml)	Total colonies	P. E. %	Transformed Colonies	
				Number	%
Control		818	18.2	0	0
BA	1.0	893	16.2	2	0.2
,,	2.5	1039	19.0	2	0.2
,,	5.0	1140	22.8	0	0
BA-epoxide	1.0	1082	19.6	3	0.3
,,	2.5	565	10.2	37	6.9
,,	5.0	0	0	—	—

TABLE 5. Toxicity and Transformation Produced in Hamster Embryo Cells by the Phenol and *cis*-Dihydrodiol of BA *(10)*

Compound	Dose (μg/ml)	Total colonies	P. E. %	Transformed Colonies	
				Number	%
Control		818	18.2	0	0
BA-diol	1.0	1320	22.0	3	0.2
,,	2.5	867	15.6	10	1.2
,,	5.0	596	12.0	39	6.5
BA-phenol	1.0	1161	21.2	3	0.3
,,	2.5	272	5.7	3	1.1
,,	5.0	0	0	—	—

TABLE 6. Transformation and Toxicity to Mouse Prostate Cells Produced by MNNG, MCA, BA, and Their Epoxides *(10)*

Compound	Dose (μg/ml)	Relative P. E.		Number of transformed colonies/dishes	
		1	2	1	2
Control	0.5% DMSO	100	100	0/5 (0)	0/7 (0)
MNNG	0.05		81		3/8 (0.38)
,,	0.10		65		4/8 (0.50)
,,	0.15	13		11/10 (1.1)	
,,	0.20		3.4		0/7 (0)
,,	0.30	5		12/8 (1.5)	
,,	0.45	2.5		12/8 (1.5)	
MCA	1.5	82	100	1/4 (0.25)	0/9 (0)
,,	10.0	74	76	1/8 (0.12)	1/9 (0.11)
MCA-epoxide	0.75 (1$\times$)	47	89	8/7 (1.1)	11/8 (1.4)
,,	0.75 (2$\times$)	45		19/12 (1.6)	
,,	1.50 (1$\times$)	25	65	5/10 (0.5)	30/8 (3.8)
,,	1.50 (2$\times$)	25		22/8 (2.8)	
BA	1.0	61	100	0/5	0/8
,,	5.0	50	84	0/10	0/8
BA-epoxide	0.5	47	57	8/10 (0.8)	1/9 (0.1)
,,	1.0 (1$\times$)	13	24	7/9 (0.8)	2/8 (0.25)
,,	1.0 (2$\times$)	2.5		12/8 (1.5)	

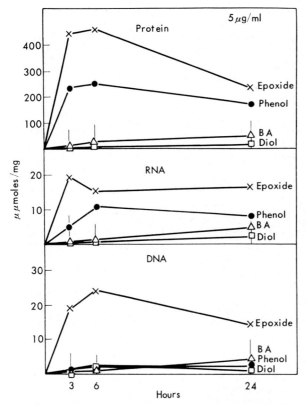

Fig. 12.   Binding of epoxide, phenol, and *cis*-dihydrodiols and benzanthracene to the DNA, RNA, and proteins of hamster embryo cells in culture.

the *cis*-dihydrodiol also produced some transformation, but was less active in other series of compounds.   The phenol was very toxic, but transformed to only a very slight extent (*10*).   Thus, with the possible exception of the *cis*-diol, which is not a metabolite (the *trans*-diol is), with BA, DBA, and MCA the epoxide was the most active compound at producing transformation in the hamster system.   Therefore, it might be considered to be eligible to be the metabolically activated form of the carcinogen.

Kuroki and I have studied the binding of labeled series of compounds to the DNA, RNA, and proteins of hamster embryo cells, as shown in Fig. 12.   In the benzanthracene series, the epoxide was bound to all three macromolecules to a much greater extent than the other derivatives, in accord with expectations based on its chemical reactivity and metabolic behavior.   This binding to DNA reached its maximum in 3 hr (Kuroki *et al.*, in preparation).

The abilities of the hydrocarbons and epoxides of MCA and BA to produce toxicity and transformation in the mouse prostate cells was studied by Dr. Marquardt, as shown in Table 6.   MNNG (methylnitrosoguanidine), which is carcinogenic and does not require metabolic activation, was included as a positive control.   The clone of prostate cells that we used metabolizes the hydrocarbons to

TABLE 7. Transformation and Toxicity in the Mouse Prostate Cell System Produced by MCA and Various *cis*- and *trans*-Dihydrodiols

	Dose (μg/ml)	P.E. (%)	Number of Tx colonies / Number dishes	Tx colonies per dish
DMSO	0.5%	22.5	0/9	0
MCA	10.0	20.5	4/8	0.50
MCA *cis*-diol	5.0	26.0	0/10	0
,,	10.0	28.0	0/9	0
MCA *trans*-diol	5.0	26.5	0/10	0
,,	10.0	27.0	1/10	0
BA *trans*-diol	5.0	26.5	0/10	0
,,	10.0	25.5	0/8	0
DBA *trans*-diol	5.0	25.0	0/10	0

TABLE 8. Toxicity and Transformation Produced by MCA in Induced and Noninduced Mouse Prostate Cells

Compounds	Dose (μg/ml)	P.E. (%)	Number of Tx colonies / Number dishes	Tx colonies per dish
No induction				
DMSO	0.5%	26.5	0/7	0
MCA	1.5	24.0	1/8	0.13
,,	10.0	24.0	4/8	0.50
Induction with BA (0.25 μg/ml)				
DMSO	0.5	26.5	0/7	0
MCA	1.5	21.5	8/7	1.1
,,	10.0	14.0	15/8	1.9
Induction with PPO (2.5 μg/ml)				
DMSO	0.5	26.0	0/7	0
MCA	1.5	21.0	11/6	1.8
,,	10.0	18.0	16/9	1.8

only a small extent; MCA produced a very low incidence of transformation, and BA produced no transformation. However, MNNG and both epoxides were very active at producing malignant transformation in this system, further emphasizing the likelihood that epoxides are the metabolically activated form of hydrocarbons (*10*).

When *trans*-dihydrodiols became available from Grover and Sims, they were tested in the prostate cells, as shown in Table 7. MCA produced some transformation in these experiments, but neither its *cis*- nor *trans*-dihydrodiols did. Moreover, the *trans*-diols of BA and DBA did not produce any transformation (Marquardt et al., in preparation). Thus, we conclude that the transformation produced by the nonmetabolic *cis*-diol in the hamster cells is an aberrant result, and that the epoxide is the most active of the compounds.

It is well known that prior treatment of cells with BA or diphenyloxazole (PPO) induces an increase in the activity of the microsomal drug-metabolizing enzymes (*20*). Since we have shown that the epoxide is produced metabolically by these enzymes, and since we believe that the carcinogenic hydrocarbons require metabolic

A: Cytotoxicity

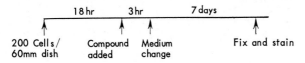

B: Mutagenesis

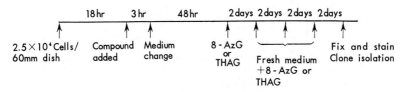

Fig. 13.   Protocol for mutagenesis experiments in Chinese hamster cells (*14*).

activation, we have tested the effect of such enzyme induction on the transformation produced by MCA in the mouse prostate system.   As shown in Table 8, a much higher frequency of transformation is produced by MCA in the induced cells.   This clearly demonstrates the necessity of metabolism for transformation (Marquardt *et al.*, in preparation).

Since the epoxides react with DNA, it became of interest to determine whether they are mutagenic.   In the past it has not been possible to develop a correlation between the mutagenic and carcinogenic activities of compounds.   The reason is that most of the test systems for studying mutagenesis involve the use of bacteria and bacteriophages, which usually do not metabolize carcinogens to their active forms.   Therefore, it seemed necessary to study the mutagenicity of these compounds in mammalian cells, and Dr. Huberman and I chose to use Chinese hamster cells, which have been developed as tools for studying mutagenesis by Chu and Malling (*6*).   The protocols of our experiments are shown in Fig. 13.   With each compound it is necessary to measure both cytotoxicity and mutagenicity.   The scheme for measuring cytotoxicity is standard and is shown in part A.   The cells were exposed to the test compound for only 3 hr.   For mutagenicity we and Chu (*6*) score for 8-azaguanine-resistance, which involves the loss of the enzyme inosinic-guanylic pyrophosphorylase, whose structural gene is probably located on the X chromosome.   In the mutagenesis tests (part B) a larger number of cells is plated.   Again the test compound is added for 3 hr, removed, the cells are allowed to grow for 48 hr, then 8-AzG is added every two days, and after 8 days of such treatment the dishes are fixed and stained, and the number of surviving colonies is counted.

The results of the experiments are shown in Fig. 14.   Again MNNG was used as a positive control, since it had been found to be highly mutagenic in these cells (*6*).   As far as cytotoxicity is concerned, MNNG was the most toxic compound, followed by the phenol (P) and then the epoxide (E) of benzanthracene.

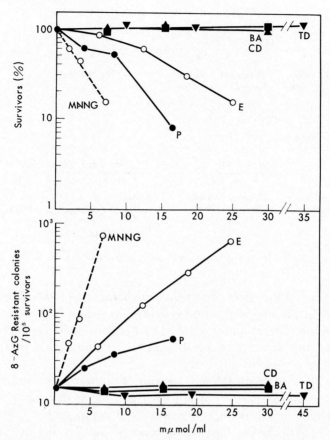

FIG. 14. Cytotoxicity and mutagenicity produced in Chinese hamster cells by MNNG and the benzanthracene series of compounds (14).

The hydrocarbon (BA) and the *cis*- and *trans*-dihydrodiols (CD and TD) exerted no toxicity to these cells. In the mutagenesis experiments, BA and the two diols were not mutagenic, the epoxide was highly mutagenic, and the phenol less so (14). Comparable results were obtained in the DBA and MCA series. It was further shown that viable 8-AzG-resistant clones could be obtained, which had the same number of chromosomes as the original clone, so that the mutations observed could not be due to a chromosomal deletion. Also, some of these clones could be back-mutated to 8-AzG sensitivity with the epoxide (14).

These findings prove that epoxides are mutagenic. They do not prove that they exert their carcinogenic activity by a mutagenic mechanism. Further studies are under way aimed at determining directly whether DNA is involved in the event(s) of malignant transformation.

We are also seeking to determine whether oncogenic viruses or their informational precursors are involved in chemical carcinogenesis; we are further studying the immunological characteristics of chemically and spontaneously transformed clones of cells; we are probing the cell-cycle characteristics of transformation; we are looking in further detail at the biochemical events essentially related to chemical carcinogenesis, and we are looking into the genetics of susceptibility to carcinogenesis by chemicals.

In summary, I have attempted to describe two systems in which studies of chemical carcinogenesis can be carried out in cultured cells.   These systems can be quantitated, and there is a tight correlation between morphological and malignant transformation.   There is an excellent quantitative correlation between the frequency of transformation produced by a compound *in vitro* and its *in vivo* carcinogenic activity.   The processes of toxicity and transformation are separate.   Studies with single cells have shown that carcinogenesis (at least in this system) does not involve the selection of pre-existing malignant cells.   Individual clones of chemically transformed cells have individually specific surface transplantation antigens.   An epoxide has been identified for the first time as an intermediate in the metabolism of a carcinogenic hydrocarbon.   Epoxides are much more active than the parent hydrocarbon, phenol, and *trans*-dihydrodiols at producing malignant transformation in both systems, and are very probably the metabolically activated and ultimately carcinogenic form of the polycyclic hydrocarbons.   Induction of the activity of the microsomal drug-metabolizing enzymes in these cells increases the frequency of transformation produced by carcinogenic hydrocarbons.   Finally, epoxides of polycyclic hydrocarbons are highly mutagenic to mammalian cells.

REFERENCES

1. Berwald, Y., and Sachs, L.   *In vitro* Transformation of Normal Cells to Tumor Cells by Carcinogenic Hydrocarbons.   J. Natl. Cancer Inst., *35*: 641, 1965.

2. Boyland, E.   The Biological Significance of Metabolism of Polycyclic Compounds. Symp. Biochem. Soc., *5*: 40, 1950.

3. Chen, T. T., and Heidelberger, C.   Cultivation *in vitro* of Cells Derived from Adult C3H Mouse Ventral Prostate.   J. Natl. Cancer Inst., *42*: 903, 1969.

4. Chen, T. T., and Heidelberger, C.   *In vitro* Malignant Transformation of Cells Derived from Mouse Prostate in the Presence of 3-Methylcholanthrene.   J. Natl. Cancer Inst., *42*: 915, 1969.

5. Chen, T. T., and Heidelberger, C.   Quantitative Studies on the Malignant Transformation of Mouse Prostate Cells by Carcinogenic Hydrocarbons *in vitro*.   Int. J. Cancer, *4*: 166, 1969.

6. Chu, E. H. Y., and Malling, H. V.   Mammalian Cell Genetics. II.   Chemical Induction of Specific Locus Mutations in Chinese Hamster Cells *in vitro*.   Proc. Natl. Acad. Sci., *61*: 1306, 1968.

7. DiPaolo, J. A., Nelson, R. L., and Donovan, P. J.   Sarcoma-producing Cell Lines Derived from Clones Transformed *in vitro* by Benzo[a]pyrene.   Science, *165*: 917, 1969.

8. Grover, P. L., Forrester, J. A., and Sims, P.   Reactivity of the K-Region Epoxides of Some Polycyclic Hydrocarbons towards the Nucleic Acids and Proteins of BHK 21 Cells.   Biochem. Pharmacol., *20*: 1297, 1971.

9. Grover, P. L., and Sims, P.   Interactions of the K-Region Epoxides of Phenanthrene and Dibenz[a,h]anthracene with Nucleic Acids and Histone.   Biochem. Pharmacol., *19*: 2251, 1970.

10. Grover, P. L., Sims, P., Huberman, E., Marquardt, H., Kuroki, T., and Heidelberger, C. *In vitro* Transformation of Rodent Cells by K-Region Derivatives of Polycyclic Hydrocarbons. Proc. Natl. Acad. Sci., *68*: 1098, 1971.

11. Heidelberger, C. Chemical Carcinogenesis, Chemotherapy: Cancer's Continuing Core Challenges—G.H.A. Clowes Memorial Lecture. Cancer Res., *30*: 1549, 1970.

12. Heidelberger, C. Studies on the Cellular and Molecular Mechanisms of Hydrocarbon Carcinogenesis. Eur. J. Cancer, *6*: 161, 1970.

13. Heidelberger, C., and Iype, P. T. Malignant Transformation *in vitro* by Carcinogenic Hydrocarbons. Science, *155*: 214, 1967.

14. Huberman, E., Aspiras, L., Heidelberger, C., Grover, P. L., and Sims, P. Mutagenicity to Mammalian Cells of Epoxides and Other Derivatives of Polycyclic Hydrocarbons. Proc. Natl. Acad. Sci., *68*: 3195, 1971.

15. Huberman, E., and Sachs, L. Cell Susceptibility to Transformation and Cytotoxicity by the Carcinogenic Hydrocarbon Benzo[a]pyrene. Proc. Natl. Acad. Sci., *56*: 1123, 1966.

16. Lasnitzki, I. Growth Pattern of the Mouse Prostate Gland in Organ Culture and Its Response to Sex Hormones, Vitamin A, and 3-Methylcholanthrene. Natl. Cancer Inst. Monograph, *12*: 381, 1963.

17. Miller, J. A. Carcinogenesis by Chemicals: An Overview—G. H. A. Clowes Memorial Lecture. Cancer Res., *30*: 599, 1970.

18. Mondal, S., and Heidelberger, C. *In vitro* Malignant Transformation by Methylcholanthrene of the Progeny of Single Cells Derived from C3H Mouse Prostate. Proc. Natl. Acad. Sci., *65*: 219, 1970.

19. Mondal, S., Iype, P. T., Griesbach, L. M., and Heidelberger, C. Antigenicity of Cells Derived from Mouse Prostate Cells after Malignant Transformation *in vitro* by Carcinogenic Hydrocarbons. Cancer Res., *30*: 1593, 1970.

20. Nebert, D. W., and Gelboin, H. V. Substrate-inducible Microsomal Aryl Hydroxylase in Mammalian Cell Culture. J. Biol. Chem., *243*: 6250, 1968.

21. Röller, M.-R., and Heidelberger, C. Attempts to Produce Carcinogenesis in Organ Cultures of Mouse Prostate with Polycyclic Hydrocarbons. Int. J. Cancer, *2*: 509, 1967.

22. Selkirk, J., Huberman, E., and Heidelberger, C. An Epoxide Is an Intermediate in the Microsomal Metabolism of the Chemical Carcinogen, Dibenz[a,h]anthracene. Biochem. Biophys. Res. Commun., *43*: 1010, 1971.

Discussion of Paper by Dr. Heidelberger

DR. SANDERS: In the experiment where you added 50 μg/ml of mouse skin H-protein attached to which methylcholanthrene was bound, have you any evidence of the amount of this protein actually taken up by the cells?

DR. HEIDELBERGER: No, but the fact that a biological effect was produced indicates that the protein entered the cells.

DR. WEISBURGER: I address two questions to Dr. Heidelberger.

Dose response in your studies appears to be satisfactory in those instances shown. In virus-added cells in the hands of Huebner and associates the lowest doses seem to transform better than higher levels. Any comment?

Could phenolic metabolites of DBA act as promoter under conditions of continuing treatment with DBA where it is a " complete " carcinogen?

DR. HEIDELBERGER: We published in the International Journal of Cancer in 1969 that transformation decreased at higher doses. This could not be accounted for by toxicity. Thus, Huebner has confirmed us.

In my opinion, and it's only an opinion based on no evidence, the hydrocarbon or epoxide produces initiation. The cell division that occurs in these cultures, I believe, corresponds to the process of promotion.

DR. PREUSSMANN: Dr. Heidelberger, have you already compared the chemical reactivity of active (in your system) K-region epoxides with inactive epoxides of phenanthrene, for example?

DR. HEIDELBERGER: We have not done this, but Grover and Sims plan to do so.

DR. MAGEE: Thinking of your remarks yesterday on the much greater potency of hydrocarbons than β-propiolactone in mouse skin carcinogenesis, I wonder if you have tested β-propiolactone in your cell culture system. This might be interesting since MNNG, which, like β-propiolactone, is an alkylating agent, was very effective at transformation in your system.

DR. HEIDELBERGER: We have not tried β-propiolactone. This would be a good idea to try. Thank you!

DR. DRUCKREY: Have you any idea about the type of reaction between the epoxide and nucleic acids?

DR. HEIDELBERGER: No. Grover and Sims will also study this.

DR. TOMATIS: Is there any evidence that epoxides are carcinogenic *in vivo* outside the skin system?

DR. HEIDELBERGER: Yes, epoxides are carcinogenic on the skin and subcutaneously but less carcinogenic than the parent hydrocarbon. I believe that this was because the epoxide reacted with keratin and other extracellular substances, before it could enter the target cells. This is why we turned to *in vitro* experiments.

DR. DAWE: In your feeder culture system, do you have information concerning the speed and completeness of binding of the epoxides within the feeder cells? Do you think it is possible that epoxides formed by feeder cells could be transferred to the test cell population?

DR. HEIDELBERGER: We have no such information now, but intend to study this matter in the future.

DR. SUGIMURA: How is the epoxide-forming enzyme distributed among various tissues? Do most normal cells have the epoxide-forming enzyme? How about the distribution of the epoxide-hydrase among various tissues?

DR. HEIDELBERGER: This is a very complicated matter, since the epoxide-forming and epoxide-metabolizing enzymes are all part of the same microsomal drug-metabolizing complex. Until they can be separated, it would be impossible to carry out the important experiments that you have proposed. I believe Gelboin is working on this.

Parameters for Malignant Transformation of Mammalian Cells Treated with Chemical Carcinogens in Tissue Culture

Hajim Katsuta and Toshiko Takaoka

Department of Cancer Cell Research, Institute of Medical Science, University of Tokyo, Tokyo, Japan

A variety of parameters have been proposed for identification of malignant transformation of mammalian cells treated with chemical carcinogens in tissue culture. However, it now appears necessary to re-evaluate and confirm their significance.

Morphological changes have been emphasized, especially by pathologists. Figures 1 and 2, respectively, represent the morphology of rat liver cells of the untreated control culture and the malignantly transformed culture by a chemical carcinogen, 4-nitroquinoline 1-oxide (4NQO). The cells in Fig. 2 produced carcinomas on back-transplantation into the peritoneal cavity of newborn rats, and the animals died from these tumors. This transformation was obtained by only a single 4NQO treatment for 30 min. However, little difference is exhibited in cell morphology between these two pictures, except that a tripolar mitosis and a little pleomorphism are observed in Fig. 2, and no distinct evidence is available for identifing the cells in this picture as malignant ones.

In primary cultures of rat liver cells, we have occasionally found very prominent nucleoli in the cells, as early as 8 days after the initiation of culture. These cells, however, were not able to grow in animals of the same strain.

Some mutant strains of liver cells derived from rats and transformed by Nagisa culture closely resemble hepatoma cells in morphology. " Nagisa culture " means the cultivation of cells in culture tubes with flattened surfaces, which are incubated, being kept slanted at 5°, without subculturing for a long period, *e.g.*, a few months or more (*8, 10*). Many mutant cell strains have been obtained by this procedure, but none of them have produced progressive tumors on back-transplantation. In morphology they appear as if they have a high activity of locomotion. By cinemicrography, however, cell locomotion has scarcely been detected.

Liver cells from normal rats occasionally exhibit a figure resembling a piling-up, but most of these cells are probably undergoing degeneration.

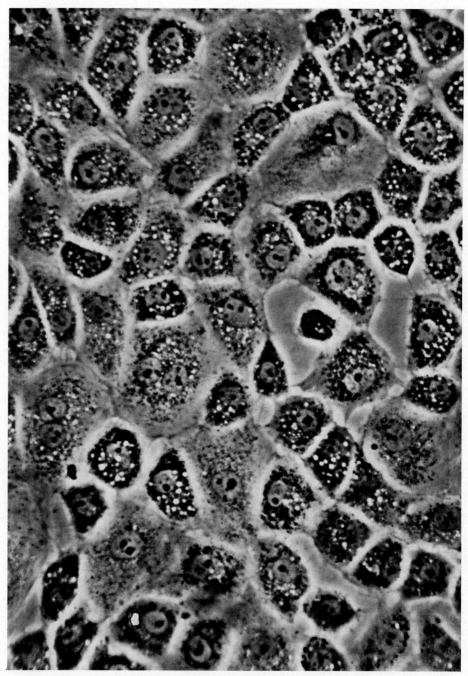

Fig. 1. Phase-contrast photomicrograph of untreated rat liver cells in tissue culture. ×10 Ocular and ×20 objective.

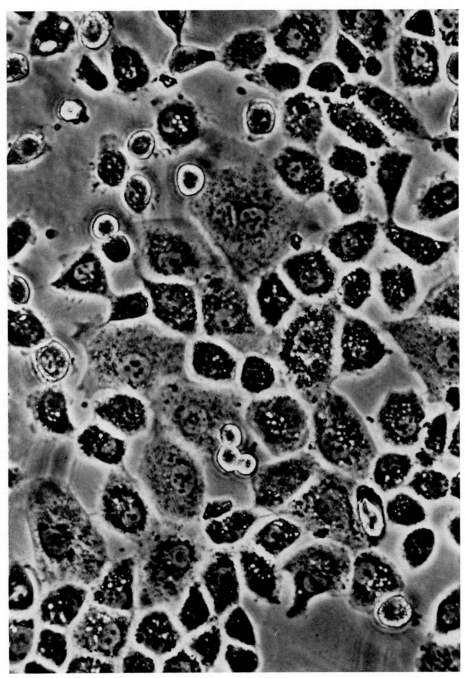

FIG. 2.   A culture of rat liver cells transformed into carcinoma cells by treatment in culture with 4NQO.   10×20.

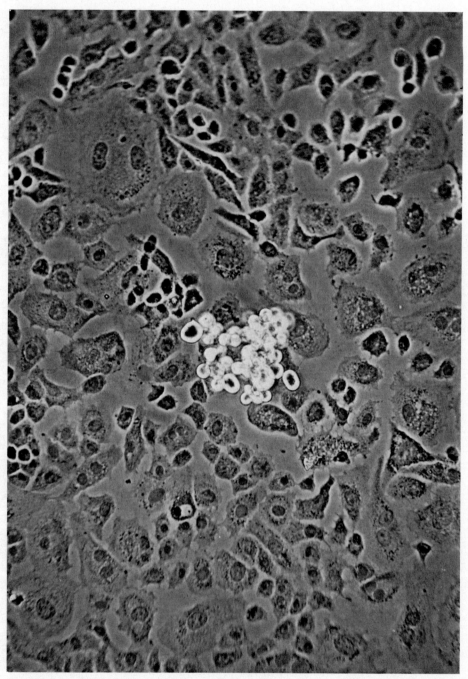

FIG. 3.   A piled-up colony on a cell sheet of rat liver cells.   This was produced after transformation by Nagisa culture.   10 × 10.

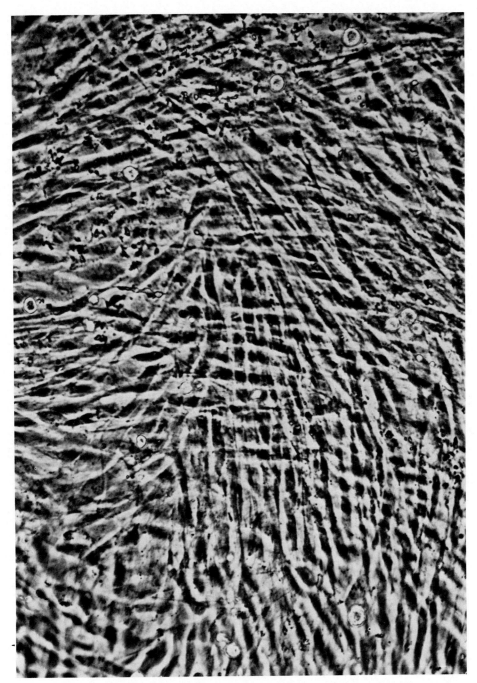

FIG. 4.   A criss-cross pattern found in an 8-day-old primary culture of fibroblasts derived from rat pancreas. 10×10.

When mutant cells were produced in Nagisa culture, we observed the formation of colonies, as shown in Fig. 3, where spherical-shaped cells were growing piled-up on each other. However, these transformed cells did not give rise to progressive tumors on back-transplantation.

A criss-cross pattern of cells was emphasized for transformed cells by some workers (1, 2, 12, 13), but it cannot necessarily be a parameter for malignant transformation. The typical criss-cross pattern shown in Fig. 4 was observed in an 8-day-old primary culture of fibroblasts from rat spleen. These cells did not give rise to tumors in animals.

As to abnormal mitoses, we have frequently found them in Nagisa cultures of rat liver cells including multipolar mitoses, unequal division of nuclei, endomitoses, and others, especially in the zone nearest to the air-liquid interface. These cells, however, produced no tumors on back-transplantation.

Changes in the modal number of chromosomes by malignant transformation have also been pointed out. We have strains of rat liver cells preserving the diploid number of chromosomes with high frequency. When these cells were transformed by Nagisa culture, the resulting mutants exhibited a marked shift in the modal numbers as shown in Fig. 5, but none of these mutant strains showed back-transplantability to animals.

Conversely, strains of rat liver cells, transformed into carcinomas by 4NQO treatment in tissue culture, have undergone little shift in their modal numbers of chromosomes, i.e., only one or two chromosomes disappeared, as illustrated in Fig. 6. But these cells produce tumors and kill the animals on back-transplantation. These findings also suggest that a shift in chromosome number cannot necessarily be a parameter for malignant transformation.

Rapid proliferation of cells is not proportional to their malignancy. A rat liver cell strain which had been transformed by Nagisa culture increased about 14-fold in cell number during 7 days, but did not produce tumors in animals.

Parabiotic culture of rat ascites hepatoma AH-130 cells with normal rat liver cells was carried out by the use of twin tubes (7, 11). It resulted in acceleration of the proliferation of hepatoma cells and degeneration or destruction of normal liver cells. A similar finding was obtained with a combination of rat ascites hepatoma AH-7974 cells and normal rat liver cells, as shown in Fig. 7 (9). However, rat liver cell strains which had been transformed by Nagisa culture also behaved similarly to these hepatoma cells in parabiotic culture with normal liver cells, and they did not produce tumors on back-transplantation into rats.

It has been a question whether or not cells acquire high resistance to a carcinogen when they have been transformed with it. From the work to date in our laboratory, such an enhancement of resistance has never been confirmed.

On the cell-to-cell adhesion, we have obtained interesting findings by cinemicrography: When rat liver cells were treated with 4NQO, they gradually lost the adhesiveness between the cells and started to move around freely as if they were swimming. This suggests that some distinct change occurred in their cell membrane.

This was also suggested by the results of cytoelectrophoretic analysis. Dr. Yamada of our research team showed that the electrophoretic mobility of hepatoma

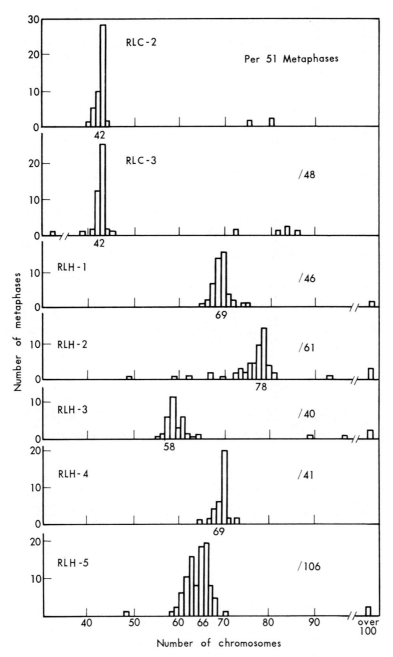

FIG. 5.   Distribution of chromosome numbers in the parent strains RLC-2 and -3 of rat liver cells and in the mutant substrains RLH-1, -2, -3, -4 and -5, transformed from them by Nagisa culture.

cells was higher than that of normal cells and was apparently decreased by treatment with neuraminidase.   The mobility of normal liver cells was low, but it was increased by neuraminidase treatment.   The mobility of Nagisa-transformed liver cells was

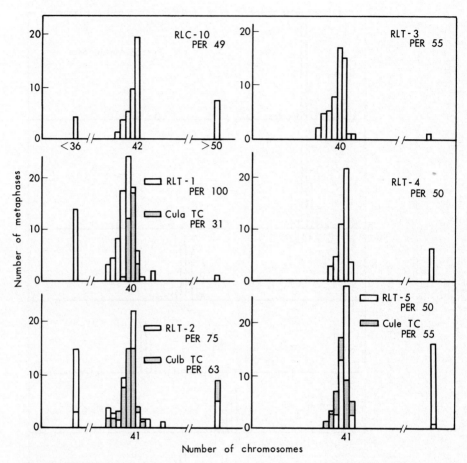

Fig. 6. Distribution of chromosome numbers in the parent strain RLC-10 of rat liver cells and in the mutant substrains RLT-1, -2, -3, -4, and -5 transformed into malignant cells by treatment with 4NQO in culture. Dotted columns represent the chromosome numbers of recultured cells from tumors produced in rats by back-transplantation of these substrains.

scarcely changed by the same treatment. Liver cells transformed into malignant cells by treatment with 4NQO exhibited a similar electrophoretic pattern to that of hepatoma cells, *i.e.*, mobility and response to neuraminidase (*15*).

JTC-25·P3 cells were derived from rat liver cells and transformed by Nagisa culture, and they have been cultured for three years in protein- and lipid-free synthetic medium (*14*). They showed a typical electrophoretic pattern as Nagisa cells. When these cells were treated twice with 4NQO, their pattern became similar to that of hepatoma cells. However, these cells did not produce tumors on back-transplantation.

Concanavalin A (Con A) has been described as agglutinating leukemic cells and cells transformed by oncogenic viruses, chemical carcinogens, and X-irradiation, whereas it does not agglutinate normal cells under the same conditions (*4–6*). We examined 19 kinds of cells, including transplantable and nontransplantable cells,

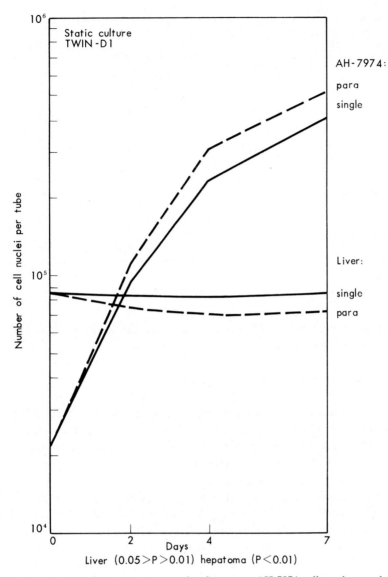

FIG. 7. Interaction between rat ascites hepatoma AH-7974 cells and normal rat liver cells on parabiotic culture in twin tubes. The proliferation of AH-7974 cells was accelerated, whereas normal liver cells were destroyed by the action of certain metabolites excreted from hepatoma cells into the culture medium.

but only 2 of them exhibited distinct agglutination with Con A. These findings indicate that some change may be induced in the cell membrane by malignant transformation but that is not essential for malignancy, in other words, for back-transplantability.

The capacities of cells to grow in soft agar medium were compared with their abilities to grow in animals on back-transplantation. As illustrated in Table 1, a strain of the rat liver cells which had been transformed in Nagisa culture showed

TABLE 1.   Comparison of the Capacities of Cultured Cells to Grow in Soft Agar Medium with Their Abilities to Grow in Animals on Back-Transplantation

Origin	(TC-days)	Back-transplantation		Soft agar	
		Cell number	Death	Inoculum	P. E. (%)
Normal tissues :					
Hamster whole embryos	(22 d)	—	—	10^6	0
Same line	(294 d)	—	—	9×10^4	0
Rat subcutaneous	(61 d)	—	—	10^6	0
Rat liver	(463 d)	5×10^6	0/2	10^5	0
Same line	(ca. 1,300 d)	5×10^6	2/2	10^5	0
Same line	(1,460 d)	—	—	3.65×10^5	numerous
Transformed by Nagisa :					
RLH-4 (JTC-24)		10^6	0/2	8×10^2	38
RLH-5 (JTC-25)		10^6	0/3	8×10^2	5
Rat ascites hepatomas :					
JTC-1 (AH-130)		10^3	3/3	5×10^3	20
JTC-2 (AH-130)		10^3	2/4	6×10^3	13
JTC-15 (AH-66)		10^6	0/3	5.8×10^3	18
JTC-16-C6 (AH-7974)		6.5×10^2	4/4	7×10^2	36

the highest plating efficiency.   However, this strain did not give rise to tumors when back-transplanted into animals.

The ability of cells to grow in animals and kill them has been regarded as the most critical and essential criterion of malignancy.   When cells produce tumors on back-transplantation, they have definitely been malignantly transformed.   However, some cells produce small nodules and then later regress (3, 10, 12).   Furthermore, some cells only grow in animals which have been pretreated with cortisone or irradiated.   However, no pretreatment is required for indefinite growth of cancer cells in man.   The problem arises of whether cells which can only grow in pretreated animals can be called malignant cells.

Thus, a big question is, what is cancer.   The discrepancies between the many parameters discussed above might be due to differences between cells, i.e., fibroblasts were employed by most other workers and epithelial cells by us.   At present, it seems most important to reconsider parameters for malignancy and to find more reliable ones.   This should also be important in cultivation of human tumor cells.

This work was supported by a grant for Cancer Research from the Japanese Ministry of Education and a grant from the Japanese Ministry of Health and Welfare, Cancer Research Subsidy, 1971–22.

REFERENCES

1.   Berwald, Y., and Sachs, L.   In vitro Cell Transformation with Chemical Carcinogens. Nature, 200: 1182–1184, 1963.
2.   Berwald, Y., and Sachs, L.   In vitro Transformation of Normal Cells to Tumor Cells by Carcinogenic Hydrocarbons.   J. Natl. Cancer Inst., 35: 641–661, 1965.
3.   Borek, C., and Sachs, L.   The Number of Cell Generations Required to Fix the

Transformed State in X-Ray-induced Transformation. Proc. Natl. Acad. Sci., *59*: 83–85, 1968.

4. Burger, M. M. A Difference in the Architecture of the Surface Membrane of Normal and Virally Transformed Cells. Proc. Natl. Acad. Sci., *62*: 994–1001, 1969.

5. Inbar, M., and Sachs, L. Structural Difference in Sites on the Surface Membrane of Normal and Transformed Cells. Nature, *223*: 710–712, 1969.

6. Inbar, M., and Sachs, L. Interaction of the Carbohydrate-binding Protein Concanavalin A with Normal and Transformed Cells. Proc. Natl. Acad. Sci., *63*: 1418–1425, 1969.

7. Katsuta, H., and Takaoka, T. Parabiotic Cell Culture. IV. Interaction between Normal and Ascites Tumor Cells of Rats. J. Natl. Cancer Inst., *32*: 963–980, 1964.

8. Katsuta, H., and Takaoka, T. Cytobiological Transformation of Normal Rat Liver Cells by Treatment with 4-Dimethylaminoazobenzene after Nagisa Culture. *In*; Katsuta, H. (ed.), Cancer Cells in Culture, pp. 321–334, Univ. of Tokyo Press, Tokyo, 1968.

9. Katsuta, H., Takaoka, T., and Nagai, Y. Interaction in Culture between Normal and Tumor Cells of Rats. *In*; Katsuta, H. (ed.), Cancer Cells in Culture, pp. 157–168, Univ. of Tokyo Press, Tokyo, 1968.

10. Katsuta, H., Takaoka, T., Doida, Y., and Kuroki, T. Carcinogenesis in Tissue Culture. VII. Morphological Transformation of Rat Liver Cells in Nagisa Culture. Japan. J. Exptl. Med., *35*: 513–544, 1965.

11. Katsuta, H., Takaoka, T., Niki, H., and Ito, S. Parabiotic Cell Culture. I. Experimental Instruments and Culture Techniques. Japan. J. Exptl. Med., *31*: 215–223, 1961.

12. Kuroki, T., and Sato, H. Transformation and Neoplastic Development *in vitro* of Hamster Embryonic Cells by 4-Nitroquinoline 1-Oxide and Its Derivatives. J. Natl. Cancer Inst., *41*: 53–71, 1968.

13. Kuroki, T., Goto, M., and Sato, H. Malignant Transformation of Hamster Embryonic Cells with 4-Nitroquinoline 1-Oxide and Its Derivatives in Tissue Culture. *In*; Katsuta, H. (ed.), Cancer Cells in Culture, pp. 364–381, Univ. of Tokyo Press, Tokyo, 1968.

14. Takaoka, T., and Katsuta, H. Long-term Cultivation of Mammalian Cell Strains in Protein- and Lipid-free Chemically Defined Synthetic Media. Exptl. Cell Res., *67*: 295–304, 1971.

15. Yamada, T., Takaoka, T., Katsuta, H., Namba, M., and Sato, J. Carcinogenesis in Tissue Culture. XX: Electrokinetic Changes in Cultured Rat Liver Cells Associated with Malignant Transformation *in vitro*. Japan. J. Exptl. Med., *42*: 377–388, 1972.

Discussion of Paper by Drs. Katsuta and Takaoka

DR. SANDERS: What is your opinion of the observations that almost all the transformations of cells *in vitro* by carcinogens have given sarcomas on back-transplantation and not carcinomas?

DR. KATSUTA: In our case, we have grown epithelial cells and obtained carcinomas.

DR. WEISBURGER: In connection with the comment of Dr. Sanders, Prof. Katsuta and his associates have succeeded, in a pioneering way, in securing transformation *in vitro* of epithelial liver cells and these transformed cells have produced hepatoma on back-transplantation. We have fully confirmed these findings in our laboratory with Dr. G. Williams. The questions raised by Prof. Katsuta may be peculiar to transformation of epithelial-like cells, so important for the understanding of cancer causation in man. In contrast, other work involving transformation of fibroblast or other mesenchymal systems leads to sarcomas on back-transplantation. Such systems may present fewer problems and ones similar to those discussed by Prof. Katsuta for epithelial cells *in vitro*.

DR. KATSUTA: Thank you very much for your comments. You described just what I wished to say.

DR. STICH: The significance of Dr. Weisburger's comment on the prevalence of carcinomas in man and the virtual absence of carcinomas in experimental *in vitro* systems should not be underestimated. In this connection it is of interest to note the absence of carcinomas among neoplasms induced by various types of human and simian adeno-viruses and SV-40 in rodents. These observations may suggest a minor, if any, involvement of these DNA-viruses in the etiology of human carcinomas.

DR. KATSUTA: I suppose we can't deny the possibility that certain viruses which are not carcinogenic might play a certain role in carcinogenesis in collaboration with certain chemicals.

Changes in Cell Interrelationships during Epithelial Carcinogenesis

Clyde J. DAWE

Laboratory of Pathology, General Laboratories and Clinics, National Cancer Institute, Bethesda, Maryland, U.S.A.

Having but little experience in the field of chemical carcinogenesis, I must assume that my function in this symposium is to play one of two possible roles: (1) that of a heathen who shows possibilities of being converted, or (2) that of a heathen who shows no possibilities of being converted, and therefore is to be tossed to the lions. Since I relish neither of these alternatives, my efforts will be directed toward avoiding both by taking an ecumenical approach.

This approach will follow the tactic of addressing myself to some problems in epithelial tumorigenesis that prevail generally, regardless of whether the agent concerned is chemical, viral or physical. The reason these problems are widely prevalent is that normal epithelium, wherever it is found, (except for the crystalline lens) exists in a special interrelationship with nonepithelial cells in order to survive, regenerate, and function. In becoming neoplastic, epithelium not only changes its morphologic and biochemical characteristics; it must also change its relationship with those nonepithelial cells with which it customarily interacts.

Just how enigmatic this change of interrelationships may become will be illustrated in specific terms in the case of salivary gland tumors induced by polyoma virus; but before getting to that, I wish to cite as a historical matter some of the other problems that have been recognized. These problems have revealed themselves in part through what may be called anecdotal observations, and in part through analytical observations.

Anecdotal Evidence

In this category fall the now almost forgotten descriptions of cancers by the early microscopists, and even before them, by the ancients who devised the terms " scirrhous " and " medullary " to indicate that some cancers may be hard and others soft or brain-like. The microscope showed that these differences could be largely explained by the variable amounts of stromal cells and collagenous deposits associated with the neoplastic epithelium.   Particularly in certain mammary and gastric cancers, but also in exceptional cancers of the cervix, thyroid, gall bladder, and prostate gland, the stromal component may be so dominant as nearly to obscure the epithelial proliferations.   One can understand the rationale of the school, led by Virchow (*65*), which erroneously contended that epithelial cancers actually originated from abnormal proliferations of the connective tissue elements.

The basic mechanisms underlying the sometimes dramatic changes in the epitheliomesenchymal relationship in cancer are still unknown, but we do know that comparably dramatic, though different, changes may also occur in the connective tissues in non-neoplastic conditions controlled by steroid sex hormones, as in the growth of antlers of male deer (*6*), and in the sex skin of monkeys (*23*).   Only slightly less dramatic are the cyclic changes in the peri-ductal connective tissues of the human female mammary gland (*37*) and the changes not only in myometrium, but also in the endometrial epithelium and stroma, associated with the ovulatory cycle and pregnancy.   Differences in thickness of the epidermis of the skin in male mice as compared with female mice appear to coincide with differences in thickness in the underlying dermis.   Other differences, such as the sexual dimorphism in the submandibular salivary glands (*38*) and in the parietal glomerular capsular epithelium of mice (*21*) are not related to visible changes in the underlying supportive stroma, but may nevertheless be suspected to depend upon hormonal effects mediated or permitted by the stroma.

A second type of anecdotal evidence bearing on changes in the epithelio-mesenchymal relationship in neoplasms includes the rather frequent and disturbing observation of " mixed tumors ", on the one hand, and of neoplasms that appear to change from carcinoma to sarcoma, on the other.   The classical and most common site for mixed tumors is in the salivary glands, particularly the parotid, but they may also occur in oral mucous membranes, skin, mammary gland, and even in the lungs. Whether these tumors originate from epithelium, mesenchyme, or both has for years been subject to unresolved controversy too lengthy to review here.   Probably the most favored view is that they originate from epithelium that is able to undergo mesenchymoid changes (*19*) through mechanisms unknown.

Squamous cell carcinomas are known to undergo sarcoma-like change, and have sometimes been referred to as " carcinomas imitating sarcomas."   Kettle (*41*) as far back as 1919 observed such variants and commented: " Without going so far as to claim that the adult epithelial cell can actually become changed into a connective tissue cell, I am convinced that some carcinomata may possess such extreme powers of polymorphic growth that their cells, losing all trace of their epithelial origin, may become indistinguishable from connective tissue elements."   The evidence that these neoplasms are in fact of epithelial rather than connective tissue origin consists chiefly in the finding of foci, within either the primary or secondary deposits, in which typical epithelial morphology, such as keratinization and epithelial pearl formation, is preserved or reappears.   This sort of observation suggests that during or after carcinogenesis the cellular phenotype may change from epithelial to mesenchymal, or at least to mesenchymoid.   It warns that in experimental systems, too, one must be wary of concluding, on the basis of morphology alone, that a given neoplasm is nonepithelial in origin merely because the cells have little or no resemblance to epithelium.

Indeed, the classic principle in cancer pathology laid down by Thiersch (63), which states " *Omnis cellula e cellula ejusdem generis,*" cannot be accepted without certain reservations, even though it is a rule that finds daily valid use in the histopathologic classification of tumors.   In embryogenesis, cellular phenotype obviously changes within closely controlled and predictable patterns, otherwise coordinated differentiation and development could not occur.   There is no theoretical reason why, under proper circumstances, the phenotype of a neoplastic cell should not also be subject to change.   Indeed, a strong body of evidence now makes it evident that neoplastic cells arising from a given tissue can secrete polypeptide hormones not normally produced in detectable quantities by that tissue (4).   Critical examination of this phenomenon indicates that it is not a random event, but depends on initial proclivities of the tissues from which the neoplasm arises (3).

The reverse situation, *i.e.*, of primary sarcomas transforming into epithelial neoplasms seems to occur rarely, if ever.   Nephroblastomas, or Wilms' tumors might be thought an exception to this rule, but it must be remembered that renal epithelium normally develops through an inductive transformation of metanephric mesenchyme.   Presumably, in the nephroblastoma the neoplastic metanephric mesenchyme is merely manifesting its pre-endowment with the potential of transforming to epithelium.

Carcinomas simulating or transforming to sarcomas have been described in experimental animals as well as in man.   Perhaps the best known examples are pulmonary adenomas (62) and mammary tumors in mice (22).   Though the primaries are plainly epithelial, in the course of serial transplantation these tumors have been observed to undergo apparent change into sarcomas.   The well-known sarcoma 37 originated from a mammary epithelial neoplasm (34).   Sanford and co-workers have reviewed this topic in detail (57), and from their own observations conclude that in some instances the sarcomatous transformation results from alteration in the neoplastic epithelium, while in others it results from *de novo* neoplastic transformation of stromal cells in the epithelioma.

Finally, in the category of anecdotal evidence, are the numerous observations of morphologic change in the stroma of epithelial organs, concomitant with or sometimes even preceding the appearance of neoplasia in the associated epithelium. Wolbach (67), as early as 1909, noted the distinctive changes that occur in the upper corium of X-irradiated skin, and suggested that it might be the effects of these changes that caused the overlying epithelium to become neoplastic, rather than the direct effects of radiation on the epidermis alone.   Similarly, marked changes in the dermis are regularly associated with the development of epidermoid carcinoma following ultraviolet irradiation, both in man and in animals (10).   The dermal changes associated with papilloma and carcinoma development after skin painting with carcinogenic hydrocarbons have long been recognized (53), and prompted the experiments of Billingham, Orr and Woodhouse (7), which at first seemed to show that the dermal changes are primarily responsible for the development of epithelial tumors.

The aggregate of these bits of anecdotal evidence constitutes little more than a strong suggestion. The stromal proliferation concomitant with certain carcinomatous growths may be entirely secondary to influences of neoplastic epithelium on the connective tissues, rather than *vice versa*. The same may be true of the early stromal changes associated with experimental radiation, chemical, and viral carcinogenesis. Or, equally likely, both the stromal and epithelial changes may be induced by the oncogen, but may be of no critical significance in relation to one another. And even if we accept as fact that epithelial neoplasms may transform to a sarcoma-like morphology, there is no clue as to the mechanism of this transformation. However, as we shall see later, there is now an experimental approach that permits analysis of it.

Analytic Evidence

Prefatory to considering observations from experiments in carcinogenesis, it is essential to summarize at least briefly some of the pertinent recent discoveries contributed by developmental biologists.

Especially relevant are the works of Grobstein and collaborators, who initially concentrated their attention on the submandibular salivary gland of the mouse. By means of a trypsinization technique, Grobstein (29) was able to accomplish very clean separation of the epithelial component of submandibular salivary gland rudiments from the mesenchymal component. Applying this method he was able to show convincingly what Borghese's less perfect techniques (9) had pointed to earlier: namely, that in the absence of specific salivary gland mesenchyme, salivary epithelium is unable to grow and undergo morphogenesis in a tissue culture system. He further showed that when the previously separated epithelial and mesenchymal components are recombined, the ability of these components to interact and to lead to relatively normal morphogenesis is restored. Later experiments (30) showed that this "inductive" interaction is dependent on proximity of epithelium and mesenchyme, but not upon actual contact, since morphogenesis by the epithelial component could be maintained when it was separated from the mesenchyme by a millipore membrane of 20 μ thickness, and a pore size of 0.45 μ. The specificity of this interaction appears to be high, since morphogenesis did not occur if the salivary mesenchyme was removed and replaced by pancreatic, thymic, or various other types of mesenchyme (32). It has been reported by Auerbach (2) that even the epithelium from adult salivary gland retains the ability to undergo growth and morphogenetic development if it is placed in contact with embryonic salivary gland mesenchyme. Other investigations have shed some light on the biochemical activities involved (33, 39), but suffice it to say here that a specific, isolatable, cell-free substance capable of inducing or sustaining growth and morphogenesis of salivary epithelium has not been found.

Similar epithelio-mesenchymal induction systems have since been shown to exist for many of the late-developing organs of mice, including pancreas, thymus, teeth, lung, and mammary gland (32). The specificity of some of these interactions is of lesser degree than in the salivary gland system, however, as shown by the fact that thymus or pancreas development can be supported by "foreign" (hetero-genous) mesenchymes such as salivary mesenchyme.   In the case of pancreas, a cell-free fraction separated from whole embryo extract is capable of supporting mor-phogenesis and cytodifferentiation (55).

More illuminating with respect to abnormal developmental phenomena and perhaps to carcinogenesis are a few experiments which show that epithelium can be "forced" to undergo atypical development under artificially imposed conditions. For example, McLoughlin (48) assembled recombinations of chick limb epidermis with various heterogenous mesenchymes such as heart myoblasts, proventriculus, and gizzard.   In contact with cardiac myoblasts, the epidermis formed thin, single-layered surface sheets of squamous epithelium, while in combination with gizzard muscle, it formed a mucin-producing, sometimes ciliated, multilayered epithelial coat.   Kratochwil (42), assembling recombinations of mammary epithelium with salivary mesenchyme, found that the resulting structure of the branching epithelial tree was more similar to that of salivary gland, with rich, dichotomous branching of the ducts, as opposed to the normal sparse, monopodial type of mammary gland branching.   When mammary epithelium was placed adjacent to mammary mesenchyme and salivary mesenchyme simultaneously, no morphogenesis took place, indicating antagonistic effects of the two mesenchymes.   Hardy (35), study-ing development of vibrissal hair follicles, found that increases in the vitamin A levels in the cultures caused the follicles to develop into branched, gland-like structures which resembled to some extent salivary gland, and which secreted a mucin-like material.   Since the structures that developed from vibrissal follicles under the in-fluence of excess vitamin A were exactly similar to neither vibrissal follicles nor any known gland, it might be contended that a "neo-organ" had been artificially pro-duced, although Hardy herself applied the conventional term, metaplasia.

The purpose of citing these observations is to emphasize that the character of a given epithelium is a labile thing, continually influenced by the interactions of that epithelium with mesenchymal cells as well as with diffusible substances in the humoral milieu.   It follows that epithelium lifted out of its normal interactive set-ting, and presented with the problem of living in an entirely different microecological niche, may very well respond differently to a carcinogen than it did before such a shift.   The selectivity of carcinogens for specific organs, tissues, and cells is a familiar phenomenon, and it should be born in mind that in effect, salivary epitheli-um interacting with salivary mesenchyme represents a different target tissue than that resulting from salivary epithelium interacting with mammary mesenchyme. The latter composite might be deemed a phenotypic hybrid organ.

I will refer briefly now to a number of experimental observations which in-dicate that epithelio-mesenchymal interactions may have an important bearing on the outcome of exposure of epithelium to carcinogens, whether chemical, viral, or physical.

After some 20 years, the provocative interpretations offered by Billingham et al. (7) regarding carcinogenesis in transplanted epidermal components of skin exposed to methylcholanthrene, are still subject to debate even though the main tenet now seems to be excludable.   In the above work, it was found that split-thickness grafts of mouse skin exposed to methylcholanthrene failed to give rise to papillomas or cancers when transferred to a new dermis at a site untreated with MC. Full thickness grafts similarly treated with MC did give rise to papillomas and carcinomas, as did untreated split-thickness grafts transferred to denuded dermis of skin previously treated with MC. The postulate based on these observations was (54) that a " permutation " had been induced in the dermis by MC, and that normal epidermis coming in contact with such permutated dermis was induced to become neoplastic. The objection was subsequently raised that after removal of split-thickness grafts, the bases of hair follicles remained and it was from these that the papillomas and carcinomas arose. Steinmuller's experiments (60) making use of histocompatibility traits to differentiate between host and donor tissues validate this objection, as they show that the carcinomas arising at sites of MC-treated graft bed covered by untreated epidermal grafts actually have the recipient's histocompatibility characteristics, and therefore must arise from residual epithelium remaining in the graft bed. Steinmuller's results, taken together with those of Giovanella (28) using hairless mice, point strongly toward the hair follicle epithelium as the site of origin of MC-induced papillomas and carcinomas, and there now exists no compelling evidence that permutated dermis is able to induce cancer in epidermis not exposed to carcinogens. However, neither Steinmuller's nor Giovanella's experiments rule out a possible role of MC-altered dermis in favoring neoplastic transformation of MC-altered hair follicle epithelium. This possibility remains, and it is furthermore evident from Giovanella's work that epithelium in the myriad cysts representing involuted hair follicles in hairless mice is strangely nonresponsive to MC. This epithelium is the same epithelium or the progeny of the epithelium that previously had given rise to one hair growth cycle, yet it has become unresponsive to MC in parallel with its loss of hair-forming capacity. One theory on the mechanism of loss of this capacity is that the dermis fails in its follicle-inducing function. If this theory were proved correct, we would then have strong evidence of the importance of epithelio-mesenchymal interactions not only in maintaining normal epithelial function, but also *pari passu*, in maintaining specific susceptibility to the carcinogenic action of MC. In this connection it is necessary to note Wolbach's contention (68) that chemical carcinogen-induced papillomas in mice originate only in those follicles that have lost their dermal papillae as a result of the action of the carcinogen. If this concept is also correct, it would appear that interaction between papilla mesenchyme and follicle epithelium is at first essential during the transforming action of the carcinogen, but that this epithelial-mesenchymal interaction must then be ablated before transformation can be expressed.

Two other experiments are relevant to epithelio-stromal interactions in skin (hair follicles) during chemically induced carcinogenesis. Ashley (1) transplanted MC-exposed haired skin subcutaneously, where it formed cysts but failed to yield papillomas or carcinomas. Control grafts to topical sites gave rise to papillomas and carcinomas as expected. This result can as yet be related in only a vague and speculative way to alterations in epithelial-stromal interaction, but it is probably significant that Friedman-Kien et al. (26) found that the hair follicle growth cycle was altered in embryonic mouse skin transplanted subcutaneously into newborn mice.   The follicles grew slowly during a greatly prolonged growth phase, and then underwent atrophy.   The transplanted fetal mouse skin thus, in effect, behaved much like that of the skin of hairless mice left *in situ*.   Evidently the subcutaneous environment does not favor the continued epithelio-mesenchymal interaction necessary for perpetuation of repeated hair growth cycles.   Nevertheless, it is clear from work of Steinmuller *et al.* (*61*) that mouse skin, subcutaneously implanted together with methylcholanthrene, is able to give rise to carcinoma.

Very recently, Edwards (*24*) observed that mouse tail skin, ordinarily refractory to carcinogenesis by MC-painting, developed papillomas and cancers readily if transplanted to a body-skin area after the MC-painting was completed.   He found decreases in the quantity of collagen in the dermis of such transplanted skins, as well as qualitative differences in the composition of that collagen.

In a viral system, the observations of Noyes and Mellors (*51*) suggest the importance of epithelio-mesenchymal interaction in determining the outcome of cell-virus relationships in the Shope papilloma.   In their experiments using fluorescent antibody to locate the sites of virus replication, it was found that only the outer, keratinizing cell layers in papillomas contained complete viruses whose coat antigens could be labeled.   None of the basal cells contained antigen.   One inference possible from this observation is that basal cells, under the influence of their interaction with dermal mesenchyme, harbor the papilloma virus in an integrated state, while epidermal cells after losing contact with the basement membrane-dermis substrate allow virus to replicate and produce cytopathic effects.   Thus the dermal-epidermal interaction may well be a critical factor in papilloma growth, which occurs through proliferation of the basal cell layer.

In another virus-tumor system, that of mouse mammary tumors associated with mammary tumor virus (MTV) and nodule-inducing virus (NIV), there is also an interesting relationship between stroma and the development of tumors, as well as between stroma and development of normal mammary gland.   DeOme and associates (*18*) have nicely demonstrated the essentiality of the mammary fat pads for support of growth of normal mammary gland and of hyperplastic mammary nodules. They found that normal mammary gland removed from fat pad and transplanted to the dorsal subcutis developed and grew poorly, whereas the same type of transplants grew and developed virtually normally when placed in mammary fat pads previously cleared of mammary tissue.   Further, they found that hyperplastic nodules transplanted to dorsal subcutis rarely gave rise to mammary cancer (1 out of 80 transplants), whereas hyperplastic nodules transplanted to mammary fat pads frequently gave rise to cancers (9 out of 19), and after a much shorter period.

Studying basal cell epitheliomas in man, Van Scott and Reinertson (*64*) found that, freed of their original stroma, these neoplasms sometimes underwent keratinization and necrosis at subcutaneous transplant sites.   In a later study (*25*), it was shown that basal cell carcinoma separated from its stroma and maintained in tissue culture undergoes squamification and keratinization.   For this nonmetastasizing neoplasm, it appears that interaction between tumor cells and appropriate stroma is necessary to maintain growth and, reciprocally, to inhibit the expression of latent cytodifferentiative capabilities.

In the field of neoplastic transformation *in vitro*, we find evidence of a negative and therefore less persuasive sort, that epithelium *not* kept in its normal interactive state with mesenchyme fails to respond to oncogens as it does *in vivo*, where it *is* kept in its normal interactive state with mesenchyme, at least during the initial phases of carcinogenesis. This applies to virally induced transformations as well as to chemically induced and "spontaneous" transformations. This negative evidence comes to attention if one asks: From how many viral, chemical, or "spontaneous" transformation systems employing enzyme- or versene-dissociated cells grown in monolayer cultures have tumors unquestionably epithelial in character been derived?

In all probability I have overlooked some, but the only ones that I can summon to mind are the lines resulting from SV-40 infection of hamster kidney in monolayer cultures, as described by Black (*8*), and the MDCK line derived spontaneously from dog kidney, described morphologically by Leighton *et al.* (*45*). It is important to reiterate in connection with these tumors that renal cortical epithelium is normally derived during embryonic development from metanephrogenic mesenchyme. Therefore the occurrence of tubular epithelial structures in the tumors derived from SV-40-infected dispersed kidney cells may, as in Wilms' tumors, represent continuing expression of metanephric mesenchymal ability to transform to epithelium, rather than the ability of transformed epithelium to retain its epithelial character. This may seem a small distinction, but it is by no means insignificant. In contrast, the MDCK line as described by Leighton *et al.* (*45*) appears to be a pure epithelial line that has retained its characteristics during many years in culture. Unfortunately, the conditions under which this cell line was established in culture are not recorded (*27*).

It must also be acknowledged that many cell lines arising from transformations in dissociated cell cultures have been seen to retain characteristics, interpreted as epithelial, in their *in vitro* situation. Examples are certain of the lines derived from the action of 3'-methyl-4-dimethylaminoazobenzene on rat liver (*40*). However, none of these lines produced tumors when back-transplanted to animals, so nothing can be said of their morphologic characteristics under conditions *in vivo*. Conversely, the rat liver cells transformed by 3'-Me-DAB, which did produce tumors when back-transplanted (*58*), have not been morphologically described and confirmed to have the histologic properties of hepatomas or bile duct carcinomas. Continuous lines of cells derived from MTV-free mouse mammary cells in monolayer culture (*43*) failed to grow *in vivo* and so again, evidence of comparability to mammary cancers occurring *in vivo* is unavailable. Spontaneously transformed cultures of hamster lung cells (*52*) produced sarcomas, not epithelial tumors, when back-transplanted. Polyoma-transformed cultures of adult mouse salivary gland, even though epithelial in appearance in culture, produced fibrosarcomas with extremely abundant collagen production when back-transplanted (*56*). A number of cell lines chemically transformed *in vitro* by DiPaolo (*20*) showed epithelial appearances in culture, but none of the tumors resulting from back-transplantation had epithelial features according to illustrations and descriptions. In their early report of chemically induced neoplastic transformation in dissociated cell culture, Berwald and Sachs (*5*) reported that a small percentage of their transformed lines produced carcinomas upon back-transplantation, but examples of these particular lines were not illustrated. Even in the two-step approach (organ culture followed by monolayer culture) used by Heidelberger and associates (*36*) with mouse prostate exposed to methylcholanthrene, the tumors appearing after back-transplantation were either sarcomas or anaplastic neoplasms designated carcinoma, but lacking clear-cut epithelial features such as acinus or duct formation. As commented by Sherwin (*59*), these tumors may well be epithelial in origin, just as certain carcinomas in man are believed to simulate sarcomas. However, the proof is lacking, the phenotypic evidence is equivocal, and the resemblance of the tumors to the usual picture of prostatic adenocarcinoma is not obvious.

These examples do not exhaust the available evidence, but should be sufficient to raise serious doubts that carcinogenesis in many of our culture systems is precisely the same as carcinogenesis *in vivo*. Morphology can be deceiving, but the deception needs to be proved before it can be accepted as such.

The Polyoma-Salivary Tumor System

Briefly, now, I will review some of our own experiments that illustrate the influence of epithelio-mesenchymal interactions during oncogenesis. At the same time, these experiments indicate ways that some of the problems implicit in the discussion above can be solved.

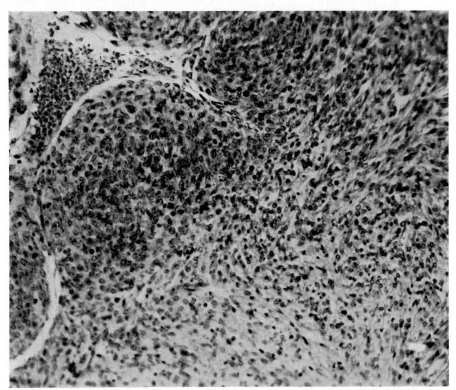

FIG. 1. Example of a polyoma virus-induced salivary gland tumor in which the histologic features are purely mesenchymoid. ×235. (Neg. 36600, NCI K-9391.)

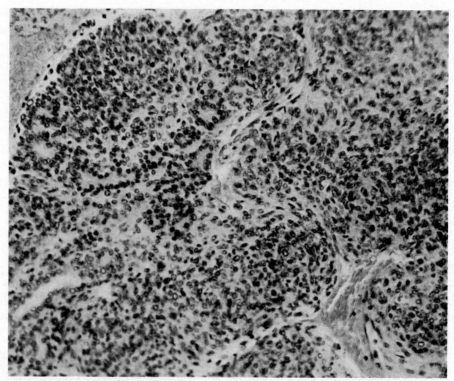

FIG. 2.   Example of a polyoma virus-induced tumor in which there is a mixture of clearly epithelial structure (duct-like structures on left) and mesenchymoid structure (spindle and round cells on right).   ×235.   (Neg. 36609, NCI K-76441.)

First the characteristics of polyoma-induced salivary gland tumors in mice must be noted.   As soon as these neoplasms were recognized to be a distinct entity, it was observed (44) that certain areas in a tumor, or even an entire tumor might be composed of closely packed round and/or elongated cells that resembled mesenchymal tissue rather than epithelium (Fig. 1).   In some areas, however, distinct gland- or duct-like structures were present, suggesting epithelial origin (Fig. 2).   Hence it was thought the polyoma salivary tumors were pleomorphic, mixed tumors, somewhat comparable to but not identical with mixed tumors of salivary gland in man. In the early transplantation work, it was observed that the mesenchymoid component often emerged in pure form after several serial transplantations (44).   All of this left open the question of whether the tumors originated from epithelium, mesenchyme, or both.

In 1959, Dawe and Law (11) reported the morphologic changes in mouse salivary gland infected with polyoma virus in organotypic cultures.   The changes induced *in vitro* closely resembled the tumors induced *in vivo* by polyoma virus (Figs. 3 and 4), and it was noted that the morphologic transformation and proliferation appeared to occur in epithelium, while the salivary mesenchyme showed chiefly a cytolytic response.   A subsequent paper by Dawe et al. (12) on the results of back-transplantation of such cultures reported that the neoplasms arising from the trans-

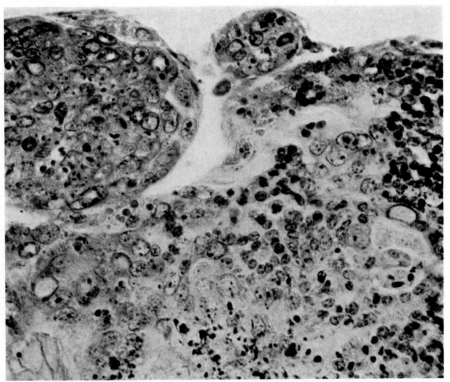

Fig. 3. Polyoma virus-induced transformation in an organotypic culture of submandibular gland. Dark, pyknotic nuclei in upper right are in nontransformed, atrophic portion of cultured gland. ×520. (Neg. 15328, NCI H-67866.)

formed organ cultures were identical with those induced *in vivo*, having both epithelial and mesenchymal features (Figs. 5 and 6).

In the period between those two publications, Vogt and Dulbecco (*66*) and subsequently many others reported the transformation of hamster embryo cells by polyoma virus acting on monolayer cultures prepared from dispersed cells. In these culture systems starting out with trypsin-versene dissociated cells, the transformed cells displayed only mesenchymal features, as did the neoplasms that developed from them after back-transplantation. The hamster cell system used by Vogt and Dulbecco was particularly useful to viral oncologists because virus disappeared early from the cultures, and transformation was more rapid than in the organotypic culture system. Most studies of polyoma-induced transformation *in vitro* have made use of dissociated hamster cell cultures.

However, we continued to study the salivary gland tumor system, both *in vivo* and in organotypic cultures, being interested in tumor genesis in an epithelial organ and in a culture system that seemed to reproduce transformations closely comparable to those *in vivo*, as judged by specific histologic features of the tumors.

To compare results *in vitro* with those *in vivo*, we devised a technique (*14, 66*) in which undissociated salivary gland tissue was infected with virus and then transplanted subcutaneously over the lower back of newborn mice (Fig. 7). Tumors

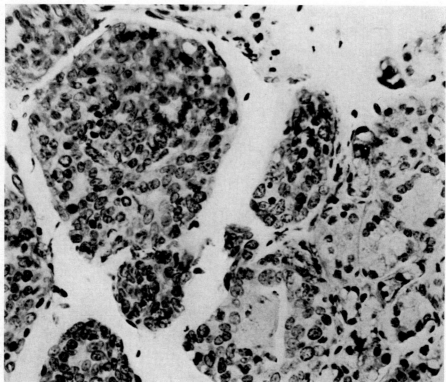

FIG. 4. Polyoma virus-induced transformation in submandibular salivary gland *in vivo*. Nodules of transformed cells on left, normal salivary gland acini on right. Transformed cells are morphologically identical with cells transformed *in vitro* (Fig. 3), but appear slightly smaller in photo because of slightly lower magnification. ×480. (Neg. 15332, NCI H-58722.)

TABLE 1. Tumor Development in Polyoma Virus-Infected Transplants of Submandibular Glands in Progressive Developmental Stages

Developmental stage of transplant	Tumors in transplants		Tumors in host's glands	
	Fraction	Percent	Fraction	Percent
Fully developed (adult)	32/41	78	28/41	68
Early functional (newborn)	18/30	60	18/30	60
Embryonic stages 4 and 5 (14 day embryos)	40/56	71	37/56	66
Embryonic stages 2 and 3 (13 day embryos)	3/28	11	19/28	68
Embryonic stage 1 and prerudimentary area	0/56	0	38/56	68

originating in such transplants were then checked histologically to determine whether they were of typical salivary gland type.

Experiments designed to determine possible differences in response of submandibular salivary gland at different stages of development (47) showed the following (Table 1): 1) Adult, newborn, or embryonic salivary gland from embryos at 14 days' gestation or older showed approximately equal responsiveness to the tumor-inducing effects of the virus. 2) Embryonic submandibular rudiments from 13-day embryos showed a decreased response, while " presumptive " tissue from the area

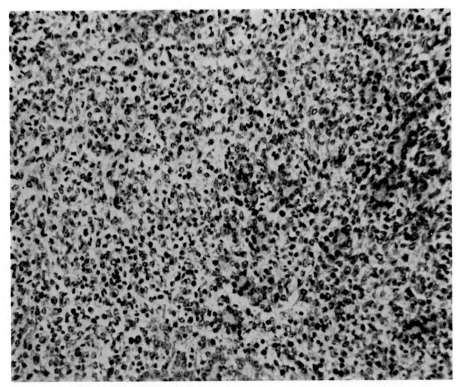

Fig. 5.   Histologic features of a tumor resulting from back-transplantation of submandibular organotypic culture after transformation *in vitro*.   Note mixture of epithelial and mesenchymoid features, typical of tumors induced *in vivo* as illustrated in Figs. 2 and 6.   ×260.   (Neg. 20624, NCI H-53403.)

where submandibular gland is expected to develop, but has not yet appeared, showed no tumor development in response to the virus, 3) Histologically the tumors that appeared were identical, and were of the typical salivary type, regardless of the stage of development of the salivary gland at time of infection.   No tumors were available, of course, from the experiments with prerudimentary embryo stages.

These findings suggested that only tissues actively involved in the epithelio-mesenchymal interaction specifically leading to salivary gland development were susceptible to the oncogenic effects of virus.

This concept could be subjected to test by applying the technique developed by Grobstein (29) for demonstrating the essentiality of epithelio-mesenchymal interaction during salivary gland morphogenesis.   In this technique, trypsin treatment followed by gentle dissection under a dissecting microscope allows a clean separation of epithelium from mesenchyme of 13- and 14-day submandibular rudiments.

Using this method (14), we separated salivary epithelium from its mesenchymal capsule, and infected each component separately (Fig. 8).   The isolated infected components were then transplanted subcutaneously into newborn mice, and development of tumors was watched for.   As one control, intact rudiments were similarly infected and transplanted, and as another the components were first separated and

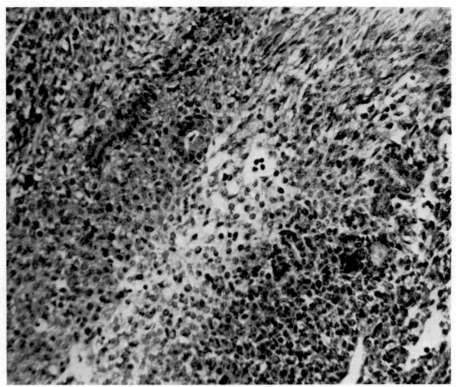

FIG. 6. Salivary gland tumor induced by polyoma virus *in vivo*. Structure is closely comparable to that of tumor derived from culture transformed *in vitro* (Fig. 5). ×260. (Neg. 19593, NCI J-6020.)

TABLE 2. Failure of Tumor Development in Isolated Epithelial and Mesenchymal Components oɪ Submandibular Rudiments Infected with Polyoma Virus *in vivo* and *in vitro*

Material in culture or transplant	Tumors in transplants		Tumors in		Response *in vitro*
			Host	Glands	
Intact submandibular rudiments (stages 2–5)	32/69	46	35/69	51	Morphogenesis. Morphologic transformation and proliferation.
Isolated submandibular epithelium	0/26	0	17/26	65	No morphogenesis. No morphologic transformation. No proliferation.
Isolated submandibular mesenchyme	0/28	0	17/28	61	Viral CPE. Few atypical cells.
Recombined epithelium and mesenchyme	11/47	23	29/47	62	Morphogenesis. Morphologic transformation and proliferation.

infected, then recombined and allowed to become coherent in tissue culture for 18 hr before transplanting to newborns. The results were (Table 2) that no tumors developed in the isolated epithelial or mesenchymal components, while tumors did

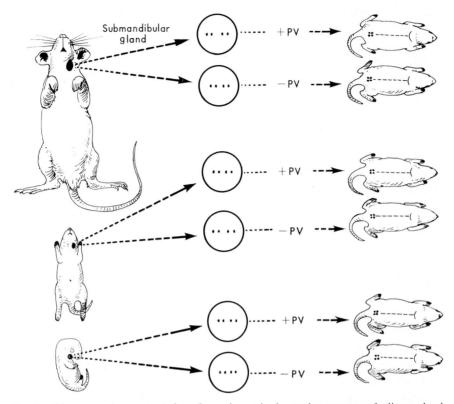

Fig. 7.   Diagrammatic representation of experiment *in vivo*, testing response of salivary glands from adult, newborn, and embryo mice following infection with polyoma virus.   After infection of excised glands or rudiments *in vitro*, the infected tissues were immediately transplanted to subcutaneous site at base of tail, by means of glass pipette introduced through incision at nape of neck.   Control glands and rudiments were not exposed to virus.   See Table 1 for results.

appear in the reassembled infected rudiments, though at only half the frequency as in unmolested, intact rudiments.

This finding, though of much interest, is difficult to interpret in its entirety for reasons discussed previously (*14*), but it showed clearly that simple exposure of the component cells of the salivary gland to polyoma virus is insufficient to cause those cells to manifest neoplastic properties.   For one reason or another, after polyoma virus infection the epithelium and mesenchyme must be allowed to interact if salivary gland neoplasms are to result.   Working with the polyoma-induced ameloblastoma system, Main (*47*) has recently made comparable observations with respect to the morphologic changes in that system *in vitro*.   In addition, he made the most interesting observation that if tooth germ mesenchyme was infected long in advance of recombining it with odontogenic epithelium, the transformation of the epithelium was accelerated.   This suggests that mesenchyme may have more than a merely supportive role during epithelial transformation.

In view of the fact that polyoma virus induces tumors in tooth rudiments (*46*) as well as in salivary gland rudiments, the temptation could not be resisted to ask

TABLE 3. Absence of Tumor Development in Reciprocal Recombinations of Epithelium and Mesenchyme from Salivary Rudiments and Dental Rudiments, Transplanted after Infection with Polyoma Virus

Rudiment or component crosses	Total number rudiments used	Av. number ruds. per recipient	Tumors in transplants		Tumors in hosts	
			Fraction	Percent	Fraction	Percent
SE × DM	262 × 276	7.3 × 7.5	0/36	0	22/36	61
DE × SM	257 × 242	7.1 × 6.7	0/36	0	25/36	70
SE × SM	188 × 188	4.0 × 4.0	11/47	23	29/47	62
Sal. Ruds.	62	2.3	17/27	63	18/27	67
Dent. Ruds.	54	2.0	0/26	0	11/26	42

SE, Submandibular rudiment epithelium; DE, dental rudiment epithelium; SM, submandibular rudiment mesenchyme; DM, dental rudiment mesenchyme

what would happen if incisor tooth bud mesenchyme were recombined with salivary epithelium, and salivary mesenchyme were recombined with tooth bud epithelium before infecting and transplanting to newborns. The experiment was done (*13*), but from neither type of recombination (Table 3) did any tumors develop, despite the fact that the same virus preparation induced tumors in controls composed of salivary epithelium recombined with salivary mesenchyme. Hence it appears that the epithelio-mesenchymal interaction in this tumor induction system has some degree of specificity. Additional experiments with combinations of salivary epithelium and various other types of heterogenous mesenchymes would be necessary to determine whether this specificity is absolute.

A complication in the experiments with PV-infected isolated salivary epithelium as well as in experiments testing salivary epithelium recombined with nonsalivary mesenchyme is that the epithelium soon ceases to grow and to undergo morphogenesis under these conditions, either *in vivo* or *in vitro*. It can be conceived that continued cell proliferation, at least for one or a few mitotic cycles, is necessary to permit expression of the oncogenic effect of the virus. Therefore it seemed imperative to find some way to support growth of salivary epithelium in the absence of interaction with its homogenous mesenchyme.

The resemblance of PV-induced tumor tissue to salivary mesenchyme suggested that the tumors themselves might serve the function of supporting salivary epithelial growth and morphogenesis. An experiment testing this possibility was done (*15*) by inserting trypsin-isolated salivary epithelium into pieces of PV-induced salivary tumor, then transplanting the combination subcutaneously into newborn syngeneic mice. After 11 to 13 days the transplants were removed and examined in serial sections for evidence of the behavior of the epithelium within the engulfing tumor. It was found that in this interaction with tumor, salivary epithelium underwent quite extensive growth and morphogenesis (Figs. 9 and 10). Further, in time-lapse cinematographic studies of normal salivary epithelium interacting with PV-induced salivary tumor cells, it was demonstrated that the epithelium underwent prolonged growth for 30 days and more in this situation (*50*). In the two-dimensional culture system, however, and in the absence of plasma clot, the salivary epithelium did not undergo morphogenesis during the course of its growth. In unpublished work in

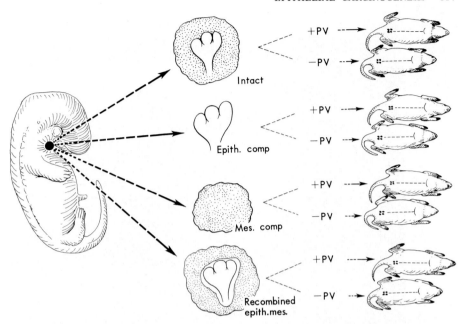

FIG. 8.   Diagrammatic representation of experiment *in vivo*, testing response of isolated epithelial and mesenchymal components respectively to polyoma virus.   Intact rudiments and rudiments reassembled from previously separated components (top and bottom series, respectively) serve as controls.   See Table 2 for results.

progress (*16*), we have also been able to demonstrate trans-filter support of salivary epithelial growth by PV-induced salivary gland tumor cells.

PV-induced tumor cells, therefore, are able to substitute for normal salivary mesenchyme as a support for salivary epithelial growth and morphogenesis.   The tumor cells are, to our knowledge, the only substrate other than homogenous mesenchyme that has been shown capable of performing this function.   Does this signify that the PV-induced tumors originate from salivary gland mesenchyme, and retain the functions of that mesenchyme?

A critical experiment was conducted (*17*) to determine whether the PV-induced tumors arise from epithelium or from mesenchyme, and thus to answer the above question.   Fig. 11 shows the design of the experiment.   Salivary gland rudiments were assembled in which either the epithelium or the mesenchyme was karyotypically marked with 2T6 chromosomes.   The opposite tissue type was left unmarked, or, in effect, negatively marked.   Tumors were then induced by infecting these reassembled glands with PV and transplanting them to newborn F_1 hybrid mice, carrying only 1T6 chromosome.   The karyotypes of the resulting tumors were the deciding factor in establishing whether the tumors arose from epithelium or from mesenchyme.   In each of eight consecutive tumors the karyotype of the tumor cells proved to be that of the epithelial component of the reassembled glands; in none of the tumors were any cells found with the karyotype of the mesenchymal component. From this evidence the conclusion follows that the PV-induced salivary tumors arise from epithelium and from epithelium alone.

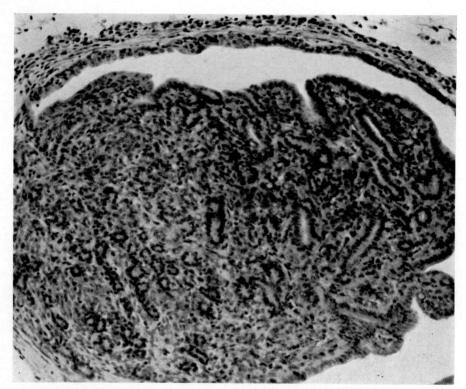

FIG. 9.   Section demonstrating extensive morphogenesis by submandibular rudimentary epithelium, freed from normal mesenchyme and inserted within a piece of salivary gland tumor before transplantation to newborn mouse.   Ducts and acini have formed from the originally solid bud of salivary rudiment epithelium.   Cells between the ducts and glands are tumor cells, substituted for normal mesenchyme.   Compare with Fig. 10.   ×200.   (Neg. 32367, NCI K-27273.)   Reproduced from Ref. 15, with permission of Williams and Wilkins Co., Baltimore.

How then do we put together the available pieces of information concerning the PV-induced salivary tumors, so that an integrated concept can be formed? Starting first from the evidence that the tumors are epithelial in origin, it follows that neoplastic transformation of salivary epithelium can give rise to cells that *appear* to be mesenchymal in origin, even though they are not.   Furthermore, these neoplastic cells of epithelial origin not only look like mesenchyme, but they behave as mesenchyme in that they support morphogenesis and/or growth of normal salivary epithelium when placed in situations permitting appropriate interaction.   It is as if, in becoming neoplastic, the tumor cells have acquired the ability to provide a factor(s) which they previously (as normal cells) depended upon homogenous mesenchyme to provide.   Thus they have achieved independence or autonomy through mechanisms still not clear but which permit drastic deviations from the epithelio-mesenchymal relationships required prior to transformation.   In effect, the transformed epithelium has taken on the quality of providing its own stromal requirements.   Whether the phenotypic changes observed are caused by the introduction

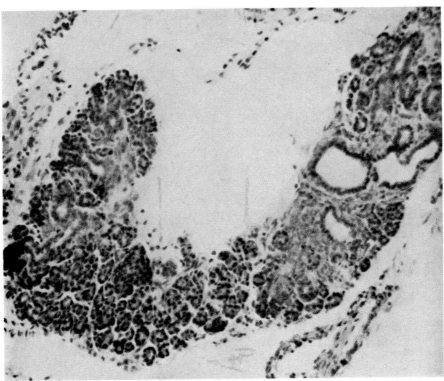

Fig. 10.   Essentially normal morphogenesis taking place in a recombination of normal salivary gland epithelium with normal salivary gland mesenchyme.   The reassembly was allowed to develop for 12 days after transplanting to subcutis of a newborn mouse.   In comparing with Fig. 9, note that ducts and acini are only narrowly separated from one another by sparse, normal mesenchyme sheaths.   ×200.   (Neg. 32632, NCI K-31535.)   Reproduced from Ref. 15, with permission of Williams and Wilkins Co., Baltimore.

of genic material by the inducing virus, or whether they result from epigenetic changes acting on the original genome of the cell cannot be stated or surmised from the data in these experiments.   It seems relevant to note in this connection none-theless, that a critical condition must be met for salivary epithelium to undergo this particular type of transformation: It must be kept in its usual interactive relation-ship with salivary mesenchyme until the transformational process has been accom-plished.   Thereafter, the transformed epithelium is no longer dependent on normal mesenchyme of any type, as proved by its ability to grow continuously in cell culture.

How do these observations and concepts bear on problems in chemical car-cinogenesis? This depends on whether it is fair to assume that epithelio-mesenchymal interactions influence chemically induced transformations of epithelium in somewhat the same way they influence the particular polyoma transformation system described above.   Perhaps they do not, but it is of fundamental importance to find out.   For, if chemical carcinogens produce identical effects on epithelium regardless of whether that epithelium is interacting " normally " with its customary mesenchyme, then it is of little importance whether tests for carcinogenicity are performed on dissociated

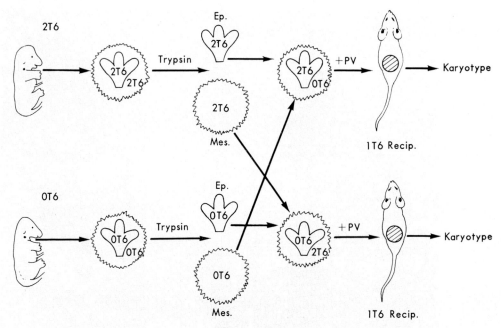

Fig. 11.   Diagrammatic representation of experiment to determine tissue type of origin of polyoma virus-induced salivary gland tumors.   Salivary rudiments are reassembled from epithelial components labeled with 2T6 chromosomes, and mesenchymal components lacking marker chromosomes, or *vice versa*.   The reassembled rudiments are then infected with virus, transplanted to newborn F_1 mice, and resulting tumors are karyotyped to determine the cell type of origin.   Reproduced from Ref. 17 with permission of editors of *Science*.

cells in culture, on nondissociated cells in organotypic culture, or on cells in undisturbed relationships in the intact animal.   If, on the other hand, epithelio-mesenchymal interactions influence transformational pathways during chemical carcinogenesis, then many of the laboratory systems in use are not going to be reliable in revealing what transpires during carcinogenesis in the intact organ.   This is not to say that studies of chemically induced transformations in dissociated culture systems are useless.   On the contrary, they are uniquely useful in that they deal with simplified systems entirely at the level of intrinsic cell regulatory mechanisms.   By isolating subcellular events from the total process involving intercellular actions and even interorgan actions, these methods may offer the best or only approach to analysis of phenomena at the subcellular level.   But the mistake must not be made of presuming that if a given carcinogen produces a given response in a dissociated cell, it is bound to produce the same response in cells residing within the community of cells that comprises a tissue, an organ, or an individual.

Grobstein (*31*) observed with reference to problems in developmental biology, that recognition of levels of regulatory activity is essential:

" Nonetheless, cells in isolation also can behave as wholes, and thus we know that cells have their own inner integrating systems.   In these terms, a central problem of cytodifferentiation is the identification and characterization of control factors extrinsic to the cell and the elucidation of the mechanism by which these impinge

TABLE 4. Karyotypes Recovered from Tumors Arising from Rudiments with Marked Components (Squash Method only)

Karyotype of comps. of transpl.		Karyotype of recipient	Number mitoses exam.	(Cases[+])			Conclusion as to cell origin
				Result (total cases)			
Ep.	Mes.			0T6	1T6	2T6	
68215 2T6	0T6	1T6	116	0/3	3/3	3/3	Epith.
78543 2T6	0T6	1T6	47	0/3	3/3	3/3	Epith.
78576 2T6	0T6	1T6	62	0/3	3/3	3/3	Epith.
80238 2T6	0T6	1T6	27	0/1	1/1	1/1	Epith.
72181 0T6	2T6	1T6	57	3/4	4/4	0/4	Epith.
76441 0T6	2T6	1T6	65	3/3	3/3	0/3	Epith.
76442 0T6	2T6	1T6	56	4/4	2/4	0/4	Epith.
80239 0T6	2T6	1T6	55	1/1	1/1	0/1	Epith.
		Total	485				

upon the cell's inner controls." His view is as applicable to principles of carcinogenesis as to principles of developmental biology. Regulatory circuits operate at humoral levels, at intercellular contact levels both homotypic and heterotypic, and at intracellular levels. Endocrinologically oriented oncologists have long recognized the importance of humoral circuitry, as exemplified in the profound influence of estrogen or prolactin levels on the response of mammary gland to carcinogens. Biochemists have demonstrated the importance of interorgan effects, as, for example, the effect of liver in inactivating estrogens or in activating carcinogens through N-hydroxylation reactions (49). Molecular biologists and geneticists are likewise accumulating great quantities of evidence relevant to the role of nucleic acids and proteins in the intracellular regulatory disorders in carcinogenesis. But perhaps because the potential of newer techniques has not been widely recognized, there have been relatively few investigations of cell-cell regulatory influences during carcinogenesis. It is timely to assert that cell phenotype is continually subject to change in response to changes in microenvironment, and to acknowledge that a basic part of microenvironment is the relationship a cell bears to its neighbor cells. As a working concept, it may be useful to adopt the attitude that a liver cell is a liver cell and a prostate cell is a prostate cell only under quite exacting conditions. After dissociation from its normal microenvironment, any cell requires phenotypic redefinition to suit its newly acquired characteristics and/or its loss of former ones.

What are some practical approaches that can be taken after adopting this attitude? Since carcinogenesis in a dissociated cell system may involve processes different from those operating in intact organ situations, experiments *in vitro* would have more meaning if designed to compare responses to carcinogens in organotypic cultures with responses to the same carcinogens in dissociated cultures. The techniques developed by embryologists for separation of epithelium from mesenchyme can be more widely applied by experimental oncologists than they have been.   Recombination experiments bringing together epithelium from one organ with mesenchyme from another should be applicable to experiments in chemical carcinogenesis, as they have been in the polyoma-salivary gland system.   Phenotypic shifts in cells can become recognizable if karyotypic markers such as the T6 and other chromosomes are used to mark cell origins, instead of depending on the time-honored but fallible method of purely phenotypic identification.   The possibility that endocrine effects on epithelial carcinogenesis may be mediated by or be dependent on stroma can be explored by studying the effects of hormones on isolated epithelium and on epithelium recombined with heterogenous stromas.

Will explorations of this type lead to a more detailed understanding of carcinogenesis, with practical value in prevention or control of cancer?   One can only answer that the principles that apply to investigations of carcinogenesis at sub-cellular or at humoral control levels are equally rational when applied to the level of cell-cell interactions.   After finding the mechanisms through which epithelium and mesenchyme regulate or influence each other's activities, investigators should be able to devise ways to modify those factors that favor neoplastic transformation, and perhaps even those that favor proliferation of already transformed cells.

SUMMARY

Although epithelio-mesenchymal interactions are essential to the processes of organogenesis, regeneration, and maintenance of normal functional state of organs, the influence of these interactions on the response of epithelium to carcinogens is still poorly understood.   For example, morphologic changes in the dermis preceding or concomitant with epidermal carcinogenesis induced by hydrocarbons, X-irradiation or ultraviolet irradiation have long been suspected to play some role in carcinogenic events, but critical evaluation of available information allows one to assign no more than a permissive or supportive role to the connective tissue component.   Currently there is no firm evidence that carcinogen-altered (permutated) stroma can compel or induce unaltered epithelium to become neoplastic.

On the contrary, there is ample evidence from studies of carcinogenesis in cell culture that neoplastic transformation *can* be induced in cells completely dissociated from normal epithelio-mesenchymal relationships.   The tumors that result, however, have with only few exceptions shown the morphologic features of sarcomas, rather than of carcinomas.   This suggests that experimental systems for transforming dissociated cells *in vitro* do not reproduce precisely those events that occur in epithelial tumorigenesis *in vivo*.   Evidently, most of the neoplasms induced in these systems either originate from nonepithelial cells or assume the morphologic characteristics of sarcomas, even though epithelial in origin.

Experiments carried out *in vivo* as well as in an organotypic culture system are described to show how polyoma virus-induced tumorigenesis has been analyzed with respect to the factor of epithelio-mesenchymal interaction.   It has been found that: (1) disruption of eipthelio-mesenchymal interaction abrogates type-specific tumor induction; (2) substitution of heterogenous mesenchyme for homogenous mesenchyme fails to restore responsiveness to the oncogen; (3) polyoma-induced salivary tumors can substitute for normal salivary mesenchyme in supporting growth and morphogenesis of normal salivary epithelium; (4) although the polyoma salivary tumors induced *in vivo* have mesenchymoid histologic features, they originate from epithelium as demonstrated by chromosome-marking experiments.

Techniques used in the polyoma experiments appear to be applicable to studies in chemical or radiation-induced carcinogenesis. In particular, the experimental method of assembling glands in which karyotypic markers are used to identify phenotypic components (epithelium vs. mesenchyme) should make it possible to identify the tissue type of origin without relying on phenotypic characteristics that have been ambiguous or misleading in the past.

This presentation represents in part a summarization of work carried out in numerous collaborations over the past 15 years. In particular I wish to acknowledge the invaluable assistance of Mr. Willie D. Morgan, and Mr. James P. Summerour, who participated in the work during that entire time. Other collaborators include Dr. Thelma B. Dunn, Dr. Lloyd W. Law, Dr. James H. P. Main, Dr. Jacqueline Whang-Peng, Mrs. Marilyn S. Slatick, and Mr. Ernest C. Hearon. I am grateful to Mrs. Jeannette E. Williams for recent technical assistance and to Mr. Ralph L. Isenburg and Mr. Gebhard Gsell for photographic assistance. The histologic material was prepared by the Pathological Technology Section, under supervision of Miss Betty Sanders and Mr. Joseph Albrecht.

REFERENCES

1. Ashley, C. A. Epithelial and Stromal Roles in Carcinogenesis. II. Tumor Development in Internal Transplants of Skin and Epithelium Treated with 3-Methylcholanthrene. J. Natl. Cancer Inst., 26: 1445–1459, 1961.
2. Auerbach, R. In; Defendi, V. (ed.), Retention of Functional Differentiation in Cultured Cells, Wistar Inst. Symp., No. 1, pp. 3–17, Wistar Inst. Press, Philadelphia, 1964.
3. Azzopardi, J. G., and Williams, E. D. Pathology of " Nonendocrine Tumors Associated with Cushing's Syndrome." Cancer, 22: 274–286, 1968.
4. Bennett, I. L., Jr. The Function of Tumors. Physiol. Physicians, 3: 1–7, 1965.
5. Berwald, Y., and Sachs, L. *In vitro* Transformation of Normal Cells to Tumor Cells by Carcinogenic Hydrocarbons. J. Natl. Cancer Inst., 35: 641–661, 1965.
6. Billingham, R. E., Mangold, R., and Silvers, W. K. The Neogenesis of Skin in the Antlers of the Deer. Ann. N. Y. Acad. Sci., 83: 491–498, 1959.
7. Billingham, R. E., Orr, J. W., and Woodhouse, D. L. Transplantation of Skin Components during Chemical Carcinogenesis with 20-Methylcholanthrene. Brit. J. Cancer, 5: 417–432, 1951.
8. Black, P. H., Berman, L. D., and Maloof, R. An Analysis of SV-40-Induced Transformation of Hamster Kidney Tissue *in vitro*. IV. Studies of the Pathology of Hamster Tumors Induced with SV-40-Transformed Hamster Cell Clones. J. Natl. Cancer Inst., 37: 495–504 1966.
9. Borghese, E. Explantation Experiments on the Influence of the Connective Tissue Capsule on the Development of the Epithelial Part of the Submandibular Gland of *Mus musculus*. J. Anat., 84: 303–318, 1950.

424   DAWE

10. Daniels, F., Jr.   Ultraviolet Carcinogenesis in Man.   Natl. Cancer Inst. Monogr., *10*: 407–422, 1963.
11. Dawe, C. J., and Law, L. W.   Morphologic Changes in Salivary-gland Tissue of the Newborn Mouse Exposed to Parotid-tumor Agent *in vitro*.   J. Natl. Cancer Inst., *23*: 1157–1177, 1959.
12. Dawe, C. J., Law, L. W., Morgan, W. D., and Shaw, M. G.   Morphologic Responses to Tumor Viruses.   Fed. Proc., *21*: 5–14, 1962.
13. Dawe, C. J., Main, J. H. P., Slatick, M. S., and Morgan, W. D.   *In*; Kirsten, W. H. (ed.), Recent Results in Cancer Research, pp. 20–33, Springer-Verlag, New York, 1966.
14. Dawe, C. J., Morgan, W. D., and Slatick, M. S.   Influence of Epithelio-Mesenchymal Interactions on Tumor Induction by Polyoma Virus.   Int. J. Cancer, *1*: 419–450, 1966.
15. Dawe, C. J., Morgan, W. D., and Slatick, M. S.   *In*; Fleischmajer, R. (ed.), Epithelial-Mesenchymal Interactions, pp. 295–312, Williams and Wilkins Co., Baltimore, 1968.
16. Dawe, C. J., Morgan, W. D., and Williams, J. E.   Unpublished work in progress.
17. Dawe, C. J., Whang-Peng, J., Morgan, W. D., Hearon, E. C., and Knutsen, T.   Epithelial Origin of Polyoma Salivary Tumors in Mice: Evidence Based on Chromosome-marked Cells.   Science, *171*: 394–397, 1971.
18. DeOme, K. B., Faulkin, L. J., Jr., Bern, H. A., and Blair, P. B.   Development of Mammary Tumors from Hyperplastic Alveolar Nodules Transplanted into Gland-free Mammary Fat Pads of Female C3H Mice.   Cancer Res., *19*: 515–520, 1959.
19. Deppisch, L. M., and Toker, C.   Mixed Tumors of the Parotid Gland.   Cancer, *24*: 174–184, 1969.
20. DiPaolo, J. A., Nelson, R. L., and Donovan, P. J.   Morphological, Oncogenic, and Karyological Characteristics of Syrian Hamster Embryo Cells Transformed *in vitro* by Carcinogenic Polycyclic Hydrocarbons.   Cancer Res., *31*: 1118–1127, 1971.
21. Dunn, T. B.   Some Observations on the Normal and Pathological Anatomy of the Kidney of the Mouse.   J. Natl. Cancer Inst., *9*: 285–301, 1949.
22. Dunn, T. B.   *In*; Homburger, F., and Hoeber, P. B. (ed.), The Physiopathology of Cancer, pp. 38–84, New York, 1960.
23. Duran-Reynals, F., Bunting, H., and van Wagenen, G.   Studies on the Sex Skin of *Macaca Mulatta*.   Ann. N. Y. Acad. Sci., *52*: 1006–1014, 1950.
24. Edwards, W. D.   Abhängichkeit chaemisch-induzierte Karzinogenese von Kollagen Ab- und Aufbauvorgängen in transplantierte Rücken- und Schwanzhaut von Mäusen.   Dissertation, Univ. of Wien, Cancer Research Institute.
25. Flaxman, B. A., and Van Scott, E. J.   Keratinization *in vitro* of Cells from a Basal Cell Carcinoma.   J. Natl. Cancer Inst., *40*: 411–422, 1968.
26. Friedman-Kien, A. E., Dawe, C. J., and Van Scott, E. J.   Hair Growth Cycle in Subcutaneous Implants of Skin.   J. Invest. Derm., *43*: 445–450, 1964.
27. Gaush, C. R., Hard, W. L., and Smith, T. F.   Characterization of an Established Line of Canine Kidney Cells (MDCK).   Proc. Soc. Exp. Biol. Med., *122*: 931–935, 1966.
28. Giovanella, B. C., Liegel, J., and Heidelberger, C.   The Refractoriness of the Skin of Hairless Mice to Chemical Carcinogenesis.   Cancer Res., *30*: 2590–2597, 1970.
29. Grobstein, C.   Analysis *in vitro* of the Early Organization of the Rudiment of the Mouse Submandibular Gland.   J. Morphol., *93*: 19–44, 1953.
30. Grobstein, C.   Morphogenetic Interaction between Embryonic Mouse Tissues Separated by a Membrane Filter.   Nature, *172*: 869–871, 1953.

31. Grobstein, C. Cytodifferentiation and Its Controls. Science, *143*: 643–650, 1964.
32. Grobstein, C. Mechanisms of Organogenetic Tissue Interaction. Natl. Cancer Inst. Monogr., 26: 279–299, 1967.
33. Grobstein, C., and Cohen, J. Collagenase; Effect on the Morphogenesis of Embryonic Salivary Epithelium *in vitro*. Science, *150*: 626–628, 1965.
34. Haaland, M. Contributions to the Study of the Development of Sarcoma under Experimental Conditions. Sc. Rep. Cancer Fund, London, *3*: 175–261, 1908.
35. Hardy, M. H. Glandular Metaplasia of Hair Follicles and Other Responses to Vitamin A Excess in Cultures of Rodent Skin. J. Embryol. Exptl. Morph., *19*: 157–180, 1968.
36. Heidelberger, C., and Iype, P. T. *In*; Katsuta, H. (ed.), Cancer Cells in Culture, pp. 351–363. Univ. of Tokyo Press, Tokyo, 1968.
37. Ingleby, H., and Gershon-Cohen, J. Comparative Anatomy, Pathology, and Roentgenology of the Breast, Univ. of Penna. Press, 1960.
38. Junqueira, L. C., Fajer, A., Rabinovitch, M., and Frankenthal, L. Biochemical and Histochemical Observations on the Sexual Dimorphism of Mice Submaxillary Glands. J. Cell Comp. Physiol., *34*: 129–158, 1949.
39. Kallman, F., and Grobstein, C. Localization of Glucosamine-incorporating Materials at Epithelial Surfaces during Salivary Epithelio-Mesenchymal Interactions *in vitro*. Dev. Biol., *14*: 52–67, 1966.
40. Katsuta, H., and Takaoka, T. *In*; Katsuta, H. (ed.), Cancer Cells in Culture, pp. 321–334, Univ. of Tokyo Press, Tokyo, 1968.
41. Kettle, E. H. On Polymorphism of the Malignant Epithelial Cell. Proc. Roy. Soc. Med., *12*: 1–32, 1919. (Sec. Path., Part 3).
42. Kratochwil, K. Organ Specificity in Mesenchymal Induction Demonstrated in the Embryonic Development of the Mammary Gland of the Mouse. Dev. Biol., *20*: 46–71, 1969.
43. Lasfargues, E. Y., and Murray, M. R. *In*; Katsuta, H. (ed.), Cancer Cells in Culture, pp. 231–240, Univ. of Tokyo Press, Tokyo, 1968.
44. Law, L. W., Dunn, T. B., and Boyle, P. J. Neoplasms in the C3H Strain and in F_1 Hybrid Mice of Two Crosses Following Introduction of Extracts and Filtrates of Leukemia Tissues. J. Natl. Cancer Inst., *16*: 495–539, 1955.
45. Leighton, J., Brada, Z., Estes, L. W., and Justh, G. Secretory Activity and Oncogenicity of a Cell Line (MDCK) Derived from Canine Kidney. Science, *163*: 472–473, 1969.
46. Main, J. H. P., and Dawe, C. J. Tumor Induction in Transplanted Tooth Buds Infected with Polyoma Virus. J. Natl. Cancer Inst., *36*: 1121–1136, 1966.
47. Main, J. H. P., and Waheed, M. A. Epithelio-Mesenchymal Interactions in the Proliferative Response Evoked by Polyoma Virus in Odontogenic Epithelium *in vitro*. J. Natl. Cancer Inst., *47*: 711–726, 1971.
48. McLoughlin, C. B. The Importance of Mesenchymal Factors in the Differentiation of Chick Epidermis. II. Modification of Epidermal Differentiation by Contact with Different Types of Mesenchyme. J. Embryol. Exptl. Morph., *9*: 385–409, 1961.
49. Miller, J. A. Carcinogenesis by Chemicals: An Overview—G. H. A. Clowes Memorial Lecture. Cancer Res., *30*: 559–576, 1970.
50. Morgan, W. D., and Dawe, C. J. Sustained Growth of Salivary Gland Epithelium during Interaction with a Polyoma Virus-induced Tumor. (A time-lapse cinematogram presented at the Annual Meeting of the Tissue Culture Association, Detroit, 1969).

51. Noyes, W. F., and Mellors, R. C. Fluorescent Antibody Detection of the Antigens of the Shope Papilloma Virus in Papillomas of the Wild and Domestic Rabbit. J. Exptl. Med., *106*: 555–562, 1957.

52. Okumura, H. *In*; Katsuta, H. (ed.), Cancer Cells in Culture, pp. 292–298, Univ. of Tokyo Press, Tokyo, 1968.

53. Orr, J. W. The Changes Antecedent to Tumour Formation during the Treatment of Mouse Skin with Carcinogenic Hydrocarbons. J. Path. Bact., *46*: 495–515, 1938.

54. Orr, J. W. The Role of the Stroma in Epidermal Carcinogenesis. Natl. Cancer Inst. Monogr., *10*: 531–537, 1963.

55. Rutter, W. J., Wessells, N. K., and Grobstein, C. Control of Specific Synthesis in the Developing Pancreas. Natl. Cancer Inst. Monogr., *13*: 51–66, 1964.

56. Sanford, K. K., Dunn, T. B., Covalesky, A. B., Dupree, L. T., and Earle, W. R. Polyoma Virus and Production of Malignancy *in vitro*. J. Natl. Cancer Inst., *26*: 331–357, 1961.

57. Sanford, K. K., Dunn, T. B., Westfall, B. B., Covalesky, A. B., Dupree, L. T., and Earle, W. R. Sarcomatous Change and Maintenance of Differentiation in Long-term Cultures of Mouse Mammary Carcinoma. J. Natl. Cancer Inst., *26*: 1139–1183, 1961.

58. Sato, J. *In*; Katsuta, H. (ed.), Cancer Cells in Culture, pp. 335–530, Univ. of Tokyo Press, Tokyo, 1968.

59. Sherwin, R. P. *In*; Katsuta, H. (ed.), Cancer Cells in Culture, p. 363, Univ. of Tokyo Press, Tokyo, 1968.

60. Steinmuller, D. Epidermal Transplantation during Chemical Carcinogenesis: A Reinvestigation. Proc. Amer. Assoc. Cancer Res., *9*: 66, 1968.

61. Steinmuller, D., Dillingham, L. A., and Prehn, R. T. Lack of Carcinogenic Activity of 3-Methylcholanthrene in the Squirrel Monkey. J. Natl. Cancer Inst., *43*: 1175–1180, 1969.

62. Stewart, H. L., Grady, M. D., and Andervont, H. B. Development of Sarcoma at Site of Serial Transplantation of Pulmonary Tumors in Inbred Mice. J. Natl. Cancer Inst., *7*: 207–225, 1947.

63. Thiersch, C. Der Epithelialkrebs, namentliche der Haut; eine anatomisch-klinische Untersuchung, Leipzig, 1865.

64. Van Scott, E. J., and Reinertson, R. P. The Modulating Influence of Stromal Environment on Epithelial Cells Studied in Human Autotransplants. J. Invest. Derm., *36*: 109–131, 1961.

65. Virchow, R. Zur Entwicklungsgeschichte des Krebses nebst Bemerkungen über Fettbildung im thierischen Körper und pathologische Resorption. Virchow Arch., *3*: 94–201, 1851.

66. Vogt, M., and Dulbecco, R. Virus-cell Interaction with a Tumor-producing Virus. Proc. Natl. Acad. Sci., *46*: 365–370, 1960.

67. Wolbach, S. B. The Pathological Histology of Chronic X-Ray Dermatitis and Early X-Ray Carcinoma. J. Med. Res., *21*: 415–449, 1909.

68. Wolbach, S. B. The Hair Cycle of the Mouse and Its Importance in the Study of Sequences of Experimental Carcinogenesis. Ann. N. Y. Acad. Sci., *53*: 517–536, 1951.

Discussion of Paper by Dr. Dawe

Dr. Mirvish: In your experiments with Millipore filters, do you think cell contact between epithelial and mesenchymal cells is needed in order to get an interaction?

Dr. Dawe: We have not attempted to determine whether actual contact is established between tumor cells on one side of the membrane and normal epithelium on the other side.   This is, of course, something that should be done.

Dr. Sugimura: I wish just to mention the information that Yoshida sarcoma which has been thought to be mesenchymal tumor underwent conversion to the form of epithelial tumor in some experimental conditions, and the converted form persisted after several transplantations.

Dr. Odashima: I saw the infiltrating pattern of cells into the sponge matrix.   Do you think this pattern is a good sign of malignant transformation?
   Do you think that your experimental system using polyoma virus is also applicapable in screening carcinogenicity of chemicals?

Dr. Dawe: In this particular system the growth pattern of morphologically altered cells does seem to correlate well with ability to grow on back-transplantation.   The pattern is, incidentally, very similar to that which occurs if one places *in vivo*-induced salivary tumor in gelatin sponge matrix cultures.
   I think this method is applicable, but must be used with caution.   Unless one can correlate morphologic transformation with back-transplantability, conclusions must be inferential.   Therefore, comparable studies with human tissues would always be open to some question, although they could be of use as a presumptive screen. It would, of course, be important to use a number of organs in addition to salivary gland as target systems.   Methods such as this may be the closest one can come to simulating conditions *in vivo*.   However, one can see where failure would occur if conversion of a compound to active form must take place in an organ other than the one placed in culture.

The Effect of Some Nonviral Oncogenic Agents on Mammalian Cells *in vitro*

F. K. SANDERS

Division of Cell Biology, Sloan-Kettering Institute for Cancer Research, New York, N.Y., U.S.A.

Treatment with oncogenic viruses *in vitro* can affect cells in many ways. Apart from cytolytic interaction, cell shape, metabolism, behavior, and the morphology of colonies consisting of cell lineages stemming from single infected cells can all be altered. The latter change is called " transformation " (*13*), and its usual manifestation is the appearance, in cultures of cells seeded at sufficiently high dilution, of colonies of a new type, topographically different from those given by untreated cells. Many colonies of untransformed cells, consisting of at most a few layers of parallel-oriented cells, are now accompanied by a few piled-up multilayered " brush heaps " of randomly oriented transformed cells. Such virus-induced morphological transformation has been linked to the ability of cells so affected to give rise to progressively growing tumors when injected into suitable hosts (*34*). Virus-transformed cells, whatever their species of origin, moreover manufacture neoantigens characteristic of the particular virus responsible for their transformation (*16*), and these virus-specific antigens also characterize tumors induced by the same virus in susceptible hosts (*2*).

Cells treated *in vitro* with nonviral oncogens, such as irradiation and chemicals, also undergo changes whose degree reflects the intensity and duration of treatment. Many of them, however, depend on the continued presence of the inducing agent, the cells reverting to normal when the latter is withdrawn, and will not be considered further here. Certain changes, however, persist in later cell generations following the removal of the inciting agent, and can be considered analogous to the virus-induced transformations already mentioned. Among such is the ability to give rise to colonies of abnormal morphology, that arise from single cells whose genetic program, or its expression, has been altered in some way by the action of the oncogen. We prefer to call this change "*morphologic conversion*", rather than transformation, since:

(a)　There is no single morphologic type of abnormal colony characteristic of these agents as there is with viruses; among the colonies formed on the hundred or so dishes comprising one experiment with ultraviolet light, at least seventeen abnormal types could be identified, each giving rise to colonies of its own bizarre morphology when recloned.

(b)   The frequency of abnormal colonies seems higher than with viruses (24).

(c)   None of these abnormalities has so far been correlated with the ability to cause tumors when the altered cells are inoculated into suitable hosts. That this state of affairs is to be expected, is suggested by the fact that chemically induced tumors, even when induced in the same animal by the same oncogen, have different antigens (22), while all cells transformed by a given virus seem to share a common antigen.

Populations of mammalian cells can undergo morphologic heritable alterations in culture following treatment with agents as diverse as polycyclic hydrocarbons (1, 6, 8, 10, 24), nitroso compounds (18, 27), 4-nitroquinoline-1-oxide (21) and its active metabolite 4-hydroxyaminoquinoline-1-oxide (31), or X-irradiation (3–5). Primary cultures consisting of mixed populations of cells of different types from rodent embryos (3–5, 21, 22), hamster cell lines (1, 31), organ cultures of mouse lung primordia (7), prostate (8), and epithelial cell strains derived therefrom (24) have all been employed in such studies.

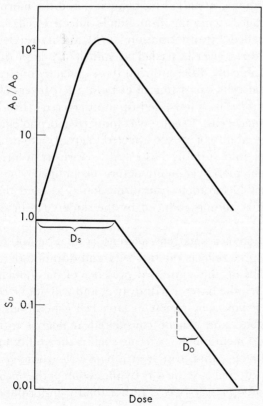

FIG. 1.   Relationship between survival (S_D), " conversion ratio " (A_D/A_O), and dose for increasing doses of a given oncogen (for explanation see text).

It is, however, difficult to compare directly the effects of different oncogenic agents on cells *in vitro*. It can be seen from the above (*1, 3–8, 10, 18, 21, 22, 27, 31*) that there has been no uniformity in either the materials or the methods by which experiments have been carried out in different laboratories, and there is so far no common criterion of cell alteration whereby different agents can be contrasted. We have thus attempted to devise a standard comparative mode of experimentation, the reasons for which, and whose details, will be discussed elsewhere (*29*), as well as to develop numerical parameters of cell conversion that can be used to compare the effects of agents as diverse as radiation, polycyclic hydrocarbons, and water-soluble carcinogens. It should, however, be stressed that all the comparisons made in this paper are based on the totality of the abnormal colonies induced. So far no attempt has been made to correlate any of the alterations with the acquisition of an ability to cause tumors when inoculated into suitable hosts, or indeed to suspect that any one morphological type might be outstandingly tumorigenic.

Type of data and method of analysis

Separate aliquots from the same batch of cells (10^6/ml) were subjected to various levels of treatment with the same oncogen; individual samples of 10^3 cells were then plated and incubated for 10–12 days prior to colony counting. Control plates, prepared from aliquots of the same batch of cells, similarly handled except for the absence of the oncogen, were included in every experiment, and the same batch of medium used throughout.

The data recorded for each treatment level then consisted of the following:

(1) *The number of cells surviving at a dose D*, as estimated by their ability to form colonies *in vitro* (N_D). From this it was possible to calculate S_D, the proportion of potential colony formers surviving the dose D, expressed as a fraction of those forming colonies at zero dose ($S_D = N_D/N_O$). When such figures were plotted against dose on a semi-logarithmic scale, we obtained survival curves like that given in Fig. 1, resembling those commonly observed in radiation biology (*15*). As with the latter, they are characterized by an initial shoulder of varying extent (D_S), presumably an indication of the extent to which damage can be repaired, followed by a descending arm (linear on a semi-logarithmic plot) whose slope is characteristic of the relative " toxicity " of the agent used; by analogy with radiation survival curves, D_O, the " *median toxic dose* " required to reduce survival by a factor $1/e$, can then be estimated from this part of the curve. There are considerable individual differences between various oncogenic agents with respect to these two parameters. However, the effects of all those studied so far can be expressed in this form, and the two parameters D_S and D_O used to compare their effects upon cell survival.

(2) *The number of cells that give rise to " abnormal " colonies at a dose D*, which will include the number of " abnormal " colony formers in the original suspension that survive at that dose, plus any " converted " but not eliminated by it. It is now possible to plot the ratio A_D/A_O (the number of abnormal colonies at dose D divided by the number of abnormal colonies at zero dose) against dose to produce curves analogous to the survival curves discussed above.

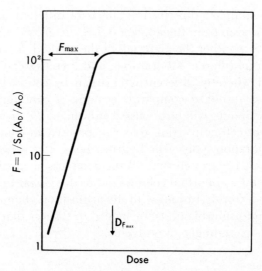

Fig. 2.   Relationship between " efficacy of cell conversion " and dose of a given oncogen (for derivation see text).

Graphs of the ratio A_D/A_O against dose have a number of interesting features. Should A_D/A_O have a value of about 1.0 at all doses, this would suggest that selection (25) by the agent being investigated of pre-existing, morphologically converted, resistant cells would be adequate to explain any effect observed; should A_D/A_O fall below 1.0, it would indicate either (a) that cells in the original suspension able to give rise to abnormal colonies were more sensitive than normal to the toxicity of the agent, or (b) that reversion to normality was being induced.

With active agents, curves of A_D/A_O (the " conversion ratio ") against dose rise to a maximum, followed by a decline (Fig. 1).   The tail of this curve tends to parallel the descending arm of the survival curve for the same agent, suggesting that converted cells have the same susceptibility to any toxic effect of the agent as do their normal counterparts.   If this is assumed to hold for all the agents tested, the surviving fraction S_D at a given dose D can be used to correct the conversion ratio A_D/A_O for that dose to obtain a quantity $F_D = 1/S_D \cdot A_D/A_O$, which is an estimate of an agent's efficacy in converting cells at that dose independently of its toxicity.   When this quantity is plotted against dose (Fig. 2), a curve is found that rises to a maximum in the case of all the active agents studied, after which it remains at a plateau level throughout the rest of the range of dose in which toxicity is not absolute.   This maximum level F_{max} is a measure of the *cell-converting capacity* of a given agent, and can be used to compare it with others.   A further comparative factor $D_{F_{max}}$ is the minimum dose at which F_D becomes equal to F_{max}.

Four parameters, (a) D_S, the width of the shoulder on the survival curve, (b) D_O, (c) F_{max}, and (d) $D_{F_{max}}$, therefore suffice to define both the toxicity and the cell-converting capacity of different oncogenic agents. D_S/D_O is a measure of the capacity of cells to repair damage by that particular oncogen to their ability to form colonies *in vitro*, and $(D_{F_{max}} - D_S)/D_O$ expresses the number of

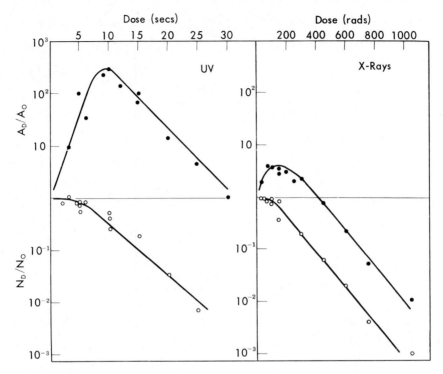

FIG. 3.   Plots of survival (N_D/N_0, ○) and conversion ratio (A_D/A_0, ●) against dose for ultraviolet radiation and X-rays.

irreparable MTD that must be suffered before maximal conversion is attained.

It should be insisted that measurements of this kind have so far been made only with one type of cell, and the mode of calculation proposed may only be valid for experiments performed in a particular way (29). In the work described in the following sections, we have attempted a direct comparison, using these methods, between (a) X-ray and ultraviolet radiation, (b) polycylic hydrocarbons, (c) nitroso compounds including nitrosoureas, as well as (d) a variety of other water-soluble substances, with regard to their effect on a single clone of Chinese hamster lung cells capable of continuous propagation *in vitro*, but unable to cause tumors in the Syrian hamster cheek pouch when 10^6 cells are injected (27).

The effects of radiation

When Chinese hamster cells are treated in suspension with either X-rays or ultraviolet irradiation, plated, and allowed to form colonies *in vitro*, it can be seen that increasing doses of both kinds of irradiation (a) reduce the total number, and (b) augment the proportion of morphologically abnormal colonies. N_D/N_0 and A_D/A_0 are shown plotted against dose for both types of irradiation in Fig. 3. Either form of treatment inhibits later colony formation, the survival curves having an initial shoulder followed by a region in which survival declines linearly with increasing

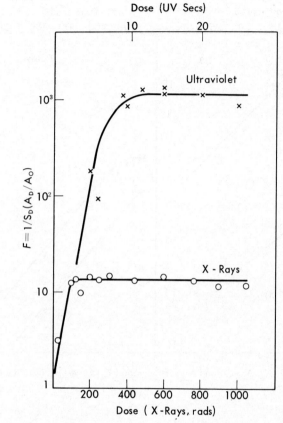

FIG. 4. Plots against dose of the efficacy of cell conversion by ultraviolet light ($\times$———$\times$) and X-rays ($\bigcirc$———$\bigcirc$).

TABLE 1. Parameters of Cell Conversion by Ultraviolet Light and X-Rays

	$F_{\max}$[a]	D_O[b]	D_S/D_O[c]	$\dfrac{D_{F\max}-D_S}{D_O}$[d]
Ultraviolet	1.1×10^3	3 secs	0.5	+2.3
X-Rays	13.5	140 rads	0.7	+0.4

[a] Maximal conversion capacity (see text). [b] Median toxic dose. [c] Number of reparable toxic doses. [d] Number of irreparable toxic doses suffered before maximal level of conversion.

dose—features which are already well known for X-irradiated Chinese hamster cells (14). Conversion frequency ratios A_D/A_O, however, rise initially to a maximum for both kinds of radiation when plotted against dose, then decline with a slope parallel to the survival curves. Figure 4 plots F, the efficacy of conversion (see previous section), against dose for both kinds of radiation. Both curves rise to a plateau, and from them the parameters $F_{\max}$ and $D_{F\max}$ can be estimated.

Table 1 gives the values of the four parameters estimated from the curves of Fig. 4. Paralleling its powerful mutagenic effect in bacteria (11), ultraviolet light is a hundred times more effective than X-rays as a cell-converting agent. This difference is to be expected, since ultraviolet light of the range of wavelengths used is strongly absorbed by nucleic acids, whereas penetrating radiations like soft X-rays are not.   A converse situation exists in multicellular organisms where ultraviolet, due to its failure to penetrate, is a less effective mutagen.   The two forms of radiation are also alike in another respect: the effects of between a half and one " median toxic dose " are reparable in each case.   With X-rays, addition of less than one MTD beyond the reparable level is required before the maximum frequency of cell conversion is attained; with ultraviolet light the figure is more than two.   However, these differences are minor compared with the great differences in the capacity to convert cells exhibited by the two forms of radiation, and may explain why many have found it difficult to consistently demonstrate cell conversion by X-rays *in vitro* under less rigidly controlled conditions (*3–5, 26*).

It will be noted from Fig. 4 and Table 1 that in both cases the *cell-converting capacity* (F_{max}) significantly exceeds unity (X-rays 10; UV 10^3).   This is direct evidence that any hypothesis involving the selection of pre-existing variants (*25*) will not suffice to explain the results obtained, and that some form of direct action of radiation on susceptible cells must be considered as an alternative.   Further experiments involving measurement of the effect on F_{max} of radio-sensitizing and cell-synchronizing agents, as well as inhibitors of protein and DNA synthesis, will be necessary before a plausible hypothesis of the mode of action of radiations can be formulated.

The effects of polycyclic hydrocarbons

To approximate the conditions used with irradiation cells were first treated briefly (2 hr) in suspension with various amounts of hydrocarbon, plated after dilution, and colonies counted.   The details of the experimental procedure employed will be described elsewhere (*28*).   However, in confirmation of the results of others (*17*), it was found in preliminary experiments that hydrocarbons, as a class, did not achieve their maximum effect unless present throughout at least one complete cycle of cell multiplication.   To achieve maximum values for the parameters described above, these compounds were accordingly added also to the dilution fluids and medium in the dishes used for plating at the same concentrations as in the original treatment vials, and were thus present to some extent for the whole duration of the experiment.

Graphs of F (the efficacy of cell conversion) against dose for three representative oncogens (benzo(a)pyrene, dimethylbenzanthracene, methylcholanthrene), control compounds (pyrene, chrysene, dibenzanthracene), and the solvent (DMSO) used to solubilize them, are given in Fig. 5.   Values for the four parameters of toxicity and cell conversion described in earlier sections are likewise given in Table 2.   Benzo-(a)pyrene and 9,12-dimethylbenzanthracene are both effective cell-converting agents, capable of increasing the frequency of appearance of converted cells to a value 5–700 times above background.   However, by this *in vitro* test BP qualifies as a superior cell-converting agent to DMBA.   While both have approximately the same cell converting capacity and D_O's of the same order of magnitude (0.75 and 0.5 μg), only one-tenth of an MTD of the damage caused by DMBA can be repaired, while the corresponding value for BP is 4.7.   In addition, $(D_{Fmax}-D_S)/D_O$ in the case of

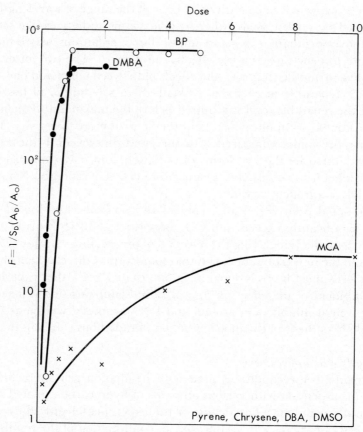

FIG. 5.   Plots against dose (μg/ml) of the efficacy of cell conversion by various hydrocarbons: benzo(a)pyrene (BP, O————O); dimethylbenzanthracene (DMBA, ●————●); methylcholanthrene (MCA, ×————×); pyrene, chrysene, dibenzanthracene (DBA), and dimethylsulfoxide (DMSO), were all without effect; numerical values in Table 2.

TABLE 2.   Parameters of Cell Conversion by Oncogenic Hydrocarbons

	F_{max}	D_O (μg/ml)	D_S/D_O	$\dfrac{D_{F\,max} - D_S}{D_O}$
Benzo(a)pyrene (BP)	7.2×10^2	0.75	4.7	−3.4
9,12-Dimethylbenzanthracene (DMBA)	5.0×10^2	0.5	0.1	+3.9
Methylcholanthrene (MCA)	20	3.7	0.9	+1.3
Pyrene	1	>10	—	—
1,2,5,6-Dibenzanthracene (DBA)	1	>10	—	—
Chrysene	1	>10	—	—
Dimethylsulfoxide (DMSO)	1	1100	0.4	—

All symbols same as in Table 1.

BP has a negative value, which means that a maximum level of cell conversion is attained well within the zone of reparable damage, while almost four MTD of irreparable damage by DMBA is incurred before the maximum level of cell conversion is reached.   Methylcholanthrene is a less active $(20\times)$ cell-converting agent than BP or DBA.   It is, however, 5–6 times less toxic than the other two compounds: about 1 MTD is reparable, and the maximum level of conversion is achieved when about 1 MTD of irreparable damage has occurred.

By contrast the other three compounds have no measurable cell-converting capacity in this system $(F_{max}=1)$, nor measurable toxicity in the range of concentrations studied.   Dimethylsulfoxide (DMSO), the solvent used to solubilize all these compounds also appears to lack the ability to convert cells morphologically. It does, however, show some toxicity, but only at concentrations 10–100 times greater than that at which it is present when used as a solvent for the other compounds discussed in this section.   None of the toxicity of DMBA or MCA can thus be ascribed to the simultaneous presence of DMSO.

The relative efficacy of cell conversion shown by the various hydrocarbons is roughly comparable to what is found when their carcinogenicity *in vivo* is assessed according to Iball's index *(20)*.   Here DMBA and BP are rated as effective carcinogens, with DMBA as the more powerful.   However, in our system, BP is rated superior, chiefly due to the high degree to which the damage it causes can be repaired, a feature which would not be revealed by conventional *in vivo* experiments. DBA was an exception since, though it had been shown to be a weak carcinogen *in vivo (30)*, it did not have any measurable cell-converting capacity for Chinese hamster cells *in vitro*.   However, it is possible that they may lack an enzyme necessary for its conversion to a proximate carcinogen that is possessed by susceptible cells *in vivo*. As will be shown in the next section, nitrosomethylmethane (DMN), an effective carcinogen *in vivo*, is also without effect on these cells in culture.

The effect of nitroso compounds

Compounds in this group had been found previously to convert cells morphologically after only a brief treatment *(27)*.   Chinese hamster cells were accordingly treated in suspension for 2 hr at 37°C with various concentrations of the compounds listed in Table 4, diluted at $+4°C$ to stop the action of the compound as well as to obtain the correct cell concentration, and then plated for later colony counting; the detailed procedure employed is discussed elsewhere *(30)*.

Eleven compounds were tested.   The various parameters of their effect on Chinese hamster cells *in vitro* are given in Table 3.   It will be noted that they vary from compounds whose toxicity was barely demonstrable, to others where an extremely low dose, briefly applied, will prevent subsequent colony formation.   Relatively little damage by any of them seems reparable, although a plateau of cell conversion is reached at dose levels only a little beyond the shoulder of the survival curve.   It should be emphasized, however, that the values given in the last two columns of Table 4 are only tentative, since in many cases of low toxicity D_O had to be estimated by extrapolation beyond the range of doses actually tested.

The efficacy of cell conversion (F) for the first eight nitroso compounds whose other parameters are given in Table 3 have been plotted against dose in Fig. 6, and provide some preliminary information regarding the possible influence of molecular structure on this quantity.   With nitrosoalkylureas, the methyl is the most active,

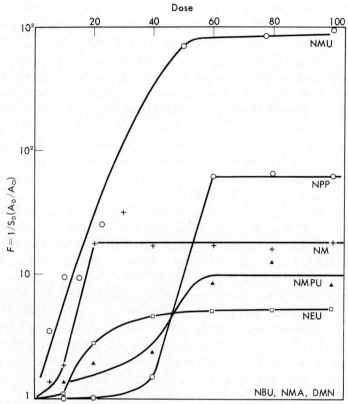

FIG. 6. Plots against dose (μg/ml) of the efficacy of cell conversion by various nitroso compounds: nitrosomethylurea (NMU, ○———○); nitrosopiperidine (NPP, ○———○; nitrosomorpholine (NM, +———+); nitrosomethylphenylurea (NMPU, ▲———▲); nitrosoethylurea (NEU, □———□); nitrosobutylurea (NBU), nitrosomethylaniline (NMA), and nitrosomethylmethane (DMN) were all without effect; numerical values in Table 3.

TABLE 3. Parameters of Cell Conversion by Nitroso Compounds

	F_{max}	D_O (μg/ml)	D_S/D_O	$\dfrac{D_{Fmax}-D_S}{D_O}$
Nitrosopiperidine (NPP)	62	>200	$\simeq$0.1	+<0.1
Nitrosomorpholine (NM)	18	>100	$\simeq$0.2	+<0.1
Nitrosomethylmethane (DMN)	1	>100	—	—
Nitrosomethylaniline (NMA)	1	>100	—	—
Nitrosomethylurea (NMU)	8.5×10^2	42	0.24	+1.0
Nitrosomethylphenylurea (NMPU)	10	>100	$\simeq$0.1	+0.2
Nitrosoethylurea (NEU)	5	30	1.7	0.0
Nitrosobutylurea (NBU)	1	>200	—	—
Nitrosobischloroethylurea (BCNU)	20	5.5	0.2	+0.3
Nitrosomethylnitroguanidine (NMNG) (S phase cells)	7.2	0.4	<0.1	+1.0
Nitrosomethylnitroguanidine (NMNG) (cells *not* in S)	20	1.4	2.3	−2.3

All symbols same as in Table 1.

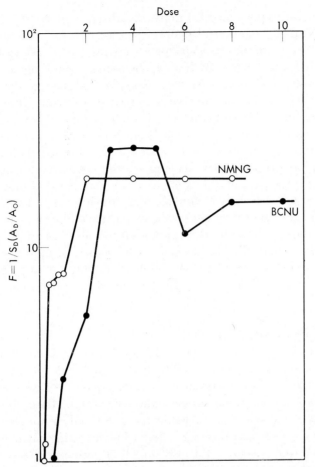

FIG. 7.   Plots of the efficacy of cell conversion against dose (μg/ml) for nitrosomethylnitroguanidine (NMNG, O———O) and nitrosobischloroethylurea (BCNU, ●———●); numerical values in Table 3.

the ethyl less so, and the butyl compound has no detectable activity in the dose range tested.   The possession of both methyl and nitroso groups on the same nitrogen atom, however, is not necessarily obligatory for a given compound to be active.   Substitution of a phenyl group for one of the hydrogens of the free amino group of nitrosomethylurea reduces its activity tenfold.   Compounds with more extreme alternatives for this part of the molecule, as in nitrosomethylmethane (DMN) or nitrosomethylaniline (NMA), are inactive with these cells, although tumorigenic *in vivo* (*23*).   The second most active compound is nitrosopiperidine (NPP), in which the alkyl group is cyclic; a minor change in this part of the molecule (nitrosomorpholine; NM) brings about a threefold reduction in activity.

Of particular interest are two further compounds, nitrosomethylnitroguanidine (NMNG) and nitrosobischloroethylurea (BCNU), whose curves of F against dose are given in Fig. 7.   Both molecules have a substituted urea structure, and although NMNG has an imino group in place of the carbonyl oxygen of urea there is no evidence that substitution at this position *per se* markedly affects activity (see thiourea in following section). NMNG, a powerful chemical mutagen (*33*), has methyl and nitroso groups on the same amino nitrogen, together with a nitro-group instead of one of the hydrogens on the other. BCNU, a chemotherapeutic agent (*35*), has alkyl radicals on both nitrogen atoms. Nevertheless, Fig. 7 shows that the two compounds behave in a very similar manner with regard to cell-converting activity, although neither approaches nitrosomethylurea in magnitude. They are also the two most toxic compounds in Table 3. It has been shown previously that nitrosomethylurea is approximately ten times more toxic for transformed than for " normal " cells, and a similar property may account for the chemotherapeutic significance of BCNU. Survival curves of cells treated *in vitro* with NMNG show that this substance is more toxic towards cells in S phase than during the rest of the cycle; this is also the reason for the small shoulder on the rising arm of the curve of F against dose. Moreover, the damage done by this compound to cells not in S phase can be more extensively repaired than damage to cells in S (Table 3), most repair being possibly undertaken during the S phase that follows removal of the compound. The cell-converting efficacy of NMNG, though, is higher during the non-S phases of the cell cycle.

The effects of other urea derivatives

Table 4 shows comparable parameters of cell conversion by a number of other urea derivatives and related compounds. Cells were treated with them in the same way as the nitroso compounds discussed in the last section. Because they all had low toxicity, D_O in almost all cases had to be found by extrapolation. The figures in the last two columns of Table 4, as with Table 3, are thus only tentative, although they show little evidence of repair processes. The cell-converting capacity of most of the compounds, moreover, was low; the only ones that perhaps can be considered active being semicarbazide and hydroxyurethane. Acetamide had an activity similar to that of X-rays, while urethane, an " incomplete " carcinogen, tetramethylurea, and

TABLE 4. Parameters of Cell Conversion by Urea Derivatives and Similar Compounds

	F_{max}	D_O (μg/ml)	D_S/D_O	$\dfrac{D_{Fmax} - D_S}{D_O}$
Urea	1	>100	—	—
Thiourea	1	75	—	—
Dimethylurea	1	>100	—	—
Tetramethylurea	10	80	<0.05	+<0.1
Hydroxyurea	5	>100	<0.05	+<0.3
Formamide	5	>100	0.05	+>0.7
Dimethylformamide	1	>100	—	—
Acetamide	13	80	<0.05	+0.3
Semicarbazide	>30	>100	<0.05	+0.2
Urethane	5	>100	—	—
Hydroxyurethane	20	>100	<0.05	+0.2

All symbols same as in Table 1.

hydroxyurea had only questionable activity under these conditions. Only in the case of hydroxyurethane, however, did the graph of F against dose have the particular features of rising phase, followed by an extended plateau, that was shown by all the active agents discussed in the previous sections. Thus the other values of F_{max} quoted in Table 4 must be interpreted with caution until further data are available regarding the effect of these compounds in other systems.

DISCUSSION

When the various oncogenic agents are compared for their efficacy in causing morphological conversion of cells by the criteria adopted in this paper, they fall into four groups whose activity roughly parallels that of their oncogenic activity *in vivo*. Ultraviolet light, NMU, BP, and DMBA, are all highly active, and the last three, are well known to easily cause a whole variety of tumors *in vivo* (*32*). NPP, MCA, NM, BCNU, are of moderate activity, and the first three have been reported to cause epitheliomas and sarcomas in the skin and respiratory tract; the last, so far as I am aware, has not been tested for oncogenic activity *in vivo*; NMPU and NEU have questionable activity, but the latter has been reported to act as a transplacental carcinogen (*12*); the inactive group of agents are mostly either inactive *in vivo*, or reported to cause tumors of the gut, liver, and accessory organs (*23*).

However, the importance of these findings does not lie only in providing a means to rank oncogens in order of potency and to screen the environment for potential cell-converting compounds in a more rapid way. Now that a valid, reproducible measure of cell-converting capacity divorced from toxicity is available, experiments on the mechanism of cell conversion by such agents can be undertaken. For example, at least five plausible hypotheses can be suggested at the present time to account for the mechanisms by which cells and their descendants become altered through the action of oncogenic agents:

1. Since chemical oncogens and radiation tend to impair the ability of cells to give rise to viable progeny, it has been suggested (*25*) that they act selectively to eliminate normal cells, and that altered cells of the type found must have been present among those originally treated; they then came to dominate the surviving population by reason of their resistance to the damaging effect of the oncogen (*9*).

2. That oncogenic agents act through the intermediary of a virus—in the case of oncogenic virus infection the action is direct (*13*) while in the case of chemicals and radiation, it takes place by the activation of viruses latent within the cells (*19*).

3. That oncogenic agents act as mutagens; *i.e.*, they permanently alter the cellular DNA, and hence its phenotypic expression.

4. A more sophisticated version of hypothesis 3: that oncogens may act by inhibiting the action of one or more enzymes concerned in the repair of DNA, so allowing the phenotypic expression of spontaneous or induced " mutations " that would otherwise be eliminated.

5. That oncogens may exert their effect by altering the pattern of expression of cellular genes, perhaps allowing the expression of growth-influencing factors that are dormant in unaffected cells.

Although the data presented in this paper would tend to rule out the first hypothesis, it is difficult at present to decide between others. In fact, there is no reason to assume that all oncogens will act in the same way, or indeed that any one of them acts through a single mechanism.

However, since we can now measure efficacy of cell conversion under different conditions, such as the presence of radio-sensitizing agents or inhibitors of protein, RNA, and DNA synthesis and repair, it should be possible to devise experiments to find the means by which different agents bring about the hereditary morphological change in cultured cells. In addition to looking for a correlation between specific types of cellular alteration *in vitro* and oncogenesis *in vivo*, it should be possible to find out whether different oncogenic agents act through a final common pathway.

REFERENCES

1. Berwald, Y., and Sachs, L. *In vitro* Transformation of Normal Cells to Tumor Cells by Carcinogenic Hydrocarbons. J. Natl. Cancer Inst., 35: 641, 1965.
2. Black, P. H. The Oncogenic DNA Viruses. A Review of *in vitro* Transformation Studies. Ann. Rev. Microbiol., 22: 391, 1968.
3. Borek, C., and Sachs, L. *In vitro* Cell Transformation by X-Irradiation. Nature, 210: 276, 1966.
4. Borek, C., and Sachs, L. Cell Susceptibility to Transformation by X-Irradiation and Fixation of the Transformed State. Proc. Natl. Acad. Sci., 57: 1522, 1967.
5. Borek, C., and Sachs, L. The Number of Cell Generations Required to Fix the Transformed State in X-Ray Induced Transformation. Proc. Natl. Acad. Sci., 59: 83, 1968.
6. Borenfreund, E., Krim, M., Sanders, F. K., Sternberg, S. S., and Bendich, A. Malignant Conversion of Cells *in vitro* by Carcinogens and Viruses. Proc. Natl. Acad. Sci., 56: 672, 1966.
7. Chan, P. C., Sanders, F. K., and Wynder, E. L. Effect of 3,4-Benzo(a)pyrene on Mouse Lung Primordia *in vitro*. Nature, 223: 847, 1969.
8. Chen, T. T., and Heidelberger, C. Quantitative Studies on the Malignant Transformation of Mouse Prostate Cells by Carcinogenic Hydrocarbons *in vitro*. Int. J. Cancer, 4: 166, 1969.
9. Diamond, L. The Interaction of Chemical Carcinogens and Cells *in vitro*. Progr. Exptl. Tumor Res., 11: 364, 1969.
10. DiPaolo, J. A., and Donovan, P. J. Properties of Syrian Hamster Cells Transformed in the Presence of Carcinogenic Hydrocarbons. Exptl. Cell Res., 48: 361, 1967.
11. Drake, J. W. The Molecular Basis of Mutation. Holden Day, San Francisco, 1970.
12. Druckrey, H., Ivankovic, S., and Preussmann, R. Teratogenic and Carcinogenic Effects in the Offspring after Single Injection of Ethylnitrosourea to Pregnant Rats. Nature, 210: 1378, 1966.
13. Dulbecco, R. Cell Transformation by Viruses. Science, 166: 962, 1969.
14. Elkind, M. M., and Sutton, H. Radiation Response of Mammalian Cells Grown in Culture. I. Repair of X-Ray Damage in Surviving Chinese Hamster Cells. Radiation Res., 13: 556, 1960.
15. Elkind, M. M., and Whitmore, G. F. The Radiobiology of Cultured Mammalian Cells, Gordon and Breach, New York, 1967.
16. Green, M. Oncogenic Viruses. Ann. Rev. Biochem., 39: 701, 1970.

17. Heidelberger, C. Chemical Carcinogenesis, Chemotherapy: Cancer's Continuing Core Challenges. G. H. A. Clowes Memorial Lecture. Cancer Res., *30*: 1549, 1970.

18. Huberman, E., Salzberg, S., and Sachs, L. The *in vitro* Induction of an Increase in Cell Multiplication and Cellular Life Span by the Water-soluble Carcinogen Dimethylnitrosamine. Proc. Natl. Acad. Sci., *59*: 77, 1968.

19. Huebner, R. J., and Todaro, G. J. Oncogenes of RNA Tumor Viruses as Determinants of Cancer. Proc. Natl. Acad. Sci., *64*: 1087, 1969.

20. Iball, J. The Relative Potency of Carcinogenic Compounds. Amer. J. Cancer, *35*: 188, 1939.

21. Kamahora, J., and Kakunaga, T. *In vitro* Transformation of Hamster Whole Embryonic Cells by 4-Nitroquinoline-1-oxide. Bikens J., *9*: 295, 1966.

22. Klein, G. Tumor-specific Transplantation Antigens. G. H. A. Clowes Memorial Lecture. Cancer Res., *28*: 625, 1968.

23. Magee, P. N., and Barnes, J. M. Carcinogenic Nitroso Compounds. Adv. Cancer Res., *10*: 163, 1967.

24. Mondal, S., and Heidelberger, C. *In vitro* Malignant Transformation by Methylcholanthrene of the Progeny of Single Cells Derived from the C3H Mouse Prostate. Proc. Natl. Acad. Sci., *65*: 219, 1970.

25. Prehn, R. T. A Clonal Selection Theory of Chemical Carcinogenesis. J. Natl. Cancer Inst., *32*: 1, 1964.

26. Sanders, F. K. Problems in the Study of Oncogens *in vitro*. Med. Clinics of N. America, *55*: 653, 1971.

27. Sanders, F. K., and Burford, B. O. Morphological Conversion of Cells *in vitro* by N-Nitrosomethylurea. Nature, *213*: 1171, 1967.

28. Sanders, F. K., and Burford, B. O. Quantitation of Morphologic Conversion of Cells by Oncogens. II. Polycylic Hydrocarbons. In preparation.

29. Sanders, F. K., Burford, B. O., and Monaghan, M. Quantitation of Morphologic Conversion of Cell Cultures by Oncogens. I. X-Rays and Ultraviolet Irradiation. In preparation.

30. Sanders, F. K., and Monaghan, M. Quantitation of Cell Conversion by Oncogens. III. Water Soluble Compounds. In preparation.

31. Sato, H., and Kuroki, T. Malignization *in vitro* of Hamster Embryonic Cells by Chemical Carcinogens. Proc. Japan Acad., *42*: 1211, 1966.

32. Schramm, T., Bielka, H., und Graffi, A. Geschwulsterzeugung durch chemische Substanzen. *In*; Experimentellen Pharmakologie, Vol. XVI, Teil 12, Springer, Berlin, 1966.

33. Singer, B., Fraenkel-Conrat, H., Greenberg, J., and Michelson, A. Reaction of Nitrosoguanidine (N-Methyl-N'-nitro-N-nitrosoguanidine) with Tobacco Mosaic Virus and Its RNA. Science, *160*: 1235, 1968.

34. Stoker, M. J., and Abel, P. Conditions Affecting Transformation by Polyma Virus. Cold Spring Harbor Symp. Quant. Biol., *27*: 375, 1962.

35. Suguira, K. Effect of 1, 3-Bis(2-chloroethyl)-1-nitrosourea (NSC-409962) and Two Related Compounds on a Spectrum of Tumors. Cancer Res., *27*: 179, 1967.

Discussion of Paper by Dr. Sanders

DR. LAWLEY: Your results immediately raise the question whether some of the nitroso compounds were metabolized in these cells; for example, do you think that nitrosopiperidine and nitrosomorpholine are acting here as the unchanged molecules?

DR. SANDERS: This interpretation is not excluded by the data. It is, however, an open question, as we have made no biochemical observations so far.

DR. MIRVISH: Are you sure that the negative result with dimethylnitrosamine was not due to its high volatility?

DR. SANDERS: Yes. Cells were treated briefly with freshly prepared solutions of DMN in closed vessels.

DR. MAGEE: There is evidence that the enzyme system which metabolizes dimethylnitrosamine may differ from that which metabolizes diethylnitrosamine. Have you tried diethylnitrosamine in your system? Would you agree that your results with nitrosomorpholine and nitrosopiperidine might be explained by their acting as the unchanged molecule?

DR. SANDERS: We have not tested diethylnitrosamine, but it would certainly be interesting to do so. The answer to your second question is that I gave to Dr. Lawley.

Prenatal Exposure to Chemical Carcinogens

L. TOMATIS, V. TURUSOV, and D. GUIBBERT

International Agency for Research on Cancer, Lyon, France, and Institut National des Sciences Appliquées, Lyon, France

The first report on the induction of tumors following prenatal exposure to a chemical carcinogen was published in 1947 by Larsen (*30*), followed by a report by Smith and Rous in 1948 (*50*) and by Klein in 1952 (*26*). In all three instances the chemical used was urethane.

Since then reports on the carcinogenic effect of a chemical administered during pregnancy on the offspring have multiplied. At least 30 chemical carcinogens have so far been reported to produce tumors following prenatal exposure (Table 1); this property is common to chemicals with different chemical structures, such as urethane, polycyclic hydrocarbons, N-nitroso compounds, etc. Among these are chemicals which are only laboratory tools and have no importance for the general population, but there are others which may represent a risk in the human environment.

TABLE 1. Chemical Carcinogens Inducing Tumors Following Prenatal Exposure

Urethane (*26, 27, 30, 47, 50, 62*)	Ethylnitrosourea (*10, 13, 18, 23, 45*) (and Ethylurea + Na-nitrite) (*23*)	1-Methyl-2-benzylhydrazine (*9*)
o-Aminoazotoluene (*16*)	Nitrosomethylurea (*2*)	1-Phenyl-3,3-dimethyltriazene (*9*)
7,12-Dimethylbenz(a)anthracene (*5, 56, 57*)	Ethylnitrosobiuret (*12*)	1-Phenyl-3,3-diethyltriazene (*9*)
Benzo(a)pyrene (*4*)	1,2-Diethylhydrazine (*11*)	1-Pyridil-3,3-diethyltriazene (*9*)
Methylcholanthrene (*48, 58, 61*)	Azoethane (*11*)	Dimethylsulfate (*9*)
Crude cycad material (*51*) (Methylazoxymethanol)	Azoxyethane (*11*) Azoxymethane (*11*)	Diethylsulfate (*9*)
Diethylnitrosamine (*31, 37, 38, 39, 40, 44, 45*)	Nitrosomethylurethane (*54*)	1,3-Propane sultone (*9*)
Dimethylnitrosamine (*1*)	Ethylnitrosourethane (*9*)	Methyl methanesulphonate (*33*)
Elasiomycin (*54*)	Aflatoxin B (*54*)	^{32}P-Phosphate (*9*)
	N-Isopropyl-α-(2-methylhydrazino)-*p*-toluamide·HCl (Natulan) (*22*)	Stilbestrol (*17, 20, 21*)

In these studies the chemicals were administered by different routes in the late period of pregnancy as it has been noted that administration in the first period of pregnancy mainly results in embryotoxicity and/or teratogenicity. Napalkov (*41, 42*) has very well illustrated the different types of receptiveness of the rat embryo and fetus at different stages of development. In this respect, pregnancy can be divided into three periods: (1) from day 1 to day 10, with two peaks on days 3 to 5 and on day 9, in which the chemical produces embryotoxicity; (2) from day 8 to day 11, with a peak on days 9 to 10, when the chemical produces a teratogenic effect; and (3) from day 10 to delivery, when the chemical exerts its carcinogenic effect. The embryotoxic and teratogenic periods overlap between days 8 and 11, and the teratogenic and carcinogenic periods overlap between days 10 and 11. However, by increasing the dose given to the pregnant animals, a teratogenic effect can be observed even if the chemical is administered within a few days prior to delivery (*41*). Moreover, there are a few experimental (*16, 48*) and human data (*17*) indicating that a carcinogenic effect can be observed when the exposure to a chemical carcinogen is limited to the first period of pregnancy. The partition of pregnancy into three periods merely indicates, therefore, the periods in which the three possible effects of a chemical, namely, embryotoxicity, teratogenicity, and carcinogenicity, are shown experimentally with maximum efficiency.

The absence of a carcinogenic effect in the first period of pregnancy may be related to the lack of an adequate metabolic system in the developing fetus. This is particularly relevant in the case of chemicals requiring a metabolic activation in order to exert their carcinogenic effect. Druckrey (*9, 11*) reported in experiments with dialkylnitrosamines and dialkylhydrazines in particular the methyl derivatives, that carcinogenesis occurs only when exposure takes place in very late pregnancy, indicating that a proximate carcinogen must be formed in the fetus and that metabolic activation occurs only in the last days of fetal development. In keeping with this hypothesis are the recent observations reported by Magee (*33*) that a definite peak of radioactivity corresponding to 7-methylguanine was found in fetal rats exposed on the 21st day of pregnancy to ^{14}C-dimethylnitrosamine (DMN). No methylation was observed in fetuses exposed on the 15th day of pregnancy. These data are consistent with the finding (*1*) that transplacental carcinogenesis by DMN can occur when treatment is given within two days from birth and not before. It has been shown, however, that fetal tissues lack the capacity to metabolize certain, but not all, drugs (*8, 15, 19*) and that some hepatic drug-metabolizing enzymes can be stimulated also in fetuses. Arhyl hydrocarbon hydroxylase, for instance, can be induced in several fetal tissues of the hamster and the rat (*43*).

Sensitivity of Fetal Tissues

In the present report only the carcinogenic effect observed following prenatal exposure to a chemical carcinogen will be discussed. From a practical point of view the main importance of this type of exposure is that it has shown the existence of a risk not only for the individuals exposed, but also for their descendants. In addition, fetal tissues may be more sensitive than adult tissues and therefore be affected by a dose level which is ineffective in adults; and exposure during pregnancy to minimal doses of a carcinogen, which *per se* are not sufficient to produce tumors, may sensitize the progeny to exposure later in life to the same or to another carcinogen at a dose which normally does not result in an increased incidence of tumors (*41*).

Until now studies on the effect of prenatal exposure have been carried out with recognized carcinogens, and all chemicals which have been proved to result in an increased incidence of tumors in the offspring following their administration to pregnant animals were already known to produce tumors in adult or newborn animals. At present we may only speculate that prenatal exposure will reveal a carcinogenic effect of chemicals which otherwise would not have been revealed, in the same way as neonatal exposure revealed a carcinogenic effect of chemicals which were ineffective when given to adults.

The term " ineffective " obviously means that no effect could be observed in the number of animals normally employed in experimental carcinogenesis. The effectiveness of neonatal exposure does not indicate therefore that something different is happening to the newborn as compared to the adult, but that the newborn, being, at least in certain respects, more sensitive, reveals an effect that might have been observed only by using a much larger and uneconomic number of adult animals. A study on newborn animals somehow miniaturizes in certain instances a study on adult animals.

While in a few instances the neonatal animal model has revealed the carcinogenicity of a compound which in adult animals was not carcinogenic, it was not consistently shown to be a more sensitive test. For most of the carcinogens the dose required to produce a similar incidence of tumors, calculated on a body weight basis, was finally shown to be very similar for adult and newborn animals (*6, 60*).

In so far as prenatal exposure is concerned, some evidence exists to indicate that fetal tissues are markedly more sensitive than adult tissues. Druckrey *et al.* (*14*) have reported that fetal nervous tissue is 50 to 100 times more sensitive than that of adults. Moreover, prenatal exposure to urethane has allowed the observation of tumors after a latency period which is probably the shortest recorded in chemical carcinogenesis. Smith and Rous (*50*) have reported the occurrence of lung adenomas in mice killed 3 and 10 days after birth following the administration of urethane to pregnant mice. Shabad (*47*) reported the occurrence of adenomas in organ cultures of fetal mouse lungs 11 and 14 days after explantation following the administration of urethane during the last 10 days of pregnancy.

Studies of Exposure Levels in Fetuses

Very little is known of how much of a carcinogen administered to the pregnant actually reaches the fetus and its target organ, or if fetal cells interact with the carcinogen in the same way as adult cells. We have recently tried to clarify the first of these two points. Part of the data has been, or will soon be, published elsewhere in detail (*58, 61*).

Methylcholanthrene (MCA) was given by stomach tube to CF-1 mice in the late period of pregnancy at doses of 8.3, 1.0, and 0.1 mg for the long-term studies,

TABLE 2.   Tumor Incidence in CF-1 Mice Following Prenatal Exposure to 8.3 mg MCA

		Number at start	Tumor-bearing animals
8.3 mg MCA during pregnancy	Mothers	34	34
	Offspring nursed by their mothers	99	97
	Offspring foster-nursed by untreated mothers	68	68

TABLE 3.   Tumor Incidence in CF-1 Mice Following Prenatal Exposure to 1 mg MCA

		Number at start	Tumor-bearing animals
1 mg MCA during pregnancy	Mothers	35	34
	Offspring nursed by their mothers	107	106

and 3.3, 1.0, and 0.1 mg for the biochemical studies.   The long-term observations are now completed for 8.3 and 1.0 mg, while many offspring of pregnant mice given 0.1 mg are still alive.

Following the administration of 8.3 or 1.0 mg of MCA to pregnant mice, both the treated mothers and all the offspring developed tumors (Tables 2 and 3).   In both instances, the most frequent tumor types were lymphomas and lung tumors. The average age at death was lower for the offspring than for their mothers, but the number of animals bearing more than one tumor was higher in the mothers than in their offspring.   As in the experiment of Bulay and Wattenberg (4, 5) with 7,12-dimethylbenz(a)anthracene (DMBA) and benzo(a)pyrene (BP), the mice were foster-nursed immediately after birth to verify that MCA could actually reach the fetuses in sufficient quantities to exert its carcinogenic effect and to disregard the possible effect of MCA which could have reached the mice after birth via the mothers' milk and/or the mothers' excreta.

In parallel with the long-term biological studies, an evaluation of MCA levels present in the fetus was carried out.   For this purpose, inert and ^{14}C-MCA were used.   MCA was dissolved in olive oil at a concentration which allowed the administration of the desired dose in 0.2 ml.   The administration was always given on the 17th day of pregnancy by stomach tube and the mothers were killed at 3 hr, 6 hr, 20 hr and 34 hr.   The fetuses were obtained through Caesarian section, minced, homogenized in benzene and then extracted in a Soxhlet apparatus with hot benzene.   The crude extracts were then subjected to thin layer chromatography (TLC) and an aliquot of the material eluted from the plate was analyzed by gas liquid chromatography with an ionization detector.   Details of the method are given in a previous paper (58).   Results are indicated in Table 4.

The analyses carried out on the fetuses at 3 hr indicate the existence of a linear relationship between the dose administered to the mother and the levels found in the respective litters.   The average levels of MCA in fetal tissues were 1090 ng/g,

TABLE 4. Levels of MCA in Total Litters at Various Times Following the Administration of MCA to Pregnant Mice

MCA to pregnant mice	Time after administration	Number of		Total fresh tissue (g)	Total MCA (ng)	MCA ng/g tissue	MCA ng/fetus
		Litters	Fetuses				
3.3 mg	3 hr	2	8+9=17	5.2+5.2=10.4	11.300	1090	665
	6 hr	2	10+4=14	11.2+5.7=16.9	1970⎫	117⎫	140⎫
		2	7+8=15	9.2+9.4=18.6	5610⎬4573	300⎬243	375⎬285
		2	10+7=17	10.9+8.8=19.7	6140⎭	310⎭	360⎭
	20 hr	2	11+11=22	10.5+8.2=18.7	630⎫ 665	34⎫ 37	29⎫ 30
		3	5+9+9=23	3.7+7.7+6.2=17.6	700⎭	40⎭	31⎭
	34 hr	9	92	85.2	2480	40	27
1 mg	3 hr	1	13	7.7	1530⎫	199⎫	118⎫
		2	5+2=7	3.7+1.6= 5.3	907⎬1067	171⎬213	130⎬112
		1	13	7.9	834⎪	106⎪	64⎪
		1	10	4.1	1493⎭	364⎭	149⎭
	6 hr	1	12	9.9	468⎫	47⎫	39⎫
		1	11	10.3	2764⎬1693	268⎬140	251⎬128
		1	12	10.8	1154⎭	106⎭	96⎭
0.1 mg	3 hr	1	9	8.5	398⎫	47⎫	44⎫
		1	8	6.5	58⎬ 198	9⎬ 22	7⎬ 19
		1	12	9.7	50⎪	5⎪	4⎪
		1	12	9.7	287⎭	30⎭	24⎭
	6 hr	1	9	8.2	644⎫	79⎫	72⎫
		1	9	7.4	31⎬ 447	4⎬ 48	3⎬ 44
		1	6	5.6	44⎪	8⎪	7⎪
		1	13	10.2	1070⎭	104⎭	82⎭
	20 hr	1	13	10.7	0.3	negligible	negligible
		1	13	8.9	8.3	0.93	0.65
		1	8	5.9	0.9	0.15	0.11
		1	11	8.9	1.2	0.13	0.10

213 ng/g, and 22 ng/g when the dose of MCA given to the mothers was, respectively 3.3 mg, 1 mg, and 0.1 mg.

When ^{14}C-MCA was used, the tissues were divided into two portions. One was dissolved in sodium hydroxide and used for counting the total radioactivity. The other was extracted in benzene as previously described and purified on thin layer chromatography. An estimation of the unchanged free MCA was made by calculating the difference between the total radioactivity counted from the tissues digested in sodium hydroxide and the radioactivity counted after benzene extraction and TLC purification. Details of the method are given in a previous paper (58). Results are given in Table 5. An average of 11% and 4% of the total radioactivity counted could be attributed to free unchanged MCA at 3 and 6 hr, respectively, following the administration of 1 mg MCA to the mothers. The remainder must be water-soluble metabolites, either free or firmly bound to cellular constituents. Following the administration of 0.1 mg MCA to the mother an average of 13% of the total radioactivity counted in the fetuses, both at 3 and 6 hr, could be attributed to unchanged MCA.

TABLE 5. Total Radioactivity and Radioactivity Attributable to Unchanged MCA in Fetuses Following ^{14}C-MCA Administration to Pregnant CF-1 Mice

^{14}C-MCA to pregnant mice	Time after administration	Total radioactivity dpm/g tissue	MCA radioactivity dpm/g tissue	% of total radio-activity attribu-table to MCA
1 mg (0.52 mCi/mmole)	3 hr (15)	6427 (4740–7880)	897 (450–1560)	11 (8–21)
1 mg (0.44 mCi/mmole)	6 hr (6)	10730 (7000–14000)	510 (172–974)	4 (2–8)
0.1 mg (4.5 mCi/mmole)	3 hr (4)	4990 (1750–7740)	735 (168–1525)	13 (7–20)
	6 hr (4)	8835 (1810–17040)	1588 (137–3400)	13 (7–20)
	20 hr (4)	4050 (1400–8400)	—	—

TABLE 6. Total Radioactivity and Radioactivity Attributable to Unchanged MCA in Maternal Blood and in the Corresponding Litter Following the Administration of 1 mg ^{14}C-MCA to the Mother

Time after administra-tion	Total radioactivity dpm/g		Radioactivity attributable to unchanged MCA dpm/g		% of total radioactivity attributable to unchanged MCA	
	Maternal blood	Litter	Maternal blood	Litter	Maternal blood	Litter
3 hr	17.200	7.880	11.300	850	66	11
6 hr	8.600	11.200	4.200	970	49	9

Specific activity: at 3 hr, 0.52 mCi/mmole; at 6 hr, 0.44 mCi/mmole.

A preliminary investigation on the nature of the different metabolites present in the fetal tissues was carried out. A tentative identification of the metabolites was done according to the method and data reported by Sims (49). The largest part the radioactivity was found in the zone $Rf=0$, which corresponds to the hydroxylated derivatives of MCA: 1,2-dihydroxy-3-MCA and 11,12-dihydro-11,12-dihdroxy-3-MCA, and in the zone $Rf=0.45$, which corresponds to the ketonic derivatives.

An attempt was also made to estimate the levels of MCA present in the maternal blood and in the litter at two different times following the administration of 1.0 mg of ^{14}C-MCA to the mothers. The results are given in Table 6.

The total radioactivity was higher in the maternal blood than in the fetus at 3 hr, but the reverse was observed at 6 hr following administration to the mothers. The percentage of unchanged MCA was much higher in the maternal blood than in the fetus. Although these data could indicate that fetal tissues on the 17th and 18th day of fetal life are able to metabolize MCA and/or to firmly fix it to cellular constituents, other possibilities must also be considered: (a) the placenta itself metabolizes MCA; (b) the permeability of the placenta to the metabolites from the mothers' blood to the fetus is greater than to the unchanged MCA and therefore more of the metabolites than of the MCA pass from the mother to the fetus; (c)

TABLE 7. Distribution in the Uterus and Weight of Fetuses and Placentas in CF-1 Mothers Given 0.1 mg MCA

Right horn		Left horn
$f=736$ $p=107$ 4		4′ $f=793$ $p=120$
$f=713$ $p=127$ 3		3′ $f=726$ $p=109$
$f=705$ $p=89$ 2		2′ $f=689$ $p=105$
$f=736$ $p=96$ 1	1′ $f=643$ $p=119$	

f, Weight of fetus in mg; p, weight of placenta in mg.

TABLE 8. Levels of MCA in Individual Fetuses and Respective Placentas 6 hr Following the Administration of 0.1 mg MCA to a Pregnant CF-1 Mouse

Position in the uterus	Total MCA (ng)			MCA ng/g tissue		
	Fetus	Placenta	Fetus and placenta	Fetus	Placenta	Fetus and placenta
1	9.0	3.3	12.3	12.2	34.4	14.8
2	5.2	3.7	8.9	7.4	41.6	11.2
3	8.7	2.8	11.5	12.2	22.0	13.7
4	15.9	6.4	22.3	21.6	59.8	26.4
1′	17.2	5.3	22.5	26.7	44.5	29.5
2′	12.9	5.0	17.9	18.7	47.6	22.5
3′	1.2	6.0	7.2	1.6	55.0	8.6
4′	14.3	3.2	17.5	18.0	26.7	19.6

MCA circulates easily from the mother to the fetus and back, while the metabolites can less easily cross back through the placenta.

In an additional experiment we tried to evaluate the amount of MCA present in individual fetuses, and the corresponding placentas of the same litter. The dose of 0.1 mg ^{14}C-MCA was given by stomach tube on the 17th day of gestation. The specific activity was 20.3 μCi/mg (32,500 dpm/μg). The mother was killed 6 hr after the administration and the fetuses with their respective placentas were carefully dissected, note being taken of their respective positions in the uterine horns (Table 7). These results are summarized in Table 8.

The absolute quantity of MCA was always higher in the fetuses than in their respective placentas, but the relative quantity appeared to be three times higher in the placentas than in the fetuses. There were conspicuous individual variations in MCA levels both in the fetuses and in the placentas, as has already been observed in the evaluation of the fetal and placental levels of DDT and metabolites in CF-1 mice (59). The relative proportion of unchanged MCA was calculated and it appeared that the average percentage of unchanged MCA was similar in fetuses (8.1%) and placentas (7%). The individual variations of the total radioactivity and of the radioactivity attributable to unchanged MCA corresponded to those observed in the biochemical analysis of MCA levels. As all preceding experiments were carried out on CF-1 outbred mice, we investigated whether individual variations in MCA levels would be different in a pure inbred strain of mice. For this purpose, a C57/B1 female was administered 0.1 mg of ^{14}C-MCA on the 17th day of pregnancy and sacrificed 6 hr later. The individual fetuses and placentas were analyzed as previously described. The quantities found were surprisingly low compared to those found with CF-1 fetuses. There was a total of 6 fetuses, 4 in the right horn and 2 in the left horn. In one fetus of the left horn the level of MCA was estimated as 0.5 ng, while in the others it was lower than 0.4 ng, which was the limit of sensitivity of the method. In contrast, the level of MCA was estimated in 4 of the 6 placentas and varied between 0.5 and 1.4 ng. It appears, therefore, that in the case of C57/B1 the placentas had a higher absolute level of MCA than the corresponding fetuses. In spite of the large difference in MCA absolute levels found in the two strains, individual variations among fetuses and respective placentas pertaining to the same litter were present in both strains.

Comparison between the dose given to pregnant mice and the dose which actually reached the fetus can so far only be attempted in the group where the mothers were given 1 mg of MCA, as the experimental group where mice received 0.1 mg of MCA is still in progress. The dose of 1 mg to a pregnant mouse roughly corresponds to 22 mg/kg. On the basis of our finding at 3 hr after administration, the average level of MCA found in the fetuses was 213 ng/g or 2.13 mg/kg, and at 6 hr the average level of MCA was 140 ng/g or 1.4 mg/kg. However, since these levels correspond only to the levels of free unchanged MCA and/or of the MCA which is loosely bound to the tissues and can be easily removed by extraction methods, we must take into account the data resulting from radiochemical evaluations. From this data it appears that only an average of 11% at 3 hr and an average of 4% at 6 hr of the total radioactivity recovered from the tissues was attributable to free unchanged MCA. Therefore if we adjust tentatively the above quantities to these percentages we may conclude that the level of MCA which may actually have reached the fetuses is rather high and approaches, expressed in mg/kg, the level given to the mothers (Table 9).

TABLE 9. Estimated Relationship between Dose Administered to Mothers and Absolute Exposure Levels of Fetuses

Dose of MCA given to mothers	Level of unchanged MCA in fetal tissues at 3 hr	% of unchanged MCA at 3 hr	Estimated level of MCA to which fetuses were actually exposed at 3 hr
1 mg = 22 mg/kg	213 ng/g = 2.13 mg/kg	11	19 mg/kg

Therefore in the present experiment it cannot be stated that fetuses were more sensitive than their mothers to the carcinogenic effect of MCA, as both mothers and fetuses were probably exposed to similar levels of MCA.

The studies of Druckrey (14) indicate a much higher sensitivity of the fetus, and, in particular, of the fetal nervous tissue, to a series of alkylating agents. It is worthwhile mentioning here the recent observations made by Magee (33) that, following NMU administration to pregnant rats, fetal DNA was methylated on the 7-position-guanine to about half the extent of that observed in the organs of adult rats and in the livers of mother rats.   In addition, no preferential alkylation was found in the brain, which is the choice target organ of NMU, of newborns the mothers of which were exposed to NMU in late pregnancy.   Further studies are required to better quantify these observations and also to verify if the case of water-soluble compounds is different from the case of lipid-soluble compounds.

Effect of Prenatal Exposure on F_1 and F_2 Generation Descendants

It is clear from the above data that a chemical carcinogen administered during pregnancy can reach the fetus, interact with the fetal cells, and induce tumors in the offspring.   While these findings already represent *per se* a warning that exposure to an environmental carcinogen may result in a risk not only for the individuals exposed but also for their descendants, experimental evidence has indicated that the risk may be persistent for at least two generations.

The experiments quoted here are all published except one (*54*), which is at present in press.   They are difficult to compare as they were carried out at different times and with different experimental procedures, however, they point to the same evidence.

Although somewhat different from the other reports mentioned, reference should be made to the extensive work of Strong (*53*) who supported the hypothesis that " the effects of methylcholanthrene upon somatic tissue cells as well as upon the germ cells may be in the direction of malignant changes or an increased susceptibility to them."

In 1952 Shay *et al.* (*48*) reported that the repeated administration of MCA to rats before and shortly after a successful mating, resulted in an increased incidence of tumors in the first generation and in the second untreated generation.   In 1961 Gel'shtein (*16*) reported that liver tumor incidence was increased in both F_1 and F_2 descendants of C3HA mice receiving *o*-aminoazotoluene (*o*-AAT) during pregnancy.   In 1965 and 1969 Tomatis (*56*) and Tomatis and Goodall (*57*) reported an increased incidence of tumors in F_1 and F_2 descendants of mice given DMBA during pregnancy.   In 1968 Shabad (*47*) referred to previous work where an increased incidence of lung tumors was observed in F_1 and F_2 untreated descendants of mice which had been exposed to repeated skin paintings with tar.   Tanaka has recently reported (*54*) an increased incidence of tumors both in F_1 and F_2 descendants of pregnant rats receiving nitrosomethylurethane during pregnancy.

As in all these experiments where direct exposure of the F_2 descendants to the original carcinogen can be reasonably excluded, one must speculate that the effect observed in the second generation might be due to the effect of the carcinogen on the germ cells of the first generation animals which were exposed during fetal life.   It is of interest to mention in this context that Tanaka has, in fact, observed a toxic effect of nitrosomethylurethane on the ovaries of fetal rats, the mothers of which received nitrosomethylurethane between the 12th and 16th day of pregnancy (*54*), and that DMBA is known to exert a direct toxic effect on the mouse ovary (*28, 29*).   Moreover, Röhrborn recently reported the induction of dominant lethal mutations in F_1 descendants of C3H mice treated during pregnancy (46).

Human Studies

The human risk consequent on the prenatal exposure to a hazardous chemical has recently ceased to be hypothetical. Two reports have been published indicating that the treatment of pregnant women with diethylstilbestrol is followed by an increased risk in their daughters of developing vaginal adenocarcinomas (17, 20). The first report included eight cases, the second five cases, and a third preliminary report indicates that about 20 more cases of vaginal carcinomas in young women have been found, and that for most of them a stilbestrol treatment of their mothers has been documented (21). The general rarity of adenocarcinomas of the vagina, especially in women of under 30 years of age, and the clustering of the cases at one hospital, certainly helped to stimulate a search for a possible common environmental factor.

From the available experimental evidence it appears that tumors in the offspring do not always have a shorter latency period than in their mothers. Therefore, one cannot exclude the possibilities that: (1) additional cases of adenocarcinoma of the vagina may appear at a later age, and (2) some of the treated mothers may also develop cancer. The absence of reports on increased tumor occurrence in women, particularly mothers, who underwent stilbestrol therapy when adult, indicates a higher sensitivity of human fetuses than of adults to the carcinogenicity of stilbestrol. However, a few more years may be needed before this observation can be confirmed. In addition, it is of vital importance that a follow-up study of children whose mothers received stilbestrol therapy during pregnancy be initiated, in order to reveal possible correlation between stilbestrol exposure and the occurrence of other cancers.

While stilbestrol is the first chemical known to produce cancer in man following prenatal exposure, it was already known that human fetal tissues are susceptible to cancer induction by transabdominal X-irradiation during pregnancy (32, 52). It is rather puzzling that this finding was not confirmed in the offspring of women exposed to the atomic bomb in Hiroshima and Nagasaki (25, 35).

The fact that in the case of both stilbestrol and X-irradiation exposure was in some instances limited to the first period of pregnancy is of major concern. It is, in fact, during the first period of pregnancy that working women are more liable to be exposed to hazardous chemicals because of their occupation.

It is certainly extremely difficult at present to identify and list potential carcinogenic chemicals, and not only in respect to transplacental carcinogenesis. For this purpose the IARC is carrying out a program on the compilation of Monographs for the Evaluation of the Potential Carcinogenic Risk of Chemicals to Man, and on the basis of this series of monographs an evaluation of the risk represented by environmental chemicals will be made. At present, however, as suggested by Miller (36), a survey should be made of cancer occurrence in people in whom malformations induced transplacentally by chemicals were found. The possible relation between childhood cancer and congenital defects has in fact been reported (*34*). Although not all carcinogens are necessarily teratogens, and certainly not all substances exerting a teratogenic effect have been proven to be carcinogenic, some correlation exists and most of the 29 carcinogens (see Table 1) which have been experimentally proven to induce tumors in animals following prenatal exposure have also shown a teratogenic effect (*1, 7*).

The establishment of a record system, as recently suggested by Miller (*36*), which would allow the linkage of maternal records during pregnancy where environmental exposure to chemical, physical, or viral agents are indicated (obviously occupational and medical exposures are the most easily recorded) with subsequent records of cancer occurrence in the child would be of extreme value.

SUMMARY

At least 30 chemical carcinogens have been proved to produce a high incidence of tumors in the progeny when administered to animals during late pregnancy. For a number of them it has been shown that exposure *in utero* is, *per se*, sufficient to produce tumors in the offspring. In many cases tumors appear earlier in the offspring of treated mothers than in their mothers. In some instances, however, tumors appear at the same or at a later age, thus indicating that offspring of treated mothers must always be observed for life span, particularly if prenatal exposure is used in carcinogenicity testing. It has been evaluated that the susceptibility of fetuses is greater than adult animals, and Druckrey *et al.* (*14*) report a 50 to 100 times higher sensitivity of fetal nervous tissue than adults. Data will be presented here on attempts to determine the levels of 3-methylcholanthrene present in fetuses following its administration to pregnant mice. Preliminary results indicate that, expressed on a body weight basis, fetuses are exposed to a level of MCA similar to that to which the pregnant mice were exposed. The levels of MCA found in individual fetuses of the same litter are far from being homogenous, the differences among individual fetuses being up to 8-fold.

Several published reports indicate that prenatal exposure to a chemical carcinogen may result in an increased incidence of tumors in the F_1 and F_2 generation descendants, and this possibility is discussed.

Evidence of the prenatal origin of cancer in man has been suspected for a long time and recent reports have shown that in the case of at least one drug the occurrence of tumors could be linked with treatment given to mothers during pregnancy.

It is suggested that a monitoring system be established by means of which maternal exposures to a chemical, whether for medical, occupational, or accidental reasons, could be linked to the occurrence of cancer in the child. Furthermore, a follow-up of children born of exposed mothers should be established.

REFERENCES

1. Alexandrov, V. A. Blastomogenic Effect of Dimethylnitrosamine on Pregnant Rats and Their Offspring. Nature, *218*: 280–281, 1968.

2. Alexandrov, V. A.   Transplacental Blastomogenic Action of N-Nitrosomethylurea on Rat Offspring.   Vopr. Onkol., *15*: 55–61, 1969 (in Russian).

3. Alexandrov, V. A.   The Characteristics of Embryotoxic and Teratogenic Reactions of the Embryo to the Effect of Chemical Carcinogenic Agents.   *In*; Transplacental Carcinogenesis.   IARC Scientific Publication.   In press.

4. Bulay, O. M., and Wattenberg, L. W.   Carcinogenic Effects of Subcutaneous Administration of Benzo(a)pyrene during Pregnancy on the Progeny.   Proc. Soc. Exptl. Biol. Med., *135*: 84–86, 1970.

5. Bulay, O. M., and Wattenberg, L. W.   Carcinogenic Effects of Polycyclic Hydrocarbon Carcinogen Administration to Mice during Pregnancy on the Progeny.   J. Natl. Cancer Inst., *46*: 397–402, 1971.

6. Della Porta, G., and Terracini, B.   Chemical Carcinogenesis in Infant Animals.   Progr. Exptl. Tumor Res., *11*: 334–363, 1969.

7. DiPaolo, J. A., and Kotin, P.   Teratogenesis-Oncogenesis: A Study of Possible Relationships.   Arch. Path., *81*: 3–23, 1966.

8. Dixon, R. L., and Willson, V. J.   Metabolism of Hexobarbital and Zoxazolamine by Placental and Fetal Liver Supernatant Fraction and Response to Phenobarbitol and Chlordane Treatment.   Arch. Int. Pharmacodyn., *172*: 453–465, 1968.

9. Druckrey, H.   Chemical Structure and Action in Transplacental Carcinogenesis and Teratogenesis.   *In*; Transplacental Carcinogenesis.   IARC Scientific Publication.   In press.

10. Druckrey, H., Ivankovic, S., and Preussmann, R.   Teratogenic and Carcinogenic Effects in the Offspring after Single Injection of Ethylnitrosourea to Pregnant Rats.   Nature, *210*: 1378–1379, 1966.

11. Druckrey, H., Ivankovic, S., Preussmann, R., Landschütz, C., Stekar, J., Brunner, U., and Schagen, B.   Transplacental Induction of Neurogenic Malignomas by 1,2-Diethyl-hydrazine, Azo- and Azoxy-ethane in Rats.   Experientia, *24*: 561–562, 1968.

12. Druckrey, H., und Landschütz, C.   Transplacentare und neonatale Krebserzeugung durch Äthylnitrosobiuret (ÄNBU) an BD IX-Ratten.   Z. Krebsforsch., *76*: 45–58, 1971.

13. Druckrey, H., Landschütz, C., und Ivankovic, S.   Transplacentare Erzeugung maligner Tumoren des Nervensystem.   II.   Äthyl-nitrosoharnstoff an 10 genetisch definierten Rattenstammen.   Z. Krebsforsch., *73*: 371–386, 1970.

14. Druckrey, H., Preussmann, R., Ivankovic, S., und Schmähl, D.   Organotrope carcinogene Wirkungen bei 65 verschiedenen N-Nitroso-Verbindungen an BD-Ratten.   Z. Krebsforsch., *69*: 103–201, 1967.

15. Fouts, J. R., and Hart, L. G.   Hepatic Drug Metabolism during the Prenatal Period.   Ann. N.Y. Acad. Sci., *123*: 245–251, 1965.

16. Gel'shtein, V. I.   The Incidence of Tumors among Offspring of Mice Exposed to Orthoaminoazotoluene.   Vopr. Onkol., *7*: 58–64, 1961.

17. Greenwald, P., Barlow, J. J., Nasca, P. C., and Burnett, W. S.   Vaginal Cancer after Maternal Treatment with Synthetic Estrogens.   New England J. Med., *285*: 390–392, 1971.

18. Grossi-Paoletti, E., Paoletti, P., Schiffer, D., and Fabiani, A.   Experimental Brain Tumours Induced in Rats by Nitrosourea Derivatives.   Part 2.   Morphological Aspects of Nitrosoethylurea Tumours Obtained by Transplacental Induction.   J. Neurol. Sci., *11*: 573–581, 1970.

19. Hart, L. G., Adamson, R. H., Dixon, R. L., and Fouts, J. R.   Stimulation of Hepatic

Microsomal Drug Metabolism in the Newborn and Fetal Rabbit. J. Pharmacol. Exp. Ther., *137*: 103–106, 1962.

20. Herbst, A. L., Ulfelder, H., and Poskanzer, D. C. Adenocarcinoma of the Vagina. Association of Maternal Stilbestrol Therapy with Tumour Appearance in Young Women. New England J. Med., *284*: 878–881, 1971.

21. Herbst, A. L., Ulfelder, H., and Poskanzer, D. C. Registry of Clear-cell Carcinoma of Genital Tract in Young Women. New England J. Med., Letter to the Editor, *285*: 407, 1971.

22. Ivankovic, S. Experimental Prenatal Carcinogenesis. *In*; Transplacental Carcinogenesis. IARC Scientific Publication. In press.

23. Ivankovic, S., und Druckrey, H. Transplacentare Erzeugung maligner Tumoren des Nervensystems. I. Äthyl-nitroso-harnstoff (ÄNH) an BD IX-Ratten. Z. Krebsforsch., *71*: 320–360, 1968.

24. Ivankovic, S., und Preussmann, R. Transplazentare Erzeugung maligner Tumoren. Naturwissenschaften, *57*: 460, 1970.

25. Jablon, S., and Kato, A. Childhood Cancer in Relation to Prenatal Exposure to Atomic-bomb Radiations. Lancet, *2*: 1000–1003, 1970.

26. Klein, M. The Transplacental Effect of Urethan on Lung Tumorigenesis in Mice. J. Natl. Cancer Inst., *12*: 1003–1010, 1952.

27. Kommineni, V. R. C., Greenblatt, M., Mihailovitch, N., and Vesselinovitch, S. D. The Significance of Perinatal Age Periods and the Dose of Urethan on the Tumour Profile in the MRC Rat. Cancer Res., *30*: 2552–2555, 1970.

28. Krarup, T. Effect of 9,10-Dimethyl-1,2-benzanthracene in the Mouse Ovary: Ovarian Tumorigenesis. Brit. J. Cancer, *24*: 168–186, 1970.

29. Kuwahara, I. Experimental Induction of Ovarian Tumours in Mice Treated with a Single Administration of 7,12-Dimethylbenz(a)anthracene and Its Histopathological Observation. Gann, *58*: 253–266, 1967.

30. Larsen, C. D. Pulmonary Tumor Induction by Transplacental Exposure to Urethan. J. Natl. Cancer Inst., *8*: 63–69, 1947.

31. Likhachev, A. Y. Transplacental Blastomogenic Action of N-Nitroso-diethylamine in Mice. Vopr. Onkol., *17*: 45–50, 1971 (in Russian).

32. MacMahon, B. Prenatal X-Ray Exposure and Childhood Cancer. J. Natl. Cancer Inst., *28*: 1173–1191, 1962.

33. Magee, P. N. Mechanisms of Transplacental Carcinogenesis by Nitroso Compounds. *In*; Transplacental Carcinogenesis. IARC Scientific Publication. In press.

34. Miller, R. W. Relation between Cancer and Congenital Defects: An Epidemiologic Evaluation. J. Natl. Cancer Inst., *40*: 1079–1085, 1968.

35. Miller, R. W. Cancer Research by the Atomic Bomb Casualty Commission. Editorial. J. Natl. Cancer Inst., *47*: V–VII, 1971.

36. Miller, R. W. Prenatal Origins of Cancer in Man: Epidemiological Evidence. *In*; Transplacental Carcinogenesis. IARC Scientific Publication. In press.

37. Mohr, U., und Althoff, J. Mögliche Diaplacentar-carcinogene Wirkung von Diäthylnitrosamin beim Goldhamster. Naturwissenschaften, *51*: 515, 1964.

38. Mohr, U., und Althoff, J. Die diaplacentare Wirkung des Cancerogens Diäthylnitrosamin bei der Maus. Z. Krebsforsch., *67*: 152–155, 1965.

39. Mohr, U., Althoff, J., and Authaler, A. Diaplacental Effect of the Carcinogen Diethylnitrosamine in the Golden Hamster. Cancer Res., *26*: 2349–2352, 1966.

40. Mohr, U., Althoff, J., und Wrba, H. Diaplacentare Wirkung des Cancerogens Diäthylnitrosamine beim Goldhamster. Z. Krebsforsch., *66*: 536–540, 1965.

41. Napalkov, N. P. Transplacental Carcinogenesis. *In*; Transplacental Carcinogenesis. IARC Scientific Publication. In press.

42. Napalkov, N. P., and Alexandrov, V. A. On the Effects of Blastomogenic Substances on the Organism during Embryogenesis. Z. Krebsforsch., *71*: 32–50, 1968.

43. Nebert, D. W., and Gelboin, H. V. The *in vivo* and *in vitro* Induction of Arhyl Hydrocarbon Hydroxylase im Mammalian Cells of Different Species, Tissues, Strains and Developmental and Hormonal States. Arch. Biochem. Biophys., *134*: 76–89, 1969.

44. Pielsticker, K., Wieser, O., Mohr, U., und Wrba, H. Diaplazentar induzierte Nierentumoren bei der Ratte. Z. Krebsforsch., *69*: 345–350, 1967.

45. Rice, J. M. Transplacental Carcinogenesis in Mice by 1-Ethyl-1-nitrosourea. Ann. N.Y. Acad. Sci., *163*: 813–827, 1969.

46. Röhrborn, G. Correlation between Mutagenesis and Carcinogenesis. *In*; Transplacental Carcinogenesis. IARC Scientific Publication. In press.

47. Shabad, L. M. Organ Culture of Lung Tissue, as a Method of the Study of Lung Tumours and the Blastomogenic Action of Substances That Can Induce Them. Z. Krebsforsch., *70*: 198–203, 1968.

48. Shay, H., Gruenstein, M., and Weinberger, M. Tumor Incidence in F_1 and F_2 Generations Derived from Female Rats Fed Methylcholanthrene by Stomach Tube Prior to Conception. Cancer Res., *12*: 296, 1952.

49. Sims, P. The Metabolism of 3-Methylcholanthrene and Some Related Compounds. Biochem. J., *98*: 215–228, 1966.

50. Smith, W. E., and Rous, P. The Neoplastic Potentialities of Mouse Embryo Tissues. IV. Lung Adenomas in Baby Mice as a Result of Prenatal Exposure to Urethane. J. Exptl. Med., *88*: 529–554, 1948.

51. Spatz, M., and Laqueur, G. L. Transplacental Induction of Tumors in Sprague-Dawley Rats with Crude Cycad Material. J. Natl. Cancer Inst., *38*: 233–245, 1967.

52. Stewart, A., and Kneale, C. W. Radiation Dose Effects in Relation to Obstetric X-Rays and Childhood Cancer. Lancet, *1*: 1185–1188, 1970.

53. Strong, L. C. Genetic Analysis of the Induction of Tumors by Methylcholanthrene. IX. Induced and Spontaneous Adenocarcinomas of the Stomach in Mice. J. Natl. Cancer Inst., *5*: 339–362, 1945.

54. Tanaka, T. Transplacental Induction of Tumours and Malformations in Rats Treated with Some Chemical Carcinogens. *In*; Transplacental Carcinogenesis. IARC Scientific Publication. In press.

55. Thomas, C., und Bollmann, R. Untersuchungen zur diaplacentaren krebserzeugenden Wirkung des Diäthylnitrosamins an Ratten. Z. Krebsforsch., *71*: 129–134, 1968.

56. Tomatis, L. Increased Incidence of Tumors in F_1 and F_2 Generations from Pregnant Mice Injected with a Polycyclic Hydrocarbon. Proc. Soc. Exptl. Biol. Med., *119*: 743–747, 1965.

57. Tomatis, L., and Goodall, C. M. The Occurrence of Tumours in F_1, F_2 and F_3 Descendants of Pregnant Mice Injected with 7,12-Dimethylbenz(a)anthracene. Int. J. Cancer, *4*: 219–225, 1969.

58. Tomatis, L., Turusov, V., Guibbert, D., Duperray, B., Malaveille, C., and Pacheco, H. Transplacental Carcinogenic Effect of 3-Methylcholanthrene in Mice and Its Quantitation in Fetal Tissues. J. Natl. Cancer Inst., *47*: 645–651, 1971.

59. Tomatis, L., Turusov, V., Terracini, B., Day, N., Barthel, W. F., Charles, R. T., Collins, G. B., and Boiocchi, M. Storage Levels of DDT and Metabolites in Mouse Tissues Following Long Term Exposure to Technical DDT. Tumori, *52*: 377–396, 1971.
60. Toth, B. A Critical Review of Experiments in Chemical Carcinogenesis Using Newborn Animals. Cancer Res., *28*: 727–738, 1968.
61. Turusov, V., Tomatis, T., and Guibbert, D. The Effect of Prenatal Exposure of Mice to Methylcholanthrene Combined with the Neonatal Administration of Diethyl-nitrosamine. *In*; Transplacental Carcinogenesis. IARC Scientific Publication. In press.
62. Vesselinovitch, S. D., Mihailovich, N., and Pietra, G. The Prenatal Exposure of Mice to Urethan and the Consequent Development of Tumors in Various Tissues. Cancer Res., *27*: 2333–2337, 1967.

Discussion of Paper by Drs. Tomatis et al.

DR. LAWLEY: Did you obtain evidence that polycyclic hydrocarbon was bound to the DNA and protein of fetal tissues?

DR. TOMATIS: These studies are in progress, but I can already say that we have evidence of binding to DNA, RNA, and proteins in various fetal tissues.   We have, in fact, found a comparable level of binding in the lung, which is target organ of choice but not in the kidney where we have never observed tumors, and these findings are now under a further investigation.

DR. NAKAHARA: What do you think of the possibility of the carcinogen administered to the maternal organism reaching the fetus in the form of more activated metabolites?   This without any intention of controverting Prof. Druckrey's result that fetuses are far more susceptible to the action of carcinogens than adults.

DR. TOMATIS: It is certainly possible; however, I don't think it is necessary. There is an old report indicating that the injection of MCA into the amniotic fluid results in tumors in the offspring.

DR. NISHIZUKA: Do you find any relationship between the day or period of administration of carcinogens and the types of tumors thus induced?   You have mentioned lung tumors and lymphoma.   Both of these tumors develop spontaneously in various strains of mice.   Do you find any other types of tumors in your animals?

DR. TOMATIS: We have found a variety of tumors occurring at different sites but we did not find a significant difference in their frequency whether MCA was given 5 days or 3, 2 or 1 day before delivery.

DR. DRUCKREY: As I understood it, you did not observe any neurogenic tumors in your transplacental experiments with methylcholanthrene.   As a second question I may ask what was the proportion between malignant and benign tumors?

DR. TOMATIS: We did not observe any neurogenic tumors in our mice following the administration of MCA.   About the malignancy of the other tumors, the lymphoid tumors were always malignant lymphomas; of the lung tumors, about 30% were clearly adenocarcinomas.

I shall also mention here that the tumors I reported previously as occuring after a very short latency period, as was reported by Smith and Rous, were lung adenomas, and not carcinomas.

Prenatal Carinogenesis

S. Ivankovic

The Institute of Experimental Toxicology and Chemotherapy, German Cancer Research Center, Heidelberg, West Germany

Malignant tumors in children between the age of 8 and 15 years are very important for practical and theoretical oncology. According to international statistics, cancer in children has been increasing in recent years. In Germany as well as in some other European countries childhood cancer is the second most frequent cause of death, accidents being the most frequent one. Leukoses and lymphomas have the first place among the malignancies, next are tumors of the nervous system and the kidney. According to Peller (*15*), leukoses, lymphomas, and malignant tumors of the nervous system and the kidney account for more than 80% of all tumors in children between the age of 8 and 15 years.

These malignancies are not so frequent in adults between 45 and 60 years of age. At that age tumors of the gastrointestinal and the respiratory tract and of the genitals are predominant. These differences in the tumor spectrum between the two age groups could be explained by the different development of biological receptors and, therefore, by their different " reactivity " with the carcinogen.

The relatively short latency period of tumors in young people suggests that the cause of childhood cancer may be effective already during the prenatal, intrauterine life. This hypothesis is quite old and has been offered by different authors. Nevertheless, nothing is known about carcinogenesis in man via the transplacental route. There have also been only a few experiments: Larsen (*13*), and later Smith and Rous (*19*) as well as Klein (*11, 12*) tried to find an experimental model to investigate this important question. They observed an increased incidence of lung adenomas in young mice, when the mothers had been treated with urethane during pregnancy. The induced tumors, however, were not malignant tumors, but benign adenomas. Such tumors also occur spontaneously in mice, as is well known.

In 1962 Druckrey and Steinhoff (*2*) described a diffuse carcinomatosis of the liver in a young guinea pig whose mother had been treated with diethylnitrosamine during pregnancy. The authors suggested that this might be a case of transplacental tumor induction.   Mohr and colleagues (*14*) have shown that treatment of Syrian hamsters leads to metaplasia in the epithelium of the tracheobronchus of the *offspring* and also to papillomas in the trachea.   Pielsticker *et al.* (*16*) described malignant kidney tumors in 2 out of 186 rats whose mothers had been treated with diethylnitrosamine during pregnancy.

In the spring of 1965 we succeeded in inducing a high incidence of malignant tumors in rats with transplacental application of a chemical carcinogen.   For several years we investigated this problem systematically and developed optimal experimental models for the confirmation of a prenatal causation of cancer.   Here now I will report on transplacental carcinogenesis in rats with ethylnitrosourea (ENU), diethylnitrosamine (DEN), and procarbazine®.

Prenatal Carcinogenetic Effect of Ethylnitrosourea (ENU)

We used BD rats as experimental animals since they have a very low rate of " spontaneous " malignant tumors.   Malignant tumors can be induced regularly in these animals with chemical carcinogens.

A single dose of ethylnitrosourea (ENU), between 80 and 5 mg/kg body wt., given intravenously or orally during the second half of pregnancy (from days 13 to 23 post coitum) induced in practically all offspring malignant tumors in the brain, the spinal cord, and the nervous system at an age of 4 to 10 months.   More than 800 young animals died with these tumors.   A very high sensitivity of the nervous system during the second half of prenatal development was found.   This high sensitivity can be very easily demonstrated by comparing the results of the experiments mentioned with dose-response experiments in adult animals.   The latter develops a significant yield of malignant tumors of the nervous system only when sublethal doses of 140–200 mg/kg are given.   Prenatal carcinogenesis leads to an almost quantitative tumor yield with the 50-fold lower dose of 5 mg/kg.   A single dose of this concentration is absolutely ineffective in adult rats.   This shows that the fetal nervous system is approximately 50 times more sensitive towards the action of carcinogens than that of adult animals (*5–7*).

During the experiment malignant neurinomas of the brain nerves appeared first.   Almost all of the tumors (175 out of 197) were located in the nervi trigemini or the ganglion Gasseri.   The latency period was 190 days.   Rapid growth and infiltration of nearby tissue and the brain often was the cause of death.

Malignancies in the other brain nerves, for example in the nervus vagus, nervus facialis, nervus hypogolossus and nervus acusticus, were much less frequent.   Malignancies in the bulbus olfactorius and the other brain nerves were never seen.   The observed high incidence of tumors in the nervus trigemius can perhaps be explained by the size of the nerve.   However it also seems probable that its intensive development in the fetal phase in comparison with the other brain nerves plays a decisive role.

Peripheral nerve tumors have been observed in 38% of the progeny.   The median latency period of these tumors was 215 days.   They were frequently situated in the plexus lumbosacralis, plexus brachialis, nervus ischiaticus, or nervus femoralis.

According to their localization, these cancers cause characteristic clinical symptoms.   At first motoric weakness is observed in the respective extremities, which continuously increases to complete paralysis.   Nearby muscles are regularly atrophic and infiltrated by malignant growth.   Histologically the tumors are malignant neurinomas or mixed malignomas containing also sarcomatous parts besides a neurogenic component.

Approximately 13% of all tumors observed in the progeny were found in the spinal cord.   The median latency period was 210 days, practically the same as with the tumors in the peripheral nerves.   The malignant growth was seen from the cervical to the lumbal region.   Frequently they were localized only in a sector of the medulla.   The clinical symptoms showed all forms from slight motoric weakness to monoplegy and paraplegy.   Tumors in the cervical region caused tetraplegy.   The histological investigations showed a series of different tumor types, most of them also

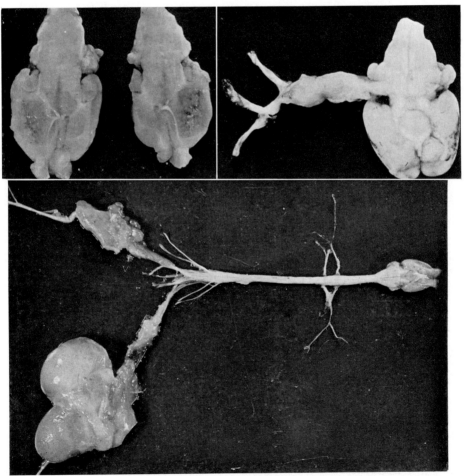

Fig. 1.   Transplacental induction of tumors by ethylnitrosourea in the offspring of rats. Mother animals were treated in the second half of pregnancy with single doses of ethylnitrosourea.   Malignant tumors of the nerves and in the brain in the progeny.

known from human pathology.   Most frequently seen were gliomas.   Also we frequently saw in the same animal several histologically different tumors.   Besides
oligodendrogliomas and astrozytomas we often saw malignant ependymomas.   The
cells were isomorphic, very often lightly packed.

The median induction time of brain tumors was 250 days and was therefore
longer than that of the other neurogenic tumors.   The growth of brain tumors could
be easily recognized in the offspring.   At first increased irritability, then apathy
and uncontrolled movements were seen long before death.   Some time before death
the animals refused to eat and drink; shortly afterwards they were in a deep coma.
In a few cases, however, death occurred rather rapidly.   These differences can be explained by the localization of the tumor in the brain and by its malignancy.   We had
a total of 207 brain tumors.   A survey as to their localization and distribution in
the different regions of the brain is given in Fig. 2.   It is evident that the majority
are situated in the temporal region of the brain (ammonshorn).   At the present moment we can offer no explanation for this experimental result.   It is known that the
chemoarchitecture is different in different parts of the brain.   Especially in the
region of the ammonshorn a special biochemical situation is known: There are re-

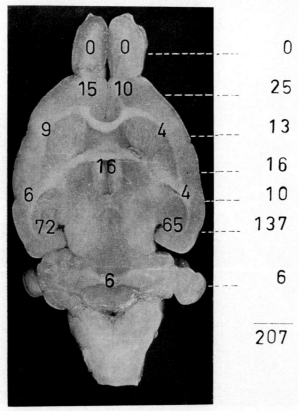

FIG. 2.   Localization of malignant tumors in the brain of rats.   Mother animals were treated
in pregnancy with single doses of ethylnitrosourea.   Striking accumulation occurred in the
area of the ammonshorn.

ports in the literature that in the ammonshorn especially, zinc is frequently present, and that in the pallidum umless ruber, in substantia nigra striatum and thalamus iron is frequently found. Furthermore, the ammonshorn is rich in sulfhydryl compounds (*8*).

In our published work (*4, 5, 7*) we have mentioned already that an enzymatic activation of ethylnitrosourea as well as a catalytic effect of cell constituents might be possible. We therefore investigated *in vitro* and *in vivo* whether trace amounts of heavy metals have such a catalytic effect or not.

It could be shown that the addition of copper ions to aqueous solutions of methyl-, ethyl-, *n*-propyl-, and *n*-butyl-nitrosourea resulted in immediate gas evolution. This effect was much reduced when ethylnitrosourea and other heavy metal ions such as nickel, cobalt, zinc, manganese and iron were used. The gas evolution was compared with an untreated control.

In vivo experiments with BD rats showed that 10% of the LD_{50} of ethylnitrosourea, that is, $25\,mg/kg$, were lethal for almost half of the experimental animals when copper was added to the injected solution. That shows a tenfold increase of the toxicity of ethylnitrosourea. In control experiments it was shown that the quantities of metal salts added were not toxic by themselves. The addition of cystine to solutions of ethylnitrosourea did not result in an increase of acute toxicity. Experiments are being performed now in our laboratory to show whether traces of heavy metals have an effect also on the selective occurrence of tumors in certain regions of the brain.

The majority of brain tumors histologically were mixed gliomas, consisting of oligodendroglia and astroglia. With a frequency of approximately 15% we found ependymomas in the offspring of ENU treated mothers. They were situated mainly in the cerebrum.

Histologically they appeared as more or less differentiated ependymomas. It is known from human pathology that similar ependymomas are the most frequent gliomas in human childhood cancer. This striking similarity of our experiments to the situation in man is further support for the hypothesis that such tumors may have a prenatal causation in man too.

In the rat, transplacental carcinogenicity is not confined to ENU. Up to now we have investigated about 30 different compounds in systematic experiments. It could be shown that not only N-nitroso compounds, but also certain hydrazo-, azo-, and azoxyalkanes and triazenes are carcinogenic for the progeny by the transplacental route. It was striking that the ethyl derivatives of these groups of compounds were always significantly more active than the corresponding methyl compounds. Even though such methyl derivatives as methylnitrosourea, 1,2-dimethylhydrazine, azoxymethane, and 1-phenyl-3,3-dimethyltriazene show powerful carcinogenic activity in adult experimental animals, in transplacental experiments they showed low or even no activity at all. The reasons for this surprising fact remain to be investigated.

Diethylnitrosamine, on the other hand, had a hepato-carcinogenic effect only when given at the end of pregnancy. The results of these investigations will be reported here.

Prenatal Induction of Malignant Liver Tumors in Rats with Diethylnitrosamine (DEN)

The carcinogen diethylnitrosamine (DEN) very likely is not active as such (it is in a " transport form "), but requires enzymatic activation *in vivo* to form the proximate and ultimate carcinogen, probably an alkylating agent. This metabolic activation is effected mainly by microsomal hydroxylases, mainly of the liver. Isolated liver microsomal fraction of the adult rat oxidatively dealkylates diethylnitrosamine. Microsomal preparations of fetal liver or of the whole rat fetus, however, did *not* show the dealkylating activity reported by v. Hodenberg and Preus-

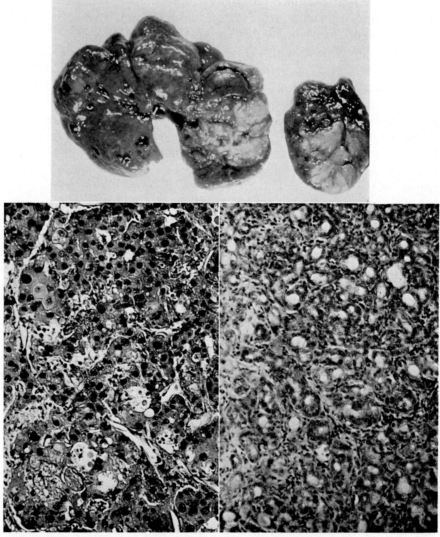

Fig. 3.   Prenatal induction of malignancies in the liver of the young.   Mother animals were treated on day 23 p.c. with 150 mg/kg diethylnitrosamine p.o. Hepatocellular and bile duct carcinomas in the offspring.

smann (*3*) in unpublished results.   It is known from the literature that microsomal hydroxylases in rat or guinea pig liver develop only shortly before the end of pregnancy or even after birth.

The missing or the low capacity for activation in the fetus may explain why all former experiments which have been performed by us and other authors produced practically no malignant tumors in the progeny.   A very high single oral dose of 150 mg/kg DEN, given on the 22nd day of pregnancy, however, induced in 14 out of 23 BD rat offspring tumors which after a median induction time of 800 days histology showed to be malignant hepatocellular carcinomas and bile duct carcinomas respectively (Fig. 3).

Such 2 experiments show that it is also possible to induce malignant tumors in organs other than the neurogenic tissue by way of transplacental carcinogenesis. The rather long induction time of 800 days indicates that tumors that arise even at the end of the normal life span may have been caused by prenatal effects.   A third example of prenatal cancer induction will now be demonstrated for the case of a hydrazine derivative, procarbazine or Natulan®.

Prenatal Induction of Malignancies with Procarbazine

The carcinogenic activity of some 1,2-disubstituted hydrazines in experimental animals is well known.   Procarbazine (Natulan) is a derivative of 1-methyl-2-benzylhydrazine; it is a valuable drug in the chemotherapy of malignant lymphogranulomatosis, bronchus carcinoma, and of malignant melanomas.   In recent

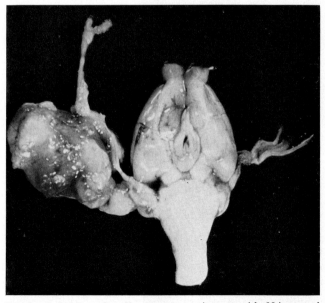

Fig. 4.   Induction of malignant tumors in rats with N-isopropyl-α-(2-methylhydrazino)-*p*-toluamide·HCl, procarbazine, Natulan.   Mother animals were treated on day 22 of pregnancy with 1×125 mg/kg procarbazine intravenously.   Malignant neurinoma in the nervus trigenimus.

years it has been used more and more in the therapy of such dissimilar diseases as chronic hepatitis, lupus erythematoides visceralis, hemolytic anemias, and also the Dupuytren contracture.

Since the compound is a potent carcinogen (*9, 10*)—even single-dose experiments induce tumors in experimental animals—it was considered necessary to investigate a possible transplacental carcinogenic effect. Recently a case was published in England where procarbazine was given to pregnant women because of an error in the names: The drug Natabec should have been given, Natulan was actually given (*1*).

BD rats recieved a single dose of 125 mg/kg of Natulan intravenously on the 22nd day of pregnancy. This is a rather high dose, approximately 25% of the LD_{50} in rats. Twenty-two young were born; after a medium induction time of 325 days 12 died with malignant tumors of the brain, the spinal cord, and the nerves (Fig. 4) (*4*). Macroscopically and histologically these tumors appeared like the tumors produced by ENU as described earlier.

Formation of N-Nitroso Compounds from Precursors

Sanders (*17, 18*) has shown that secondary amines and amides can react with nitrite in human stomach juice and in the stomach of experimental animals to form

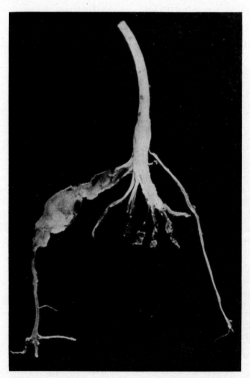

Fig. 5.   Prenatal induction of malignant neurinomas in the offspring of rats.   Mother animals were fed ethylurea and sodium nitrite between days 13 and 23 of pregnancy.   All offspring died with malignant neurinomas, mainly of the peripheral nervous system.

carcinogenic nitrosamines and nitrosamides.   Such a synthesis from inactive precursors may be of special importance for cancer in man.

We have therefore recently undertaken some experiments showing that without exception the progeny of rats died of leukemia and malignant neurogenic tumors when the mothers were treated orally with ethylurea and sodium nitrite (Fig. 5). Neither ethylurea nor sodium nitrite, given alone, were carcinogenic in corresponding control experiments.

SUMMARY

Our extensive experiments lead to the following conclusions.   The main result is that for the first time the induction of malignant tumors by prenatal exposure to certain carcinogens could be demonstrated experimentally.   In the majority of cases malignancies of the nervous system have been induced in the progeny after treatment with ENU or Natulan during sensitive periods of pregnancy.   The treatment with DEN, however, when given at the end of pregnancy, induced bile duct and liver carcinomas.   This showed that carcinomas could also arise in other organs.

The relevance of prenatal carcinogenesis for man should not be underestimated. The results show clearly the necessity to protect man from carcinogens and this is of special importance in the case of children and pregnant women.   Adequate precaution can open important improvements in cancer prevention.

Finally I want to thank Prof. K. J. Zülich and Dr. Mennel for their histological evaluation of the neurogenic tumors.   I also want to thank the Deutsche Forschungsgemeinschaft for supporting our work.

REFERENCES

1. Daw, R. G.   Procarboside in Pregnancy.   Lancet, 2: 934, 1970.
2. Druckrey, H., und Steinhoff.   Erzeugung von Leberkrebs an Meerschweinchen. Naturwiss., 49: 497–498, 1962.
3. Hodenberg, v. G., and Preussmann, R.   Unpublished.
4. Ivankovic, S.   Erzeugung von Malignomen bei Ratten nach transplazentarer Einwirkung von N-Isopropyl-α-2-(methyl-hydrazino)-p-toluamid·HCl Natulan. Arzneim. -Forsch.   In press.
5. Ivankovic, S.   Selektive Erzeugung von Geschwülsten im Gehirn und Nervensystem. Deutscher Krebskongress, München, 24–26, February, 1966.   Krebsforschung und Krebsbekämpfung, VI, 97, 1967.
6. Ivankovic, S., und Druckrey, H.   Transplazentare Erzeugung malignen Tumoren des Nervensystems.   I.   Äthyl-nitrosoharnstoff (ÄNH) an BD IX-Ratten.   Z. Krebsforsch., 71: 320–360, 1968.
7. Ivankovic, S., Druckrey, H., und Preussmann, R.   Erzeugung neurogener Tumoren bei dem Nachscommen nach einmaliger Injection von Äthylnitrosoharnstoff an schwangere Ratten.   Naturwiss., 53: 410, 1966.
8. Ivankovic, S., und Preussmann, R.   Transplazentare Erzeugung malignen Tumoren nach oraler Gabe von Äthylharnstoff und Nitrit an Ratten.   Naturwiss., 57: 460, 1970.

9. Kelly, M. G., and O'Gara, R. W. Carcinogenic Activity of N-Isopropyl-α-(2-methylhydrazino)-*p*-toluamide·HCl. Proc. Amer. Ass. Cancer Res., *6*: 134, 1965.
10. Kelly, M. G., O'Gara, R. W., Gadekar, S. D., Yancey, S. D., and Oliverio, V. T. Carcinogenic Activity of a New Antitumor Agent, N-Isopropyl-α-(2-methylhydrazino)-*p*-toluamide·HCl. Cancer Chemoth. Rep., *19*: 77–80, 1964.
11. Klein, M. The Transplacental Effect of Urethane on Lung Tumorigenesis in Mice. J. Natl. Cancer Inst., *12*: 1003–1010, 1952.
12. Klein, M. Induction of Lung Adenomas Following Exposure of Pregnant, Newborn, and Immature Male Mice to Urethane. Cancer Res., *14*: 438–440, 1954.
13. Larsen, C. D. Pulmonary Tumor Induction by Transplacental Exposure to Urethane. J. Natl. Cancer Inst., *8*: 63–69, 1947.
14. Mohr, U., Althoff, J., und Wrba, H. Diaplazentare Wirkung des Carcinogens Diäthylnitrosamins beim Goldhamster. Z. Krebsforsch., *66*: 536–540, 1965.
15. Peller, S. Cancer in Childhood and Youth, John Wright Sons Ltd., Bristol, 1960.
16. Pielsticker, K., Wiese, O., Mohr, U., und Wrba, H. Diaplazentar induzierte Nierentumoren bei der Ratte. Z. Krebsforsch., *69*: 345–350, 1967.
17. Sanders, J. Kann Nitrit in der menschlichen Nahrung Ursache einer Krebsentstehung dursh Nitrosaminbildung? Arch. Hyg. Bak., *151*: 22, 1967.
18. Sanders, J., und Bürkle, G. Induktion malignen Tumoren bei Ratten durch gleichzeitige Verfütterung von Nitrit und sekunderen Aminen. Z. Krebsforsch., *73*: 54, 1969.
19. Smith, W. E., and Rous, P. The Neoplastic Potentialities of Mouse Embryo Tissue. IV. Lung Adenomas in Baby Mice as Result of Placental Exposure to Urethane. J. Exptl. Med., *88*: 529–555, 1948.

Discussion of Paper by Dr. Ivankovic

DR. DAWE: Before opening the discussion on your paper, Dr. Ivankovic, I would like to comment that your excellent dissection of the central and peripheral nervous systems are most helpful in giving us an appreciation of the location and size of the tumors.

DR. MAGEE: What was the earliest day of pregnancy on which tumors were induced transplacentally by diethylnitrosamine? Have you ever observed tumors of the brain or other parts of the nervous system in untreated control rats?

DR. IVANKOVIC: Tumors appeared only in the offspring when diethylnitrosamine was given on the 22nd day of pregnancy. Administration before that day never gave tumors in the offspring.

In more than 10,000 neurogenic sections of untreated rats we have never seen brain tumors.

DR. HEIDELBERGER: It is interesting to me that the compounds that do *not* require metabolic activation produce tumors of the central nervous system, where metabolic activation would not be expected to occur.

DR. IVANKOVIC: This is true. Methylnitrosourea, however, which also does not need metabolic activation probably, in transplacental experiments hardly ever induced tumors of the nervous system.

DR. WEISBURGER: I wonder whether the careful expression by Dr. Ivankovic that brain tumors may be suspected of being due to transplacental action is not too conservative. We know that biochemical DNA synthesis and mitosis are required for blocking the information reflecting transformation by carcinogens. This is characteristically very low or zero in brain and nervous tissue. Thus, one can say that virtually all human brain and nervous tissue cancers may be due to transplacental action.

DR. IVANKOVIC: Brain tumors in man are rather rare. It might very well be that these tumors have a prenatal origin. Of course this is speculative.

DR. DRUCKREY: In answering the comment of Dr. Heidelberger, I want to mention that 1,2-diethylhydrazine as well as azo- and azoxyethane, although metabolic activation is needed, did produce neurogenic malignomas in almost all offspring.   In contrast to that, the corresponding methyl-compounds, when given to pregnant rats at the 15th day of gestation, were neither teratogenic nor carcinogenic to the fetus. Accordingly, the metabolic activation of the methyl- and ethyl- compounds by the fetus is different, and occurs at different periods of development.

DR. DAWE: Dr. Ivankovic, as you know, there are some recorded examples of neuroblastomas in man that have shown well-documented evidence of differentiation into ganglioneuromas, a much more benign type of neoplasm.   I wonder if you have seen any histologic evidence to suggest that some of your ganglioneuromas (neurinomas) may have evolved from a neuroblastoma phase?

DR. STICH: Did you observe an elevated frequency of congenital anomalies among the offspring of rats exposed to various carcinogens?

DR. IVANKOVIC: Between days 9 and 13 post coitus teratogenic effects are regularly seen, when the mothers are treated with *high* doses of nitrosoureas and certain other carcinogens.

DR. HIGGINSON: Do you know anything about the age at which the blood-brain barrier develops in the rat embryo?
    In contrast to mature nerve cells, there are some tumors in glial cells, so they should not be regarded as completely inert.
    There is a difference between the maturity of the human and rat brain.   At birth, the human brain is almost completely developed, whereas the number of cells in the rat brain increases as has been shown by experiments on protein deficiency.

DR. IVANKOVIC: I do not have data on the blood-brain barrier development for the rat.

DR. SUGIMURA: Did you find meningioma which is of mesenchymal origin as well as glioblastoma, neuroblastoma, and ependymoma which are of neurodermal origin, in your experiments with ethylnitrosourea?

DR. IVANKOVIC: We observed only a few meningioma among the many brain tumors.

DR. TOMATIS: Regarding the induction of liver tumor following the administration of DEN, you said that DEN was given on the 22nd day of pregnancy and your rats have a duration of pregnancy of 22 days+10 hr.   Were the offspring of the treated mothers foster nursed?

DR. IVANKOVIC: The offspring were not foster nursed.   This was in view of the rapid metabolism of DEN *in vivo*.

DR. NISHIZUKA: Dr. Takizawa (Hiroshima Univ.) has done an experiment in which he gave N-butylnitrosourea by oral route to rats.   His results show that about 30% of the animals have brain tumors which show similar histological patterns to those you have shown in your series induced by transplacental route.

Leukemogenic Effect of N-Nitroso-N-butylurea in Rats

Shigeyoshi ODASHIMA

Department of Chemical Pathology, National Institute of Hygienic Sciences, Tokyo, Japan

A tool for the induction of leukemia in experimental animals as a model disease of myelogenous leukemia in human beings has not yet been established. Many murine leukemias are induced by viruses, but the patterns of these diseases differ from those of leukemias in human beings, especially in orientals. Thus a long-standing requirement has been an experimental system capable of producing myelogenous leukemias in rats and mice. Several chemicals, such as 3-methylcholanthrene, 7,12-dimethylbenz(a)anthracene (*3, 5*), 2-acetylaminophenanthrene (*4*), N,N'-2,7-fluorenylenebisacetamide (*7*), *p*-nitroso(methylamino)azobenzene (*6*), and N-ethyl-N-nitrosourea (*1*), have been reported to be leukemogenic, but the incidence of leukemia induced by them was only 36–56%, except in Huggins and Sugiyama's experiment (*5*) using 7,12-dimethylbenz(a)anthracene. These authors reported an incidence of 100% leukemia in rats after 4–7 intravenous injections of the compound.

According to Druckrey *et al.*, among 65 N-nitroso derivatives tested only N-nitroso-N-ethylurea showed a leukemogenic effect in their rats (*1*). They observed leukemia in 9 of 16 rats after intravenous injections of a total of 250 mg of this compound in doses of 10 mg/kg body weight.

The carcinogenicity of N-nitroso-N-butylurea (NBU), the chemical employed in the present experiments, was also tested by these authors in their rats and found to induce sarcomas at the site of injection (*2*). There were no other reports of tests on the carcinogenicity of NBU in experimental animals before the present author described its highly leukemogenic effect when given to female Donryu rats in their drinking water (*8, 9*). Subsequently, the carcinogenic effect of this compound has been studied by several investigators in Japan (*10*).

This paper describes the results of two series of experiments. In the first experiment Donryu rats, which are a closed colony of rats commonly used in cancer research in Japan, were used to determine the effect of the concentration of NBU by administration of solutions of 0.01 to 0.04% as drinking water.   In the second experiment, the effects at periods of administration of a 0.04% NBU solution from 5 to 20 weeks were studied in Sprague-Dawley rats.   In both experiments, the NBU used (mp 81–82°C) was synthesized and supplied by Dr. Y. Sakurai of the Cancer Institute, Tokyo, and was kept refrigerated at 5°C before use.   The rats were separated into groups of 4 animals at 11 weeks of age and kept in hanging metal cages. Each day, 60 ml of freshly prepared solution of NBU in distilled water was placed in the drinking bottle of each cage so that approximately 15 ml of the solution was given to each rat as drinking water.   The drinking bottle was completely covered with black vinyl tape to exclude light.

Incidence of Leukemia and Other Tumors

1)   Effect on female Donryu rats of various concentrations of NBU solution as drinking water (Fig. 1 and Tables 1 and 2).

Three groups, I, II, and III, each containing 32 female Donryu rats, were given 0.04, 0.02, and 0.01% NBU solution for 18, 24, and 46 weeks, respectively.   Therefore, the animals in the three groups received approximately 6, 3, and 1.5 mg of NBU per day or totals of 756, 504, and 338 mg, respectively (Table 1).

Animals that died within 19 weeks were not included in the results because blood smears were not made during this period of the experiment.   However, most of these animals had hepatosplenomegaly.

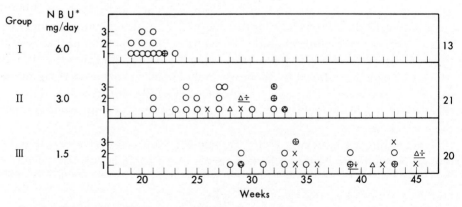

FIG. 1.   Tumors in various organs and leukemias.
*, N-Nitroso-N-butylurea; ○, leukemia; ÷, esophagus; ↑, small intestine; ↓, mammary glands; △, ear duct; ×, no tumor

TABLE 1.   Groups and Treatments

Groups	Number of rats	Concentration of NBU (%)	Daily dose (mg)	Duration of treat. (weeks)	Total dose (mg)
I	32	0.04	6	18	756
II	32	0.02	3	24	504
III	32	0.01	1.5	46	338

TABLE 2.   Localization of Tumors

Group	Daily dose (mg)	Number of rats	Number of rats with tumors	Target organs				
				Leukemia	Esopha-gus	Ear duct	Mammary gland	Small intestine
I	6.0	13	13 (100)	13 (100)	1 (8)	0	0	0
II	3.0	21	19 (90)	17 (90)	2 (10)	3 (16)	0	1 (5)
III	1.5	20	14 (70)	12 (86)	4 (28)	3 (21)	1 (7)	0
Total		54	46 (85)	42 (91)	7 (15)	6 (13)	1 (2)	1 (2)

TABLE 3.   Experimental Groups

Group	Number of rats	Treatment (weeks)	Total dose (mg)	Number of rats killed for PFC count[a]	Number of rats examined for tumors
1	32	5	210	12	20
2	32	10	420	9	23
3	32	15	630	6	26
4	32	20	840	3	29

[a]   Carried out by Y. Hashimoto, Tokyo Biochemical Research Institute.

In Group I, all of the 13 rats developed leukemia and were killed for autopsy between the 19th and 24th weeks, the average being the 20th week.   In Group II, leukemia was found in 17 of 21 rats (81%) after an average of 27 weeks.   In Group III, 12 of 20 rats (60%) developed leukemia after an average of 33 weeks.   The non-hematopoietic tumors found were: 1 esophageal tumor in Group I; 2 esophageal tumors, 3 ear duct carcinomas, and 1 intestinal tumor in Group II; and 4 esophageal tumors, 3 ear duct carcinomas, and 1 mammary tumor in Group III.   These non-hematopoietic tumors were found in animals that were killed in the later part of the experimental period (Table 2).   In addition to these tumors, small papillomatous lesions were found in the forestomach of most animals in all three groups.

2)   Effect on female Sprague-Dawley rats at various periods of administration of a 0.04% NBU solution as drinking water.

Four groups (1–4) of thirty-two 11-week-old rats were given 15 ml of a 0.04% NBU solution daily for 5, 10, 15, and 20 weeks, respectively.   Thus they received totals of approximately 210, 420, 630, and 840 mg of NBU, respectively (Table 3).

To study the immunosuppressive effect of NBU, three rats each were killed immediately after NBU treatment and every 5th week thereafter until the 25th week.   These animals were used by Dr. Yoshiyuki Hashimoto of the Tokyo Biochemical Research Institute to determine the number of cells in the spleen capable of forming plaques against sheep blood cells.   Consequently, the numbers of rats observed for tumor development were reduced to 20, 23, 26, and 29 rats in Groups 1, 2, 3, and 4 respectively.

The localizations and times of appearance of tumors in the rats in each group are shown in Fig. 2 and the cumulative percentages of tumors in the various organs

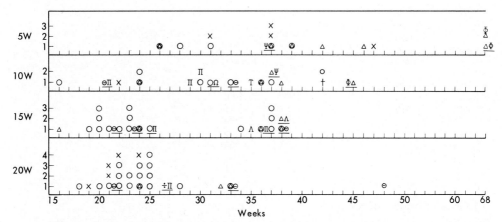

FIG. 2.   Localization of tumors in the rat given a 0.04% NBU solution for 5, 10, 15, and 20 weeks.

◯, Leukemia; △, mammary gland; *II*, ear duct; ⊖, small intestine; *Φ*, uterus; *Ψ*, liver; *Ω*, esophags; *γ*, salivary gland; †, larynx; ×, no tumor; *Λ*, glandular stomach; ÷, tongue

TABLE 4.   Localization of Tumors in the Rat Given a 0.04% NBU Solution for 5, 10, 15, and 20 Weeks, Respectively, in Their Drinking Water

Group	Treat. (weeks)	Number of rats	Number of rats with tumor	Tumors					
				Leuke-mia	Mammary gland	Small intestine	Ear duct	Uterus	Others[a]
1	5	14	10 (71)	5 (50)	7 (70)	0 (0)	0 (0)	2 (20)	1 (10)
2	10	18	17 (94)	8 (47)	5 (29)	3 (18)	3 (18)	1 (6)	4 (24)
3	15	20	20 (100)	17 (85)	5 (25)	3 (15)	2 (10)	0 (0)	1 (5)
4	20	25	20 (80)	17 (85)	3 (15)	3 (15)	1 (5)	0 (0)	1 (5)
Total		77	67 (88)	47 (70)	20 (30)	9 (13)	6 (9)	3 (4)	7 (10)

[a]   One each in the liver in Group 1, liver, esophagus, salivary gland and larynx in Group 2, glandular stomach in Group 3, and tongue in Group 4.

Numbers in parentheses indicate percentage.

are indicated in Table 4.   Among the 10 rats with tumors in Group 1, 5 rats, or 50%, developed leukemia after an average of 31 weeks, and nonhematopoietic tumors were found in 8 rats (80%) after an average of 42 weeks.   In Group 2, leukemia developed in 8 of 17 rats (47%), and other types of tumors in 13 rats (76%).   The average induction time was 30 weeks for leukemia and 35 weeks for other tumors.   In Group 3, leukemia and nonhematopoietic tumors developed in 85% and 45%, respectively, of 20 rats, with an average induction time of 23 weeks for leukemia and 25 weeks for other tumors.   In Group 4, among 20 rats 85% developed leukemia after an average of 24 weeks, and 30% developed other tumors after an average of

30 weeks.   Among the 67 nonhematopoietic tumors, most were of the mammary gland (30%), small intestine (13%), and ear duct (9%).

This second experiment showed that NBU, when given continuously as drinking water for more than 15 weeks, caused an incidence of leukemia in female Sprague-Dawley rats of as high as about 85% in an average period of as short as 23 weeks. Treatment for less than 10 weeks also induced leukemia but the incidence was less, about 50%, and the induction time was longer, averaging 31 weeks.

Plaque-forming Cells

The numbers of cells in the spleen capable of forming plaques against sheep blood cells are shown in Fig. 3.   Plaque-forming cells were very rare in all the rats in each group killed immediately after NBU treatment.   In the rats that received NBU treatment for 5 weeks, the count recovered gradually thereafter, and was about 60% of the control level at the end of the 25th week.   In the other three groups, however, the count remained zero throughout the experiment.   Therefore, it was apparent that leukemic cells and the other tumor cells proliferated, finally killing the host animals that were in a highly immunosuppressed state so far as was indicated by the number of plaque-forming cells.

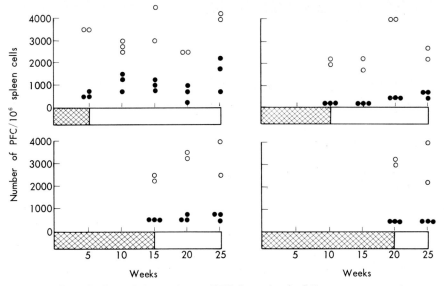

FIG. 3.   Effect of NBU administration on PFC formation in S.D. rats.

⊠ NBU Administration, o Control, ● Treated

Macroscopic Findings on Leukemic Animals

Anemia and diffuse enlargement of the liver, spleen, adrenal glands and cysternal group of lymph nodes, due to intensive proliferation of leukemic cells, were commonly observed in leukemic rats (Fig. 4).   Swelling of the systemic lymph nodes or

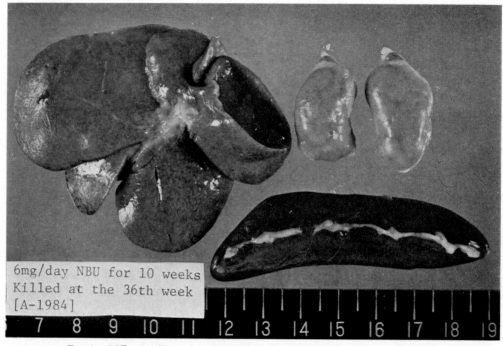

FIG. 4.   Diffuse swelling of the liver (20.51 g), spleen (8.08 g), kidneys, and adrenal glands are shown.   The leukemia was a chronic myelogenous type and the white blood cell count was 452×10^3 at autopsy.

the thymus was very rare.   The average weights of the liver and spleen of leukemic rats were 23.7 g and 2.3 g, respectively, both being two times the normal weights.

White Blood Cell Count

The change of the white blood cell count in rats that received 0.04% NBU solution continuously is shown in Fig. 5.   The numbers of red and white blood cells in the circulating blood decreased gradually until about the 10th week, when they were about 50% of the normal level, and then the white blood cells increased rather rapidly.   Leukemic cells began to appear in the circulating blood from the 15th week.   The white blood cell counts in leukemic animals varied greatly in different animals from the normal level to as high as one million at the time the animals were killed for autopsy.   Usually, however, the count was 20 to 60 thousand.

Classification of NBU Leukemias

It is still too early to make any definite classification of NBU leukemias in rats because of the complexity and variety of pathological findings in these diseases. However, they can be classified roughly as aleukemic and leukemic leukemias. Aleukemic leukemia includes cases in which leukemic lesions were found in one of the blood-forming organs, such as the bone marrow, liver, spleen, or thymus,

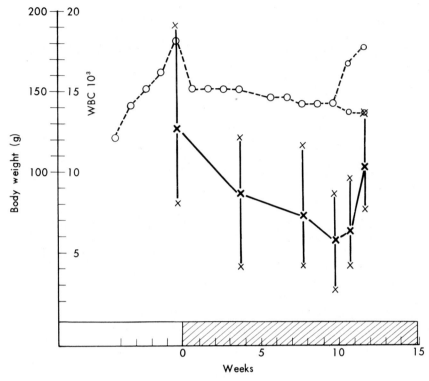

FIG. 5.   Body weight and WBC count of rats given 0.04% N-nitrosobutylurea in their drinking water.

⫿⫿⫿⫿, 0.04% N-Nitrosobutylurea;   O---O, body weight;   ×——×, WBC count.

although leukemic cells were not detected in the circulating blood.   This type could be further subdivided into thymic and nonthymic types, depending on whether the thymus was swollen or not.

Leukemic leukemia designates cases in which leukemic cells were detected in the circulating blood and leukemic lesions were also seen in various organs.   This type could also be further subdivided into granulocytic and nongranulocytic leukemias, depending on whether the azurophilic granules were seen in the cells or not.   The former contained various amounts of azurophilic granules in the cytoplasm and gave a positive peroxidase reaction.   Both the number and size of the granules were much larger than in normal neutrophils.   These granules were sometimes even found in mitotic cells.   The nucleus was oval, kidney-shaped, or lobular and consisted of a fine network of karyoplasm and several small nucleoli.   These cells resembled promyelocytes, myelocytes, or metamyelocytes.   Many cases of granulocytic leukemia showed cells at various levels of maturation as in chronic myelogenous leukemias (Fig. 6).   In the other cases, however, the bone marrow and tumor nodules were a characteristic greenish color resembling that in chloroleukemia in human beings.

The nongranulocytic leukemic cells of the second type had large, oval, bean-

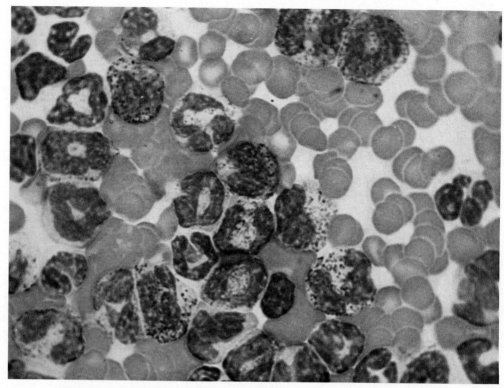

Fig. 6.   Leukemic cells in the peripheral blood of a rat that had received a 0.04% NBU solution for 15 weeks and was killed after 37 weeks.   The white blood cell count was 208×10^3. Cells have a large number of azurophilic granules in the cytoplasm and lobulated or kidney-shaped nuclei with a few large nucleoli resembling myelocytes or metamyelocytes.   This case was diagnosed as granulocytic leukemia.

TABLE 5.   Incidence of Various Types of Leukemia in S.D. Rats Given a 0.04% NBU Solution for 5, 10, 15, and 20 Weeks, Respectively

NBU treatment (weeks)	Number of cases	Aleukemic		Leukemic		Unclassified
		Thymic	Nonthymic	Granulo-cytic	Nongranulo-cytic	
5	5	0	0	2	2	1
10	8	0	0	5	2	1
15	17	1	1	4	10	1
20	17	1	3	2	8	3
Total	47	2 (4%)	4 (9%)	13 (28%)	22 (47%)	6 (13%)

shaped, or lobulated nuclei which consisted of fine networks of karyoplasm and a few large nucleoli.   Most of these cells, particularly those that had an oval or round nucleus, had a narrow rim of very basophilic cytoplasm with a white halo (Fig. 7). There were no azurophilic granules and neither the peroxidase nor the PAS reaction was positive.   These cells resembled undifferentiated hemocytoblasts or sometimes erythroblasts.   Further studies are required to determine the origin of this type of cell.

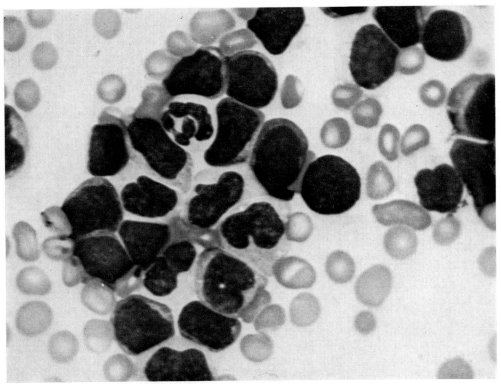

FIG. 7.   The leukemic cells in the peripheral blood of a rat that had received a 0.04% NBU solution for 15 weeks and was killed after 27 weeks.   The white blood cell count was 64×10^3. There were no azurophilic granules in the cytoplasm and neither the PAS nor peroxidase reaction was positive.   This case was classified as nongranulocytic leukemia.

TABLE 6.   WBC Count and Types of Leukemia

WBC count (10^3)	Aleukemic	Leukemic	
		Granulocytic	Nongranulo-cytic
− 10	3	0	2
− 20	1	0	5
− 30	0	0	3
− 40	0	0	3
− 70	0	2	0
−150	0	3	2
−300	0	3	0
−600	0	2	0
Total	4	10	15

The incidences of various types of leukemias found in the second experiment are summarized in Table 5.   Animals in which blood smears were not examined are indicated as unclassified.   Among the 47 leukemias, only 6 (13%) were aleukemic and 35 (75%) were leukemic.   Among the 35 leukemic leukemias, 13 were granulocytic

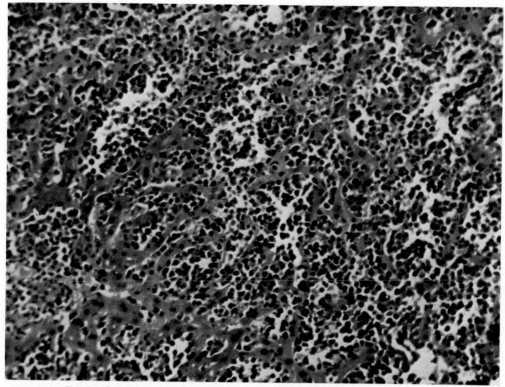

FIG. 8.   Leukemic lesions in the liver of a rat that had received a 0.04% solution for 20 weeks and was autopsied after 23 weeks.   Abundant leukemic cells have proliferated in the sinuses of the liver and the liver cell cords are atrophic.   This pattern was seen in most cases of nongranulocytic leukemia.

and 22 were nongranulocytic.   Most leukemias in rats that received NBU for 5 or 10 weeks were chronic granulocytic leukemias and most leukemias in rats which received NBU for 15 or 20 weeks were of an undifferentiated blastic type.

There was a close relationship between the type of leukemia and the number of white blood cells in the circulating blood, as shown in Table 6.   The white blood cell count was in the normal range in all 4 rats with aleukemic leukemias and was between 10 and 40 thousand in 13 of 15 rats with nongranulocytic leukemias, while it was more than 70 thousand in all 10 rats with granulocytic leukemias.

There were two different patterns of leukemic lesions in the liver.   One was diffuse, extensive proliferation of leukemic cells in the sinuses.   In these cases, the liver cell cords were highly atrophic and the normal architecture of the liver was not seen in any part, due to proliferation of leukemic cells (Fig. 8).   The other was localized proliferation of leukemic cells arround the Glisson's capsules.   In these cases, only a few leukemic cells were seen in the sinuses (Fig. 9.)   The former pattern was seen in 19 of 22 cases of nongranulocytic leukemia and the latter was seen in 8 of 13 cases of granulocytic leukemia (Table 7).   In general, the weight of the liver was much larger in the former than in the latter.

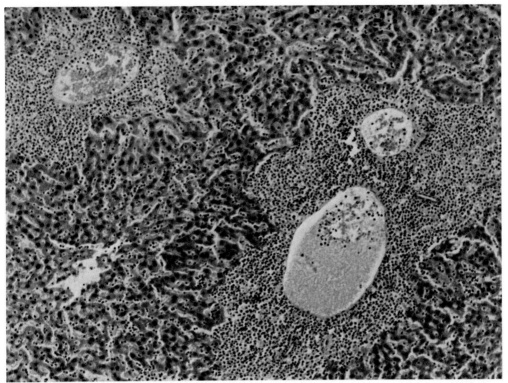

FIG. 9.   Leukemic infiltration in the liver of a rat that had been given a 0.04% NBU solution for 5 weeks and was killed after 26 weeks.   Although there are few leukemic cells in the sinuses, the leukemic lesions are most prominent around the Glisson's capsule.   This pattern was seen in many cases of granulocytic leukemia.

TABLE 7.   Types of Leukemia and Their Invasive Patterns in the Liver

	Aleukemic		Leukemic		Unclassified	Total
	Thymic	Nonthymic	Granulo-cytic	Nongranulo-cytic		
Sinusoid	0	3	4	19	4	30 (64%)
Glisson's	1	1	8	2	2	14 (30%)
Invasion negative	1	0	1	1	0	3 (6%)
Total	2 (4%)	4 (9%)	13 (28%)	22 (47%)	6 (13%)	47

DISCUSSION

The present two experiments showed several interesting results on the carcinogenicity of N-nitroso-N-butylurea (NBU): 1) NBU has a strong leukemogenic effect on rats when given continuously in their drinking water.   This is very interesting because Druckrey *et al.* did not find any tumors in tissues remote from the site of injection of this chemical in their animals (2).   Further studies employing various routes of administration are required to determine the target organs of this chemical. 2) Higher doses of NBU, *i.e.*, either higher concentrations in the drinking water or longer periods of administration of a certain concentration in the drinking water, resulted in a high incidence of leukemia early in the experimental period. A lower dose induced some tumors in nonhematopoietic organs in the later part of the experimental period. The incidence of leukemia was as high as 85%, and the average induction period was as short as 23 weeks in rats receiving a 0.04% NBU solution for more than 10 weeks. In contrast, tumors in nonhematopoietic organs, especially the mammary glands, ear duct, and small intestine, were found in 77% of the animals that were given a 0.04% NBU solution for less than 10 weeks. These tumors appeared in the later part of the experimental period. In addition to this relationship between the dose and the organs in which tumors developed, there was a slight difference in strain susceptibility, the incidence of leukemia being slightly higher in Donryu rats than in Sprague-Dawley rats. Therefore, more strains of rats should be examined to determine the oncogenic effects of NBU.

The types of leukemias found in Donryu and Sprague-Dawley rats differed. In the former 97% of the leukemias were nongranulocytic and in the later only 72%. Moreover, most of the leukemias found in rats that received a 0.04% NBU solution for 5 and 10 weeks were granulocytic, resembling chronic myelogenous leukemias in human beings. This seems very important in understanding the development of various types of leukemias, especially acute and chronic myelogenous leukemias and the acute conversion of the latter. However, more detailed cytologic and cytochemical studies are required before the induced leukemias can be classified morphologically.

In addition to its oncogenic effect, NBU showed a strong immunosuppressive effect in Sprague-Dawley rats so far as was indicated by the number of spleen cells capable of forming plaques against sheep red blood cells. It is uncertain whether this was entirely or partly the cause of the development, proliferation, and invasion of leukemic cells in the NBU-treated animals. The effects of immunosuppressants and of transplantation of bone marrow cells are being studied in NBU-treated rats in relation to the appearance of leukemia.

Much further work is required on various aspects of this problem, but the present results show that leukemias induced in animals by NBU provide excellent models of leukemias in human beings.

SUMMARY

Solutions of 0.01 to 0.04% NBU were administered continuously to female Donryu rats as drinking water and a 0.04% solution of NBU was given to female Sprague-Dawley rats in the same way for 5 to 20 weeks. The results were as follows: 1) NBU had a strong leukemogenic effect on rats. 2) Higher doses of NBU resulted in higher incidences of leukemia early in the experimental period both in Donryu and Sprague-Dawley rats. With the highest dose the incidence of leukemia was as high as 85%, and the average induction period was as short as 23 weeks. 3) There was a slight difference in strain susceptibility, the incidence of leukemia being slightly higher in Donryu rats than in Sprague-Dawley rats. 4) Donryu rats mainly developed blastic and erythroblastic leukemias, and Sprague-Dawley rats developed more chronic myelogenous leukemias when they were treated with NBU for 5 or 10 weeks.   5) In addition to these oncogenic effects, NBU had a strong immunosuppressive effect.

The author wishes to thank Dr. Y. Sakurai of the Cancer Institute, Tokyo, for synthesizing and supplying N-butyl-N-nitrosourea, Dr. Y. Hashimoto and Miss Y. Oshima of the Tokyo Biochemical Research Institute, Tokyo, for performing the plaque-forming cell counts, and Miss S. Yamazaki of the Sasaki Institute, Tokyo, for technical assistance in animal experiments.

This work was supported by Grant DRG-96At from the Damon Runyon Memorial Fund for Cancer Research, Inc., New York, U.S.A., and a grant-in-aid for scientific research from the Japanese Ministry of Education, Japan.

REFERENCES

1. Druckrey, H., Preussman, R., Ivankovic, S., und Schmähl, D.   Organotrope carcinogene Wirkungen bei 65 verschiedenen N-Nitroso-Verbindungen an BD-Ratten. Z. Krebsforsch., 69: 103–201 1067.
2. Druckrey, H., Preussmann, R., Ivankovic, S., So, B. T., Schmidt, C. H., und Bucheler, J.   Zur Erzeugung subcutaner Sarkome an Ratten.   Carcinogene Wirkung von Hydrazodicarbonsäurebis(methyl-nitrosamid), N-Nitroso-N-n-butylharnstoff, N-Methyl-N-nitroso-N′-nitroguanidine, und N-Nitroso-imidazolidon. Z. Krebsforsch., 68: 87–102, 1966.
3. Fukunishi, R.   Studies on Tumor Induction in Rats with 7,12-Dimethylbenz(a)-anthracene, with Special References to the Morphogenesis and Fine-structural Changes in the Target Organs.   Acta Path. Jap., 18: 51–72, 1968.
4. Hartmann, H. A., Miller, E. C., Miller, J. A., and Morris, F. K.   The Leukemogenic Action of 2-Acetylaminophenanthrene.   Cancer Res., 19: 210–216, 1959.
5. Huggins, C. B., and Sugiyama, T.   Induction of Leukemia in Rats by Pulse Doses of 7,12-Dimethylbenz(a)anthracene.   Proc. Natl. Acad. Sci., 55: 74–81, 1966.
6. Ivankovic, S.   Übertragung einer Ratten Leukämie durch peripheres Blut. Arzneim.-forsch., 14: 836–837, 1964.
7. Morris, H. P., Wagner, B. P., Ray, F. E., Snell, K. C., and Stewart, H. L.   Comparative Studies of Cancer and Other Lesions of Rats Fed N,N′-2,7-Fluorenylenebisacetamide or N-2-Fluorenylacetamide.   Natl. Cancer Inst. Monogr., 5: 1–54, 1961.
8. Odashima, S.   Development of Leukemia in Rats by Oral Administration of N-Nitrosobutylurea in the Drinking Water.   Gann, 60: 237, 1969.
9. Odashima, S.   Leukemogenesis of N-Nitrosobutylurea in the Rat.   I.   Effect of Various Concentrations in the Drinking Water to Female Donryu Rats.   Gann, 61: 239–244, 1970.
10. Yokoro, K., Imamura, N., Takizawa, S., Nishihara, H., and Nishihara, E.   Leukemogenic and Mammary Tumorigenic Effect of N-Nitrosobutylurea in Mice and Rats. Gann, 61: 295–296, 1970.

Discussion of Paper by Dr. Odashima

DR. STICH: Oncogenic virus preparations and potent cell-free filtrates were repeatedly obtained from murine leukemias induced by physical and chemical carcinogens.   Have you been able to isolate viruses or prepare oncogenic cell-free filtrates from the NBU-induced leukemias of rats?

DR. ODASHIMA: Cell-free transmission was negative, electron microscopic studies by Dr. Sugano of the Cancer Institute, and group-specific cell surface antigen studied by Dr. Yokoro were also negative.

DR. STICH: The chronic myelogenic leukemia that you obtained in rats appears to be more comparable to the human situation than the chemically induced thymic lymphosarcomas of mice.

DR. ODASHIMA: I think that NBU can give you the model disease of leukemia in human beings based on hematological studies.

DR. DAWE: The tendency for leukemias to appear in those animals showing the greatest degree of immunosuppression suggests that incipient leukemias may have occurred, but were suppressed in those animals with lesser degrees of, or a fluctuating pattern of, immune suppression.   Did you see any hemotologic or histologic evidence that in some cases leukemias may have started to develop, but regressed?

DR. ODASHIMA: No,   I didn't have such evidence.   However, it requires further detailed studies before we can give any conclusions.

DR. IVANKOVIC: Have you differentiated your leukosis cytochemically, and what methods were used?

DR. ODASHIMA: Wright-Giemsa stain and peroxidase reactions were routinely used.

DR. NAKAHARA: In referring to the question raised by Dr. Stich, I would point out that no rat leukemia is now known to be associated with virus.   This is confirmed by consultation with Dr. Weisburger seated next to me.

DR. HASHIMOTO: Referring to Dr. Dawe's question, besides NBU, N-nitroso-N-methylurea and N-nitroso-N,N'-dimethylurea, which give rise to tumors in organs other than lymphoid organs, showed a potent immunosuppressive effect.   Butyl-butanol-nitrosamine, which induces bladder tumor, showed no immunosuppressive effect.   Therefore, immunosuppression caused by NBU may play some role in the leukemogenic process but not a major role.   Reconstitution by normal bone marrow cells of NBU-immunosuppressed rats inhibited the suppression, but thymocytes did not.   Thus, it is assumed that NBU specifically affects the bone marrow cells, especially in their immunological function.

DR. DRUCKREY: In comparative tests with the homologous series of alkyl-nitroso-ureas in rats we found that the methyl-, propyl-, and pentyl- compounds were only weakly leukemogenic, whereas with ethyl- and n-butyl-nitrosourea about 50% of treated rats died with leukemias.   Accordingly, it may play a role whether the C-atoms in the alkyl-chain are even or odd-numbered.

Leukemogenesis in Thymectomized Mice Induced by N-Butyl-N-nitrosourea

Yasuaki Nishizuka and Hayase Shisa

Laboratory of Experimental Pathology, Aichi Cancer Center Research Institute, Nagoya, Japan

In the mouse, chemical leukemogenesis may differ from chemical carcinogenesis in various organs in at least two ways. One is that Type C virus, a possible causative agent, has frequently been demonstrated in leukemic tissues in electron microscopic and bioassay studies (*3, 4, 6, 17*). Secondly, as in the case of tumorigenesis in organs and tissues of the endocrine system, endogenous and exogenous factors may greatly influence development of leukemia. The incidence, pathological patterns, and sometimes the latent periods of chemically induced leukemias can be modified by alteration of thymus function (*11, 16*). Moreover, inoculation of normal hematopoietic cells before or after exposure to carcinogenic chemicals may reduce the incidence of chemically induced leukemia (*2*).

In connection with the latter phenomenon, this paper reports studies on leukemogenesis by N-butylnitrosourea (NBU) in mice. Some additional studies on leukemogenesis by 7,12-dimethylbenz(a)anthracene (DMBA) are also presented. The thymus may have critical significance in the development of mouse leukemia of viral etiology (*9*). Thus, in order to compare the leukemogenic responses to these chemicals with those to Gross virus, these chemicals were also tested in thymectomized mice.

Induction of Leukemia by NBU

Continuous oral administration of NBU in drinking water to young adult mice for a period of about 60 days is the most effective method for rapid induction of leukemia. This method was used to induce leukemia in rats by Odashima (*12*). For induction of leukemia with DMBA, a single subcutaneous injection of DMBA as a fat emulsion into newborn or young adult animals is the best method (*11, 16*).

Table 1 shows that many strains of mice are susceptible to the leukemogenic action of NBU. This is in contrast to the leukemogenic activities of other chemicals,

TABLE 1.   Strain Difference in Susceptibility to NBU Leukemogenesis[a]

Strain	Number of mice used	Leukemia[b]			
		Number	%	Latent period (days)	Thymic leukemia
Swiss/Ms	20	20	100.0	73	17
C57Bl/6J	19	18	94.7	103	15
C3Hf/Bi	19	18	94.7	114	15
A/Jax	16	15	93.7	99	11
BALB/c	21	14	66.6	185	12

[a]   Oral administration of NBU (total 45–72 mg) from 35 days after birth was continued for 60 days.
[b]   BALB/c strain mice were killed within 240 days after birth and other strains within 180 days after birth.

TABLE 2.   Effect of NBU Administration on Leukemogenesis of High-Leukemia Strains[a]

Strain	Number of mice used	Leukemia[b]			
		Number	%	Latent period (days)	Thymic leukemia
AKR/Ms	18	18	100.0	90	17
SL/Ms	41	41	100.0	102	28

[a]   NBU was administered as described in Table 1.
[b]   All animals were killed within 180 days after birth. The incidences of spontaneous leukemias in AKR and SL strain mice of the same age were approximately 8% and 4%, respectively (10).

such as DMBA and urethane, which differ from strain to strain (8, 11, 14).   For example, Swiss mice are highly susceptible to DMBA and urethane leukemogenesis, whereas C57Bl and A/Jax mice are rather refractory.

Most of the leukemias induced by NBU were typical lymphocytic leukemias with marked involvement of the thymus, as shown in Table 1.   This type of leukemia is the most commonly induced in mice by chemicals or other agents such as Gross virus and X-ray.   However, some mice treated with NBU did not show thymic involvement but showed the histological features of poorly differentiated lymphocytic leukemia.   Observation of the hematopoietic organs showed that the histological sequences leading to development of thymic leukemia after treatment with NBU or DMBA were fundamentally similar to those observed in X-ray or viral leukemogenesis.   Depletion of lymphocytes from the thymic cortex seemed to be a clearly noticeable and essential preceding event, and this usually took place in only one lobe. After thymic neoplasm has been established, the leukemic cells rapidly spread to the opposite lobe and may also disseminate to other tissues.

NBU treatment resulted in more rapid development of thymic leukemias than that observed in control animals of high-leukemia strains, such as AKR and SL mice (Table 2).   The SL strain is an inbred strain established by Tsuchikawa in the National Institute of Genetics, Mishima.   In this strain, the incidence of spontaneous lymphocytic leukemias and reticulum cell sarcomas, type A and type B, is approximately 70% (10).   In other words, NBU accelerates the appearance of virus-induced spontaneous leukemias.   Table 3 shows the leukemogenic effects of NBU when ad-

TABLE 3.   Incidence of Tumors in Mice Treated with NBU or DMBA during the Fetal Period

| Strain | Carcinogen[a] | Dose (mg) | Number of animals | Leukemia[c] | | | | Lung adenoma | Ovarian tumor | Mammary cancer |
				Number	%	Latent period (days)			
Swiss/Ms	—	—	55	1	1.8	240	1	0	4/29[d]
Swiss/Ms	NBU	13[b]	39	12	30.8	157	37	2/20[d]	3/20[d]
C57B1/6J	NBU	11[b]	18	4	22.2	207	13	0	0
Swiss/Ms	DMBA	3	14	1	7.1	109	10	1/7[d]	0

[a] NBU was given to mothers by the oral route from the 11th day of pregnancy to the day of delivery.   DMBA in a single dose was given to mothers subcutaneously on the 11th day of pregnancy.

[b] Total dose given throughout pregnancy.

[c] All animals were killed within 240 days after birth.

[d] No. of mice with tumors/total no. of female mice used.

ministered prenatally to Swiss and C57B1 mice.   In this experiment, NBU was given to mothers from the 11th day of pregnancy to the day before delivery.   Leukemias developed in 20–30% of the mice given a rather small amount of NBU by the transplacental route.

It must be mentioned here that Yokoro and his associates (*18*) have recently demonstrated the presence of leukemogenic Type C virus in the leukemic tissues of NBU-treated C57B1 mice.   Thus it seems that the mechanisms of DMBA and NBU leukemogenesis in mice are similar, since there is ample evidence of the presence of leukemogenic virus in DMBA leukemias (*3, 4, 17*).   NBU seems to be more effective than DMBA, since a wider range of animals, including rats and hamsters, are susceptible to it (*15*) and it has a greater leukemogenic effect when given by the transplacental route.

Leukemias in Thymectomized Mice

It is well known that the thymus is of critical importance in determining the susceptibilities of mice to induction of leukemia by X-ray and Gross virus (*9*).   Thymectomy at various ages, even when it is performed shortly before the clinical appearance of the disease, can prevent the occurrence of leukemia.   Hence, information on the effect of thymectomy on chemical leukemogenesis would be of great interest.   Table 4 shows the effects of thymectomy on NBU leukemogenesis in C57B1 and Swiss mice.   It is obvious that thymectomy of young adult mice had no marked inhibitory effect.   In addition, thymectomy caused only a slight decrease in the incidence of DMBA leukemia.   Therefore, the frequent occurrence of leukemias in thymectomized mice is a distinctive feature of chemically induced leukemia.   This is in sharp contrast to X-ray and viral leukemogenesis where the incidence of leukemia in thymectomized mice is low, usually being less than 10% (*9*).

The pathology of leukemias in thymectomized mice seems to differ from that in intact animals.   In the former, gross examination showed moderate or slight splenomegaly with systemic enlargement of the lymph nodes in all cases.   Histologically, typical lymphocytic leukemia was not seen, and the " starry sky " feature, commonly

TABLE 4.   Incidence of Leukemias Induced by NBU and DMBA in Thymectomized Mice

Strain	Chemicals	Number of mice used	Leukemia[e]		
			Number	%	Latent period (days)
Swiss/Ms[a]	NBU[c]	7	7	100	97
C57Bl/6J[a]	NBU[c]	16	13	81	155
Swiss/Ms[b]	DMBA[d]	53	32	60	116
Swiss/Ms (Non-thymectomized)	DMBA[d]	22	18	82	126

[a]   Thymectomy was performed at 32 days.
[b]   Thymectomy was performed at 3 days.
[c]   Chemicals were administered as described in Table 1.
[d]   A single subcutaneous injection of DMBA (50 μg/g) was given 35 days after birth.
[e]   All animals were killed within 180 days after birth.

TABLE 5.   Theta Antigen in Leukemic Cells in NBU-Induced Leukemias

Thymus involvement	Leukemic cells	Host	Theta antigen
Yes	Well-differentiated lymphocytic	Normal	+
No	Poorly diff. (undiff.) lymphocytic	Normal	−
—	Poorly diff. (undiff.) lymphocytic	Thymectomized	−
Yes	Well-differentiated lymphocytic	Thymectomized with thymus-grafts	+

seen in leukemic tissues in both viral and chemical leukemias in intact mice, was not observed in most thymectomized, leukemic mice.   Tumor cells are generally large and polygonal or irregular in shape, and tend to aggregate.   Nodular infiltration of leukemic cells into various organs, especially the liver and spleen, is seen as one of the characteristic histological patterns.   This type of leukemia, which is referred to as " poorly differentiated " (undifferentiated) lymphocytic leukemia, can be distinguished from thymic, " well-differentiated " lymphocytic leukemias developing in nonthymectomized hosts.

It is of interest that neoplastic cells in thymectomized, leukemic mice had no theta antigen, which is a specific cell surface antigen detectable by a cytotoxicity test in thymus-derived lymphocytes (13).   Table 5 summarizes our results on theta antigen of leukemic cells in hosts of primary and transplanted leukemias (5).   This table shows that theta-positive leukemic cells were detected in nonthymectomized leukemic animals in which the thymus usually contained many well-differentiated lymphocytic leukemic cells.   Theta-negative cells were found in both thymectomized and intact mice with no histological evidence of involvement of the thymus by leukemic processes.   Theta-positive cells were frequently detected in leukemias developing in thymectomized mice that received subsequent subcutaneous grafts of thymic tissues from neonatal isologous mice.   In these mice, the grafted thymic tissues were markedly enlarged and occupied by well-differentiated, lymphocytic leukemic cells.

It is well known that, in viral leukemogenesis, a remarkable restoration of

TABLE 6. Effect of Thymus Grafting on DMBA Leukemogenesis in Thymectomized Swiss Mice[a]

Age at DMBA injection[b] (days)	Age at thymus grafting[c] (days)	Number of mice used	Leukemia[d]		
			Number	%	Latent period (days)
3	—	22	7	32	157
3	7	13	4	31	176
35	—	53	32	60	116
35	40	17	11	65	111

[a] Thymectomy was performed at 3 days.
[b] Single subcutaneous injection of DMBA (50 μg/g).
[c] The whole thymus taken from intact isologous neonatal mice was grafted into the #4 fat pads.
[d] All animals were killed within 180 days after birth.

susceptibility to development of leukemia in thymectomized mice is observed when the subsequent grafting of thymic tissue is performed (9). In contrast, in chemical leukemogenesis, no increase in the incidence of leukemia was noticed even when grafting of thymic tissue was done shortly after exposure to DMBA. The result of two sets of experiments on this line are shown in Table 6. Here again, it appeared that leukemic cells invaded the grafted thymic tissue, and there they may have changed into well-differentiated cells of the lymphatic series carrying theta antigen. No direct action of Type C virus on target cells was demonstrated in this particular system, but it seems possible that DMBA may provide chances of neoplastic transformation of presumably undifferentiated lymphoid cells outside the thymus shortly after chemical exposure. These transformed cells may proliferate and maintain their nature as poorly differentiated lymphocytic cells unless thymic tissue, which seems to be a suitable tissue for proliferation of neoplastic or preneoplastic cells and which also allows maturation of the neoplastic cells and their expression of theta-antigenicity, is present. Therefore, we propose the hypothesis that shortly after injection of a chemical carcinogen, cells of hematopoietic tissues, most probably the bone marrow, are transformed by a leukemic virus which is otherwise ineffective. The transformed cells may then migrate into the thymus and form a mass which results in marked enlargement of the thymus. Previously we found a close relationship between the incidence of leukemias and the rates of acute chromosomal aberration of bone marrow cells, but not of thymus and spleen cells, within 48 hr after exposure to DMBA (7). This also suggests that the carcinogen acts on the bone marrow. This concept is supported by the demonstration that bone marrow cells from mice exposed to DMBA show leukemia-inducing activity when given to syngeneic mice (1).

Thus, differences in responses of thymectomized mice and in the possible processes leading to the development of frank leukemia can be pointed out between chemical and viral leukemogenesis. However, it is impossible at present to give any positive evidence that leukemia can develop in mice by the direct action of carcinogenic chemicals on hematopoietic cells without any relation to viral activity.

SUMMARY

Experiments were made on the induction of mouse leukemia by oral administration of N-butylnitrosourea (NBU) with the following results: (1) NBU is a potent leukemogen capable of inducing thymic lymphocytic leukemias in mice of all the strains tested and in the progeny when given to pregnant females.   NBU also accelerates development of leukemias of viral etiology in high-leukemia strains.   (2) Administration of NBU induces leukemias in thymectomized mice in almost the same frequency as in nonoperated mice.   This is in sharp contrast to leukemogenesis by Gross virus where thymectomized mice are highly refractory to development of leukemia.   (3) A distinctive feature of chemical leukemogenesis seems to be that lymphoid cells both inside and outside the thymus can be transformed shortly after chemical exposure and proliferate to develop frank thymic leukemia.   However, the thymus may play some role in determining the pathological patterns of the leukemias induced by the chemical.

This work was supported in part by a grant-in-aid from the Japanese Ministry of Education and from the Princess Takamatsu Fund for Cancer Research.

REFERENCES

1.   Ball, J. K.   Role of Bone Marrow in Induction of Thymic Lymphoma by Neonatal Injection of 7,12-Dimethylbenz(a)anthracene.   J. Natl. Cancer Inst., *41*: 553–558, 1968.
2.   Ball, J. K.   Depressive Effect of Bone Marrow on the Yield of 7,12-Dimethylbenz-(a)anthracene Induced Thymic Lymphomas.   J. Natl. Cancer Inst., *44*: 439–445, 1970.
3.   Ball, J. K., and McCarter, J. A.   Repeated Demonstration of a Mouse Leukemia Virus after Treatment with Chemical Carcinogens.   J. Natl. Inst. Cancer, *46*: 751–762, 1971.
4.   Haran-Ghera, N.   A Leukemogenic Filtrable Agent from Chemically Induced Lymphoid Leukemia in C57BL Mice.   Proc. Soc. Exptl. Biol. Med., *124*: 697–699, 1967.
5.   Hiai, H., Shisa, H., and Nishizuka, Y.   Unpublished data.
6.   Irino, S., Ota, Z., Sezaki, T., and Suzaki, K.   Cell-free Transmission of 20-Methylcholanthrene-induced RF Mouse Leukemia and Electron Microscopic Demonstration of Virus Particles in Its Leukemic Tissue.   Gann, *54*: 225–237, 1963.
7.   Kurita, Y., Shisa, H., Matsuyama, M., Nishizuka, Y., Tsuruta, R., and Yoshida, T. H.   Carcinogen-induced Chromosome Aberrations in Hematopoietic Cells of Mice.   Gann, *60*: 91–95, 1969.
8.   Matsuyama, M., and Suzuki, H.   The Role of Repeated Administration of Suckling Mice with Urethan on Carcinogenesis.   Nagoya Med. J., *16*: 105–111, 1970.
9.   Metcalf, D.   The Thymus: Its Role in Immune Responses, Leukemia Development and Carcinogenesis, Springer-Verlag, Berlin, Heidelberg, New York, 1966.
10.   Nakakuki, K.   Pathology of Mouse Leukemia.   Role of Thymus in Its Morphogenesis.   Mie Med. J., *14*: 1–35, 1964.
11.   Nishizuka, Y., and Shisa, H.   Enhancement of 7,12-Dimethylbenz(a)anthracene

Leukemogenesis in Mice by Neonatal Injection of Cortisone Acetate. Brit. J. Cancer, *32*: 290–295, 1968.

12. Odashima, S. Leukemogenesis of N-Nitrosobutylurea in the Rat. I. Effect of Various Concentrations in the Drinking Water to Female Donryu Rats. Gann, *61*: 245–253, 1970.

13. Reif, A. E., and Allen, J. M. The AKR Thymic Antigen and Its Distribution in Leukemias and Nervous System. J. Exptl. Med., *120*: 413–433, 1964.

14. Shisa, H. Studies on the Mechanism of 7,12-Dimethylbenz(a)anthracene Leukemogenesis in Mice. I. Strain Difference in Susceptibility of DMBA Leukemogenesis. Mie Med. J., *19*: 89–99, 1969.

15. Shisa, H. Unpublished data.

16. Shisa, H., and Nishizuka, Y. Determining Role of Age and Thymus in Pathology of 7,12-DMBA-Induced Leukemia in Mice. Gann, *62*: 407–412, 1971.

17. Toth, B. Development of Malignant Lymphoma by Cell-free Filtrates Prepared from a Chemically Induced Mouse Lymphoma. Proc. Soc. Exptl. Biol. Med., *112*: 873–875, 1963.

18. Yokoro, K., and Imamura, S. Personal communication.

Discussion of Paper by Drs. Nishizuka and Shisa

DR. NAKAHARA: Here the question raised by Dr. Stich becomes important, because many of the mouse leukemias are supposed to be associated with viruses. Have you tried any cell-free transmission of your chemically induced leukemia, or attempted to demonstrate the presence of C-particles electron microscopically?

DR. NISHIZUKA: Dr. Yokoro and his co-workers have demonstrated the presence of a leukemogenic virus in NBU-induced leukemias.   So far as DMBA-induced rat leukemias are concerned, demonstration of C-Type virus has been unsuccessful to date both in electron microscopic studies and in bioassay studies with cell-free filtrates from leukemic tissues.

DR. HASHIMOTO: You showed that some lines of the leukemia cells have θ antigen, but others not.   Are the θ antigen-negative leukemia cells derived from bone marrow cells?

DR. NISHIZUKA: I have no direct evidence that θ-negative cells come from bone marrow.   But I think this is the most likely possibility.   In the cases of SL lymphocytic leukemias in which no histological evidence of thymus involvement is present, leukemic cells do not carry θ antigen.

DR. STICH: Dr. Yokoro, you described the induction of leukemias in rats with cell-free extracts obtained from chemically induced leukemias of mice.   Can you produce a cell-free extract from these rat leukemias that has the capacity of producing leukemias in rats?   Or expressed in other words, did you succeed in adapting a mouse leukemia virus to rat tissues?

DR. YOKORO: We are able to transmit NBU-induced mouse leukemias into both mice and rats by neonatal inoculation of a leukemic cell-free supernatant.   Cell-free transmitted leukemia in rats could be serially passaged by cell-free inoculation both in rats and mice.

Metabolism of N-Nitroso-N-butylurea

Yoshiyuki Hashimoto and Keizo Tada

Tokyo Biochemical Research Institute, Tokyo, Japan [Y.H.]; Kyoritsu Pharmaceutical College, Tokyo, Japan [K.T.]

Druckrey *et al.* (*2*) injected N-nitroso-N-butylurea (NBU) subcutaneously into rats and observed sarcomas induced at the sites of injection. However, Odashima (*5*) and Yokoro *et al.* (*9*) recently found that when a solution of NBU dissolved in the drinking water was administered to rats and mice, leukemia developed in many of the animals. These findings prompted us to study the relationship between the metabolic fate of NBU and the biological effects of this compound.

This paper is on the metabolism of NBU and the tissue distribution of radioactivity of ^{14}C-labeled NBU in C57BL mice. The products obtained on decomposition of NBU in alkaline solution, the reaction of NBU with proteins and nucleic acids, and its cytotoxic effects on tumor cells in tissue culture are also reported.

Chemicals

N-Nitroso-N-butylurea was synthesized by nitrosation of *n*-butylurea, which was obtained from *n*-butylamine hydrochloride and potassium cyanate. ^{14}C-Labeled NBU was prepared by the same method. N-Nitroso-N-butylurea[butyl-1-^{14}C] and N-nitroso-N-butylurea [carbonyl-^{14}C] were synthesized from butylamine [butyl-1-^{14}C] hydrochloride and potassium cyanate-^{14}C, respectively. The specific radioactivity of both compounds was 340 μCi/mmole.

N-Nitroso-N-methylurea and N-nitroso-N,N'-dimethylurea were synthesized by nitrosating methylurea and N,N'-dimethylurea, respectively. The purity of these compounds was proved by determination of their melting points and UV spectra, and by thin layer chromatography.

In vitro Decomposition of N-Nitroso-N-butylurea and Its Products

NBU was dissolved in 1/15 M buffer solutions of various pH values and incubated at 37°C. The amount of NBU remaining in solution was measured from the absorbancy at 399 nm. As shown in Fig. 1, NBU decomposed rapidly at neutral or alkaline pH values. Urea was isolated from the solution after decomposition of NBU.

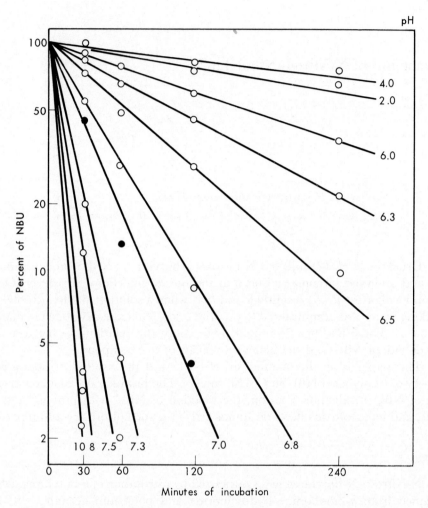

FIG. 1.   Decomposition of N-nitroso-N-butylurea at various pH values.   N-Nitroso-N-butyl-urea (NBU) was dissolved in 1/15 M Michaelis' buffer solutions of various pH values and incubated at 37°C.   The amount of NBU was calculated from the absorbancy at 399 nm.

A peak identical to *n*-butanol was detected by direct gas chromatography of the solution.   Following addition of acetic acid to an ether extract of the solution, the reaction mixture was subjected to gas chromatography and gave a peak corresponding to butyl acetate, suggesting that diazobutane was produced on decomposition of NBU in alkali.

Jones and Muck (3) showed that the reaction of N-nitroso-N-alkylurea with the base proceeds by an attack of the base on the nitroso nitrogen followed by cleavage of the N-CO bond to give cyanic acid and diazoalkane.   Decomposition of NBU in alkaline solution may proceed by this mechanism.   Urea may be formed from cyanic acid and ammonia, which is produced by hydrolysis of the acid.   The cyanate ions may be stable for several hours in alkaline solution, because if an amine such as

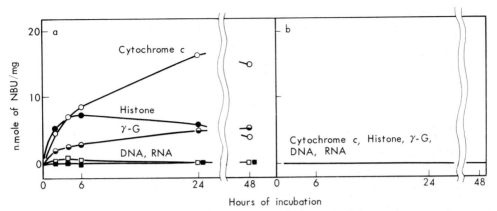

F<small>IG</small>. 2.   Reaction of ¹⁴C-labeled N-nitroso-N-butylurea with proteins and nucleic acids.   For experimental conditions see text.   a, Carbonyl-¹⁴C-NBU;   b, butyl-¹⁴C-NBU.

methylamine or aniline is added to the solution 5 hr after complete decomposition of NBU, methylurea or phenylurea can be isolated from the reaction mixture.

In vitro Reaction of N-Nitroso-N-butylurea with Proteins and Nucleic Acids

The reaction of labeled NBU with protein and nucleic acids was examined by the method of Sugimura *et al.* (7).   Cytochrome *c*, calf thymus histone, human γ-globulin, calf thymus DNA, or yeast RNA was dissolved in 0.1 M cacodylate buffer, pH 7.2.   Labeled NBU in aqueous solution was added to the solution of a biological material, and the mixture was incubated at 37°C.   Periodical determination of the radioactivity remaining on an acid-washed biological material showed that proteins were labeled with carbonyl-¹⁴C-NBU but not with butyl-¹⁴C-NBU, whereas nucleic acids were not labeled with either (Fig. 2).   This suggests that the carbamoyl group of NBU binds with the amino groups of protein to form urea residues, while the alkyl group of NBU does not bind with proteins or nucleic acids to any detectable extent under these conditions.

Cytotoxic Activity of N-Nitroso-N-alkylurea Derivatives

As demonstrated above, NBU is unstable at physiological pH values and on decomposition gives chemically active products such as cyanic acid and diazoalkane. These active products may be cytotoxic by reacting with cell constituents.   Accordingly, the cytotoxicities of NBU on 5 strains of mouse and rat ascites tumor cells were examined *in vitro*.   The cytotoxicities of N-nitroso-N-methylurea and N-nitroso-N,N'-dimethylurea were also examined for comparison.   Solutions of the test compounds in physiological saline were added to tumor cell suspensions containing 250×10^3 cells per ml of RPMI 1640 medium supplimented with 15% calf serum, and the suspensions were incubated at 37°C.   The concentration of the compounds required to inhibit growth of the tumor cells by 50% in 24 hr are listed in Table 1. The cytotoxicities of NBU and N-nitroso-N-methylurea were much less than that of

TABLE 1.   Cytotoxicity of N-Nitroso-N-alkylurea Derivatives on Tumor Cells

$$CH_3—N—CONH_2 \ (NMU) \qquad CH_3—N—CONH—CH_3 \ (NDMU)$$
$$\qquad | \qquad\qquad\qquad\qquad\qquad\qquad | $$
$$\qquad NO \qquad\qquad\qquad\qquad\qquad\qquad NO$$

Tumor cells (1×10^5/ml)	IC_{50} (mM)		
	NBU	NMU	NDMU
YS	1.4	1.2	0.2
DBLA1	0.6	0.1	0.1
RADA1	1.0	0.7	0.1
BALB/c RL2	1.3	1.5	0.1
Meth A	>1.4	>1.9	0.1
Half-life at pH 7.2, 37°C	12 min	12 min	18 hr

IC_{50}:   Concentration of compound inhibiting growth of tumor cells by 50%.

TABLE 2.   Cytotoxic Effects of N-Nitroso-N-alkylurea Derivatives on Yoshida Sarcoma Cells in Tissue Culture When Given in Single and Divided Doses

Compound	Living tumor cells as percentage of control	
	200 μg/ml single	12.5 μg/ml$\times$16 30 min intervals
NBU	43	10
NMU	23	7
NDMU	3	0

Figures show living tumor cells as percentages of those in the control after 24-hr incubation. NMU, N-nitroso-N-methylurea, NDMU, N-nitroso-N,N'-dimethylurea.

N-nitroso-N,N'-dimethylurea.   NBU and N-nitroso-N-methylurea differ from N-nitroso-N,N'-dimethylurea in being very unstable in alkaline solution (2).   Under our conditions the half-lives of the former two compounds were both 12 min in solution at pH 7.2 at 37°C, whereas that of the latter compound was 18 hr.   In consideration of the instability of these compounds, a known amount of NBU or N-nitroso-N-methylurea was divided into 16 portions which were then added to the suspension of Yoshida sarcoma cells at 30-min intervals for 8 hr.   As shown in Table 2, many fewer tumor cells survived after treatment in this manner than after treatment with single doses of these compounds.   These results suggest that N-nitroso-N-alkylurea has a cumulative cytotoxic effect.

Metabolic Fate of N-Nitroso-N-butylurea in C57BL Mice

Solutions of 0.3 to 0.4 mg of labeled NBU in 0.4 ml of water were given to mice by stomach tube.   Then the radioactivity in the expired air and urine, and in various organs and tissues was measured.   Expired CO_2 was trapped in a mixture of monoethanolamine and methylcellosolve (1 : 2, v/v).   Tissues and excreted materials were digested with Soluene TM 100 (Packard Instrument Inc., U.S.A.).   The radioactivities of the samples were measured in a liquid scintillation photometer with toluene-base scintillator.

The time-course of the excretion of the radioactivity in the expired air is illustrated in Fig. 3. The excretion of the radioactivity of both butyl-[14]C- and car-
bonyl-^{14}C-NBU was almost complete within 5 hr after administration, and about
60% of the dose was recovered in the expired air in 24 hr.

The distribution of radioactivity in tissues and organs 24 hr after administration
of labeled NBU is summarized in Table 3. When butyl-^{14}C-NBU was given, radioactivity per unit wet weight of tissues was slightly higher in the liver and digestive
organs than elsewhere, while in the case of carbonyl-^{14}C-NBU it was slightly higher in

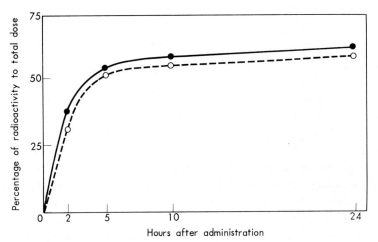

FIG. 3. Excretion of radioactivity in expired air. For experimental conditions see text.
●———●, Carbonyl-^{14}C-NBU; ○·········○, butyl-^{14}C-NBU.

TABLE 3. Deposition of Radioactivity in Organs and Tissues

Organ and tissue	dpm/g tissue ($\times 10^3$)	
	*Bu-NBU	*CO-NBU
Brain	2.8	6.0
Lymph nodes	8.1	9.7
Thymus	6.2	5.7
Spleen	7.3	12.6
Heart	3.5	13.1
Lung	7.5	8.0
Liver	16.1	11.4
Stomach	11.9	8.2
Intestine	15.8	5.6
Colon	15.3	8.4
Kidney	7.7	10.8
Bladder	8.1	9.4
Testis	3.2	3.3
Muscle	2.6	4.1
Adipose	1.6	1.1
Dose of ^{14}C-NBU	1177×10^3 dpm	1833×10^3 dpm

C57BL mice, weighing about 30 g, were given butyl-^{14}C-NBU (*Bu-NBU) or carbonyl-^{14}C-NBU (*CO-
NBU) and killed 24 hr later.

TABLE 4.   Excretion and Deposition of Radioactivity in Mice Given ^{14}C-Labeled Compounds

Sample	Percentage of radioactivity administered to mouse				
	*Bu-NBU	*CO-NBU	*Bu-BU	*Urea	H*CNO
Urine	17	13	71	82	12
Expired air	60	61	12	11	ND
Blood cells	0.1	2.0	0.2	ND	2.3
Plasma	0.5	0.2	0.2	ND	0.5

Urine and expired air were collected for 24 hr.   Blood was obtained 24 hr after administration of the ^{14}C-labeled compound.   Asterisks indicate the position of ^{14}C in the molecule.   BU, butylurea; ND, not determined.

the heart, liver, and spleen.   However, in both cases there were no large differences in the distribution of radioactivity in different organs.   The total retention of radioactivity in whole organs and tissues after 24 hr was about 4% of the given dose. The radioactivity in the feces and contents of digestive organs constituted only 1% of the total dose.   Much more radioactivity of carbonyl-^{14}C-NBU than of butyl-^{14}C-NBU was bound to blood cells, as shown in Table 4.   When ^{14}C-labeled cyanic acid was given to a mouse, it bound to blood cells to an extent similar to carbonyl-^{14}C-NBU, so the carbamoyl group of NBU seems to react with blood cell components, such as hemoglobin, in the way deduced from *in vitro* experiments.

The radioactivities excreted by mice in the urine and expired air after administration of ^{14}C-labeled NBU, butylurea, urea, and potassium cyanate are also shown in Table 4.   When either butyl-^{14}C, or carbonyl-^{14}C-NBU was given, about 15% of the radioactivity was excreted in the urine in 24 hr.   In contrast, when butyl-^{14}C-butylurea was given, 71% of the radioactivity was excreted in the urine and 12% in the expired air during the same period.

Urinary Metabolites of N-Nitroso-N-butylurea

Urine was collected for 24 hr after oral administration of ^{14}C-labeled NBU, butylurea, urea, or potassium cyanate and subjected to paper chromatography using *n*-propanol: *n*-butanol: water (2:3:2, v/v) and *n*-butanol: acetic acid: water (4:1:2, v/v) as developing solvents.   Figure 4 shows the chromatograms of radioactive metabolites.   Four peaks (I to IV) were detected after administration of carbonyl-^{14}C-NBU.   The metabolite giving peak II was identified as urea.   Peak I had the same Rf value as the first peak of the metabolites of potassium cyanate, and may be derived from the carbamoyl group of NBU.   Peaks III and IV showed the same Rf values as the metabolites of butyl-^{14}C-butylurea.   The metabolites comprising these two peaks were isolated from the urine of mice after administration of unlabeled butylurea.   The metabolite in peak IV was purified to a crystalline state, and all its characters were identical to those of butylurea.   Purified material from peak III was a liquid, and its structure was identified as N-(3-hydroxybutyl)urea from its NMR spectrum.   Peak V was only obtained after administration of butyl-^{14}C-NBU, and its Rf value was higher in the acidic solvent than in the neutral solvent

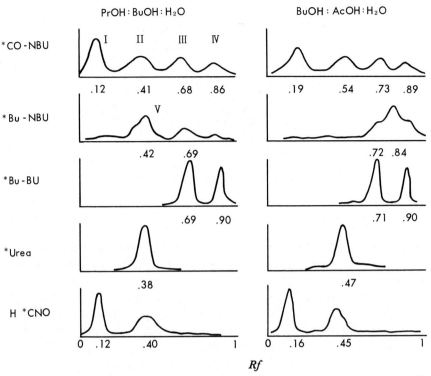

FIG. 4. Paper chromatograms of radioactive urinary metabolites. For compounds see Table 4.

suggesting that it contained a carboxyl group in the molecule. However, its structure is still unknown.

DISCUSSION

The metabolic fate of NBU in mice is summarized in Fig. 5. After administration, NBU is metabolized rapidly and is excreted in the expired air as carbon dioxide and in the urine as five metabolites. *In vitro* experiments suggest that cyanic acid and diazobutane or carbonium ion may be produced as intermediates of these metabolites. Cyanic acid or the carbamoyl group of NBU reacts with ammonia to give urea and with proteins, especially hemoglobin, giving urea residue on the molecule. Some of the NBU is denitrosated and excreted in the urine as butylurea and its ω-1 hydroxylated product, N-(3-hydroxybutyl)urea. Kawachi *et al.* (*4*) reported that when N-methyl-N'-nitro-N-nitrosoguanidine is given to rats, it is mainly excreted in the urine as the denitrosated product, N-methyl-N'-nitroguanidine, and they suggested that the denitroso reaction is the main metabolic pathway of this compound. However, in the case of NBU, this seems to be a minor one, at least in mice, since the denitroso product of NBU in the urine accounted for only 5% of the dose administered, whereas when butylurea was administered to mice, more than 70% of the dose was excreted in the urine as butylurea itself and its hydroxylated

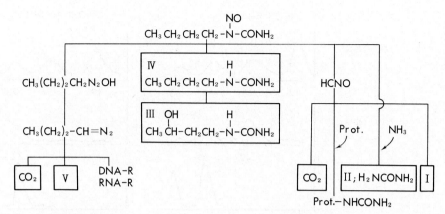

Fig. 5.   Metabolic pathway of N-nitroso-N-butylurea in C57BL mice.

product.   The butyl group of NBU may be converted to diazoalkane or the carbonium ion, and some of it was excreted in the urine as an unknown metabolite V. Some diazoalkane may bind to nucleic acids.   In a preliminary experiment, nucleic acid of liver was isolated by the method of Caldwell et al. (1) 1 and 24 hr after administration of labeled NBU.   The specific radioactivities of DNA and RNA 24 hr after administration of butyl-^{14}C-NBU were significantly higher than those obtained after administration of carbonyl-^{14}C-NBU.

Continuous administration of NBU in the drinking water is known to cause severe damage of the bone marrow in animals.   NBU is very unstable at physiological pH values, so very little NBU must actually reach the bone marrow.   Damage of bone marrow cells by such a minute amount of NBU may be explained by the cumulative cytotoxic effect of the compound: When a certain dose of NBU is added in small portions to a cell suspension over a long period, its cytotoxic effect is much higher than when it is given as a single dose.   In relation to bone marrow damage, it has been demonstrated that NBU has a strong immunosuppressive effect in animals (6).

It is still uncertain why lymphoid cells are the target of NBU.   However, recent studies by Yokoro et al. (9) and Takizawa et al. (8) have shown that the age and strain of animals affect the target organs of NBU.   Mammary and brain tumors were induced by NBU under some conditions.   Further comparative studies on the metabolic fate of NBU in these conditions and of those of other N-nitroso-N-alkylurea derivatives which have target organs other than lymphoid tissue are required to clarify the mechanism of NBU leukemogenesis.

SUMMARY

The tissue distribution and metabolic fate of a potent leukemogenic compound, N-nitroso-N-butylurea (NBU) in mice were studied using butyl-^{14}C-NBU and carbonyl-^{14}C-NBU.   The products obtained on its decomposition in alkaline solution, its reaction with nucleic acids and proteins, and its cytotoxicity on tumor cells were also examined.

1) When isotope-labeled NBU was administered orally to mice, irrespective of the position of the ^{14}C in NBU, 60% of the radioactivity was excreted in the expired air and about 15% in the urine within 24 hr. Lymphoid organs did not contain more radioactivity than other organs. Blood cells of mice given carbonyl-^{14}C-NBU retained higher radioactivity than those of mice given butyl-^{14}C-NBU. Five radio-active metabolites of NBU were detected from 24 hr urine specimens. They were urea, a substance derived from the carbamoyl group of NBU which had an identical *Rf* value to one of the two metabolites of cyanic acid, an acidic substance derived from the butyl group of NBU, and two denitroso metabolites which were identified as butylurea and N-(3-hydroxybutyl)urea.

2) Incubation of labeled NBU with proteins and nucleic acids *in vitro* shows that the carbamoyl group of NBU binds to proteins but not to nucleic acids, while no binding of the alkyl group to proteins or nucleic acids was observed.

3) The cytotoxic effect of NBU on tumor cells in tissue culture was equal to that of N-nitroso-N-methylurea, but was much weaker than that of N-nitroso-N,N'-dimethylurea. However, when NBU was added to a cell suspension in divided doses over a long period, its cytotoxicity increased.

This work was supported in part by a grant-in-aid for cancer research from the Ministry of Education.

REFERENCES

1. Caldwell, I. C., and Henderson, J. F. Isolation of Nucleotides, Nucleic Acids, and Protein from Single Tissue Samples by a Phenol Technique. Anal. Biochem., *34*: 303, 1970.
2. Druckrey, H., Preussmann, R., Ivankovic, S., und Schmähl, D. Organotrope carcinogene Wirkungen bei 65 verschiedenen N-Nitroso-Verbindungen an BD-Ratten. Z. Krebsforsch., *69*: 103, 1967.
3. Jones, W. M., and Muck, D. L. The Mechanism of the Alkoxy-induced Conversion of N-Nitroso-N-alkylamine Derivatives to Diazoalkane. J. Amer. Chem. Soc., *88*: 3798, 1966.
4. Kawachi, T., Kogure, K., Kamijo, Y., and Sugimura, T. The Metabolism of N-Methyl-N'-nitro-N-nitrosoguanidine. Biochim. Biophys. Acta, *222*: 409, 1970.
5. Odashima, S. Leukemogenesis of N-Nitrosobutylurea in the Rat. I. Effect of Various Concentrations in the Drinking Water to Female Donryu Rats. Gann, *61*: 245, 1970.
6. Odashima, S. Leukemogenic Effect of N-Nitroso-N-butylurea. *In*; Nakahara, W. (ed.), Topics in Chemical Carcinogenesis, p. 473, Univ. of Tokyo Press, Tokyo, 1972.
7. Sugimura, T., Fujimura, M., Nagao, T., Yokoshima, T., and Hasegawa, M. Reaction of N-Methyl-N'-nitro-N-nitrosoguanidine with Proteins. Biochim. Biophys. Acta, *170*: 427, 1968.
8. Takizawa, S., and Nishihara, H. Induction of Tumors in the Brain, Kidney, and Other Extra-mammary Gland Organs by a Continuous Oral Administration of N-Nitroso-N-Butylurea in Wistar / Furth Rats. Gann, *62*: 495, 1971.
9. Yokoro, K., Imamura, N., Takizawa, S., Nishihara, H., and Nishihara, E. Leukemogenic and Mammary Tumorigenic Effects of N-Nitrosobutylurea in Mice and Rats. Gann, *61*: 287, 1970.

Discussion of Paper by Drs. Hashimoto and Tada

Dr. Preussmann: In your first slide you showed a reaction scheme for the alkaline degradation of NBU according to a paper by Jones *et al.*   In this mechanism the OH⁻ attacks at the N=O bond.   I think this is extremely unlikely.   In N-nitroso compounds the double bond is more between the N—N bond, and not between the N—O bond.   It is known that the oxygen of the nitroso group bears a partial negative charge and, in fact, is nucleophilic.

$$>N-N=O \rightleftharpoons >\overset{+}{N}=N-O^-$$

There is much more convincing evidence that the first attack of OH⁻ on nitrosamides is on the $>C=O$ double bond.

Dr. Hashimoto: It has been shown by Jones and Muck (J. Amer. Chem. Soc., *88*: 3798, 1966) that attack of OH⁻ to nitrosoalkyl-urea takes place on NO-nitrogen, but in the case of other nitroso compounds, such as nitrosoalkylurethan, the position is $>C=O$ double bond.

Dr. Druckrey: The mechanism of breakdown of alkylnitrosourea compounds is probably different under neutral and alkaline conditions.   What was the pH in your experiments?

Dr. Hashimoto: pH 7.2 or pH 8.0.

Dr. Magee: Have you studied the interaction of ¹⁴C-butylnitrosourea with tissue nucleic acids at other times after injection as well as at 24 hr?
    Do you know what is the half-life of NBU in the animal after injection?

Dr. Hashimoto: It is hard to predict, but *in vitro*, the half-life of NBU at pH 7.2–7.4 is shorter than 20 min.

Dr. Mirvish: You showed two urinary metabolites of cyanate.   One was urea. What was the other one?

Dr. Hashimoto: It has not been identified yet, but it is not cyanic acid itself.

The Role of Environmental Biology in Chemical Carcinogenesis

John Higginson

International Agency for Research on Cancer, Lyon 6, France

The great contributions made by Japanese scientists to the field of chemical carcinogenesis since the days of Yamagiwa are too well known to require repetition. It must not be forgotten, however, that experimental carcinogenesis originated in the simple epidemiological observations of a London surgeon almost 200 years ago and that Japanese scientists have also significantly contributed to this field. Thus, it should occasion no surprise that a paper on the program be directed to the environmental problems of chemical carcinogenesis in man.

Present Situation

In Table 1, the relative developments of chemical carcinogenesis and epidemiology are compared. In spite of the success of the epidemiological method in communicable disease and although the significance of Pott's work had long been recognized, cancer epidemiology has developed comparatively slowly. Thus, while mortality rates of varying accuracy had been available in certain areas for some 100 years, by the nineteen-forties morbidity data were only available from two countries. During the last decade however, the situation has changed and today there are approximately 70 cancer registries which are engaged in the nonprestigious but basic work of collecting descriptive data on human cancer. In addition, successful analytical studies undertaken during the last two decades have also demonstrated the value of the epidemiological method. In a recent report to the U.S. Congress (*13*), high priority is given to expanding epidemiological research as a necessary part of cancer control. Such developments have resulted from the recognition that geographical differences in cancer patterns almost certainly represent variations in environment, many of which are probably chemical in nature, and that genetic factors appear of limited significance in man. Moreover, the rapidly occurring environmental changes seen in industrial communities increasingly emphasize that a

TABLE 1.   Historical Developments in Chemical Carcinogenesis in Man and Animals

PHASE I	
1775– Potts; Stern	Clinical observations: identified high-risk populations, *e.g.*, chimney sweeps, uranium miners, unmarried females, *etc.*
PHASE II	
1900– Yamagiwa *et al.* Kennaway *et al.* Hoffman	1) Early vital statistics on deaths; recognition of geographical differences; occupational cancers. 2) Early chemical carcinogenic experiments.
PHASE III	
1930– Dorn; Clemmesen Cook *et al.* Berenblum; Yoshida Lacassagne	1) Organization of morbidity surveys, *e.g.*, Connecticut, Denmark, 10 cities; occupational studies expanded. 2) Pure carcinogens isolated, *e.g.*, 3,4 benz(α)pyrene. 3) Principle and theory of experimental carcinogenesis established.
PHASE IV	
1945–present Segi Doll & Hill Watson & Crick	1) Retro- and prospective case history studies, *e.g.*, cigarettes and lung cancer; modern morbidity surveys (58 registries); cohort and correlation studies. 2) Large scale screening of chemicals for carcinogenic activity. 3) Biochemical carcinogenesis, molecular biology.
PHASE V	
? Future	1) Systematic registration and measurement in key areas: a) cancer; b) environmental stimuli. 2) Record linkage and monitoring systems. 3) Chemical and biological studies on a comparative basis permitting rational extrapolation from animals to man.

legislative approach to cancer control based on inadequate human data will be insufficient to meet the needs of a modern society.   It is apparent that many of the proposed modifications of the environment will have socio-economic implications of great magnitude necessitating rational practical solutions in which hazards are weighed against benefits.   Thus, the modern chemical oncologist must have a width of knowledge of his society beyond that of his immediate laboratory if he is to play a significant role, either in protecting the community from exposure to new compounds which are potentially toxic, or in avoiding unnecessary socio-economic disruption resulting from decisions based essentially on political expediency and legislative definition rather than on scientific fact.

Geographical variations in cancer patterns will not be discussed here, since they have been adequately covered in numerous reviews (*2, 3, 16*).   Discussion will rather be directed to the principles by which geographical pathology may contribute to studies in chemical carcinogenesis and the need for integrating laboratory and epidemiological studies in a multidisciplinary approach.

Chemical Environment in an Industrial State

In recent years, the term " industrialization " has been subconsciously equated with a common chemical environment, although in fact, industrial societies may differ very widely.   The term essentially reflects a way of life in modern energy-dependent societies.   In fact, no clear association of cancer patterns with indices of industrialization has been found so far.   Thus, the pattern of cancer in New Zealand, for example, is not dissimilar from that seen in the United Kingdom and the United States of America despite the marked differences in industrial development.

TABLE 2. Characteristics of Human Tumors According to Suspected Causative Stimuli

	High-risk group identifiable	Dose response	Geographical variations	Nature of agent	Examples	Usual type of cancer
1. Cultural						
a) Direct	Yes	Yes	Varies according to habit, e.g., cigarettes, betel chewing	Probably chemical but most agents not identified	Lung, esophagus, buccal cavity, skin, etc.	Epithelial
b) Indirect	Sometimes	No, but (?) penis	Geographic and intracommunity variations	Mechanisms unknown. Cultural habits may modify host's response, e.g., hormones, or exposure to agent	Penis, breast, uterus	Epithelial
2. Occupational	Yes	Yes	Usually marked intracommunity differences	Chemicals	Paranasal, sinuses, lung, bladder, skin, etc.	Epithelial
3. Iatrogenic	Yes	Usually	No	Drugs, ionizing radiation, etc.	Leukemia, sarcomas, bladder, vagina	Blood-forming organs, epithelial
4. Congenital (including familial)	Sometimes	Sometimes	Usually slight	Includes possible viral or chemical damage in intra-uterine life	Brain, leukemia, retinoblastoma, nasopharynx (?)	Mesenchymal, blood-forming organs, C.N.S.
5. Idiopathic						
a) Suspected chemical	Only in a geographic sense	Theoretically yes	Marked	Numerous possibilities	Most epithelial tumors (?) chronic lymphatic leukemia	Epithelial, blood-forming organs
b) Suspected viral	Doubtful	(?) No	Usually not marked (but note Burkitt's lymphoma)	i. Specific virus ii. Nonspecific virus	(?) Acute leukemia, lymphomas	Lymphoid tissue, blood-forming organs, soft tissues

After Higginson (4).

At the level of individual environment, variations may be less marked, for example in the consumption of processed foods, high protein diets, *etc.*, which may be more immediately concerned with neoplasia.

TABLE 3. Approximate Estimate (%) of Theoretical Potential of Prevention According to Present Etiological Hypotheses[a]

Site[b]	Cultural	Occupational	Iatrogenic	Congenital (familial or acquired)	Miscellaneous	Unknown	Remarks
	(a)	(b)	(c)	(d)	(e)	(f)	
Mouth (140, 141, 143, 145)	90	1	—	—	5	<10	(a) In India almost 100% due to betel chewing.
Salivary gland (142)	—	—	—	—	—	100	
Esophagus (150)	80	—	—	—	4	±15	(a) Alcohol and tobacco major factors in France, USA *etc.*, not in Caribbean, S. Africa, Kazakhstan. (e) Iron deficiency in Scandinavia.
Stomach (150)	4	—	—	—	1	96	(a) Role of tobacco at cardia.
Colon and rectum (153–154)	—	—	—	<1	1	99	(e) Mineral oil possible factor.
Liver (155.1) W. Industrial	70	—	—	—	1	30	(a) Alcohol predominant factor.
Liver (155.1) Africa	—	—	—	—	—	100	
Lung (162)	90	1–2	—	—	±5	<10	(b) Doll estimates up to 50% of cigarette-caused cancer may also be dependent on synergistic effect of atmospheric pollution.
Breast (170)	—	—	—	—	—	100	The eventual possibility of prevention through diet, child-bearing control, and good hygiene at present difficult to assess.
Female genital system (171–176)	—	—	—	—	—	100	
Prostate and testis (177 and 178)	—	—	—	—	—	100	
Penis (179)	—	<1	—	—	95	<5	(e) Adequate circumcision and cleanliness.
Bladder (180) W. industrial	50	10	<1	—	—	40	(a) and (b) Based on chemical exposure and possible role of cigarettes.
Bladder (180) Africa	—	—	—	—	50	50	(e) Schistosomiasis in Africa.
Skin (191)	—	2	—	10	80	<5	(b) Excludes outdoor workers who are classified as miscellaneous. (d) Refers to melanoma.
Brain tumors (192, 193)	—	—	2	<1	—	98	(d) Maternal radiation.
Leukemia and lymphoma -children	—	—	<7	1	—	94	(c) Refers to effect of ionizing radiation in embryonic and adult life.
-adults	—	—	<1	—	—	99	

[a]   Unless stated these estimates refer predominantly to a western-type industrial population.   After Higginson (4).

[b]   The figures in parenthesis refer to the 7th I.C.D. list.

While few responsible individuals would expose man unnecessarily today to carcinogenic chemicals of doubtful benefit, the confusion and conflicting views regarding environmental control of carcinogenic factors in industrial states are well known. Major factors responsible for this confusion include the absence of agreed scientific criteria for extrapolation of results from experimental animals to man, which in many cases still remains a calculated estimate by experts. Further, disagreement remains as to whether tolerance limits can be established for reasonably safe use of chemicals which animal experimentation would indicate are potential carcinogens. This has become an increasing problem with improved analytical techniques, whereby the concept of "zero" levels has largely disappeared. These disagreements illustrate the difficulties of establishing rational standards and control procedures both at a national and at an international level. The absence of an internationally agreed policy on such chemicals may sometimes cause significant socio-economic disruption out of all proportion to the potential health hazard. Thus, the economy of an African state whose external income predominantly depends on peanuts collected in a peasant culture, is highly vulnerable to aflatoxin levels set by its customers. Conversely, an economic advantage may pertain to a country which avoids environmental industrial control. Chemical pollution by one country may affect others, since such pollution is no respecter of national boundaries. Thus the gases from the high anti-pollution smokestacks of England are said to cause ecological damage in Scandinavia. Since cancer is one of the feared hazards of environmental pollution, efforts to obtain satisfactory decisions here may offer a fruitful example for international agreements on other forms of environmental pollution with possible health hazards.

In Table 2 the geographic and biological characteristics of the major groups of human tumors are shown classified according to their probably etiology. In Table 3, the proportion of certain common tumors is shown for which the nature of the etiological stimulus has already been identified. It will be observed that the majority fall into the occupational or cultural group where association with a specific factor could most easily be identified. In some cases a specific chemical has been identified, in others, circumstantial evidence strongly suggests a chemical. In most cases the tumors are epithelial in nature. Previously, we presented evidence indicating that 80% of tumors in North America are conditioned by our present environment and thus theoretically preventable (4), although for the majority of sites the stimuli remain to be identified.

Role of Epidemiology in Cancer Control

Epidemiological studies may help to clarify the following areas of environmental chemical carcinogenesis.
1. The identification of agents already present in the environment.
2. The monitoring of changes in cancer incidence indicating the entry of new agents in the human environment.
3. Provision of data on the biology of human cancer which can be used:
   a) to identify the nature of suspected environmental stimuli;

b) to determine the requirements of animal models best approximating to the situation in man;

c) to study the application of laboratory techniques to field studies on human cancer.

4. Calculations of safe levels for potential carcinogenic stimuli already present in the environment.

Simple risk situations

The most successful applications of the epidemiological methods of cancer have been in relation to simple high-risk situations such as cultural or occupational cancers, *e.g.*, cigarette smoking, where the existence of a carcinogenic agent in the environment is already suspected. Figures 1 and 2 present in set form the essential difference between prospective and retrospective studies whereby a hypothesis is tested by the investigator. This situation is comparable to that seen in the laboratory experiment. The technique is also useful in identifying simple additive risks, *e.g.*, the synergistic effect of asbestos and cigarette smoking on lung cancer (Fig. 3) (*17*).

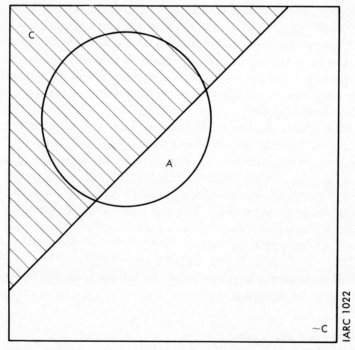

FIG. 1. Retrospective case history study. Diagram illustrating that individuals showing a cancer have a greater exposure to the suspected risk factor. The Venne Diagrams illustrate the various relationships which may exist between certain cancers and an environmental hazard. A further set should be added to illustrate the selected sample, but this has been excluded to avoid confusion. C, Cancer patients (lung); ~C, general population; A, risk factor (smoking).

$$\frac{A \cap C}{C} > \frac{\sim C \cap A}{\sim C}$$

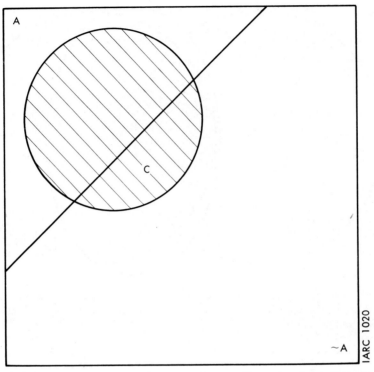

Fig. 2. Prospective case history study. Diagram illustrating that individuals exposed to the risk factor show a higher frequency of cancer.

A, Risk (smoking); C, cancer patients (lung).

$$\frac{A \cap C}{A} > \frac{\sim A \cap C}{\sim A}$$

As far as I know, this still remains one of the few proven additive risk situations for man although liver is another possibility. However, case history studies have so far proved unsuccessful in identifying the etiological background for such common cancers as colon, rectum, breast, corpus uteri, stomach and prostate.

A relatively recent example indicating that such studies are not necessarily applicable only to man has been shown in Kenya. Thus, Plowright, Linsell and Peers (11) found that approximately 10% of all cattle in an isolated valley in Kenya developed rumenal cancer, the incidence being approximately 1,500 per 100,000 *per annum*. Such cancers were not seen in the surrounding valleys, but the Masai cattle owners stated that other cattle brought into the valley were affected. It was found on further study that the cattle in this valley, in contrast to the neighboring valleys, were often forced to feed in the surrounding forest. The significance of forest feeding was further supported by the demonstration of rumenal cancer in two giant forest hogs (*Hylochoerus meinertzhageni, Thomas*) killed in the same forest. Preventive methods are now obviously possible. Of course, if the actual carcinogenic plant can be identified, the situation will certainly be academically more satisfying.

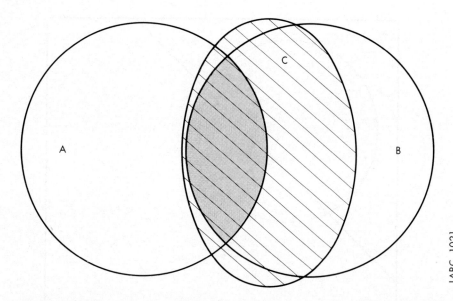

FIG. 3.   Diagram illustrating the situation when two factors may be both additive and synergistic, *e.g.*, the combination of asbestos and cigarette smoking may be a more harmful carcinogen
than smoking alone.

A∩B⊂C

A, Asbestos;   B, smoking.

Complex risk situations and correlation studies

In an industrial society, several factors may be suspected to be of etiological
significance for certain cancers.   A possible approach is to test whether a significant association can be demonstrated between cancer incidence and level of exposure to the suspected stimulus.   Such studies differ from case history studies in that
the investigation is made on groups rather than on individuals, and they lack the
statistical strength of the former.   So far such studies have not proved successful in
identifying etiological agents, but they have been of value in testing hypotheses by
comparing, for example, the level of cigarette consumption and lung cancer incidence (*2*).

There are several possible reasons for this lack of success.   These include:

1)   Exposure of a population to approximately similar levels of a diffusely distributed carcinogen or carcinogens.   Since only susceptible individuals would develop cancers, the appearance of a tumor might appear as a random event, no
difference in exposure between individuals with and without cancer being demonstrable.   Since high-risk groups do not exist, prospective or retrospective case history
studies would not be possible.   The situation with a multifactorial etiological background, which would include both additive and subadditive risks, would be even
more difficult to investigate (Figs. 4 and 5).   Similarly this would the method of
illustrating the carcinogenic effect of two compounds noncarcinogenic *per se*.

2)   Cancers at a specific site might represent a group of cancers caused by

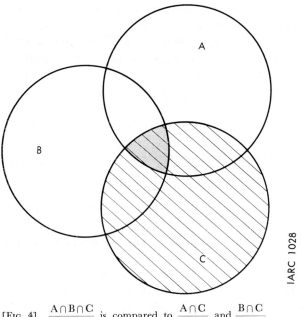

[Fig. 4]. $\dfrac{A \cap B \cap C}{A \cap B}$ is compared to $\dfrac{A \cap C}{A}$ and $\dfrac{B \cap C}{B}$

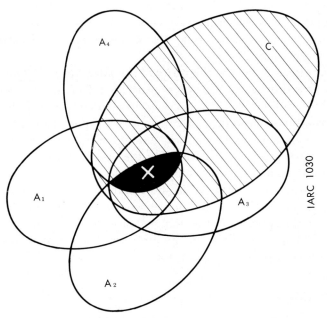

[Fig. 5] $\dfrac{A_1 \cap A_2 \cap A_3 \cap A_4 \cap C}{A_1 \cap A_2 \cap A_3 \cap A_4} = X \quad X > \dfrac{A_i \cap A_j \cap A_k \cap C}{A_i \cap A_j \cap A_k} > \dfrac{A_i \cap A_j \cap C}{A_i \cap A_j} > \dfrac{A_i \cap C}{A_i}$

Figs. 4 and 5. Diagram illustrating the problems of dissociating many additive and subtractive risks as possibly occurring in an industrial society.
A, Exposed to risk A; B, exposed to risk B; C, cancer cases.

several different stimuli.   Accordingly, the significance of any single factor would be diluted out if the whole group was examined.   If, however, high-risk groups could be identified as in certain occupations, the etiology in this group could be established. Cancer of the bladder is an example of such a situation.   Fortunately, in man the frequency with which a second cancer develops at another site within the body would suggest no extensive exposure to non-organ specific carcinogens (15) nor diffuse susceptibility to carcinogens at several sites.   Since, however, cancer occurs relatively infrequently in man, this possibility cannot be completely excluded.

3)   The long latent period of most human cancers is believed to be between 20 and 40 years.   Thus the cancer patterns observed today represent the initiating action of agents which entered the environment many years ago and are most unlikely to reflect the effects of the newer chemicals of the last two decades.   Accordingly, correlations based on present levels would be meaningless unless the latter had not changed.

These limitations are equally applicable to any monitoring system for environmental carcinogens.

Further, animal experimentations in this area are inadequately developed. Thus, experiments involving combinations of different carcinogens are surprisingly few despite the frequency with which a multifactorial mechanism is evoked as important in human cancer.   This is probably due to logistic reasons, as at least six groups of experimental animals are necessary for testing for a synergistic effect between two compounds.   The role of enzyme induction in human carcinogenesis is unknown and the possibility of either a detrimental or beneficial effect cannot be excluded.   Animal experimentation is also poorly developed on the effects of exposure to chemicals at very low dose levels.

4)   Nonspecific effects.   Due to the rarity of human cancer as compared to experimental tumors, it is difficult to identify nonspecific effects which modify tumor incidence only slightly, although a 20% decrease in incidence would clearly be important in terms of absolute numbers of cancer cases.   For example, the role of nutrition is unknown in man and attention among oncologists has largely been directed to specific nutritional deficiencies.   On the other hand, there is considerable work indicating that malnourished animals are less susceptible to cancer than the well fed.   Since large areas of the world show both poor dietary levels and low frequency of certain cancers, this observation is worthy of further study and again correlation studies would appear to offer the best approach.   However, the difficulty of expressing non-specific effects in quantitative terms makes this approach very defficult in practice and hard to quantitate.

Separation of Risks by Extension to Several Geographical Areas

For the majority of so-called idiopathic cancers, high-risk groups have not been demonstrated.   However, striking geographical differences in incidence are known, suggesting that populations are exposed at different risk levels.   Thus, extension of epidemiological studies on specific cancers to cover several geographical areas of varying environments and with different cancer frequencies could be of value in

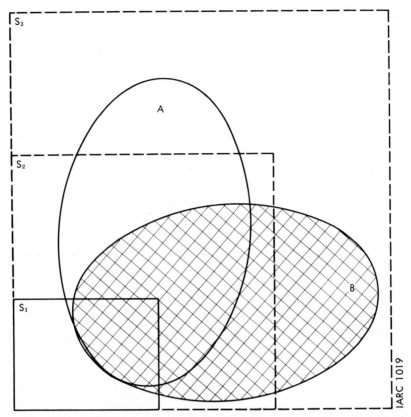

Fig. 6. Diagram illustrating how separation of risk factors might be produced by investigation in different geographical areas. "S_1" represents areas in a relatively homogeneous society where the dissociation of the risk factors "A" and "B" may be impossible. Where several non-homogeneous societies are examined, S_3, separation of "A" and "B" may be demonstrated.

$$S_1 \cap A \cap B \simeq S_1 \cap A \simeq S_1 \cap B$$
$$\text{BUT:} \quad S_3 \cap A \cap B < \frac{S_3 \cap A}{S_3 \cap B}$$

separating risks and permitting their possible identification (Fig. 6). Where a hypothesis has been proposed a case history study can be used to test its accuracylater.

Aflatoxin, for example, an experimental hepatocarcinogen, has been linked to a primary liver cancer in man. On the assumption that diets in certain developing countries may not have changed significantly in recent decades, Linsell and Peers (9) have investigated the amount of aflatoxin actually ingested by a rural population in Kenya. A statistically significant correlation between the amount of aflatoxin ingested and the incidence of liver cancer is present. If this observation is found to be reproducible in other areas of varying aflatoxin exposure, legislative action to reduce dietary aflatoxin would be justified although a definite causal relationship had not been established.

For the moment, however, hasty legislative action should be avoided as there are several inherent sources of bias. Furthermore, it has been too often concluded prematurely in the past that the cause of liver cancer in Africa has been discovered. Thus, histopathological and circumstantial evidence suggested previously that a hepatitis virus was almost certainly an etiological factor in liver cancer in Africa (5) and this evidence has never been refuted. Recently, Au/SH antigen has been found to be very frequent in Africa and the antigen also is present in a higher proportion of patients with liver cancer than in the general population (12). Similar results have now been reported from Asia (6). However, if the antigen is related to primary carcinoma of the liver, it is not a simple association. This illustrates the inherent weakness of correlation studies in identifying etiology.

A similar situation has been found in attempts to correlate the incidence of colon and rectal cancer and level of industrialization. Thus, it was found that a better association occurred with meat ingestion which is, of course, higher in industrial societies. When this factor was held steady, the correlation with industrialization disappeared.

In Iran, Kmet (8) has shown a 20- to 30-fold variation in the incidence of esophageal cancer along the Caspian Littoral. Preliminary case history studies have excluded a probable role for alcohol or tobacco. In the absence of suitable hypotheses, correlations must be established with as many environmental factors as possible. While the logistic problems are great, for the moment such studies seem to be the only logical approach. Further, this is an unusual opportunity to study the value of such techniques in a clear-cut situation.

Correlation Studies as Demonstrating Possible Tolerable Levels

The greatest value of correlation studies may eventually be in indicating possible safe levels of exposure. Thus, evidence that a cancer is rare in an area where exposure to a suspected carcinogen is high would suggest that it was not a carcinogen for man or that the exposure levels were relatively innocuous, provided that a marked change in exposure in recent years could be excluded. This technique is probably the only method of answering the perennial question as to whether or not a noneffect or tolerance level of a potential carcinogen exists for man. It has been suggested that a level of less than one case per million per year would be acceptable for practical purposes, since such levels could not be detected and would approximate to the spontaneous cancer rate. The value of such studies would be strengthened if they could be supplemented by data from certain high-risk groups, e.g., malarial sprayers of DDT. For rare cancers even this level would be insufficient, e.g., mesothelioma.

The Potential Value of a Cancer Monitoring System

The studies indicated above have been largely concentrated on the past entry of a carcinogen into the environment, but there is now increasing interest in the possibility of developing a monitoring system for environmental carcinogens similar to that which has been reported as feasible for identifying environmental teratogens (7). The requirements for developing such a system are discussed below.

Cancer registration

The establishment of long-term cancer registration systems in certain key geographic areas is essential in determining the temporal changes in incidence which would indicate the presence of a potential risk. Association with a record linkage system enhances the value of such registries (*1*).

Registries for environmental carcinogens

Quantitative data must be made available regarding potential environmental carcinogens. However, the latter are now so numerous that priorities must be selected, based either on the degree of human exposure or level of potential risk as suggested by animal experimentation. Problems will be least where the factor is specific and readily measurable with available technology. It will be difficult, however, to relate future changes in cancer patterns to a past event unless there is a very clear indication as to the factor involved and level of exposure, such as a single exposure to ionizing radiation. Indices of previous exposure, such as asbestos bodies within the lung, or DDT levels in body fat, represent another approach. Where exposure may be of short duration and the chemical rapidly metabolized, *e.g.*, nitrosamines, no marker of exposure may be available. The situation is even more complicated if a carcinogen is formed *in vivo* by the interaction of two noncarcinogenic agents, as has been suggested for secondary amines and nitrites (*14*).

Latent period

Contrary to the case of congenital malformations, where the lesion can be referred back to an event occurring during the previous few months, human cancers have latent periods of over 20 years, thus reference must be made to events many years earlier. The most hopeful situation relates to children's cancers with their relatively short latent periods, *e.g.*, cancers induced by maternal diagnostic radiation or a transplacental carcinogen. Few registries have been in operation sufficiently long to permit such studies. In Tables 4 and 5, the trends in cancer patterns for children's cancers are shown. It will be observed that these changes are in general not very prominent, nor in general do geographical variations show the same wide range as seen in cancer in adults (Table 6).

Munoz and Asvall have demonstrated that for stomach cancer, at least, it is possible that modification of promoting factors may affect incidence quite rapidly (*10*).

TABLE 4. Incidence of Children's Cancer in Connecticut 1935–1962 Age-specific Rates per 100,000 *per annum*

All sites	Males			Females		
	0–4	5–9	10–14	0–4	5–9	10–14
1935–39	10.5	12.1	4.3	10.6	5.1	8.1
1940–44	13.0	9.6	7.9	11.4	6.4	7.9
1945–49	16.9	11.2	8.8	12.3	8.7	8.7
1950–54	16.8	12.5	7.7	20.7	10.2	7.2
1955–59	17.2	12.5	11.5	15.8	8.5	9.1
1960–62	17.2	10.6	13.6	18.9	7.9	10.3

TABLE 5. Incidence of Cancer in Connecticut 1935–1962 Age-specific Rates per 100,000 *per annum* (0–14 years)

	Males	Females
All sites	Increase up to 1955 then perhaps slight fall except in the 10–14 age group	
Kidney	No increase	No increase
Eye	No increase	No increase
Brain	Slight increase up to 1955 then fall, except the 10–14 age group	Slight increase up to 1950
Bone	No increase	No increase
Conn. tissue	No increase	No increase
Lymphatic system	Steady increase in the 10–14 age-group but number small	No increase
Leukemia	Slight increase up to 1955	Slight increase up to 1950

TABLE 6. Cancer Incidence in Male Children 0–4 Years Rate/100,000 *per annum*

	US	UK	Norway	S. Africa Bantu	India	Israel All Jews	Israel Afro-Asian Jews
Digestive system	0.2	0.0	0.0	0.0	0.0	0.0	0.0
Liver	0.5	1.0	0.0	0.0	0.0	0.0	0.0
Respiratory system	0.0	0.0	0.0	0.0	0.0	0.2	0.0
Kidney	1.2	2.4	1.2	1.1	1.2	0.7	0.0
Eye	0.2	1.1	1.2	3.4	0.9	0.7	0.0
C.N.S	2.8	4.0	4.9	2.1	0.7	4.1	8.7
Lymphosarcoma	0.7	0.8	0.6	0.0	0.8	2.4	8.7
Leukemia	9.6	4.1	6.6	5.0	2.2	5.0	4.4
All sites	18.8	14.6	16.1	13.3	6.9	15.4	30.5

Variations in cancer incidence

In Table 7, the change in cancer incidence that must occur over a period to permit identification of trends is given. The necessity to continue studies for periods up to 15 years, and the possibility that factors causing both increases and decreases may be present simultaneously would indicate that interpretation will be difficult unless the effect of the agent is very marked or unless it produces an unusual cancer, *e.g.*, mesotheliomas due to asbestos or vaginal adenocarcinoma in the offspring of diethyl stilbestrol-treated mothers.

TABLE 7. Average Percentage Change in Rate Which Must Occur Each Year to Indicate a Significant Trend Over Either 5- or 15-Year Period

Absolute number of cases p.a.	5 yr[a]	5 yr[b]	15 yr[a]	15 yr[b]
500	4.5	8.4	0.5	0.8
50	14.2	26.4	1.6	2.4

Significance test
[a] A one-sided test at 0.05% level.
[b] A two-sided test at 1% level.

Consistency

Any association between a suspected etiological factor and an environmental carcinogen must be consistent with the known biological data. Further, geographical pathology investigations should indicate similar associations in several geographical areas.

Probably the greatest value of a monitoring system will lie in the potential of demonstrating marked changes in cancer patterns thus providing a warning that some significant change has occurred in the environment. Its value as an identifying system will be much less satisfactory and will probably be only successful in the following situations.

1. Childhood cancers with their relatively short latent periods as in transplacental carcinogenesis.
2. High-risk groups exposed to marked changes in the environment of a cultural or occupational nature, involving either an initiating or promoting agent.
3. Large populations exposed to an unusual concentration of a carcinogen, *e.g.*, atomic bomb.
4. Changes in rare cancers whose incidence may be rapidly appreciated, *e.g.*, mesothelioma.
5. In providing additional evidence for safety of compounds to which man is exposed.
6. While the relationship between mutagenesis, teratogenesis and carcinogenesis is far from absolute, a registry for teratogenic effects may give some indication of a possible later carcinogenic effect.

FUTURE DEVELOPMENTS

I believe that sufficient has been said regarding the potential developments of geographical pathology and its limitations. Many of the latter have in the past been related to the absence of quantitative data on the environment, and others are theoretically soluble provided the logistic difficulties covering manpower and cost can be overcome. The improvement in analytical technology during the last decade and the coordination of international efforts is now becoming of increasing importance. Certainly there are hypotheses at present available for such cancers as colon and rectum which can be tested.

However, I believe that the greatest problems in environmental carcinogenesis in the immediate future lie in the absence of rational methods for extrapolation from animal to man, an area which will continue to be bedevilled with contradiction and confusion and for which I see no immediate solution. The spectra of spontaneous tumors in most rodents differ from those seen in humans. Further, many experimental models are clearly not applicable to the human situation except for morphological comparisons. It is still unknown to what extent a tumor in one organ in a rodent, *e.g.*, hepatoma, can be regarded as an index of carcinogenic potential in another organ in man. Thus it is true, on one hand, that asbestos produces mesotheliomas in both man and rodents whereas beta-naphthylamine causes hepatomas in mice but bladder cancer in man. (The human liver may be able to detoxify the low levels of compounds as found in the human environment.)

There will be strong support, notably by experimentalists, for complete avoidance by man of exposure to any potential carcinogens and, on the other hand, pressure from agricultural and other interests for continued use of new and old compounds where significant sociological or economic benefits can be demonstrated. Thus, the modern oncologist clearly has to face up to the problem of calculated risk.

Figure 7 summarizes the possible legislative actions that in the absence of better methods of extrapolation testings might be taken based on observations in animals and man.

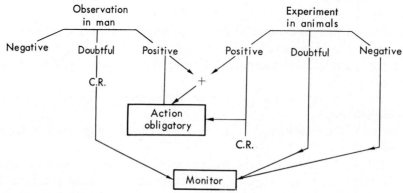

Fig. 7. Possible schema on which to base legislative action in man for useful or necessary compounds. C.R.: Calculated risk implying some form of legislative control.

REFERENCES

1. Acheson, E. D. Medical Record Linkage, Oxford University Press, 1967.
2. Clemmesen, J. Statistical Studies in the Aetiology of Malignant Neoplasms. I. Review and Results, Munksgaard, Copenhagen, 1965.
3. Doll, R., Muir, C., and Waterhouse, J. A. H. (eds.) Cancer Incidence in Five Continents. A Technical Report, Vol. II, Springer Verlag, Berlin, Heidelberg, New York, 1970.
4. Higginson, J. Present Trends in Cancer Epidemiology. Proceedings of the Eighth Canadian Cancer Conference, Honey Harbour, Ontario, 1968; pp. 40–75, 1969.
5. Higginson, J., and Svoboda, D. J. Primary Carcinoma of the Liver as a Pathologist's Problem. *In*; Sommers, Sheldon C. (ed.), Pathology Annual, *1970*: 61–89.
6. Hiroyama, T. Personal communication.
7. Kallén, B., and Winberg, J. A Swedish Register of Congenital Malformations. Experience with Continuous Registration during 2 Years with Special Reference to Multiple Malformations. Pediatrics, *41*: 765, 1968.
8. Kmet, J. A Technical Report. Annual Report, International Agency for Research on Cancer, pp. 24–27, Lyon, 1970.
9. Linsell, C. A., and Peers, F. G. A Technical Report. Annual Report, International Agency for Research on Cancer, pp. 84–89, Lyon, 1970.
10. Munoz, N., and Asvall, J. Time Trends of Intestinal and Diffuse Types of Gastric Cancer in Norway. Int. J. Cancer, *8*: 144–157, 1971.

11. Plowright, W., Linsell, C. A., and Peers, F. G. A Focus of Rumenal Cancer in Kenyan Cattle. Brit. J. Cancer, *25*: 72–80, 1971.

12. Prince, A. M., Leblanc, L., Krohn, K., Masseyeff, R., and Alpert, M. E. Detection of SH Antigen in Sera from Patients with Chronic Active Hepatitis, Cirrhosis and Carcinoma of the Liver. Lancet, *2*: 717–718, 1970.

13. Report of the National Panel of Consultants on the Conquest of Cancer Authorized by S. Res. 376, Prepared for the Committee on Labor and Public Welfare, United States Senate, U.S. Govt. Printing Office, Washington, 1971.

14. Sander, J. Kann Nitrit in der menschlichen Nahrung Ursache einer Krebsentstehung durch Nitrosaminbildung sein. Arch. Hyg. Bakt., *151*: 22–28, 1967.

15. Schottenfeld, D., Berg, J. W., and Vitsky, B. Incidence of Multiple Primary Cancers. II. Index Cancers Arising in the Stomach and Lower Digestive System. J. Natl. Cancer Inst., *43*: 77–86, 1969.

16. Segi, M., Kurihara, M., and Matsuyama, T. Cancer Mortality for Selected Sites in 24 Countries, No. 5 (1964–1965). Department of Public Health, Tohoku University School of Medicine, Sendai, Japan, 1969.

17. Selikoff, I. J., Hammond, E. C., and Churg, J. Asbestos Exposure, Smoking and Neoplasia. J. Amer. Med. Assoc., *204*: 106–112, 1968.

Discussion of Paper by Dr. Higginson

DR. DRUCKREY: Carcinogens are in our environment.   We have to live and even to work with them.   However, the potential risk should be considered not only versus economic benefit but also, and in first line, versus the necessary measures for protection of men and animals.   The greatest obstacle in endeavoring cancer prevention is ignorance about what and where carcinogens are in the human environment.   In order to overcome this, systematic and planned research work is needed.   The most promising and economic way would be a close cooperation between epidemiologists, experimental cancerologists, and chemists.

DR. HIGGINSON: I completely agree that future epidemiology must combine field epidemiologists and laboratory research workers.

DR. MIRVISH: Presumably two chemical factors in our environment can interact in two ways.   They might interact biologically, *e.g.*, as initiator and promoter, or they might interact chemically, *e.g.*, nitrite from one food might react in the stomach with secondary amines from another food to give nitrosamines.   Would you comment please?

DR. HIGGINSON: That is of course highly possible and we are exploring the possibility in the Caspian Littoral.

DR. HIRAYAMA: In connection with Dr. Higginson's presentation, I just wish to indicate that fruitful results have been obtained by our ongoing population prospective study.   In addition to the effect of cigarette smoking on most of the causes of death, both for males and females, a significant reduction of mortality rate for gastric cancer was observed in daily drinkers of 360 cc of milk.   A significant combined effect was also recognized as follows: smoking and alcohol drinking on cancer of the esophagus, smoking and daily intake of meat on cancer of the pancreas and lung, and smoking and frequent intake of hot green tea on most of the gastrointestinal tract cancers.   These results are expected to give fresh stimulus to experimental oncologists in the future.

Closing Remarks

Dr. J. H. WEISBURGER

Ladies and gentlemen, I did not wish to have the last word, but the next to the last word, before the statement by our genial key organizer, Professor Nakahara. As we have said, cancer is international, disease is international, we cancer researchers are international. We do not feel that we belong to any one nation.

Nonetheless, I think it would not be polite on our part, as foreign guests, to come from abroad, after having been invited to take part in this really extensive, very valuable, and very important symposium in the host country that pioneered in carcinogenesis studies, and not to thank the Princess Takamatsu Fund, Princess Takamatsu, and the Imperial Family who have honored us by their presence and participation. We are all indebted to the organizers of the Second International Symposium of the Princess Takamatsu Cancer Research Fund, Professor Nakahara, and Doctors Sugimura, Odashima, Takayama, and indeed all of the many other Japanese colleagues, including the secretarial staff, who have made our stay so enticingly wonderful professionally, intellectually, and socially. Professor Nakahara, may we please thank you. Kindly transmit our deep appreciation to all your colleagues for a superb reception, for a fine significant meeting which will be recognized as a marker and permanent keystone in the annals of worldwide cancer research.

Dr. WARO NAKAHARA

The three days of this symposium have come to an end, and it seems that now I am to close the symposium by some appropriate remarks. First and foremost, allow me to express my cordial thanks to the gracious patronage of Her Imperial

Highness Princess Takamatsu, the generous support of the Princess Takamatsu Cancer Research Fund, and the active cooperation of the participants. Without these the symposium could not have achieved the success that I sincerely believe it has.

Our original plan was to limit the scope of the symposium to carcinogenesis by nitro and nitroso compounds, but from the very nature of the topics, discussions extended to other carcinogens, and, in fact, to the carcinogenic mechanism in general.

Very many interesting and exciting experimental results marked this symposium, altogether forming a really substantial contribution to our knowledge of chemical carcinogenesis. Transplacental carcinogenicity of some nitrosamines that were administered to maternal organisms during pregnancy; questions centering around the detection of weak carcinogens and the so-called promoters; problems in chemical reaction biology in the carcinogenic mechanism, such as those of the proximate carcinogenic metabolites of nitrosamines and the formation of epoxides and free radical reaction; the possible role of nitrosamines as a carcinogenic hazard for man, with due regards to the injudiciousness of easy going extrapolation of the results *in vitro* experiments and of animal experiments to the case of man. These are a few of the numerous points of interest we have discussed. There were some differences of opinion as to the interpretation of some of the results, which were natural and very welcome. Without differences of opinions, no progress in science can be expected. In this connection, I may be permitted to say that the unavoidable absence from this meeting of Professor Schmähl was very unfortunate for us. Professor Schmähl's paper was unique in being concerned with means of counter acting the carcinogenic action of nitrosamine. This aspect of the problem has not been considered by any other investigator. Years ago, I showed that hepatocarcinogenesis by aminoazo dyes can be prevented by dietary supplement of beef liver powder. Liver feeding, however, had no effect on hydrocarbon carcinogenesis. It might be of importance to look for some agent that might prevent the formation of nitrosamine from nitrite and amines or so detoxicate nitrosamines as to render them noncarcinogenic.

It is good indeed that there are so many different carcinogens and different ways of using them experimentally. Every investagator is free to choose his pet carcinogen, pet experimental methods, and pet theory. All roads may lead to Rome, but it is very likely that some roads may lead us there much more quickly than other roads. If everybody uses the same carcinogen and the same guiding theory of carcinogenesis, then the outlook for our reaching " Rome " may not be so good.

Now that the symposium is ended, let us go back to our laboratories and follow the road to " Rome " as seems most promising. I hope that in a few years time we may be in a position to look back upon this symposium and find that many constructive suggestions emerged out of it.